Pediatric Body MRI

Edward Y. Lee, MD, MPH
Editor

Mark C. Liszewski, MD
Michael S. Gee, MD, PhD
Pedro Daltro, MD, PhD
Associate Editors

Ricardo Restrepo, MD
Associate Imaging Editor

Heron Werner Junior, MD, PhD
Assistant Imaging Editor

Pediatric Body MRI

A Comprehensive, Multidisciplinary
Guide

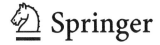 Springer

Editor
Edward Y. Lee, MD, MPH
Division of Thoracic Imaging
Department of Radiology
Boston Children's Hospital
Harvard Medical School
Boston, MA, USA

Associate Editors
Mark C. Liszewski, MD
Division of Pediatric Radiology
Departments of Radiology and Pediatrics
The Children's Hospital at Montefiore and
Montefiore Medical Center Bronx,
New York, NY, USA

Pedro Daltro, MD, PhD
Alta Excelência Diagnóstica and
Department of Radiology
Clínica Diagnóstico por Imagem (CDPI)
Rio de Janeiro, Brazil

Michael S. Gee, MD, PhD
Division of Pediatric Imaging
Department of Radiology
Massachusetts General Hospital
Harvard Medical School
Boston, MA, USA

Ricardo Restrepo, MD
Department of Interventional Radiology
and Body Imaging
Nicklaus Children's Hospital
Miami, FL, USA

Assistant Imaging Editor
Heron Werner Junior, MD, PhD
Alta Excelência Diagnóstica and
Department of Radiology
Clínica Diagnóstico por Imagem (CDPI)
Rio de Janeiro, Brazil

ISBN 978-3-030-31988-5   ISBN 978-3-030-31989-2   (eBook)
https://doi.org/10.1007/978-3-030-31989-2

This Springer imprint is published by the registered company Springer Nature Switzerland AG
The registered company address is: Gewerbestrasse 11, 6330 Cham, Switzerland

*To my parents, Kang-Ja and Kwan-Pyo, for instilling in me the values of hard
    work and dedication*
To my family for their constant support, love, and encouragement
*To my editorial team for contributing their time and expertise in this project.
    There is absolutely no better group to be with*

Edward Y. Lee, MD, MPH

To my supportive wife, Jiwon, and our wonderful children, James and Emily
To my loving parents, Kathleen and Steven

Mark C. Liszewski, MD

*To my parents, Elizabeth and Stanley, and my brother Brian, for their love
    and support*

Michael S. Gee, MD, PhD

*To my family, especially to my wife Leise and to my four kids, Pedro, João,
    Maria and Isabel*
*To the my pediatric radiology team, with whom I have proudly been working
    for so many years*

Pedro Daltro, MD, PhD

*To my parents, Jairo and Helena, for providing the inspiration that guided me
    throughout my career*
*To LBS for his support and for constantly reminding me that life is beautiful
    and to be enjoyed in all aspects*

Ricardo Restrepo, MD

To my family for their constant support, love, and encouragement

Herone Werner Junior, MD, PhD

Preface

Ever since its first development approximately four decades ago, MR imaging has undergone rapid growth and technological advancement in screening, diagnosis, and follow-up assessment of various medical disorders. Particularly in recent years, the advancement to 3T and 7T magnets combined with many newer and faster MR imaging sequences and multichannel coils with parallel imaging capabilities has substantially improved the quality of MR imaging and allowed 3D imaging while reducing imaging acquisition time. In addition, due to its many advantages, including lack of harmful ionizing radiation, superb soft tissue characterization, and capacity to obtain functional information, MR imaging is currently being increasingly utilized as an integral component of noninvasive imaging assessment in many clinical circumstances in the pediatric population. Therefore, a clear understanding of pediatric MR imaging techniques and characteristic MR imaging findings of various pediatric disorders is essential for practicing pediatric and general radiologists, who encounter pediatric patients in their clinical practice to ensure optimal pediatric patient care.

The initial idea of this book arose from trainees, pediatric radiologists, general radiologists, and various specialists whom I have encountered as a pediatric radiologist at Boston Children's Hospital, chair of the pediatric radiology section of the Core Examination for radiology residents and Online Longitudinal Assessment (OLA) Committee for practicing pediatric radiologists at the American Board of Radiology (ABR), and visiting professor to more than 50 different countries around the world for the past 15 years. Everyone from these groups was looking for an up-to-date single volume practical resource for learning and reviewing the fundamentals and essentials of pediatric body MR imaging. However, there was no such book currently available. From this came my desire to write a pediatric body MR imaging textbook.

This book is organized into 17 main chapters based on organ systems in addition to a last chapter dedicated to whole body MR imaging. The organization and presentation of this book are structured to provide accessibility to both common and less common but clinically important pediatric body disorders that can be currently evaluated with MR imaging. Each chapter included in this book is designed to provide up-to-date information on current as well as emerging MR imaging techniques and outline methods to specifically tailor MR imaging for each individual pediatric patient. Practical strategies including pre-imaging pediatric patient preparation are highlighted. Developmental embryology, normal anatomy and variants, and characteristic MR imaging findings are reviewed. In addition, the discussion of each disorder includes the clinical features, characteristic MR imaging findings, and up-to-date management information in some selected cases. Given its focus on disorders affecting the pediatric population, we have emphasized how to differentiate between normal variants and abnormal pathology and how to determine whether certain MR imaging findings are related to age or a genetic or malformation syndrome. Furthermore, current information on optimizing performance, analysis, and interpretation of MR imaging is highlighted along with practical tips on navigating technical and interpretative pitfalls that occur in pediatric body MR imaging.

This book is intended primarily for radiology trainees and practicing pediatric and general radiologists. However, other physicians in different specialties as well as MR technologists and physicists who encounter the pediatric patient for MR imaging may derive valuable clinical MR imaging and some patient management information that can be used to optimize their pediatric patient care.

For a book such as this one, which requires an extensive collaborative effort for preparation, I am a strong believer that we are only as good as the people that we work with. This book has greatly benefited from the tireless work of gifted associate and assistant editors whom I can proudly call my true "academic brothers." No word can adequately thank associate editors, Mark C. Liszewski, Michael S. Gee, and Pedro Daltro, for sharing their boundless enthusiasm and depth of knowledge in pediatric disorders. I am especially appreciative of Ricardo Restrepo, image associate editor, and Heron Werner Junior, image assistant editor, for their careful attention to detail in image acquisition and preparation. I would also like to thank the contributing authors of this book for their superb work, all of whom are experts or rising stars in the field of pediatric body MR imaging. Lastly but also importantly, I would like to acknowledge Margaret Moore and her colleagues at Springer for understanding the importance of a book such as this one for pediatric patient care, turning our initial ideas into a reality, and providing their superb administrative and editorial assistance from beginning to end.

It is understandable that writing a book such as this can be often challenging because it is trying to catch a moving target in the field of rapid technical advancement in MR imaging. However, our overarching hope is that the contents of this book will increase interest and understanding of pediatric body MR imaging that can enhance the care of pediatric patients with various congenital and acquired disorders. Then, we will have accomplished our overarching goal that we have set with this edition. We truly look forward to feedback from readers that can be incorporated into the next edition. Until then, we sincerely hope that all readers enjoy this book and learn as much as we did in preparing and writing it.

Boston, MA, USA   Edward Y. Lee, MD, MPH

Contents

Editors and Contributors

Editor

Edward Y. Lee, MD, MPH Division of Thoracic Imaging, Department of Radiology, Boston Children's Hospital, Harvard Medical School, Boston, MA, USA

Associate Editors

Mark C. Liszewski, MD Division of Pediatric Radiology, Departments of Radiology and Pediatrics, The Children's Hospital at Montefiore and Montefiore Medical Center, Bronx, NY, USA

Michael S. Gee, MD, PhD Division of Pediatric Imaging, Department of Radiology, Massachusetts General Hospital, Harvard Medical School, Boston, MA, USA

Ricardo Restrepo, MD Department of Interventional Radiology and Body Imaging, Nicklaus Children's Hospital, Miami, FL, USA

Pedro Daltro, MD, PhD Alta Excelência Diagnóstica and Department of Radiology, Clínica Diagnóstico por Imagem (CDPI), Rio de Janeiro, Brazil

Assistant Imaging Editor

Heron Werner Junior, MD, PhD Alta Excelência Diagnóstica and Department of Radiology, Clínica Diagnóstico por Imagem (CDPI), Rio de Janeiro, Brazil

Contributors

Sudha A. Anupindi, MD Department of Radiology, The Children's Hospital of Philadelphia, Perelman School of Medicine, University of Pennsylvania, Philadelphia, PA, USA

Susan J. Back, MD Department of Radiology, The Children's Hospital of Philadelphia, University of Pennsylvania, Philadelphia, PA, USA

Gerald Behr, MD Department of Radiology, Memorial Sloan Kettering Cancer Center, New York, NY, USA

James M. Brian, MD Department of Radiology, Penn State Hershey Children's Hospital, Penn State College of Medicine, Hershey, PA, USA

Juan S. Calle Toro, MD Department of Radiology, The Children's Hospital of Philadelphia, University of Pennsylvania, Philadelphia, PA, USA

Pierluigi Ciet, MD, PhD Department of Radiology and Nuclear Medicine; Department of Pediatric Pulmonology, Sophia Children's Hospital Erasmus Medical Center, Rotterdam, The Netherlands

Monica Epelman, MD Department of Radiology, Nemours Children's Health System, Nemours Children's Hospital, University of Central Florida College of Medicine, Orlando, FL, USA

Michael S. Gee, MD, PhD Division of Pediatric Imaging, Department of Radiology, Massachusetts General Hospital, Harvard Medical School, Boston, MA, USA

Sharon W. Gould, MD Department of Medical Imaging, Nemours Children's Health System, A. I. DuPont Hospital for Children, Wilmington, DE, USA

Mary-Louise C. Greer, MBBS, FRANZCR Department of Diagnostic Imaging, The Hospital for Sick Children, University of Toronto, Toronto, ON, Canada

Samantha G. Harrington, MD, MSc Department of Radiology, Massachusetts General Hospital, Boston, MA, USA

Alison R. Hart, MD Diagnostic Imaging, Rhode Island Hospital, Brown University, Providence, RI, USA

Nathan C. Hull, MD Department of Radiology, Mayo Clinic, Rochester, MN, USA

Monica Johnson, MD, MPH Department of Radiology, Massachusetts General Hospital, Harvard Medical School, Boston, MA, USA

Kyung Rae Kim, MD Division of Interventional Radiology, Department of Radiology, UNC Medical Center/University of North Carolina School of Medicine, Chapel Hill, NC, USA

Benjamin M. Kozak, MD Department of Radiology, Massachusetts General Hospital, Harvard Medical School, Boston, MA, USA

Rekha Krishnasarma, MD Department of Radiology, Boston Children's Hospital, Harvard Medical School, Boston, MA, USA

Jessica Kurian, MD Department of Radiology, Montefiore Medical Center, Albert Einstein College of Medicine, Bronx, NY, USA

Edward Y. Lee, MD, MPH Division of Thoracic Imaging, Department of Radiology, Boston Children's Hospital, Harvard Medical School, Boston, MA, USA

Teresa Liang, MD Department of Radiology, Boston Children's Hospital, Harvard Medical School, Boston, MA, USA

Department of Radiology, University of Alberta/Stollery Children's Hospital, Edmonton, AB, Canada

Mark C. Liszewski, MD Division of Pediatric Radiology, Departments of Radiology and Pediatrics, The Children's Hospital at Montefiore and Montefiore Medical Center, Bronx, NY, USA

Archana Malik, MD Department of Radiology, St. Christopher's Hospital for Children, Drexel University College of Medicine, Philadelphia, PA, USA

Amirkasra Mojtahed, MD Division of Pediatric Imaging, Department of Radiology, Massachusetts General Hospital, Harvard Medical School, Boston, MA, USA

Michael M. Moore, MD Department of Radiology, Penn State Hershey Children's Hospital, Penn State College of Medicine, Hershey, PA, USA

Katherine Nimkin, MD Division of Pediatric Imaging, Department of Radiology, Massachusetts General Hospital, Harvard Medical School, Boston, MA, USA

Harriet J. Paltiel, MD Department of Radiology, Boston Children's Hospital, Harvard Medical School, Boston, MA, USA

Daniel J. Podberesky, MD Department of Radiology, Nemours Children's Health System, Nemours Children's Hospital, University of Central Florida College of Medicine, Orlando, FL, USA

Anil G. Rao, MBBS, DMRD, DNB Desert Radiology, Las Vegas, NV, USA

Ricardo Restrepo, MD Department of Interventional Radiology and Body Imaging, Nicklaus Children's Hospital, Miami, FL, USA

Gary R. Schooler, MD Department of Radiology, Duke University Medical Center, Durham, NC, USA

Abdusamea Shabani, MB BCh FRCR Division of Body and Diagnostic Imaging, Sidra Medicine, Doha, Qatar

Raja Shaikh, MD Division of Interventional Radiology, Department of Radiology, Boston Children's Hospital, Harvard Medical School, Boston, MA, USA

Jennifer K. Son, MD Division of Pediatric Radiology, Russell H. Morgan Department of Radiology and Radiological Sciences, Johns Hopkins University School of Medicine, Baltimore, MD, USA

Jeffrey J. Tutman, MD Division of Pediatric Radiology, Department of Radiology, Children's Hospital of Colorado, University of Colorado School of Medicine, Aurora, CO, USA

Lung and Pleura

Mark C. Liszewski, Pierluigi Ciet, and Edward Y. Lee

Introduction

Disorders of the lungs and pleura are common in children and are a frequent indication for medical imaging. Over the past decade, a combination of advances in magnetic resonance (MR) imaging scanner technology and increased concern about the effects of ionizing radiation has led to increased utilization of MR imaging in the pediatric population. Despite this general trend, there has been slower adoption of MR imaging to evaluate the lungs and pleura due to technical limitations including motion artifact, low signal-to-noise ratios, and signal dephasing at air-tissue interfaces. As MR imaging technology advances, many of these technical hurdles are being overcome, and MR imaging of the lungs and pleura has begun to be a feasible option for evaluation of many pediatric pleuropulmonary conditions. Therefore, an up-to-date understanding of these emerging applications is important to practitioners performing MR imaging in infants and children.

In this chapter, an overview of MR imaging techniques to evaluate the lungs and pleura in children is discussed. Normal anatomy and development of the lungs and pleura are described, and the MR imaging findings in a spectrum of pediatric lung and pleural disease are illustrated.

M. C. Liszewski (✉)
Division of Pediatric Radiology, Departments of Radiology and Pediatrics, The Children's Hospital at Montefiore and Montefiore Medical Center, Bronx, NY, USA

P. Ciet
Department of Radiology and Nuclear Medicine, Department of Pediatric Pulmonology, Sophia Children's Hospital Erasmus Medical Center, Rotterdam, The Netherlands

E. Y. Lee
Division of Thoracic Imaging, Department of Radiology, Boston Children's Hospital, Harvard Medical School, Boston, MA, USA

Magnetic Resonance Imaging Techniques

A main advantage of MR imaging is the ability to obtain cross-sectional images with high-contrast resolution without requiring ionizing radiation. Because of technical challenges when imaging the lungs and pleura, the key to successful MR imaging of the thorax lies in appropriate patient preparation and use of optimized pulse sequences and protocols.

Patient Preparation

MR imaging is an imaging modality that is highly sensitive to motion artifact, and successful MR imaging of the chest depends on appropriate patient selection and preparation prior to imaging. Selection of a successful technique largely depends on the age of the child and the assessment of the child's ability to follow instructions.

Infants are often able to undergo successful MR imaging utilizing a "feed and wrap" technique, in which the child is fed and swaddled prior to MR imaging [1]. After infancy, nearly all children under 5 years of age are not able to hold still or adequately follow breathing instructions and therefore require moderate sedation or general anesthesia for successful MR imaging. Examinations performed under moderate sedation must utilize sequences that are optimized for quite free breathing. Examinations performed under general anesthesia may utilize sequences that require apnea. Children as young as 5 years of age may be candidates for MR imaging without sedation or anesthesia but must be carefully assessed prior to imaging to gauge their ability to cooperate for the examination. In order for an examination to be successful, preparation and coaching are essential prior to the MR imaging. Children must practice breathing maneuvers and become familiar with the scanner prior to the examination, ideally in a mock scanner environment with the assistance of child life specialists. During practice sessions, children learn to hold their breaths at end-inspiration and end-expiration, rapidly breathe in and out, and perform coughing maneuvers.

© Springer Nature Switzerland AG 2020
E. Y. Lee et al. (eds.), *Pediatric Body MRI*, https://doi.org/10.1007/978-3-030-31989-2_1

MR Imaging Pulse Sequences and Protocols

Historically, MR imaging of the lungs and pleura has been hampered by technical factors inherent to these organ systems including respiratory motion artifact, low signal-to-noise ratios, and signal dephasing at air-tissue interphases. However, in recent years, technological advances have helped to overcome many of these impediments, and diagnostic MR imaging of the lungs and pleura can now be achieved on MR imaging scanners currently in use at many medical centers. MR imaging protocols of the lungs and pleura mainly consist of spin-echo and gradient-echo sequences which can often produce image qual-ity that approaches that of CT [2]. Newer techniques including ultra-short (UTE) or zero echo time (ZTE) sequences provide even better image quality which is on par with CT [3, 4]. When pediatric patients are unable to cooperate with breathing instructions, respiratory gating can be employed by utilizing a pneumobelt or navigator echo sequence [2]. Specialized sequences, which minimize motion artifact, can be used to obtain images during free breathing, including helicoidal (PROPELLER@GE) or radial (STARVIBE@SIEMENS) k-space acquisition schemes [5, 6]. MR imaging also has the ability to provide information about ventilation, inflammation, perfusion, and structure, under the acronym VIPS [7–10].

Table 1.1 MR imaging sequences for ventilation, inflammation, perfusion, and structural (VIPS) MR imaging of the lung and pleura

SEQUENCE	ACRONYMS	MR IMAGING SYSTEM	AVERAGE ACQUISITION TIME (FOR THE ENTIRE CHEST COVERAGE)	SPATIAL RESOLUTION	TEMPORAL RESOLUTION	SCAN PARAMETERS
Ventilation						
2D gradient echo	SSFP (GE) TruFISP (SIEMENS) bFFE (PHILIPS)	1.5 T	3–9 min	FOV = 450 × 450 mm SL = 12 mm Matrix = 128 × 128	3.33 images/s acquisition	TE/TR 0.67 ms/1.46 ms FA = 65° BW = 2056 Hz/pixel
2D gradient echo	2D SPGR (GE) 2D FLASH (SIEMENS) 2D FFE	1.5 and 3 T	3–9 min	FOV = 500 × 500 mm SL = 15 mm Matrix = 256 × 192	3.08 images/s acquisition	TE/TR 1.04 ms/3 ms FA = 5° BW = 1500 Hz/pixel
Inflammation						
2D single-shot echo- planar imaging sequence (EPI)	EPI-DWI (SIEMENS/GE/ PHILIPS)	1.5 T	5–7 min	FOV SL = 5 mm Matrix	Low	TE/TR 83 ms/5632 ms FA = 90° B = 0 and 600 s/mm²
2D single-shot echo- planar imaging sequence (EPI)	EPI-DWI	1.5 T	5–7 min	Voxel size 2.5 × 2.5 × 6 mm³	Low	TE/TR 54 ms/4800 ms FA = 90° BW = 1644 Hz/pixel B = 0, 10, 20, 30, 50, 70, 100, 150, 200, 400, 800 s/mm²
2D T2-weighted Turbo spin echo	TSE (SIEMENS) FSE (GE) TSE (PHILIPS)	1.5 T and 3 T	5–7 min	FOV = 400 mm SL = 5–7 mm Matrix = 256 × 192	Low	TE/TR 80 ms/2000–4000 ms FA = 90° BW = 1644 Hz/pixel Fat suppression mode = SPAIR
Perfusion/Angiography						
2D gradient echo	SSFP (GE) TruFISP (SIEMENS) bFFE (PHILIPS)	See scan parameters above				
2D gradient echo	2D SPGR (GE) 2D FLASH (SIEMENS) 2D FFE	See scan parameters above				
3D gradient echo T1-weighted	FLASH 3D (SIEMENS) SPGR (GE) FFE (PHILIPS)	1.5 and 3 T	12–20 s	FOV = 460 mm matrix = 40 × 192 × 256 (isotropic voxel as low as 1 mm³)	Low	TR = 2.5–3 ms TE = 1.0–1.5 ms FA = 30°–40°
3D gradient echo T1-weighted	Twist(SIEMENS) TRICKS (GE) TRACK (PHILIPS)	1.5 and 3 T	Breath-hold (end-expiratory)/ shallow breathing	FOV = 460 mm matrix = 32 × 96 × 128	High, 0.5–1 s/ volume	TR = 2.0–2.5 ms TE = 0.8–1.0 ms FA = 30°–40°

Table 1.1 (continued)

SEQUENCE	ACRONYMS	MR IMAGING SYSTEM	AVERAGE ACQUISITION TIME (FOR THE ENTIRE CHEST COVERAGE)	SPATIAL RESOLUTION	TEMPORAL RESOLUTION	SCAN PARAMETERS
Structure						
2D	T2-weighted BLADE (SIEMENS) T2-weighted PROPELLER (GE) T2-weighted MultiVane (PHILIPS) ± FAT suppression	1.5 and 3 T	End-expiratory with navigator echo triggering 3 to 7 min according respiratory pace and pattern	FOV: 380–400 mm Matrix = 200 × 200 SL = 5–6 mm, axial and coronal	Low	TR = 1000–2000 TE = 27–60 ms FA = 90°–150°
2D	TRUFISP (SIEMENS) SSFP (GE) Balanced FFE (PHILIPS)	1.5 T	12–20 s	FOV = 400 mm Matrix = 160 × 160 SL 2.5–5 mm	High	TR = 1.08 ms TE = 0.42 ms FA = 20° BW = 1776 Hz/pixel
3D	SPACE (SIEMENS) CUBE (GE) VISTA (PHILIPS)	1.5 T–3 T	End-expiratory with navigator echo triggering 5 min	FOV = 320 mm Matrix = 160 × 160 SL = 2 mm	Low	TR = 940 ms TE = 60 ms FA = 90° BW = 355 Hz/pixel Echo train length = 120
3D	VIBE(SIEMENS) SPGR (GE) THRIVE (PHILIPS)	1.5 T–3 T	Breath-hold 10–12 s (inspiratory and expiratory)	FOV = 400 mm Matrix = 200 × 200 SL = 2 mm	High	TR = 1.7 ms TE = 0.7 ms FA = 2° BW = 862 Hz/pixel
3D	STARVIBE (SIEMENS) Not available for GE and PHILIPS	1.5 T–3 T	Free-breathing 3–5 min	FOV = 400 mm Matrix = 320 × 320 SL = 4 mm	Low	TR = 7.46 ms TE = 2.46 ms FA = 9° BW = 820 Hz/pixel
3D	LAVA FLEX (GE)	1.5 T–3 T	Breath-hold (10 s)	FOV = 260 mm Matrix = 128 × 128 SL = 3 mm	High	TR = 3.7 ms TE = min full ms FA = 1°
3D	PETRA(SIEMENS) ZTE(GE) MULTIVANE-XD (PHILIPS)	1.5 T–3 T	Free-breathing 7–10 min	FOV = 360 mm³ Matrix size = 416 mm³	Low	TR = 4.1 ms TE = 0.07 ms

Adapted from Liszewski et al. [11], with permission
GE General Electric, Boston, Massachusetts, USA, *Siemens* Munich, Germany, *Philips* Amsterdam, Netherlands

Table 1.1 provides an outline of MR imaging sequences commonly used to image the lungs and pleura [11].

Anatomy

Embryology

Lung Development The development of the lung begins in the first gestational month and continues after birth into childhood. The development is divided into five phases: embryonic, pseudoglandular, canalicular, saccular, and alveolar.

Phases of Prenatal Lung Development During the fourth week of gestation, lung development begins when the laryn-

gotracheal groove arises from the foregut endoderm and forms the lung bud. The embryonic phase begins when the lung bud divides into the right and left bronchial buds [12]. In the embryonic phase, the bronchial buds lengthen and divide into three branches on the right and two branches on the left and further subdivide into the pulmonary segments. By the end of the embryonic phase, a vascular plexus begins to form within the lung mesenchyme [13] (Fig. 1.1).

The pseudoglandular phase begins at week 5 and ends at week 17. In this phase, the bronchi further divide, and by week 17, the entire air-conducting portion of the lung has developed to the level of the terminal bronchiole. On the cellular level, ciliated, goblet, and neuroendocrine cells develop, and the terminal bronchioles contain cuboid columnar cells (see Fig. 1.1).

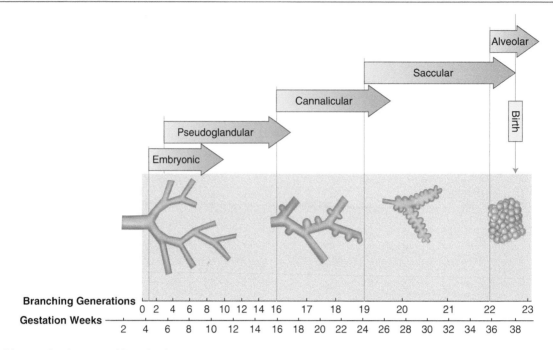

Fig. 1.1 Diagram showing prenatal lung development

The canalicular phase begins at week 17 and ends at week 28. The portion of the lung involved in oxygen exchange develops during this phase, including the respiratory bronchioles, alveolar ducts, and alveoli. Type I pneumocytes begin to develop in this phase, and Type II pneumocytes contain surfactant proteins but do not secrete them. The alveolar capillary bed begins to form at this stage. By the end of the canalicular phase, gas exchange is possible, and survival outside the uterus is feasible, but only with intensive medical care, exogenous surfactant therapy, and mechanical ventilation (see Fig. 1.1).

The saccular phase begins at week 29 and ends at week 36. Alveolar sacculi proliferate during this phase, and the basal lamina of the distal respiratory epithelium fuses with the basal lamina of the alveolar capillary endothelium, allowing for improved gas exchange. Surfactant begins to be excreted during this phase, but its production is not yet at the levels of a full-term newborn, and children born at this phase usually require exogenous surfactant therapy [14] (see Fig. 1.1).

The alveolar phase begins at week 36 and continues through 18 months of age. Throughout this phase, more alveoli form, leading to approximately 50 million alveoli soon after birth and 300 million alveoli by the time the lung is fully mature. With alveolar development, the pulmonary alveolar capillary network also grows, leading to increased capacity for gas exchange [15] (see Fig. 1.1).

Fetal Lung Fluid and Surfactant Fetal lung fluid fills the airways and alveoli while in utero. Although it mixes with amniotic fluid, the composition of fetal lung fluid is differ-

ent than that of amniotic fluid. Fetal lung fluid is produced by the respiratory epithelium. At term, approximately 5 mL/kg/hour. of lung fluid is produced [16]. During labor and immediately after birth, fetal lung fluid is cleared by pulmonary lymphatics [17].

Surfactant is composed of phospholipids, protein, neutral lipids, and cholesterol and is found within fetal lung liquid in the later stages of gestation. Intracellular surfactant is present within Type II pneumocytes in the canalicular phase at 20–24 weeks gestation and can be found within fetal lung fluid starting in the saccular phase [17]. Surfactant produced before 35 weeks gestation is present in smaller amounts and is more susceptible to inactivation than after 35 weeks [17, 18]. Surfactant allows alveoli to expand during inspiration by reducing surface tension [19, 20]. Surfactant is essential to lung function, and a major complication of pre-term birth is surfactant deficiency disorder (SDD). When a pre-term birth is imminent, pregnant mothers can be treated with glucocorticoids to speed up endogenous surfactant production by the fetus. After birth, exogenous surfactant may be administered via endotracheal tube to treat SDD.

Pleural Development The pleura begins development before the lungs at 3 weeks gestation. At this time, the pleura begins to form from the mesoderm along with the pericardium and peritoneum [21]. At 9 weeks gestation, the pleura separates from the pericardium and peritoneum. The pleura is comprised of the visceral pleural, which covers the lung, and the parietal pleura, which covers the chest wall and diaphragm [21] (Fig. 1.2).

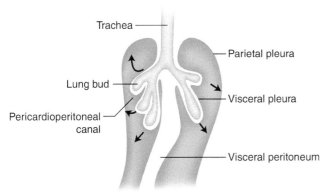

Fig. 1.2 Diagram showing pleural development

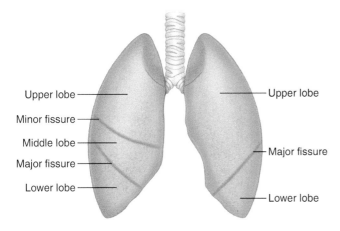

Fig. 1.3 Diagram of lobar anatomy: sections of normal lung

Table 1.2 Lung lobes and segments

Lobes	Segments
Right upper	Apical, posterior, and anterior
Right middle	Lateral and medial
Right lower	Superior, medial basal, anterior basal, lateral basal, and posterior basal
Left upper	Apicoposterior, anterior, superior lingular, and inferior lingular
Left lower	Superior, medial basal, anterior basal, lateral basal, and posterior basal

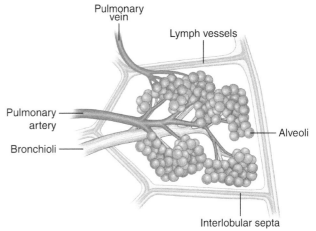

Fig. 1.4 Diagram of lung parenchyma: secondary pulmonary lobule

Normal Development and Anatomy

Lobar Anatomy The right lung is composed of three lobes (upper, middle, and lower), and the left lung is composed of two lobes (upper, which includes the lingua, and lower) (Fig. 1.3). Each lobe is separated by a pleura-lined fissure. Each lobe is further divided into segments, which are defined by segmental bronchi and not divided by fissures. Table 1.2 describes the segments in each lobe.

Lung Parenchyma

Secondary Pulmonary Lobule The secondary pulmonary lobule is the smallest structural unit of the lung that may be visible on MR imaging; smaller structures such as the pulmonary acini and alveoli are too small to be visualized as discrete structures. Each secondary pulmonary lobule has a polyhedral shape and is bordered by connective tissue septations called interlobular septa (Fig. 1.4). At birth, secondary pulmonary lobules have a mean diameter of 3 mm and are therefore not visible on most conventional MR imaging sequences. However, they are visible in older children and adults on MR imaging, and they reach a diameter of 13–20 mm in adulthood

[22]. A lobular bronchiole is in the center of each secondary pulmonary lobule and communicates with up to 25 terminal bronchioles and their acini [23, 24].

Acini and Alveoli Acini and alveoli are the functional units of the lung where gas exchange occurs. These structures are too small to be visualized as discrete structures on MR imaging. Each lobular bronchiole communicates with up to 25 terminal bronchioles, which communicate with acini and alveoli [23, 24] (Fig. 1.5). When filled with air, groups of acini and alveoli appear uniformly hypointense, and when filled with fluid or other material, they appear uniformly intense because the alveolar walls are beyond the spatial resolution of MR imaging.

Vascular Anatomy Deoxygenated blood moves through the lungs to the alveolar capillaries via the pulmonary arteries, which travel along with bronchi and bronchioles in bronchovascular bundles. The smallest pulmonary arterial branch that can be visualized on MR imaging is the lobular artery which travels in the center of the secondary pulmonary lobule along with the lobular bronchiole. Lobular arteries branch into intralobular and acinar arteries which are beyond the spatial resolution of MR imaging. These small pulmonary artery branches supply an extensive alveolar capillary bed, where gas exchange occurs. Oxygenated blood then enters pulmonary venules,

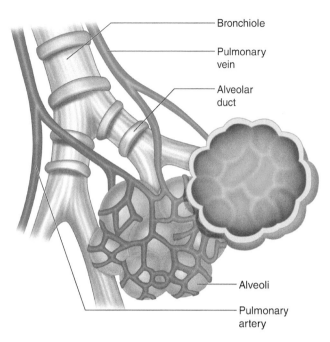

Fig. 1.5 Diagram of acini and alveoli: structure of the lung

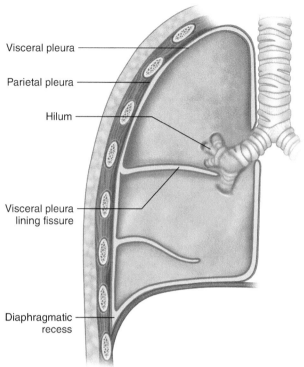

Fig. 1.6 Diagram of pleural anatomy: parietal and visceral pleura

which are located within the interlobular septa, separate from the bronchovascular bundles. Pulmonary arteries and veins therefore travel separately, except in the hila where they are adjacent to one another.

A small amount of oxygenated blood is supplied to the lung via bronchial arteries to provide oxygen to the metabolically active tissues in the trachea, bronchi, and pulmonary arteries [9]. Venous drainage of these structures is primarily via systemic bronchial veins, which continue to the right side of the heart via hemiazygous and azygous veins.

Lymphatic Anatomy Pulmonary lymphatics are comprised of a deep plexus and superficial plexus [25]. The deep plexus is located within the bronchovascular bundles in the center of the secondary pulmonary lobule. The superficial plexus travels alongside pulmonary venules within the interlobular septa [23, 25].

Pleural Anatomy

Parietal and Visceral Pleura The pleural space is formed by two pleural membranes: the parietal pleura and the visceral pleura (Fig. 1.6). Each is comprised of a single layer of mesothelial cells, a basement membrane, and a layer of connective tissue which contains blood vessels and lymphatics [21]. The arterial supply to the parietal pleura is via the intercostal arteries, and the visceral pleura is supplied by bronchial arteries. Normal pleural fluid is produced from systemic pleural arteries in both the visceral and parietal pleura [21].

The visceral and parietal pleura both have extensive lymphatic channels. Fluid within the pleural space drains via parietal pleural lymphatics, but not visceral pleural lymphatics [21].

Pleural Fissures The visceral pleura is tightly adherent to the surface of the lung parenchyma and forms the pleural fissures where it invaginates between lobes of the lung (see Fig. 1.6). The right lung contains a major fissure which separates the right lower lobe from the right upper and middle lobes and a minor fissure, which separates the right upper lobe and the right middle lobe. The left lung contains only a major fissure, which separates the left upper lobe and left lower lobe.

Anatomic Variants

Accessory Pleural Fissures and Lobes Accessory pleural fissures and lobes are relatively common normal variants, seen in approximately 30% of the population [26, 27]. Accessory fissures include (in order of frequency) inferior accessory fissure (12–21%), left minor fissure (8–9%), superior accessory fissure (1–5%), fissure between the medial and lateral segments of the right middle lobe (2–5%), fissure between the superior and inferior segments

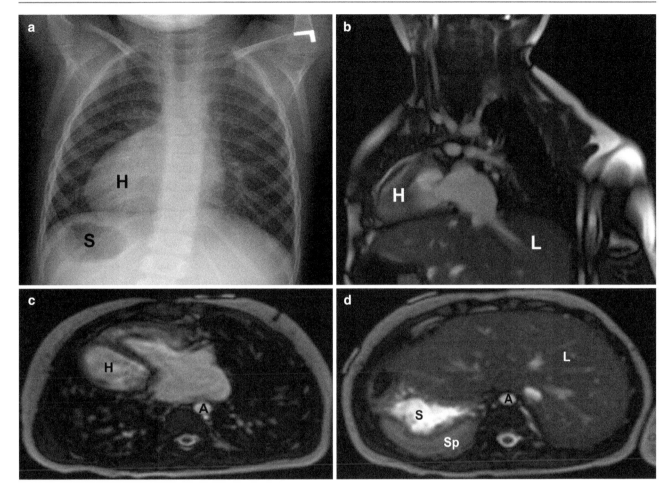

Fig. 1.7 Heterotaxy syndrome in a 4-year-old girl. (**a**) Frontal chest radiograph shows a right-sided heart (H) and stomach (S). (**b**) Coronal oblique non-enhanced bright-blood MR image shows right-sided heart (H) and left-sided liver (L). (**c**) Axial non-enhanced bright-blood MR image shows right-sided heart (H) and left-sided descending thoracic aorta (A). (**d**) Axial non-enhanced bright-blood MR image shows left-sided liver (L), right-sided stomach (S), right-sided spleen (Sp), and midline abdominal aorta (A)

of the lingula (1–5%), and fissure between the anterobasal and laterobasal lower lobe segments (2.5–3%) [26, 27].

The azygous fissure is another type of accessory fissure, but it has a different origin than the other accessory fissures. An azygous fissure forms when the azygous vein takes an anomalous lateral course during development and bisects the right upper lobe. Therefore, the azygous fissure is lined by parietal and visceral pleura, unlike the other fissures, which are composed of only visceral pleura.

Heterotaxy Syndromes Heterotaxy syndromes are a group of conditions in which the location and laterality of structures is altered (Fig. 1.7). The simplest example is situs inversus totalis, where all structures are flipped from left to right. In the lungs, situs inversus totalis manifests as a three-lobed left lung and two-lobed right lung. More complex heterotaxy syndromes may occur in which both lungs have three lobes (right isomerism) or both lungs have two lobes (left isomerism). Right isomerism is associated with asplenia and left isomerism is associated with polysplenia.

Spectrum of Lung and Pleural Disorders

In the following sections, the MR imaging findings in a spectrum of congenital and acquired lung and pleural disorders affecting children are presented. Pertinent clinical features and current treatments are also discussed.

Congenital and Developmental Lung Disorders

Bronchial Atresia Bronchial atresia is a congenital thoracic lesion characterized by developmental interruption, or atresia, of a bronchus. There are two main theories about the underlying etiology of bronchial atresia. The first proposes that an ischemic event after bronchial development leads to obliteration of the bronchus. The second proposes a primary disruption of proximal bronchial bud development affecting only the proximal portion of the bronchus but not affecting the distal portion. In either case, the lung distal to the atretic bronchus does not communicate with the central airway. Pulmonary secretions are unable to pass through the atretic bronchus, and the bronchus distal to the atresia eventually fills with fluid, forming a bronchocele. The lung distal to the atretic bronchus becomes hyperinflated due to a check-valve mechanism or air drift via collateral pathways of aeration [28]. The air within the hyperinflated lung becomes deoxygenated, and the vascularity decreases due to hypoxia-induced vasoconstriction.

Bronchial atresia may be detected on prenatal ultrasound, and prenatal MR imaging may be utilized to characterize the lesion. In utero, amniotic fluid rather than air becomes trapped within the lung distal to the atretic bronchus, and prenatal MR imaging characteristically demonstrates hyperintense hyperexpanded region of the lung on T2-weighted imaging due to trapped fluid [28]. If not detected on prenatal imaging, bronchial atresia may be first detected on chest radiographs. Chest radiograph demonstrates a round or oval perihilar opacity representing the bronchocele often with adjacent lucent overinflated segment of the lung.

Whether detected in utero or on chest radiograph, postnatal cross-sectional imaging is often obtained to further evaluate and confirm bronchial atresia, especially when surgical resection is being considered. In current practice, this is most often achieved with contrast-enhanced CT; however, MR imaging has also been described for this indication. MR imaging depicts the bronchocele as a tubular perihilar structure which is hyperintense on T1- and T2-weighted images and does not enhance on post contrast images [29, 30]. Hyperinflation within the distal lung is not as easily depicted on MR imaging as on CT due to the proton-poor environment within the air-filled hyperexpanded lung [31].

When symptomatic, bronchial atresia is treated with surgical resection. Management of small asymptomatic bronchial atresia is currently controversial, with some recommending resection due to risk of superinfection and others favoring a conservative approach [32, 33].

Congenital Lobar Emphysema Congenital lobar emphysema (CLE) or also known as congenital lobar overinfla-

tion is characterized by hyperexpansion of a lobe of the lung due to narrowing of a lobar bronchus. CLE occurs in certain lobes more frequently, occurring in the left upper lobe > right middle lobe > right upper lobe > right or left lower lobe [34]. It can also affect more than one lobe. CLE often produces symptoms soon after birth due to progressive lobar hyperexpansion, and treatment consists of lobectomy.

CLE may be detected on prenatal ultrasound, and prenatal MR imaging may be utilized to characterize the lesion. In utero, amniotic fluid rather than air becomes trapped within the hyperexpanded lobe, and prenatal MR imaging characteristically demonstrates hyperintense hyperexpanded lobe of lung on T2-weighted imaging due to trapped fluid. CLE and bronchial atresia have similar findings on fetal MR imaging, and differentiating between the two is often difficult. If not detected on prenatal imaging, CLE may be detected on chest radiographs in the newborn period demonstrating progressive hyperexpansion of a lobe of the lung.

Whether detected in utero or on chest radiograph, postnatal cross-sectional imaging is often obtained to further evaluate, characterize, and confirm CLE, especially when surgical resection is being considered. In current practice, this is most often achieved with CT. MR imaging has a limited role for this indication, because the proton-poor hyperexpanded lung is not as well characterized on MR imaging. With newer imaging techniques that improve MR imaging resolution (such as UTE and ZTE sequences), MR imaging may play a larger role in the future. On MR imaging, CLE appears as a hypointense hyperexpanded lobe of the lung, often with accompanying mediastinal shift and ground-glass signal abnormality within the adjacent lobes due to compressive atelectasis.

Currently, asymptomatic children or those with only mild symptoms are often managed conservatively with continuous follow-up to assess possible interval resolution or stability, whereas lobectomy by open or thoracoscopic approach is employed for symptomatic pediatric patients.

Bronchogenic and Other Foregut Duplication Cysts
Bronchogenic cysts are a type of foregut duplication cyst that occurs due to abnormal budding of the ventral lung bud or abnormal branching of the tracheobronchial tree during lung development. Most bronchogenic cysts develop in close proximity to the central tracheobronchial tree, and most are located within the mediastinum, but approximately 15% are located within the lung parenchyma (Fig. 1.8) [35]. Esophageal duplication cysts and neurenteric cysts are other types of foregut duplication cysts, which are related to

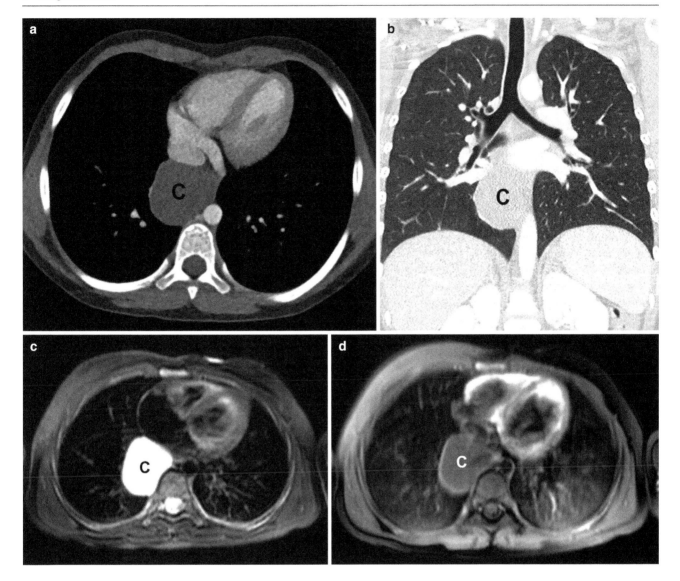

Fig. 1.8 Bronchogenic cyst in a 7-year-old girl. (**a**) Axial enhanced soft tissue window setting CT image shows a thin-walled cyst (C) in the right posterior mediastinum containing simple fluid density. (**b**) Coronal enhanced lung window setting CT image shows the thin-walled cyst (C). (**c**) Axial non-enhanced bright-blood short tau inversion recovery (STIR) MR image shows hyperintense signal within the cyst (C). (**d**) Axial enhanced T1-weighted fat-suppressed MR image shows the cyst (C) with a thin enhancing wall and no central enhancement

bronchogenic cysts (Fig. 1.9). Esophageal duplication cysts arise from the dorsal bud of the primitive foregut, and neurenteric cysts occur due to incomplete separation of the endoderm and notochord. Although often treated as distinct lesions, foregut duplication cysts frequently contain elements of more than one foregut tissue, and hybrid lesions are common.

Bronchogenic and other foregut duplication cysts are most often detected as incidental findings in asymptomatic infants and children. They may be diagnosed on prenatal imaging, and fetal MR imaging typically demonstrates a unilocular thin-walled hyperintense cyst within the mediastinum on T2-weighted sequences (Fig. 1.10) [36–38]. If not detected prenatally, bronchogenic and other foregut duplication cysts may be detected on chest radiograph as a mediastinal or pulmonary mass. Cross-sectional imaging is often performed to evaluate the finding of a mass. Although this is most typically achieved with CT, MR imaging is an excellent modality to characterize bronchogenic and other foregut duplication cysts. MR imaging

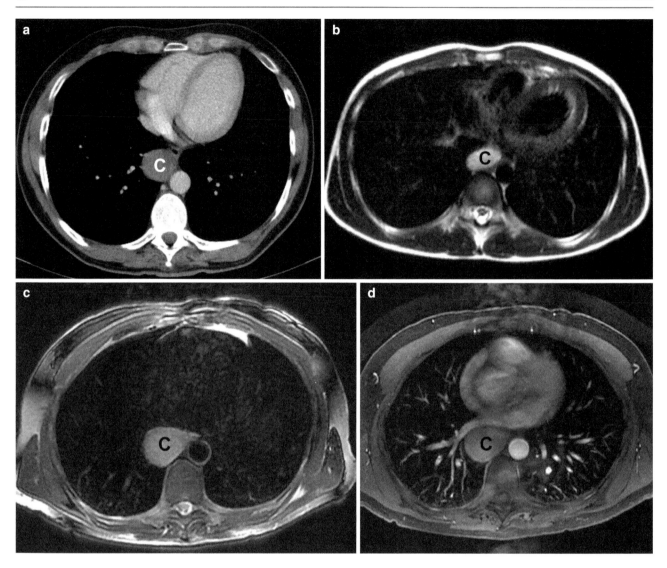

Fig. 1.9 Esophageal duplication cyst in a 12-year-old boy. (**a**) Axial enhanced soft tissue window setting CT image shows a cyst (C) adjacent to the esophagus which is greater than simple fluid density due to proteinaceous contents. (**b**) Axial non-enhanced SSFSE T2-weighted MR image shows hyperintense signal within the cyst (C). (**c**) Axial non-enhanced black-blood T2-weighted MR image shows hyperintense signal within the cyst (C). (**d**) Axial enhanced T1-weighted fat-suppressed MR image shows the cyst (C) with internal hyperintensity due to intrinsically hyperintense proteinaceous material rather than due to enhancement

typically demonstrates a cyst that is hyperintense on T2-weighted images and has variable intensity on T1-weighted images and does not enhance on contrast-enhanced images, except for a thin rim of wall enhancement [34]. Bronchogenic cysts within the mediastinum rarely communicate with the airway, but more peripheral cysts may communicate with the airway and contain an air-fluid level [39]. Bronchogenic cysts may become infected, especially when there is communication with the airway. When superinfected, cysts may develop a thick enhancing wall with irregular borders [40].

Currently, both asymptomatic and symptomatic bronchogenic and other foregut duplication cysts are typically treated with surgical resection [40].

Congenital Pulmonary Airway Malformation Congenital pulmonary airway malformations (CPAMs), previously known as cystic adenomatoid malformations (CCAMs), are a group congenital lung lesions composed of large cysts or microscopic cysts, bronchiolar overgrowth, and abnormal connection with the airway [39, 40]. Classically, CPAMs have conventional pulmonary vascular anatomy,

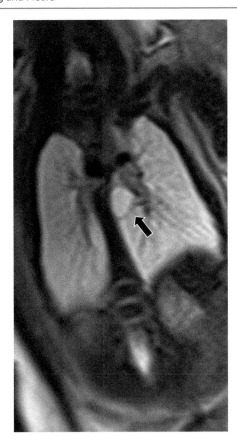

Fig. 1.10 Bronchogenic cyst on prenatal MR imaging. Coronal non-enhanced T2-weighted image shows a thin-walled cyst (*arrow*) adjacent to the left bronchus

Table 1.3 Congenital pulmonary airway malformation (CPAM) modified Stocker classification

Type	Characteristics
Type 0	Diffuse acinar dysgenesis
	Incompatible with life and rarely seen in clinical practice
Type 1	Large cyst or cysts measuring >2 cm
Type 2	Cyst or cysts measuring <2 cm
Type 3	Tiny "microcysts" measuring <5 mm
	Appears as a solid mass on imaging and gross inspection
Type 4	Large cysts in the periphery of the lung
	Difficult to differentiate from type 1

receiving blood from the pulmonary artery and draining to the pulmonary vein [41]. However, hybrid lesions are common, and elements of CPAM are frequently present in pulmonary lesions supplied by a systemic artery [42–44]. Several classification systems have been developed to describe CPAMs, but the most commonly used system in current practice is the modified Stocker system [39, 40, 42, 44–47]. The modified Stocker system is described in Table 1.3.

CPAMs may be first diagnosed on prenatal imaging. On fetal MR imaging, CPAMs appear as hyperintense lung lesions, and depending on the type discrete cysts may or may not be visible (Fig. 1.11) [48]. Categorization of CPAMs on fetal imaging is slightly different than on postnatal imaging, largely due to the smaller size of the fetus. On fetal imaging, CPAMS are categorized as macrocystic when cysts are ≥5 mm or microcystic when cysts are <5 mm [49]. Macrocystic (≥5 mm) lesions on fetal imaging correspond to Stocker Type 1 lesions, and microcystic (<5 mm) lesions on fetal imaging correspond to Stocker Type 2 lesions [40, 48]. If not detected on prenatal imaging, CPAM may be first visualized on chest radiograph as an air-filled cystic lesion or a solid mass, depending on the type [48].

Postnatal cross-sectional imaging is indicated to further assess CPAM especially when surgical resection is considered. Currently, CT is the modality most often utilized for this indication, but MR imaging can be utilized as an alternative. Because pulmonary sequestration and hybrid lesions are often a differential consideration, MR angiography is indicated to evaluate the vascular supply. MR imaging findings of CPAMs depend on the type. Cysts in type 1, 2, and 4 lesions are air-filled or fluid-filled and have a thin hyperintense wall that enhances on contrast-enhanced images (Fig. 1.12) [31]. Type 3 lesions appear as solid enhancing masses on contrast-enhanced MR images.

If a CPAM is causing symptoms, surgical resection is indicated. Management of asymptomatic CPAM is more variable. Many advocate surgical resection due to small risks of superinfection and associated malignancy, but others recommend a conservative approach due to the small incidence of these complications [50–55].

Pulmonary Sequestration Pulmonary sequestration was defined by Pryce in 1946 as "disconnected bronchopulmonary mass or cyst with an anomalous arterial supply" [56]. Twenty-five percent of lesions are defined as extralobar, with their own pleural covering and venous drainage to a systemic vein [39–41]. Seventy-five percent of lesions are defined as intralobar, sharing a pleural covering with the normal lung and with venous drainage to the left atrium [39–41]. Extralobar sequestration may occur in the lower lobes, within the diaphragm, in the abdomen, or within the mediastinum, and intralobar sequestration most often occurs in the lower lobes [39–41].

Sequestration is often diagnosed on prenatal ultrasound. Fetal MR imaging may be performed to further characterize lesions, which typically demonstrates a lesion that is hyper-

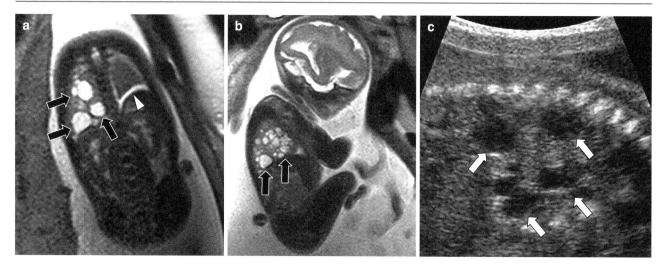

Fig. 1.11 Macrocystic congenital pulmonary airway malformation (CPAM) on prenatal MR imaging. (**a**) Coronal non-enhanced T2-weighted MR image shows several hyperintense cysts (*arrows*) in the right lung. A left pleural effusion (*arrowhead*) is also present. (**b**) Sagittal non-enhanced T2-weighted MR image shows several hyperintense cysts (*arrows*) in the lung. (**c**) Sagittal ultrasound image shows several hypoechoic cysts (*arrows*) in the lung

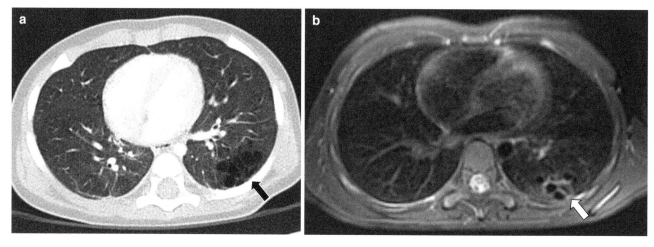

Fig. 1.12 Congenital pulmonary airway malformation (CPAM) type 2 in a boy at 7 months old and 9 years old. (**a**) Axial enhanced lung window setting CT image at 7 months of age shows multiple cysts (*arrow*) measuring <2 cm in the left lower lobe. (**b**) Axial enhanced T1-weighted fat-suppressed PROPELLER MR image at 9 years of age shows multiple cysts (*arrow*) measuring <2 cm in the left lower lobe

intense on T2-weighted images (Figs. 1.13 and 1.14). A flow-void might be seen arising from the aorta, indicating the systemic arterial supply, but this is often difficult to visualize. Therefore, the MR imaging appearance may be similar to other lesions including CPAM, bronchial atresia, and congenital lobar emphysema [48, 49, 57].

After birth, cross-sectional imaging is often indicated, especially when surgical resection is considered. CTA is most often performed for this indication given its excellent temporal and spatial resolution and ability to visualize anomalous vasculature. MRA may be appropriate in certain cases, such as if there is heightened concern about the effects of ionizing radiation. The key to imaging pulmonary seques-

tration is defining the arterial supply and the venous drainage. On conventional fluid-sensitive MR imaging sequences, sequestration typically appears as a cystic or solid lesion within the lung [31]. MRA demonstrates the systemic feeding artery (usually from the aorta) and the venous drainage to the left atrium (intralobar sequestration) or a systemic vein (extralobar sequestration) [31].

If symptomatic, pulmonary sequestration is treated with surgical resection. Similar to CPAM, management of asymptomatic pulmonary sequestration is somewhat controversial. Treatment may include resection due to concern about superinfection and small risk for malignancy or a watchful waiting strategy [58, 59].

Fig. 1.13 Intralobar pulmonary sequestration on prenatal imaging. (**a**) Coronal non-enhanced T2-weighted MR image shows hyperintense lesion (S) replacing the right lower lobe and crossing the midline. (**b**) Sagittal non-enhanced T2-weighted MR image shows hyperintense lesion (S) replacing the right lower lobe. (**c**) Sagittal ultrasound image with color Doppler shows an anomalous systemic artery (*arrow*) arising from the descending thoracic aorta. (**d**) 3D reconstructed ultrasound image shows an anomalous systemic artery (*arrow*) arising from the descending thoracic aorta

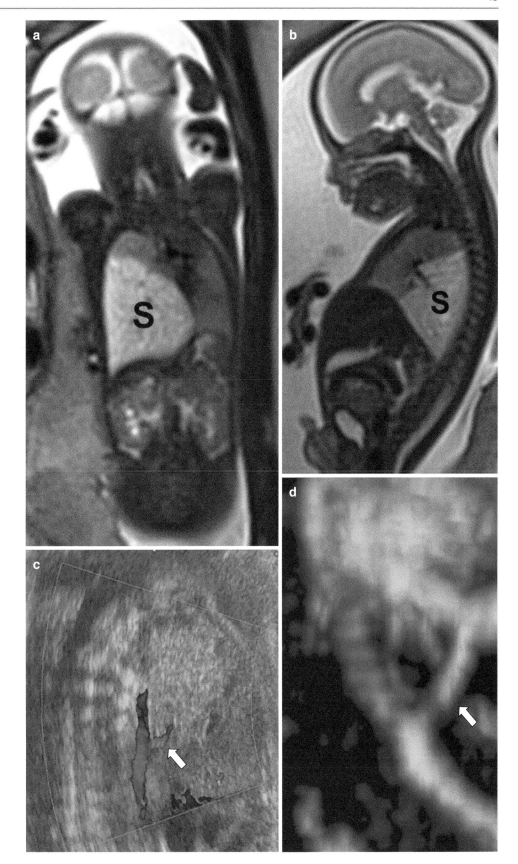

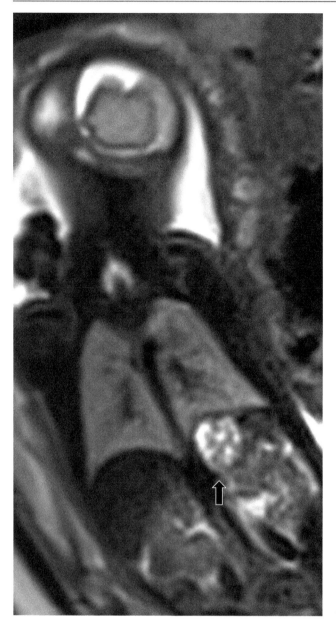

Fig. 1.14 Extralobar infradiaphragmatic pulmonary sequestration on prenatal MR imaging. Coronal non-enhanced T2-weighted MR image shows hyperintense lesion (*arrow*) inferior to the left diaphragm

Infectious Lung and Pleural Disorders

Infections of the lungs and pleura are among the most common reasons for children to require medical attention [60, 61]. Imaging is often performed in these children, most commonly beginning with chest radiographs. When complicated infection is suspected, cross-sectional imaging tests are often performed, frequently CT. With increased concern about the potentially harmful effects of ionizing radiation, and technical advances allowing for diagnostic MR imaging imaging of the thorax, MR imaging has begun to gain attention as a potential alternative to CT in this scenario. A large number of different infections may affect the lungs and pleura, and there is overlap in the

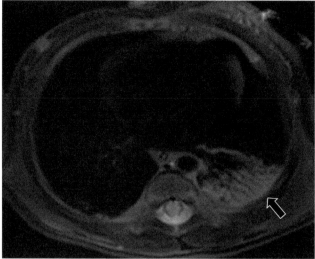

Fig. 1.15 Aspiration pneumonia in a 3-week-old girl who presented with fever and respiratory distress. Axial non-enhanced T2-weighted fat-suppressed MR image shows left lower lobe consolidation (*arrow*)

imaging features of different infections. In this section, the most frequently encountered pediatric infections of the lungs and pleura are described, and common MR imaging patterns of these infections are illustrated.

Bacterial Infection Bacterial infection of the lung causes pneumonia. Pleural effusion may occur in association with bacterial pneumonia, and empyema occurs if infection spreads to the pleural space. The two most common pathogens to cause bacterial pneumonia in the pediatric population are *Streptococcus Pneumoniae and Staphylococcus Aureus*. Less common pathogens include *Haemophilus Influenzae, Bordetella Pertussis*, and *Klebsiella Pneumoniae*. Other pathogens may occur in specific scenarios, for example, *Group B Streptococcus* infection in newborn children of colonized mothers, *Pseudomonas Aeruginosa* infection in pediatric patients with cystic fibrosis, and anaerobic organisms in aspiration pneumonia.

Three main patterns have been recognized in bacterial pneumonia. These include pulmonary consolidation, bronchopneumonia, and atypical pneumonia. Pulmonary consolidation occurs when alveoli fill with exudate, inflammatory cells, and fibrin (Fig. 1.15) [62]. In children consolidation may be lobar or spherical, resulting in "round pneumonia" [63, 64]. Bronchopneumonia describes a pulmonary infection characterized by peribronchial inflammation affecting multiple lobes and may result in patchy peribronchial consolidation and ground-glass signal (Fig. 1.16). Atypical pneumonia is a condition in which imaging may show only mild pulmonary findings such as mild reticular or patchy opacities without a focal region of consolidation, and symptoms may include headache and sore throat [65]. In current clinical practice, these three patterns are most often seen on chest radiograph or CT, but the findings may also be seen on MR imaging. Detailed descriptions of the specific MR imaging findings (e.g., consolidation and ground-glass signal) are covered in a subsequent section.

Pleural effusion may occur in association with bacterial pneumonia and is called parapneumonic effusion (see Fig. 1.16). Empyema occurs when infection spreads to the pleural space, resulting in thickening and hyperemia of the pleural membranes, complex fluid within the pleural space, and loculated pockets of infected fluid. These findings may be appreciated on MR imaging and include hyperintense non-enhancing complex fluid within the pleural space and hyperenhancing thickened parietal and visceral pleura. Rarely, a condition called empyema necessitans can occur when empyema spreads from the pleural space to the chest wall (Fig. 1.17). Empyema

necessitans is most often caused by *Actinomyces israelii* or *Mycobacterium tuberculosis* infection.

Viral Infection Viral respiratory infections include bronchiolitis and viral pneumonia and occur when airborne viruses infect the respiratory mucosa. Infection leads to bronchial wall thickening, inflammation, and mucous production. Mucous plugging and bronchial wall thickening often lead to air trapping and atelectasis. Pleural effusions may accompany viral lower respiratory tract infection. Although these imaging findings are more often described on chest radiograph and CT, the finding may also be appreciated on MR imaging (Fig. 1.18).

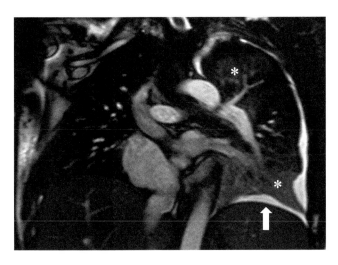

Fig. 1.16 Bacterial bronchopneumonia in a 16-year-old girl who presented with fever and cough. Coronal non-enhanced TruFISP/FIESTA MR image shows peribronchial ground-glass signal abnormality in the left upper and left lower lobes (*asterisks*) and a simple left pleural effusion (*arrow*)

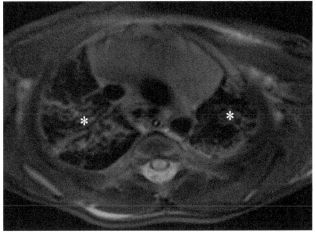

Fig. 1.18 Respiratory syncytial virus infection in a 1-week-old girl who presented with respiratory distress. Axial non-enhanced T2-weighted fat-suppressed MR image shows bilateral peribronchial interstitial thickening (*asterisks*)

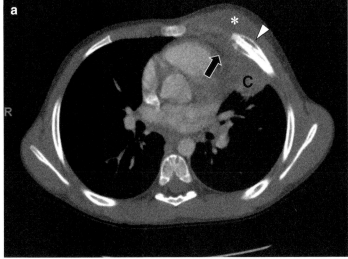

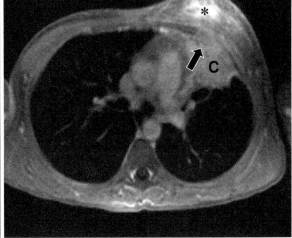

Fig. 1.17 Empyema necessitans in a 17-year-old boy who presented with fever and chest swelling. (**a**) Axial enhanced soft tissue window setting CT image shows consolidation (C) in the lingua, dense pleural fluid and soft tissue density (*arrow*), and left chest wall soft tissue thickening and inflam-

mation (*asterisk*) with periosteal reaction (*arrowhead*) in the adjacent rib. (**b**) Axial enhanced T1-weighted fat-suppressed MR image shows consolidation (C) in the lingua, pleural soft tissue thickening (*arrow*), and left chest wall soft tissue thickening and inflammation (*asterisk*)

A large number of different viruses may cause lower respiratory tract infection in children. Respiratory syncytial virus (RSV) is the most common cause of viral bronchiolitis in infants and young children (see Fig. 1.18). Other viruses that may result in lower respiratory tract infection include human metapneumovirus, parainfluenza virus, rhinovirus, influenza, adenovirus, and cytomegalovirus, among others.

Fungal Infection Fungal infection of the lungs is uncommon in immunocompetent children but is relatively frequent in immunocompromised children [66]. The most common pulmonary fungal infections are aspergillosis, coccidioidomycosis, and histoplasmosis in the pediatric population. Pulmonary infection most often occurs when airborne fungi enter and disseminate through the lung via endobronchial spread, resulting in multiple pulmonary nodules distributed in a tree-in-bud pattern (Figs. 1.19 and 1.20) [65]. Hematogenous spread also occurs, leading to a pattern of small randomly distributed pulmonary nodules in a "miliary" pattern. Pulmonary nodules in fungal infection often

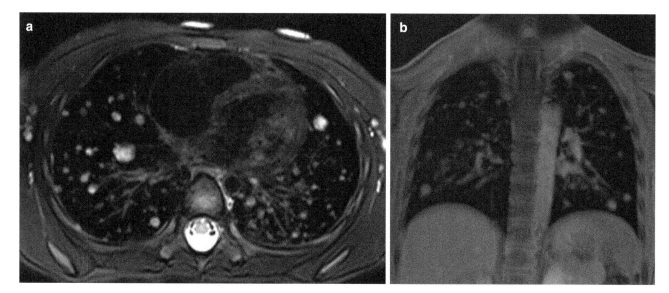

Fig. 1.19 Pulmonary coccidioidomycosis infection in a 5-year-old girl who presented with fever, cough, and headache. (**a**) Axial non-enhanced T2-weighted fat-suppressed MR image shows numerous bilateral hyperintense pulmonary nodules. (**b**) Coronal enhanced T1-weighted fat-suppressed MR image shows numerous bilateral hyperintense pulmonary nodules

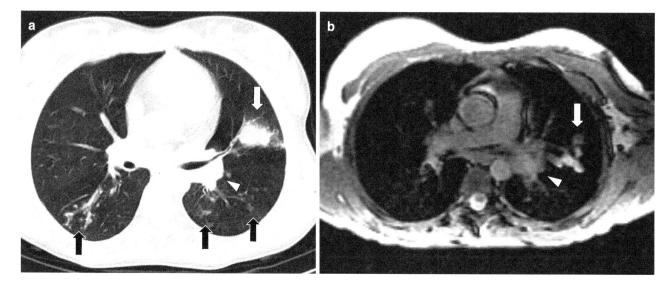

Fig. 1.20 Pulmonary *Aspergillus* infection in 14-year-old girl with cystic fibrosis. (**a**) Axial enhanced lung window setting CT image shows tree-in-bud nodularity (*black arrows*) in bilateral lower lobes, a larger nodule (*white arrow*) with ground-glass halo in the left upper lobe, and left hilar adenopathy (*arrowhead*). (**b**) Axial non-enhanced SSFP T2/T1-weighted MR image shows left upper lobe nodule (*arrow*) and left hilar adenopathy (*arrowhead*)

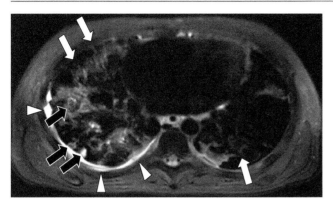

Fig. 1.21 Mycobacterium tuberculosis infection in 13-year-old boy with immunosuppression. Axial non-enhanced T2-weighted MR image shows multiple hyperintense and ground-glass pulmonary nodules (*black arrows*), bilateral interstitial thickening (*white arrows*), and small right pleural effusion (*arrowheads*)

have a solid center (which may cavitate) surrounded by a rim of ground-glass signal intensity, producing a "halo" sign [67]. These findings are most often described on chest radiograph and CT, but they can also be seen on MR imaging as described in a following section.

Mycobacterial Infection (Tuberculosis) In the developing world, tuberculosis (TB) continues to be a significant cause of community-acquired illness and, in the developed world, TB primarily affects patients who are immunocompromised or patients who emigrate from the developing world (Fig. 1.21) [68–70]. Although chest radiograph and CT are the most commonly used imaging modalities to assess TB infection, MR imaging may be considered in certain scenarios. For example, MR imaging may be utilized in immunocompromised pediatric patients receiving multiple imaging studies in order to mitigate exposure to ionizing radiation.

The most common primary mode of transmission for TB infection is through inhalation of infected droplets, and the initial infection is termed primary TB. In children, primary infection most often causes mild symptoms with no findings on imaging studies [71]. Less often, primary infection may cause more significant symptoms and be accompanied by mediastinal and hilar lymphadenopathy and pulmonary parenchymal opacity (see Fig. 1.21) [72, 73]. Lymphadenopathy is most often mild, but in a minority of cases, lymph nodes can become significantly enlarged and cause significant bronchial obstruction [74, 75]. Pleural effusion occurs in approximately 22% of children with primary TB infection (see Fig. 1.21) [76]. In pri-

mary infection, MR imaging may be normal or demonstrate pulmonary consolidation, pulmonary nodules, pleural effusion, or lymphadenopathy (see Fig. 1.21) [77, 78].

Dormant infection may become active at a time after primary infection, referred to as reactivation TB. Symptoms typically include fever, night sweats, productive cough, and hemoptysis. Imaging findings in reactivation TB typically include upper lobe consolidation with cavitation [79]. MR imaging may demonstrate upper lobe consolidation as a region of increased signal on fluid-sensitive sequences and show central necrosis as a region of relatively lower signal intensity within the consolidation [78].

Hematogenous spread of TB infection can lead to innumerable small nodules scattered throughout the lungs, liver, and spleen, termed miliary infection [73]. Young children and immunocompromised pediatric patients are at higher risk for miliary disease. In miliary infection, MR imaging shows innumerable 1–3 mm nodules within the lungs, liver, and spleen.

Parasitic Infection (e.g., Hydatid Disease) Pulmonary hydatid disease is caused by infection with *Echinococcus granulosus*, a parasite whose definitive host is the dog or other canids and intermediate host is sheep, goats, pigs, cattle, horses, or camels. Children may become infected by ingesting the eggs of the parasite located within feces of infected canids. After ingestion, the eggs hatch in the child's gastrointestinal tract and larvae enter the bloodstream. By hematogenous spread, larvae can then form cysts throughout the body; the two most common locations are the liver and the lung. Although most hydatid infections occur during childhood, the hydatid infection is often indolent, and affected patients may not present until adulthood [80]. Pulmonary hydatid disease is rare in many regions of the world, but, in endemic regions, it is a common differential diagnosis for a cystic lung lesion [81]. Hydatid cysts are composed of three layers (pericyst, laminated layer, and germinal layer) with membranes between them [82].

Pulmonary hydatid disease may first be detected on chest radiograph as a single (81%) or multiple (19%) round densities ranging in size from 1 to 20 cm [83–85]. On CT, these lesions demonstrate internal fluid density and a smooth wall that is higher density than fluid (Fig. 1.22). If cyst communicates with the airway an "air-crescent" sign may be seen and a "water lilly" sign may be seen when a collapsed endocyst floats within a cyst [85, 86]. MR imaging may help differentiate pulmonary hydatid disease from other cystic lung lesions by showing characteristic hypoin-

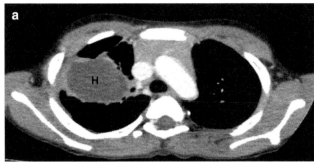
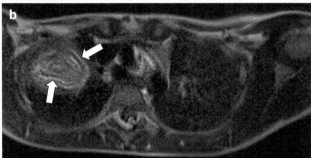
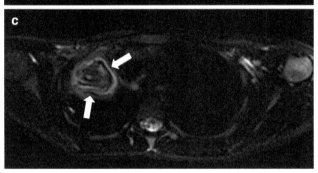

Fig. 1.22 Pulmonary hydatid disease in a 10-year-old boy who presented with chest pain and cough. (Courtesy of Kushaljit Singh Sodhi, MD, PhD, Department of Radiodiagnosis, Postgraduate Institute of Medical Education and Research, Chandigarh, India). (**a**) Axial enhanced soft tissue window setting CT image shows cystic lesion (H) with peripheral enhancement in the right upper lobe. (**b**) Axial non-enhanced T2-HASTE-weighted MR image shows internal folded membranes (*arrows*) within the cystic lesion. (**c**) Axial non-enhanced T2-BLADE-weighted MR image shows internal folded membranes (*arrows*) within the cystic lesion

tense folded membrane within the cyst and a hypointense rim surrounding the cyst (see Fig. 1.22) [81]. Recent prospective study which compared MR and contrast-enhanced MDCT for evaluation of pediatric pulmonary hydatid disease showed that fast MR imaging without contrast material is comparable to contrast-enhanced MDCT for accurately diagnosing lung cysts in pediatric patients with pulmonary hydatid disease. However, added diagnostic value demonstrating internal membranes of cysts, which is specific to pulmonary hydatid disease, was provided by MR imaging in comparison to MDCT [87].

MR imaging Findings of Infectious Disorders of the Lung and Pleura Pulmonary infection may produce a number of different findings on MR imaging. The following section illustrates these MR imaging findings.

Lung Consolidation Pulmonary consolidation is common in bacterial pneumonia. On CT, pulmonary consolidation appears as opacified lung which obscures pulmonary vessels, often with air bronchograms [88]. On MR imaging, homogenous signal intensity fills the normally hypointense lung and obscures pulmonary vessels (Fig. 1.23 and see Fig. 1.15) [88]. On T2-weighted sequences, the signal within pulmonary consolidation is typically greater than the signal in skeletal muscle. On contrast-enhanced T1-weigthed images with fat suppression, the region of consolidation typically enhances homogenously, unless there is necrosis.

Ground-Glass Signal Pulmonary infection may lead to ground-glass abnormalities within the lungs. On CT, ground-glass opacities are defined as opacities which are denser than the air-filled lung, but not dense enough to obscure the pulmonary vasculature. On MR imaging, ground-glass signal is defined as hyperintense signal within the lungs that is more intense than the air-filled lung

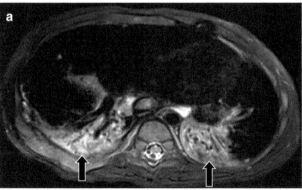
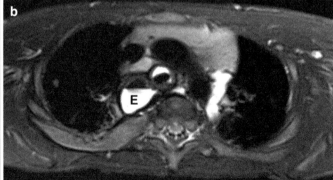

Fig. 1.23 Aspiration-related bilateral lower lobe consolidation in a 3-year-old boy with esophageal atresia repair. (**a**) Axial non-enhanced T2-weighted fat-suppressed MR image shows bilateral lower lobe con-

solidation (*arrows*). (**b**) Axial non-enhanced T2-weighted fat-suppressed MR image shows a dilated fluid-filled esophagus (E)

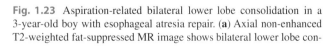

but does not obscure the pulmonary vasculature (Fig. 1.24 and see Fig. 1.16) [88]. Pulmonary infection may lead to ground-glass signal within the lungs, or areas of mixed consolidation and ground-glass signal. Ground-glass signal can also be seen surrounding a central nodule, producing a "halo" sign seen in fungal and other infections [67].

Lung Abscess and Necrosis Pulmonary infection can progress from consolidation and ground-glass abnormalities to pulmonary necrosis and abscess if there is interruption of the blood supply to the lung. Pulmonary necrosis describes devitalized lung which loses its normal architecture and often contains irregularly shaped pockets of air and coalescing fluid. Pulmonary necrosis evolves into pulmonary abscess when a wall forms around a region of devitalized lung (Fig. 1.25) [65, 89, 90]. On MR imaging,

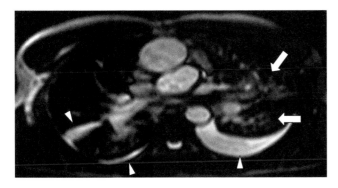

Fig. 1.24 Bronchopneumonia causing ground-glass signal abnormality in a 13-year-old boy who presented with fever and cough. Axial non-enhanced bright-blood T2-weighted MR image shows peribronchial ground-glass signal abnormality (arrows) in the left upper and left lower lobe and bilateral pleural effusions (*arrowheads*)

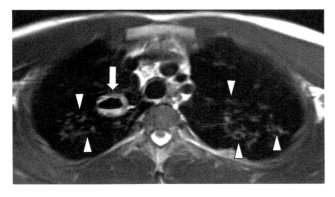

Fig. 1.25 Pulmonary abscess in a 17-year-old girl with cystic fibrosis, fever, and cough. Axial non-enhanced bright-blood MR image shows a cavity (*arrow*) containing an air-fluid level within the right upper lobe and bilateral bronchiectasis (*arrowheads*) with bronchial wall thickening

pulmonary necrosis is defined as an area of lung consolidation without enhancement on contrast-enhanced images. On T2-weighted images, necrosis may be appreciated as a region of lower signal centered within a higher-signal region of consolidation. Like on chest radiograph and CT, irregularly shaped locules of air may be seen within a region of pulmonary necrosis, and an air-filled cavity or a cavity with an air-fluid level may be seen in pulmonary abscess (see Fig. 1.25) [91].

Internal Membrane (e.g., Hydatid Disease) Hydatid cysts are composed of three layers: the outermost pericyst, the middle laminated layer sometimes called the ectocyst, and the innermost germinal layer also known as the endocyst [82]. Each of these layers is separated by a membrane, and visualization of these membranes may aid in the diagnosis of pulmonary hydatid disease (see Fig. 1.22).

Pulmonary hydatid cysts appear as smooth-walled cystic masses, which contain fluid that is hyperintense on T2-weighted images and does not enhance on contrast-enhanced images. MR imaging may be helpful for differentiating hydatid cysts from other cystic masses by demonstrating a characteristic hypointense rim surrounding the cyst and a folded hypointense membrane within the cyst (see Fig. 1.22) [81, 87].

Bronchiectasis Bronchiectasis may occur as a complication of pulmonary infection and is defined as irreversible dilation of a bronchus or bronchiole. Bronchiectasis may also occur in the setting of cystic fibrosis or ciliary dyskinesia [86, 92–96]. Bronchiectasis can be diagnosed on MR imaging when the diameter of a bronchus is greater than the diameter of the pulmonary artery adjacent to it [65]. Because bronchi are air-filled structures surrounded by a thin wall, CT is often better at depicting bronchiectasis than MR imaging. However, the bronchial walls are often thickened and inflamed in bronchiectasis, and these bronchial walls are often hyperintense and visible on T2-weighted MR images (see Fig. 1.25).

Pleural Effusion Simple pleural effusions may occur in cases of pulmonary infection. In these cases, infection may not spread to the pleural space, but the pleural effusion is reactive to the adjacent inflammatory process. In these cases, pleural fluid is homogenous and hyperintense on T2-weighted images and hypointense on T1-weighted images, and pleural membranes are thin without thickening or hyperenhancement on contrast-enhanced MR images (see Figs. 1.16 and 1.24) [97]. Thoracentesis and chest tube placement may be performed for symptom relief when simple effusions are large or to sample fluid in cases of suspected empyema.

Empyema When infection spreads from the lung into the pleural space, an empyema occurs. The appearance of an empyema differs from the appearance of a simple pleural effusion. In empyema, MR imaging may show heterogeneous signal within the pleural space on T2-weighted images due to septations or complex material (see Fig. 1.17) [91]. On contrast-enhanced images, the pleural membranes are typically thickened and hyperenhancing. Empyema may be treated with one of two strategies: antibiotics, chest tube placement, and infusion of fibrinolytics to the pleural space or video-assisted thoracoscopic surgery (VATS)-assisted drainage [98, 99].

Neoplastic Lung and Pleural Disorders

Primary neoplasms of the lungs and pleura are rare and metastatic disease is much more common in the pediatric population [100, 101]. Most neoplasms of the lungs and pleura are first detected on chest radiographs and then further evaluated with CT. MR imaging may be utilized in select scenarios where radiation exposure is a concern or as a part of whole-body MR imaging [102]. The MR imaging appearance of pulmonary and pleural neoplasms is discussed in the following sections.

Benign Primary Neoplasms of Lung and Pleura Benign primary neoplasms of the lung and pleura are rare in children. Benign neoplasms that may occur in children include pulmonary hamartoma, pulmonary chondroma, respiratory papillomatosis, pulmonary sclerosing pneumocytoma, pulmonary inflammatory myofibroblastic tumor, and pleural fibrous pseudotumor [103]. Given the rarity of these entities, there is little in the medical literature describing the MR imaging appearance of many of these entities, though some have been described.

Pulmonary hamartomas are smooth or slightly lobulated solitary pulmonary nodules which may contain fat or calcification. On MR imaging, hamartomas demonstrate hyperintensity on T2-weighted images and early peripheral enhancement that becomes homogenous on delay-phase images (Fig. 1.26) [104]. Cleft-like structures separating small cystic spaces have been described within pulmonary hamartomas on T2-weighted and contrast-enhanced images [104, 105], and chemical shift MR imaging can aid in detection of fat within lesions [106].

Inflammatory myofibroblastic tumors are low-grade mesenchymal tumors that may present as solitary circum-

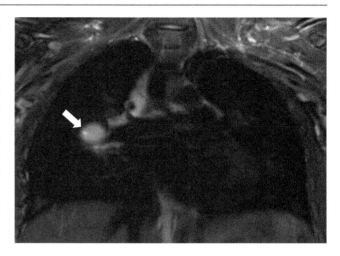

Fig. 1.26 Pulmonary hamartoma in a 13-year-old girl. Coronal non-enhanced T2-weighted fat-suppressed MR image shows a right perihilar hyperintense solitary pulmonary nodule (*arrow*) with a smooth margin

scribed pulmonary nodules or masses or can be infiltrative [107]. In the limited literature describing the MR imaging appearance, inflammatory myofibroblastic tumors may be heterogeneous on T2-weighted images with heterogeneous enhancement and necrosis on contrast-enhanced imaging (Fig. 1.27) [108].

Malignant Primary Neoplasms of Lung and Pleura Malignant primary neoplasms of the lung and pleura are rare in children. Entities include pleuropulmonary blastoma (PPB), pulmonary carcinoid tumor, bronchogenic carcinoma, mucoepidermoid tumor, and epithelioid hemangioendothelioma. As with the benign tumors, there is little in the medical literature describing the MR imaging appearance of many of these entities, although some have been described.

PPB is an aggressive embryonal tumor that arises from the lung or less often from the pleura. PPB is associated with a hereditary tumor predisposition syndrome which includes cystic nephroma, stromal sex-cord ovarian tumors, seminomas or dysgerminomas, intestinal polyps, thyroid hyperplasias, hamartomas, and medulloblastoma [109]. PBB and this hereditary tumor predisposition syndrome are associated with a mutation in the DICER1 gene [110]. There are three types of PPB: type I is purely cystic, type II is cystic and solid, and type III is completely solid. The median age at diagnosis for type I is 8 months, type II is 35 months, and type III is 41 months [111]. The MR imaging appearance depends on the type. In type III, masses are typically large and heterogeneous on T1- and T2-weighted images and often contain regions of necrosis which do not enhance on contrast-enhanced images (Fig. 1.28) [112].

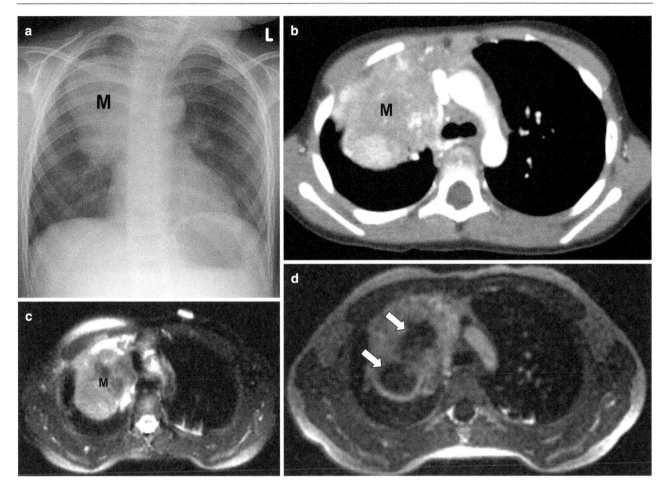

Fig. 1.27 Pulmonary inflammatory myofibroblastic tumor in a 5-year-old boy. (**a**) Frontal chest radiograph shows a large right upper lobe mass (M). (**b**) Axial enhanced soft tissue window setting CT image shows the right upper lobe mass (M) demonstrating heterogeneous enhancement. (**c**) Axial non-enhanced SSFSE T2-weighted MR image shows the right upper lobe mass (M) demonstrating heterogeneous signal intensity. (**d**) Axial enhanced T1-weighted fat-suppressed MR image shows regions of non-enhancement *(arrows)* within the mass, indicating necrosis

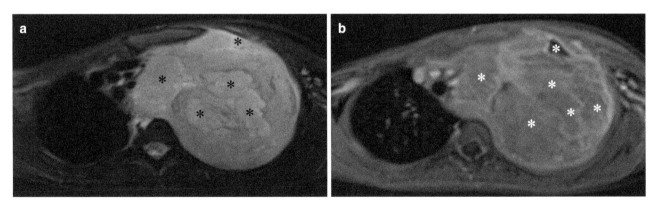

Fig. 1.28 Type III pleuropulmonary blastoma in a 5-year-old girl. (**a**) Axial non-enhanced T2-weighted fat-suppressed MR image shows a large heterogeneously hyperintense left upper lobe mass which exerts mass effect on the mediastinum. Regions of greater hyperintensity *(asterisks)* within the mass correspond to regions of necrosis. (**b**) Axial enhanced T1-weighted fat-suppressed MR image shows heterogenous enhancement within the mass with several non-enhancing regions *(asterisks)*, indicating necrosis

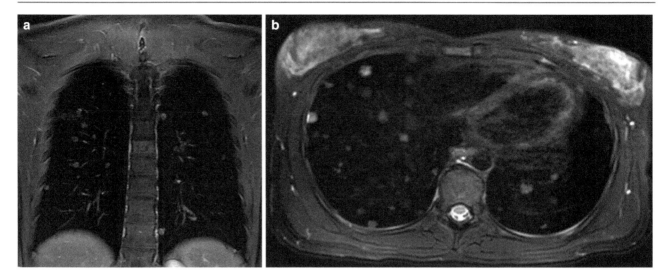

Fig. 1.29 Epithelioid hemangioendothelioma in a 16-year-old girl. (**a**) Coronal non-enhanced T2-weighted fat-suppressed MR image shows multiple bilateral hyperintense pulmonary nodules. (**b**) Axial non-enhanced T2-weighted fat-suppressed MR image shows multiple bilateral hyperintense pulmonary nodules

Epithelioid hemangioendothelioma is a rare vascular sarcoma that can occur at any age and any organ in the body including the lung and pleura [113–115]. Three patterns on imaging are described with thoracic epithelioid hemangioendothelioma: multiple pulmonary nodules, multiple pulmonary reticulonodular opacities, or diffuse infiltrative pleural thickening [116]. Although these findings have been described on CT, similar findings are seen on MR imaging (Fig. 1.29).

Metastatic Neoplasm of Lung and Pleura Metastatic disease is much more common than primary malignancy in the thorax in the pediatric population. In children, pulmonary metastatic disease is 11.6 times more common than primary pulmonary malignancy [101]. In children with a known primary malignancy, surveillance for thoracic metastases is most often achieved with CT given its excellent ability to detect pulmonary nodules with little motion artifact. MR imaging is able to reliably detect pulmonary metastases ≥5 mm [117, 118], but early identification of small pulmonary metastasis (<4 mm) has significant implications for treatment and survival; therefore, CT is currently the preferred method for evaluation of pulmonary metastatic disease. MR imaging may be considered to monitor known pulmonary metastases during therapy in select scenarios or may be used as a part of whole-body screening in patients with hereditary cancer syndromes.

On MR imaging, metastatic pulmonary nodules typically appear isointense to skeletal muscle on T1-weighted images, slightly hyperintense to skeletal muscle on T2-weighted images and demonstrate variable enhancement on contrast-enhanced images (Fig. 1.30). Because pulmonary nodules contain signal-producing protons, they are typically easily

detectible on the background of hypointense aerated lung, although respiratory motion artifact can obscure small nodules. Pulmonary metastatic disease is most often characterized by multiple pulmonary nodules but can also disseminate within the lung via the lymphatic system, in a process called lymphangitic spread (Fig. 1.31).

Pleural effusions may also occur in metastatic disease. In cases of pulmonary metastasis with reactive pleural effusions, the pleural effusions typically contain simple fluid that is hypointense on T1-weighted images and hyperintense on T2-weighted images without associated enhancement. In cases of metastatic spread to the pleura, pleural effusions are accompanied by pleural nodularity, pleural enhancement, and pleural fluid may be complex and contain septations (see Fig. 1.30).

Other Pulmonary and Pleural Conditions Which May Be Evaluated on MR imaging

Pulmonary Edema Pulmonary edema is a condition where fluid accumulates with the pulmonary interstitium and alveoli. Pulmonary edema may be cardiogenic or non-cardiogenic. Cardiogenic pulmonary edema is most commonly due to depressed left ventricular function or obstructed pulmonary venous return. Non-cardiogenic edema may be due to fluid overload, as in cases of excessive intravenous fluid administration or renal failure, or due to increased pulmonary capillary permeability, as in cases of drug toxicity, acute respiratory distress syndrome (ARDS), and neurogenic edema.

MR imaging findings of pulmonary edema are best appreciated on T2-weighted sequences. The interlobular septa are normally not visible on MR imaging, but, in cases of intersti-

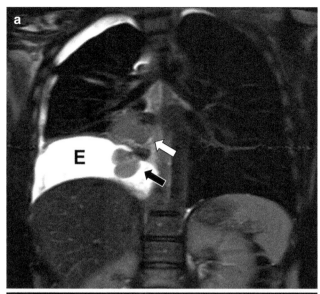

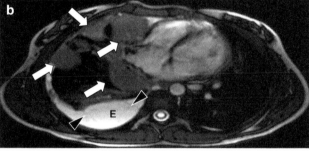

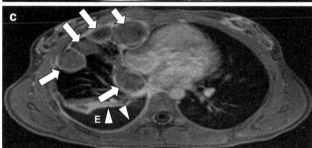

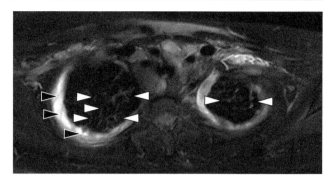

Fig. 1.31 Lymphangitic spread of metastatic disease and pleural effusion in a 12-year-old girl with metastatic renal cell carcinoma. Axial non-enhanced T2-weighted fat-suppressed MR image shows bilateral interlobular septal thickening (*white arrowheads*) due to lymphangitic spread of metastatic disease and bilateral pleural effusions containing septations (*black arrowheads*)

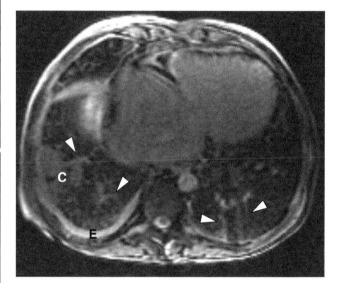

Fig. 1.30 Pulmonary and pleural metastases in a 14-year-old girl with synovial cell sarcoma of the left knee. (**a**) Coronal non-enhanced T2-weighted fat-suppressed MR image shows metastatic nodules in the right lung (*white arrow*) and pleura (*black arrow*) and pleural effusion (E). (**b**) Axial non-enhanced T2-weighted fat-suppressed MR image shows metastatic nodules in the right lung (*white arrows*), pleural effusion (E), and septations (*black arrowheads*) in the pleura. (**c**) Axial enhanced T1-weighted fat-suppressed MR image shows central hypoenhancement within metastatic nodules in the right lung (*white arrows*) and pleural effusion (E) with enhancement of the pleura (*arrowheads*)

Fig. 1.32 Pulmonary edema in a 17-year-old girl with congenital heart disease. Axial non-enhanced T2-weighted MR image shows interlobular septal thickening (*arrowheads*), small region of consolidation (C), and small right pleural effusion (E). Cardiomegaly is also seen

tial pulmonary edema, the septa become visible and hyperintense on T2-weighted images (Fig. 1.32). When fluid fills the alveoli, ground-glass signal and consolidation may be seen (Fig. 1.33 and see Fig. 1.32). MR imaging may also show pleural effusion and cardiomegaly in cases of cardiogenic pulmonary edema.

Pleural Effusion Pleural effusions may form when excess production or decreased absorption of pleural fluid leads to accumulation within the pleural space. The most common causes of pleural effusion are infection, congestive heart failure, and malignancy (see Figs. 1.16, 1.17, 1.24, 1.30, 1.31, and 1.32). Exudative pleural effusions are composed of simple clear fluid. On MR imaging, exudative pleural effusions appear as homogenous fluid that is hyperintense on T2-weighted images and hypointense on T1-weighted images. If causing symptoms, exudative pleural effusions can be treated with chest tube placement. Fibrinopurulent pleural effusions occur when infection spreads to the pleural space and cause empyema (see Fig. 1.17). Empyema is described in detail in an earlier section.

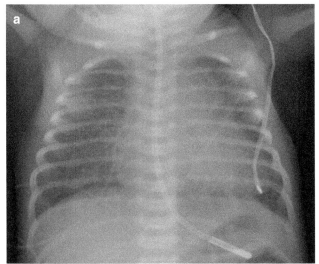

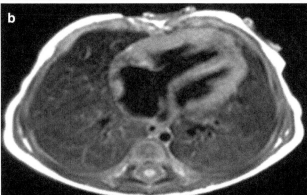

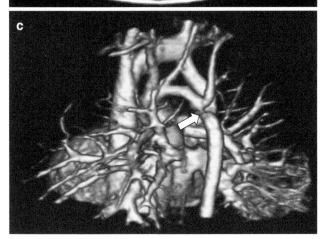

Fig. 1.33 Pulmonary edema in an 8-day-old girl with coarctation of aorta. (**a**) Frontal chest radiograph shows hazy bilateral pulmonary opacities due to pulmonary edema. (**b**) Axial non-enhanced T1-weighted MR image shows ground-glass signal intensity throughout both lungs. (**c**) Posterior projection from 3D reformatted MR image of the mediastinal vessels shows focal narrowing (*arrow*) of the aorta distal to the origin of the left subclavian artery

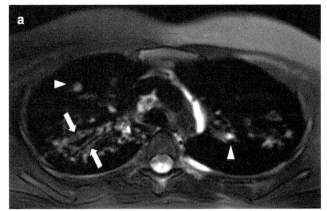

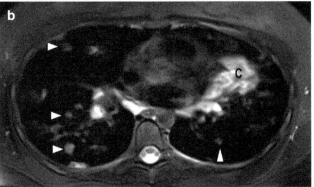

Fig. 1.34 Cystic fibrosis in a 17-year-old girl. (**a**) Axial non-enhanced T2-weighted fat-suppressed MR image shows bronchiectasis with bronchial wall thickening (*white arrows*) and hyperintense pulmonary nodules (*white arrowheads*). (**b**) Axial non-enhanced T2-weighted fat-suppressed MR image shows hyperintense pulmonary nodules (*white arrowheads*) and consolidation (C)

Cystic Fibrosis Cystic fibrosis (CF) is a multisystem genetic disease that primarily affects the lungs but also affects the gastrointestinal and genitourinary systems. CF is caused by mutations in the CF transmembrane regulator (CFTR) gene, leading to decreased transmembranous chloride transport causing secretions to be thick and viscous. In the lungs, CF causes mucus impaction, air trapping, bronchial wall thickening, and bronchiectasis [119–121].

Imaging is utilized in CF to evaluate superimposed infection but is also an important tool for monitoring disease progression. Although CT has historically filled this role, MR imaging has gained attention as an attractive alternative because repeated used of CT throughout the life of a patient with CF can lead to large cumulative radiation doses over time [122]. Many of the key imaging findings in CF produce increased signal on T2-weighted images, facilitating their detection on MR imaging (Fig. 1.34). For example, bronchiectasis with bronchial wall thickening, mucus plugs, and consolidation are detected on MR imaging with sensitivity comparable to CT [121, 123–125].

Conclusion

As MR imaging has become the primary imaging modality to assess many diseases in pediatric patients, its role in the evaluation of the lungs and pleura has lagged due to technical challenges unique to the thorax. However, in recent years, new advances in scanner, computing, and sequence technology have allowed many of these challenges to be overcome. Diagnostic imaging of the lungs and pleura is currently a feasible option for many pediatric patients in many medical centers. As practitioners become familiar with these new techniques and appreciate its potential role, MR imaging will likely be used more in the future when evaluating the spectrum of congenital and acquired pediatric pulmonary and pleural disorders.

References

1. Baez JC, Seethamraju RT, Mulkern R, Ciet P, Lee EY. Pediatric chest MR imaging: sedation, techniques, and extracardiac vessels. Magn Reson Imaging Clin N Am. 2015;23(2):321–35.
2. Ciet P, Tiddens HA, Wielopolski PA, Wild JM, Lee EY, Morana G, et al. Magnetic resonance imaging in children: common problems and possible solutions for lung and airways imaging. Pediatr Radiol. 2015;45(13):1901–15.
3. Gibiino F, Sacolick L, Menini A, Landini L, Wiesinger F. Free-breathing, zero-TE MR lung imaging. MAGMA. 2015;28(3):207–15.
4. Dournes G, Grodzki D, Macey J, Girodet PO, Fayon M, Chateil JF, et al. Quiet submillimeter MR imaging of the lung is feasible with a PETRA sequence at 1.5 T. Radiology. 2015;276(1):258–65.
5. Ciet P, Serra G, Bertolo S, Spronk S, Ros M, Fraioli F, et al. Assessment of CF lung disease using motion corrected PROPELLER MRI: a comparison with CT. Eur Radiol. 2016;26(3):780–7.
6. Kumar S, Rai R, Stemmer A, Josan S, Holloway L, Vinod S, et al. Feasibility of free breathing lung MRI for radiotherapy using non-Cartesian k-space acquisition schemes. Br J Radiol. 2017;90(1080):20170037.
7. Ciet P, Bertolo S, Ros M, Andrinopoulou ER, Tavano V, Lucca F, et al. Detection and monitoring of lung inflammation in cystic fibrosis during respiratory tract exacerbation using diffusion-weighted magnetic resonance imaging. Eur Respir J. 2017;50(1):1601437.
8. Wielputz MO, Puderbach M, Kopp-Schneider A, Stahl M, Fritzsching E, Sommerburg O, et al. Magnetic resonance imaging detects changes in structure and perfusion, and response to therapy in early cystic fibrosis lung disease. Am J Respir Crit Care Med. 2014;189(8):956–65.
9. Dournes G, Menut F, Macey J, Fayon M, Chateil JF, Salel M, et al. Lung morphology assessment of cystic fibrosis using MRI

with ultra-short echo time at submillimeter spatial resolution. Eur Radiol. 2016;26(11):3811–20.
10. Tiddens HA, Stick SM, Wild JM, Ciet P, Parker GJ, Koch A, et al. Respiratory tract exacerbations revisited: ventilation, inflammation, perfusion, and structure (VIPS) monitoring to redefine treatment. Pediatr Pulmonol. 2015;50(Suppl 40):S57–65.
11. Liszewski MC, Ciet P, Lee EY. MR imaging of lungs and airways in children: past and present. Magn Reson Imaging Clin N Am. 2019;27(2):201–25.
12. Shannon JM, Wikenheiser-Brokamp KA, Greenberg JM. Lung growth and development. In: Broaddus VC, editor. Murray & Nadel's textbook of respiratory medicine. 6th ed. Philadelphia: Elsevier; 2016. p. 22–31, 19103–2899.
13. Gebb SA, Shannon JM. Tissue interactions mediate early events in pulmonary vasculogenesis. Dev Dyn. 2000;217(2):159–69.
14. Brown LM, Duck-Chong CG. Methods of evaluating fetal lung maturity. Crit Rev Clin Lab Sci. 1982;16(2):85–159.
15. Steinhorn RH. Pulmonary vascular development. In: Martin RJ, Fanaroff AA, Walsh MC, editors. Fanaroff and Martin's neonatal-perinatal medicine: diseases of the fetus and infant. 10th ed. Philadelphia: Elsevier; 2015. p. 1198–209.
16. Bland RD. Lung epithelial ion transport and fluid movement during the perinatal period. Am J Phys. 1990;259(2 Pt 1):L30–7.
17. Jobe AH, Kamath-Rayne BD. Fetal lung development and surfactant. In: Creasy RK, Resnik R, Iams JD, Lockwood CJ, Moore TR, Greene MF, editors. Creasy and Resnik's maternal-fetal medicine: principles and practice. 7th ed. Philadelphia: Elsevier; 2014. p. 175–86.
18. Ueda T, Ikegami M, Jobe AH. Developmental changes of sheep surfactant: in vivo function and in vitro subtype conversion. J Appl Physiol (1985). 1994;76(6):2701–6.
19. Rider ED, Jobe AH, Ikegami M, Sun B. Different ventilation strategies alter surfactant responses in preterm rabbits. J Appl Physiol (1985). 1992;73(5):2089–96.
20. Kallapur SG, Jobe AH. Lung development and maturation. In: Martin RJ, Fanaroff AA, Walsh MC, editors. Fanaroff and Martin's neonatal-perinatal medicine: diseases of the fetus and infant. 10th ed. Philadelphia: Elsevier; 2015.
21. Broaddus VC, Light RW. Pleural effusion. In: Broaddus VC, editor. Murray and Nadel's textbook of respiratory medicine. 6th ed. Philadelphia: Saunders; 2016. p. 1396–424.
22. Osborne DR, Effmann EL, Hedlund LW. Postnatal growth and size of the pulmonary acinus and secondary lobule in man. AJR Am J Roentgenol. 1983;140(3):449–54.
23. Webb WR. Thin-section CT of the secondary pulmonary lobule: anatomy and the image–the 2004 Fleischner lecture. Radiology. 2006;239(2):322–38.
24. Itoh H, Murata K, Konishi J, Nishimura K, Kitaichi M, Izumi T. Diffuse lung disease: pathologic basis for the high-resolution computed tomography findings. J Thorac Imaging. 1993;8(3):176–88.
25. Albertine K. Anatomy of the lungs. In: Broaddus VC, editor. Murray & Nadel's textbook of respiratory medicine. 6th ed. Philadelphia: Elsevier; 2016. p. 3–21.
26. Yildiz A, Golpinar F, Calikoglu M, Duce MN, Ozer C, Apaydin FD. HRCT evaluation of the accessory fissures of the lung. Eur J Radiol. 2004;49(3):245–9.
27. Ariyurek OM, Gulsun M, Demirkazik FB. Accessory fissures of the lung: evaluation by high-resolution computed tomography. Eur Radiol. 2001;11(12):2449–53.
28. Alamo L, Vial Y, Gengler C, Meuli R. Imaging findings of bronchial atresia in fetuses, neonates and infants. Pediatr Radiol. 2016;46(3):383–90.
29. Ko SF, Lee TY, Kao CL, Ng SH, Wan YL, Lin JW, et al. Bronchial atresia associated with epibronchial right pulmonary artery and aberrant right middle lobe artery. Br J Radiol. 1998;71(842):217–20.

30. Naidich DP, Rumancik WM, Ettenger NA, Feiner HD, Hernanz-Schulman M, Spatz EM, et al. Congenital anomalies of the lungs in adults: MR diagnosis. AJR Am J Roentgenol. 1988;151(1):13–9.

31. Liszewski MC, Hersman FW, Altes TA, Ohno Y, Ciet P, Warfield SK, et al. Magnetic resonance imaging of pediatric lung parenchyma, airways, vasculature, ventilation, and perfusion: state of the art. Radiol Clin North Am. 2013;51(4):555–82.

32. Peranteau WH, Merchant AM, Hedrick HL, Liechty KW, Howell LJ, Flake AW, et al. Prenatal course and postnatal management of peripheral bronchial atresia: association with congenital cystic adenomatoid malformation of the lung. Fetal Diagn Ther. 2008;24(3):190–6.

33. Kunisaki SM, Fauza DO, Nemes LP, Barnewolt CE, Estroff JA, Kozakewich HP, et al. Bronchial atresia: the hidden pathology within a spectrum of prenatally diagnosed lung masses. J Pediatr Surg. 2006;41(1):61–5; discussion −5

34. Berrocal T, Madrid C, Novo S, Gutierrez J, Arjonilla A, Gomez-Leon N. Congenital anomalies of the tracheobronchial tree, lung, and mediastinum: embryology, radiology, and pathology. Radiographics. 2004;24(1):e17.

35. McAdams HP, Kirejczyk WM, Rosado-de-Christenson ML, Matsumoto S. Bronchogenic cyst: imaging features with clinical and histopathologic correlation. Radiology. 2000;217(2):441–6.

36. Alamo L, Reinberg O, Vial Y, Gudinchet F, Meuli R. Comparison of foetal US and MRI in the characterisation of congenital lung anomalies. Eur J Radiol. 2013;82(12):e860–6.

37. Rios LT, Araujo Junior E, Nardozza LM, Moron AF, Martins Mda G. Prenatal diagnosis and postnatal findings of bronchogenic cyst. Case Rep Pulmonol. 2013;2013:483864.

38. Pacharn P, Kline-Fath B, Calvo-Garcia M, Linam LE, Rubio EI, Salisbury S, et al. Congenital lung lesions: prenatal MRI and postnatal findings. Pediatr Radiol. 2013;43(9):1136–43.

39. Lee EY, Dorkin H, Vargas SO. Congenital pulmonary malformations in pediatric patients: review and update on etiology, classification, and imaging findings. Radiol Clin N Am. 2011;49(5):921–48.

40. Epelman M, Daltro P, Soto G, Ferrari CM, Lee EY. Congenital lung anomalies. In: Coley BD, editor. Caffey's pediatric diagnostic imaging. 12th ed. Philadelphia: Elsevier; 2013. p. 550–66.

41. Lee EY, Boiselle PM, Cleveland RH. Multidetector CT evaluation of congenital lung anomalies. Radiology. 2008;247(3):632–48.

42. Holder PD, Langston C. Intralobar pulmonary sequestration (a nonentity?). Pediatr Pulmonol. 1986;2(3):147–53.

43. Laurin S, Hagerstrand I. Intralobar bronchopulmonary sequestration in the newborn--a congenital malformation. Pediatr Radiol. 1999;29(3):174–8.

44. Riedlinger WF, Vargas SO, Jennings RW, Estroff JA, Barnewolt CE, Lillehei CW, et al. Bronchial atresia is common to extralobar sequestration, intralobar sequestration, congenital cystic adenomatoid malformation, and lobar emphysema. Pediatr Dev Pathol. 2006;9(5):361–73.

45. Langston C. New concepts in the pathology of congenital lung malformations. Semin Pediatr Surg. 2003;12(1):17–37.

46. Stocker JT, Madewell JE, Drake RM. Congenital cystic adenomatoid malformation of the lung. Classification and morphologic spectrum. Hum Pathol. 1977;8(2):155–71.

47. Stocker J. The respiratory tract. In: Stocker JT, LP D, editors. Pediatric pathology. 2nd ed. Philadelphia: Lippincott, Williams & Wilkins; 2001. p. 466–73.

48. Alamo L, Gudinchet F, Reinberg O, Vial Y, Francini K, Osterheld MC, et al. Prenatal diagnosis of congenital lung malformations. Pediatr Radiol. 2012;42(3):273–83.

49. Epelman M, Kreiger PA, Servaes S, Victoria T, Hellinger JC. Current imaging of prenatally diagnosed congenital lung lesions. Semin Ultrasound CT MR. 2010;31(2):141–57.

50. MacSweeney F, Papagiannopoulos K, Goldstraw P, Sheppard MN, Corrin B, Nicholson AG. An assessment of the expanded classification of congenital cystic adenomatoid malformations and their relationship to malignant transformation. Am J Surg Pathol. 2003;27(8):1139–46.

51. d'Agostino S, Bonoldi E, Dante S, Meli S, Cappellari F, Musi L. Embryonal rhabdomyosarcoma of the lung arising in cystic adenomatoid malformation: case report and review of the literature. J Pediatr Surg. 1997;32(9):1381–3.

52. Domizio P, Liesner RJ, Dicks-Mireaux C, Risdon RA. Malignant mesenchymoma associated with a congenital lung cyst in a child: case report and review of the literature. Pediatr Pathol. 1990;10(5):785–97.

53. Ozcan C, Celik A, Ural Z, Veral A, Kandiloglu G, Balik E. Primary pulmonary rhabdomyosarcoma arising within cystic adenomatoid malformation: a case report and review of the literature. J Pediatr Surg. 2001;36(7):1062–5.

54. Federici S, Domenichelli V, Tani G, Sciutti R, Burnelli R, Zanetti G, et al. Pleuropulmonary blastoma in congenital cystic adenomatoid malformation: report of a case. Eur J Pediatr Surg. 2001;11(3):196–9.

55. Burge D, Wheeler R. Increasing incidence of detection of congenital lung lesions. Pediatr Pulmonol. 2010;45(1):103; author reply: 4

56. Pryce DM. Lower accessory pulmonary artery with intralobar sequestration of lung; a report of seven cases. J Pathol Bacteriol. 1946;58(3):457–67.

57. Cannie M, Jani J, De Keyzer F, Van Kerkhove F, Meersschaert J, Lewi L, et al. Magnetic resonance imaging of the fetal lung: a pictorial essay. Eur Radiol. 2008;18(7):1364–74.

58. Eber E. Antenatal diagnosis of congenital thoracic malformations: early surgery, late surgery, or no surgery? Semin Respir Crit Care Med. 2007;28(3):355–66.

59. Laje P, Liechty KW. Postnatal management and outcome of prenatally diagnosed lung lesions. Prenat Diagn. 2008;28(7):612–8.

60. Rudan I, Tomaskovic L, Boschi-Pinto C, Campbell H. Global estimate of the incidence of clinical pneumonia among children under five years of age. Bull World Health Organ. 2004;82(12):895–903.

61. Jokinen C, Heiskanen L, Juvonen H, Kallinen S, Karkola K, Korppi M, et al. Incidence of community-acquired pneumonia in the population of four municipalities in eastern Finland. Am J Epidemiol. 1993;137(9):977–88.

62. Daltro P, Santos EN, Gasparetto TD, Ucar ME, Marchiori E. Pulmonary infections. Pediatr Radiol. 2011;41(Suppl 1):S69–82.

63. Kim YW, Donnelly LF. Round pneumonia: imaging findings in a large series of children. Pediatr Radiol. 2007;37(12):1235–40.

64. Restrepo R, Palani R, Matapathi UM, Wu YY. Imaging of round pneumonia and mimics in children. Pediatr Radiol. 2010;40(12):1931–40.

65. Eslamy HK, Newman B. Pneumonia in normal and immunocompromised children: an overview and update. Radiol Clin N Am. 2011;49(5):895–920.

66. George R, Andronikou S, Theron S, du Plessis J, Hayes M, Goussard P, et al. Pulmonary infections in HIV-positive children. Pediatr Radiol. 2009;39(6):545–54.

67. Buckingham SJ, Hansell DM. Aspergillus in the lung: diverse and coincident forms. Eur Radiol. 2003;13(8):1786–800.

68. Alami NN, Yuen CM, Miramontes R, Pratt R, Price SF, Navin TR. Trends in tuberculosis – United States, 2013. MMWR Morb Mortal Wkly Rep. 2014;63(11):229–33.

69. Lobato MN, Hopewell PC. Mycobacterium tuberculosis infection after travel to or contact with visitors from countries with a high prevalence of tuberculosis. Am J Respir Crit Care Med. 1998;158(6):1871–5.

70. de Almeida CPB, Ziegelmann PK, Couban R, Wang L, Busse JW, Silva DR. Predictors of in-hospital mortality among patients with pulmonary tuberculosis: a systematic review and meta-analysis. Sci Rep. 2018;8(1):7230.

71. Marais BJ, Gie RP, Schaaf HS, Hesseling AC, Obihara CC, Starke JJ, et al. The natural history of childhood intra-thoracic tuberculo-

sis: a critical review of literature from the pre-chemotherapy era. Int J Tuberc Lung Dis. 2004;8(4):392–402.

72. Leung AN, Muller NL, Pineda PR, FitzGerald JM. Primary tuberculosis in childhood: radiographic manifestations. Radiology. 1992;182(1):87–91.

73. Starke JR. Mycobacterium tuberculosis. In: Long SS, Pickering LK, Prober CG, editors. Principles and practice of pediatric infectious diseases. 4th ed. Philadelphia: Elsevier; 2012. p. 771–86.

74. Goussard P, Gie RP, Janson JT, le Roux P, Kling S, Andronikou S, et al. Decompression of enlarged mediastinal lymph nodes due to mycobacterium tuberculosis causing severe airway obstruction in children. Ann Thorac Surg. 2015;99(4):1157–63.

75. Goussard P, Gie R. Airway involvement in pulmonary tuberculosis. Paediatr Respir Rev. 2007;8(2):118–23.

76. Merino JM, Carpintero I, Alvarez T, Rodrigo J, Sanchez J, Coello JM. Tuberculous pleural effusion in children. Chest. 1999;115(1):26–30.

77. Rizzi EB, Schinina V, Cristofaro M, Goletti D, Palmieri F, Bevilacqua N, et al. Detection of pulmonary tuberculosis: comparing MR imaging with HRCT. BMC Infect Dis. 2011; 11:243.

78. Peprah KO, Andronikou S, Goussard P. Characteristic magnetic resonance imaging low T2 signal intensity of necrotic lung parenchyma in children with pulmonary tuberculosis. J Thorac Imaging. 2012;27(3):171–4.

79. Griffith-Richards SB, Goussard P, Andronikou S, Gie RP, Przybojewski SJ, Strachan M, et al. Cavitating pulmonary tuberculosis in children: correlating radiology with pathogenesis. Pediatr Radiol. 2007;37(8):798–804; quiz 48–9

80. Moro PL, Schantz PM. Echinococcus species (agents of cystic, alveolar, and polycystic echinococcosis). In: Long SS, Pickering LK, Prober CG, editors. Principles and practice of pediatric infectious diseases. 4th ed; 2012. p. 1356–62.

81. Tandur R, Irodi A, Chacko BR, Vimala LR, Christopher DJ, Gnanamuthu BR. Magnetic resonance imaging as an adjunct to computed tomography in the diagnosis of pulmonary hydatid cysts. Indian J Radiol Imaging. 2018;28(3):342–9.

82. Garg MK, Sharma M, Gulati A, Gorsi U, Aggarwal AN, Agarwal R, et al. Imaging in pulmonary hydatid cysts. World J Radiol. 2016;8(6):581–7.

83. Sarkar M, Pathania R, Jhobta A, Thakur BR, Chopra R. Cystic pulmonary hydatidosis. Lung India. 2016;33(2):179–91.

84. Sadrizadeh A, Haghi SZ, Masuom SH, Bagheri R, Dalouee MN. Evaluation of the effect of pulmonary hydatid cyst location on the surgical technique approaches. Lung India. 2014;31(4):361–5.

85. Turgut AT, Altinok T, Topcu S, Kosar U. Local complications of hydatid disease involving thoracic cavity: imaging findings. Eur J Radiol. 2009;70(1):49–56.

86. Westra SJ, Adler B, Yikilmaz A, Lee EY. Pulmonary infection. In: Coley BD, editor. Caffey's pediatric diagnostic imaging. 12th ed. Philadelphia: Elsevier; 2013. p. 567–81.

87. Sodhi KS, Bhatia A, Samujh R, Mathew JL, Lee EY. Prospective comparison of MRI and contrast-enhanced MDCT for evaluation of pediatric pulmonary hydatid disease: added diagnostic value of MRI. AJR Am J Roentgenol. 2019;1–6.

88. Attenberger UI, Morelli J, Henzler T, Buchheidt D, Fink C, Schoenberg SO, et al. 3 Tesla proton MRI for the diagnosis of pneumonia/lung infiltrates in neutropenic patients with acute myeloid leukemia: initial results in comparison to HRCT. Eur J Radiol. 2014;83(1):e61–6.

89. Donnelly LF, Klosterman LA. Pneumonia in children: decreased parenchymal contrast enhancement–CT sign of intense illness and impending cavitary necrosis. Radiology. 1997;205(3): 817–20.

90. Donnelly LF. Practical issues concerning imaging of pulmonary infection in children. J Thorac Imaging. 2001;16(4):238–50.

91. Peltola V, Ruuskanen O, Svedstrom E. Magnetic resonance imaging of lung infections in children. Pediatr Radiol. 2008;38(11):1225–31.

92. Osborne D, White P. Radiology of epidemic adenovirus 21 infection of the lower respiratory tract in infants and young children. AJR Am J Roentgenol. 1979;133(3):397–400.

93. Brady MT, Marcon MJ. Pseudomonas and related genera. In: Cherry JD, Harrison GJ, Kaplan SL, Steinbach WJ, Hotez PJ, editors. Feigin and Cherry's textbook of pediatric infectious diseases. 7th ed. Philadelphia: Elsevier; 2014. p. 1582–605.

94. Chu HQ, Li B, Zhao L, Huang DD, Zhang ZM, Xu JF, et al. Chest imaging comparison between non-tuberculous and tuberculosis mycobacteria in sputum acid fast bacilli smear-positive patients. Eur Rev Med Pharmacol Sci. 2015;19(13):2429–39.

95. Maffessanti M, Candusso M, Brizzi F, Piovesana F. Cystic fibrosis in children: HRCT findings and distribution of disease. J Thorac Imaging. 1996;11(1):27–38.

96. Kennedy MP, Noone PG, Leigh MW, Zariwala MA, Minnix SL, Knowles MR, et al. High-resolution CT of patients with primary ciliary dyskinesia. AJR Am J Roentgenol. 2007;188(5):1232–8.

97. Gorkem SB, Coskun A, Yikilmaz A, Zurakowski D, Mulkern RV, Lee EY. Evaluation of pediatric thoracic disorders: comparison of unenhanced fast-imaging-sequence 1.5-T MRI and contrast-enhanced MDCT. AJR Am J Roentgenol. 2013;200(6):1352–7.

98. Aziz A, Healey JM, Qureshi F, Kane TD, Kurland G, Green M, et al. Comparative analysis of chest tube thoracostomy and video-assisted thoracoscopic surgery in empyema and parapneumonic effusion associated with pneumonia in children. Surg Infect. 2008;9(3):317–23.

99. Kelly MM, Coller RJ, Kohler JE, Zhao Q, Sklansky DJ, Shadman KA, et al. Trends in hospital treatment of empyema in children in the united states. J Pediatr. 2018;202:245–51.e1.

100. Tischer W, Reddemann H, Herzog P, Gdanietz K, Witt J, Wurnig P, et al. Experience in surgical treatment of pulmonary and bronchial tumours in childhood. Prog Pediatr Surg. 1987;21:118–35.

101. Dishop MK, Kuruvilla S. Primary and metastatic lung tumors in the pediatric population: a review and 25-year experience at a large children's hospital. Arch Pathol Lab Med. 2008;132(7):1079–103.

102. Bueno MT, Martinez-Rios C, la Puente Gregorio A, Ahyad RA, Villani A, Druker H, et al. Pediatric imaging in DICER1 syndrome. Pediatr Radiol. 2017;47(10):1292–301.

103. Erasmus JJ, McAdams HP, Patz EF Jr, Murray JG, Pinkard NB. Calcifying fibrous pseudotumor of pleura: radiologic features in three cases. J Comput Assist Tomogr. 1996;20(5):763–5.

104. Alexopoulou E, Economopoulos N, Priftis KN, Tsigka A, Kelekis NL. MR imaging findings of an atypical pulmonary hamartoma in a 12-year-old child. Pediatr Radiol. 2008;38(10):1134–7.

105. Park KY, Kim SJ, Noh TW, Cho SH, Lee DY, Paik HC, et al. Diagnostic efficacy and characteristic feature of MRI in pulmonary hamartoma: comparison with CT, specimen MRI, and pathology. J Comput Assist Tomogr. 2008;32(6):919–25.

106. Hochhegger B, Marchiori E, dos Reis DQ, Souza AS Jr, Souza LS, Brum T, et al. Chemical-shift MRI of pulmonary hamartomas: initial experience using a modified technique to assess nodule fat. AJR Am J Roentgenol. 2012;199(3):W331–4.

107. Surabhi VR, Chua S, Patel RP, Takahashi N, Lalwani N, Prasad SR. Inflammatory myofibroblastic tumors: current update. Radiol Clin North Am. 2016;54(3):553–63.

108. Naime S, Bandarkar A, Nino G, Perez G. Pulmonary inflammatory myofibroblastic tumour misdiagnosed as a round pneumonia. BMJ Case Rep. 2018;2018:bcr-2017-224091.

109. Priest JR, Williams GM, Hill DA, Dehner LP, Jaffe A. Pulmonary cysts in early childhood and the risk of malignancy. Pediatr Pulmonol. 2009;44(1):14–30.

110. Hill DA, Ivanovich J, Priest JR, Gurnett CA, Dehner LP, Desruisseau D, et al. DICER1 mutations in familial pleuropulmonary blastoma. Science. 2009;325(5943):965.

111. Messinger YH, Stewart DR, Priest JR, Williams GM, Harris AK, Schultz KA, et al. Pleuropulmonary blastoma: a report on 350 central pathology-confirmed pleuropulmonary blastoma cases by the International Pleuropulmonary Blastoma Registry. Cancer. 2015;121(2):276–85.

112. Papaioannou G, Sebire NJ, McHugh K. Imaging of the unusual pediatric 'blastomas'. Cancer Imaging. 2009;9:1–11.

113. Hettmer S, Andrieux G, Hochrein J, Kurz P, Rossler J, Lassmann S, et al. Epithelioid hemangioendotheliomas of the liver and lung in children and adolescents. Pediatr Blood Cancer. 2017;64(12)

114. Siraj S, Akhter S, Rizvi N. Primary pleural epitheliod hemangioendothelioma with lung involvement. J Coll Physicians Surg Pak. 2017;27(9):S120–s1.

115. Mucientes P, Gomez-Arellano L, Rao N. Malignant pleuropulmonary epithelioid hemangioendothelioma – unusual presentation of an aggressive angiogenic neoplasm. Pathol Res Pract. 2014;210(9):613–8.

116. Kim EY, Kim TS, Han J, Choi JY, Kwon OJ, Kim J. Thoracic epithelioid hemangioendothelioma: imaging and pathologic features. Acta Radiol. 2011;52(2):161–6.

117. Hirsch W, Sorge I, Krohmer S, Weber D, Meier K, Till H. MRI of the lungs in children. Eur J Radiol. 2008;68(2):278–88.

118. Gorkem S, Coskun A, Yikilmaz A, Zurakowski D, Mulkern R, Lee E. Evaluation of pediatric thoracic disorders: comparison of unenhanced fast-imaging sequence 1.5T MRI with contrast-enhanced MDCT. AJR Am J Roentgenol. 2013;200(6):1352–7.

119. Mott LS, Park J, Murray CP, Gangell CL, de Klerk NH, Robinson PJ, et al. Progression of early structural lung disease in young children with cystic fibrosis assessed using CT. Thorax. 2012;67(6):509–16.

120. Sly PD, Gangell CL, Chen L, Ware RS, Ranganathan S, Mott LS, et al. Risk factors for bronchiectasis in children with cystic fibrosis. N Engl J Med. 2013;368(21):1963–70.

121. Wielputz MO, Mall MA. Imaging modalities in cystic fibrosis: emerging role of MRI. Curr Opin Pulm Med. 2015;21(6): 609–16.

122. Wielputz MO, Eichinger M, Puderbach M. Magnetic resonance imaging of cystic fibrosis lung disease. J Thorac Imaging. 2013;28(3):151–9.

123. Puderbach M, Eichinger M, Gahr J, Ley S, Tuengerthal S, Schmahl A, et al. Proton MRI appearance of cystic fibrosis: comparison to CT. Eur Radiol. 2007;17(3):716–24.

124. Puderbach M, Eichinger M, Haeselbarth J, Ley S, Kopp-Schneider A, Tuengerthal S, et al. Assessment of morphological MRI for pulmonary changes in cystic fibrosis (CF) patients: comparison to thin-section CT and chest x-ray. Investig Radiol. 2007;42(10):715–25.

125. Murphy KP, Maher MM, O'Connor OJ. Imaging of cystic fibrosis and pediatric bronchiectasis. AJR Am J Roentgenol. 2016;206(3):448–54.

Large Airways

Pierluigi Ciet, Mark C. Liszewski, and Edward Y. Lee

Introduction

Large airway magnetic resonance (MR) imaging is a relatively new technique in thoracic imaging, with chest radiography (CXR) and computed tomography (CT) being the most used modalities [1]. However, the lack of ionizing radiation makes MR imaging an attractive alternative to CT particularly in the pediatric population [2]. Disorders of the respiratory system are quite common and of great importance in pediatrics, including both lung and airway disorders [3]. While CXR is most often the first step for imaging disorders of the lungs, CT is the technique with the highest sensitivity to assess airway pathology [4]. The rapid improvement of MR imaging techniques has made it feasible to obtain similar image quality to CT but with the unparalleled advantage of combined structural and functional imaging without radiation exposure [5].

In this chapter, MR imaging techniques for evaluating the large airways and normal anatomy in pediatric patients are discussed. In addition, various congenital and acquired disorders commonly affecting infants and children are reviewed including clinical features, characteristic MR imaging findings, and current treatment approaches.

P. Ciet (✉)
Department of Radiology and Nuclear Medicine, Department of Pediatric Pulmonology, Sophia Children's Hospital Erasmus Medical Center, Rotterdam, South-Holland, The Netherlands
e-mail: p.ciet@erasmusmc.nl

M. C. Liszewski
Division of Pediatric Radiology, Departments of Radiology and Pediatrics, The Children's Hospital at Montefiore and Montefiore Medical Center, Bronx, NY, USA

E. Y. Lee
Division of Thoracic Imaging, Department of Radiology, Boston Children's Hospital, Harvard Medical School, Boston, MA, USA

Magnetic Resonance Imaging Techniques

Patient Preparation

Patient age is an essential factor to consider when preparing patients for large airway MR imaging. In pediatric patients who are unable to follow instructions, including most patients younger than 5 years and patients with cognitive delay, free-breathing MR imaging techniques with or without anesthesia are mandatory [6]. The risks of anesthesia should be discussed with the referring physician and the parents and weighed with the potential benefits of the MR imaging examination. Possible negative sequelae of deep sedation on the developing brain have been shown in animal models [6]. When sedated, the patient needs to be closely monitored, ensuring appropriate heart rate, blood pressure, and oxygenation. A possible alternative to sedation in neonates is the "feed and swaddle" technique [7], where the child is fed immediately before the examination and then placed in the scanner after being swaddled. This technique works well in imaging of stationary body parts such as the brain. However, for chest imaging, its use is frequently limited due to respiratory motion, which is accentuated by the high respiratory rates of neonates.

Cardiac and respiratory rate are two crucial factors that determine image quality in the neonatal patient age group [6]. Even with an optimized MR imaging protocol including sequences with low motion sensitivity, such as those with radial and of helicoidal k-space acquisitions, unexpected patient movement can make a scan non-diagnostic. To reduce respiratory motion, the anesthesiologist can hold respiration at end-inspiration or end-expiration in a controlled setting where patient's vital signs are constantly monitored [6]. Alternatively, a breath-hold state can be recreated through hyperventilation. The radiologist is responsible to keep the scan time as short as possible and at the same time to ensure diagnostic image quality. A short scan time is also important to limit the development of atelectasis, which can obscure underlying abnormalities [8]. After the MR imaging is completed, the patient is usually monitored in a controlled environment until discharge from the radiology department to ensure full recovery from anesthesia.

Older pediatric patients (usually older than 5 years), who can follow directions, may attempt to undergo MR imaging without sedation. Preparation before the MR imaging examination greatly improves the success rate in this pediatric patient group. This preparation consists of familiarizing the patient with the noisy environment of MR scanner and practicing the breathing maneuvers that will be performed during the MR imaging examination [6]. A mock scanner (Fig. 2.1) can be used to reproduce similar noises of real MR imaging sequences and the movement of the table. Moreover, the patient can understand the importance of laying still and rehearse specific maneuvers in the supine position recreating the same conditions as during the MR imaging scan [9]. Coaching and scanning with an MR imaging-compatible spirometer helps standardize lung volume assessment [9]. This device allows real-time monitoring of maximal inspiratory and expiratory volumes that can be used as references to trigger MR imaging acquisition during the scan [9]. Finally, to reduce possible anxiety related to the scan, parents should be allowed to stay in the MR imaging room with the child and distraction methods, such as projecting a movie, can be used to help the children feel comfortable [6].

MR Imaging Pulse Sequences and Protocols

Unlike lung imaging, where 1.5 Tesla (T) systems are more suitable to achieve high signal-to-noise ratio (SNR) thanks to lower T2 star (T2*) dephasing and susceptibility artifacts, large airway MR imaging is more suitable at higher magnetic fields, such as 3T or higher [2]. These systems can allow faster performance especially for dynamic imaging (because of higher SNR and slew rate). Another critical factor for better image quality in large airway MR imaging is choosing the correct receiver coil. Close-fitting, high-density, receiver phase-array coils are of key importance [2]. Phase-array coils provide higher SNR by virtue of the closer proximity to the large airways but also allow for shorter acquisition time through the use of parallel imaging [2].

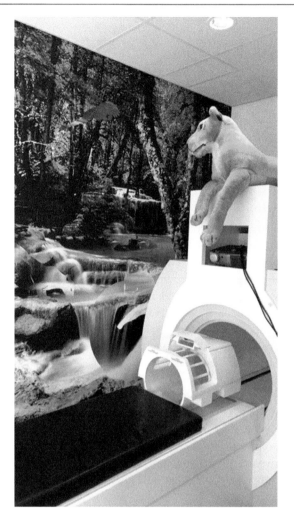

Fig. 2.1 Mock scanner for pediatric patient training. In the mock scanner, pediatric patients familiarize themselves with the noisy environment of the MR imaging scanner and can rehearse breathing maneuvers

Optimal coil designs differ depending on the patient anatomy; for thoracic MR imaging the coils most frequently used are arrays with 8–32 receiver channels. Infants and young children can benefit from the use of small flexible coils directly in contact with the target area, while older patients can be imaged using a torso or head/neck/spine (HNS) coil. A loose HNS coil design has the advantage of a small anterior coil receiver, which provides a tighter fit when imaging the upper airways compared to a torso coil (Fig. 2.2). This is especially true in older girls with fully developed breasts or muscular boys with prominent pectoral muscles. Further improvements in SNR could be obtained with dedicated cape-like coils

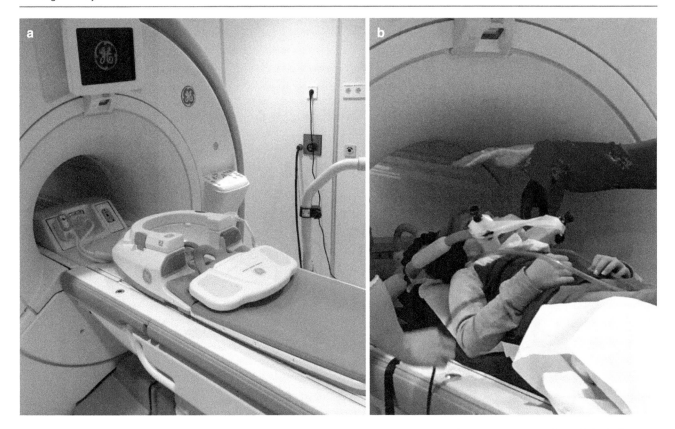

Fig. 2.2 Coil selection and placement for a 7-year-old girl. (**a**) 8-channel head/neck/spine (HNS) phase-array coil (GE), consisting of an anterior portion that is freely adaptable to variable thoracic sizes allowing for closer-fitting than standard torso coils in children. (**b**) 6-channel coil prototype for upper airway imaging built in the Erasmus Medical Center (Rotterdam, The Netherlands) in collaboration with Machnet B.V. and Flick Engineering B.V. (Winterswijk, The Netherlands)

tailored for large airway MR imaging. MR imaging techniques for large airway imaging are summarized in the following sections. A dedicated protocol for large airway MR imaging is presented in Table 2.1.

Static MR Large Airway Imaging

Complete MR airway imaging relies on both end-inspiratory and end-expiratory acquisitions. This can only be achieved in compliant pediatric patients. Breath-hold time needs to be tailored to patient's age; therefore, younger patients require shorter acquisition times in the range of 8–12 seconds. Such scan times are achievable with several two dimensional (2D) and three-dimensional (3D) sequences. In pediatric patients who cannot follow instructions, free-breathing acquisitions combined with respiratory triggering or navigation allow diagnostic image quality, though at the expense of longer acquisition times.

2D Techniques

Fast Spin-Echo Sequences Fast spin-echo (FSE) or turbo spin-echo (TSE) sequences have low sensitivity to magnetic susceptibility artifacts and can achieve sub-second acquisition times (e.g., single-shot FSE scans) [2]. A typical sequence is the 2D T2-weighted single-shot FSE scan, known under different acronyms depending on the MR imaging scan manufacturer [2]. Single-shot FSE techniques have high sensitivity and high SNR for fluid detection. As all T2-weighted sequences, they are suitable to assess bronchial wall thickening and mucus plugging (Fig. 2.3). Bronchial walls can be further highlighted with blood suppression techniques, such as those using a black blood (BB) preparation. BB preparation involves the application of two radio-frequency (RF)-inversion pulses in close succession (non-selective and selective excitation and a corresponding inversion

Table 2.1 MR imaging protocols for large airway imaging

Sequence type	Brand name (Brand)	Weighting	Acquisition setting and duration	Spatial resolution and orientation	Temporal resolution	Scan parameters	MR imaging system
Static airway evaluation							
2D Fast spin echo	PROPELLER (GE) BLADE (Siemens) MultiVane (Philips)	T2-weighted Black blood	End-expiratory with navigator echo triggering 3–7 min according respiratory pace and pattern	FOV = 380–400 mm Matrix = 200 × 200 SL = 5–6 mm Axial and coronal	Low	TR = respiratory rate (2–5 s) TE = short–medium (25–60 ms) FA = 90°/150° ± FAT saturation BW = low–medium	1.5T and 3.0T
2D SSFP	FIESTA (GE) TrueFISP (Siemens) Balanced-FFE (Philips)	T1/T2-weighted Bright blood	12–20 s Breath-hold	FOV = 400 mm Matrix = 160 × 160 SL = 2.5–5 mm Axial and coronal	High	TR = shortest (<4 ms) TE = shortest (<2 ms) FA = 40° BW = high	1.5T
3D Fast spin echo	CUBE (GE) SPACE (Siemens) VISTA (Philips)	T2-weighted Black blood	End-expiratory with pencil-beam navigator triggering 5–7 min	FOV = 320 mm Matrix = 160 × 160 SL = 2 mm Sagittal or coronal	Low	TR = respiratory rate (2–5 s) TE = medium (60 ms~) FA = 90°/variable flip train BW = medium–high Echo train length = 80–140 FAT saturation	1.5T and 3.0T
3D RF spoiled gradient echo	SPGR (GE) VIBE (Siemens) THRIVE (Philips)	PD to T1-weighted	Breath-hold 10–12 s (inspiratory and expiratory)	FOV = 400 mm Matrix = 200 × 200 SL = 2 mm Isotropic voxel, as low as 8 mm³ Sagittal or coronal	High	TR = shortest (<1.7 ms) TE = shortest (<0.7 ms) FA = 2° BW = medium–high	1.5T and 3.0T
3D RF spoiled gradient echo	StarVIBE (Siemens) Clinically not available for GE or Philips	PD to T1-weighted	Free breathing 3–5 min	FOV = 400 mm Matrix = 320 × 320 SL = 1.2–4 mm voxel (2–5 mm³) Axial	Low	TR = 7.46 ms TE = 2.46 ms FA = 9° BW = medium	1.5T and 3.0T
3D Two-point DIXON RF spoiled gradient echo	LAVA Flex (GE)	PD to T1-weighted Water-only, fat-only, in-phase, and out-of-phase contrast	Breath-hold (10 s) Free breathing (pencil-beam navigator)	FOV = 260 mm Matrix = 128 × 128 SL = 3 mm Voxel (<3 mm³) Axial	High	TR = 3.7–4.5 ms TE = min full (<2.0 ms) FA = 2°–10° BW = medium–high	1.5T and 3.0T
3D Ultra-short TE gradient echo	UTE (GE) SPIRALVIBE (Siemens) MultiVane (Philips)	PD-weighted Slight T1-weighting depending on readout flip angle chosen UTE	7–10 min Free breathing	FOV = 360 mm Voxel size = 1–8 mm³ Sagittal or coronal	Low	TR = short (<5 ms) TE = 0.07 ms BW = medium–high	1.5T and 3.0T
3D Ultra-short TE gradient echo	VNAV (GE) SPIRALVIBE (Siemens)	PD-weighted Slight T1-weighting depending on readout flip angle chosen Silent	7–10 min Free breathing	FOV = 360 mm Matrix = 360 × 360 × 360 Sagittal or coronal	Low	TR = shortest (<1.3 ms) TE = 0 ms BW = medium–high	1.5T and 3.0T

Sequence type	Brand name (Brand)	Weighting	Acquisition setting and duration	Spatial resolution and orientation	Temporal resolution	Scan parameters	MR imaging system
Dynamic airway evaluation							
2D Steady-state free precession gradient echo – SSFP	FIESTA (GE) TrueFISP (Siemens) Balanced-FFE (Philips)	T1/T2-weighted Inflow enhancement	3–4 minutes hyperventilation Coverage larynx to carina ~ 4 s per slice position	FOV = 450 × 160 mm Matrix = 128 × 128 SL = 8 mm Axial	4–5 images/s	TR = shortest (1.8 ms–2.4 ms) TE = shortest (<1.2 ms) FA = 35° BW = medium–high	1.5T
3D RF spoiled gradient echo	TRICKS (GE) TWIST (Siemens) 4D-TRAK (Philips)	PD to T1-weighted	20 s Forced expiration, free breathing, or hyperventilation	FOV = 300 mm Matrix = 80 × 100 SL = 3.2 mm Sagittal	<400 ms/ volume	TR = shortest (<2 ms) TE = minimum (<1.1 ms) FA = 2° BW = medium–high	1.5T and 3.0T

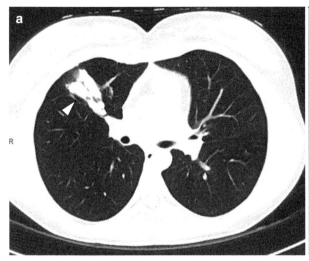 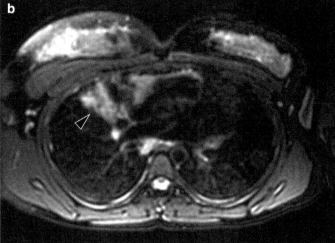

Fig. 2.3 Cystic fibrosis and allergic bronchopulmonary aspergillosis in a 16-year-old girl. (**a**) Axial nonenhanced lung window setting CT image obtained at end-expiration shows impacted mucus and bronchiectasis (*white arrowhead*) in the right middle lobe. (**b**) Axial nonen- hanced isotropic three-dimensional (3D) CUBE (GE) T2-weighted MR image obtained at end-expiration shows impacted mucus and bronchiectasis (*black arrowhead*) in the right middle lobe

time TI) in order to cancel all signal deriving from the blood. These sequences have a very high specific absorption ratio (SAR). Especially with small children, single-shot FSE requires longer wait time between slices to stay within safety norms and avoid patient heating.

Fast Spin Echo with Helical K-Space Acquisition PRO-PELLER (Periodically Rotated Overlapping ParallEL Lines with Enhanced Reconstruction) is a particular FSE non-breath-hold readout that collects imaging data using rotating k-space bands or blades, which is more resistant to respiratory and cardiac motion artifact [2]. The collection of blades oversamples the center of k-space, thus producing better SNR and reducing rotational and translational in-plane motion occurring between k-space segments collected on each blade [2]. This sequence is suitable for non-cooperative pediatric patients and can be combined with prospective respiratory-gated techniques (i.e., using pen-beam navigators or pneumobelts), to further reduce the effects of motion. Full axial chest coverage (approximately 25–30 cm craniocaudally) can be achieved in 4–7 minutes with good spatial resolution (1 × 1 × 5 mm) [2]. To enhance detection of bronchial wall thickening, bronchiectasis, and bronchial wall lesions, long TE settings are preferred in order to reduce signal from vascular structure and to increase water detection (Fig. 2.4).

Steady-State Free Precession Technique Steady-state free precession (SSFP) techniques are a group of gradient-recalled echo (GRE) sequences, which generate T2/T1 weighting with medium to high readout flip angle (FA) set- tings (>30°) using very short repetition times (TR). On these sequences tissues with water-like characteristics are hyper-intense, such as mucus plugs in the airways [2]. 2D SSFP scans allow fast acquisitions of the entire thorax in a single breath-hold with good SNR. Moreover vascular structures also appear bright on SSFP (bright blood), allowing assessment of mediastinal vessels for possible compression of large airways. A limitation of this sequence is its sensitivity to magnetic field inhomogeneities, which can become problematic at higher magnetic field strengths (i.e., 3T). SSFP also has an intensive SAR profile (though much less than single-shot FSE), which with high flip angles and at higher field strengths can exceed the maximal safety level allowed in MR imaging.

3D Techniques

Gradient Recalled Echo Sequences Short and ultra-short echo time GRE sequences are typically considered as the most robust sequence for chest MR imaging [2]. These sequences when used with short or ultra-short echo times can minimize the signal loss created by air-tissue interfaces thus providing high SNR. GRE are usually collected with minimum TR and TE settings to achieve the best SNR possible and the shortest acquisition time. For isotropic voxel sizes between 2 and 3.5 mm, a capable MR imaging system can provide a TE ranging from 0.4 to 0.7 ms with an acquisition time around 10 seconds for full chest coverage (Fig. 2.5). Such short acquisition time is critical for children, who are unable to accomplish long breath-holds (>10 seconds), especially if in respiratory distress [2].

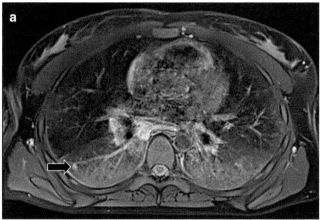

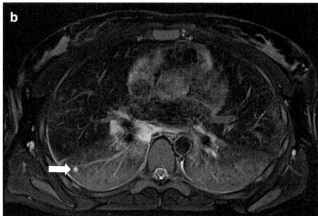

Fig. 2.4 Differing appearance of lungs and pulmonary nodule on black blood MR images in patient with systemic sclerosis. (**a**) Axial nonenhanced BLADE (Siemens) proton density-weighted MR image (1 × 1 × 5 mm, echo time of 28 ms) shows a nodule (*black arrow*) in the right lower lobe. (**b**) Axial nonenhanced BLADE (Siemens) T2-weighted MR image (1 × 1 × 5 mm, echo time of 87 ms) again shows the nodule (*white arrow*) in the right lower lobe which is more conspicuous than on the proton density-weighted MR image despite an overall lower signal-to-noise ratio on the T2-weighted MR image

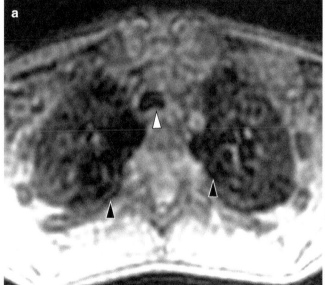

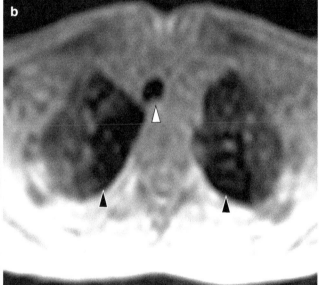

Fig. 2.5 Differing resolution of 3D SPGR MR imaging of the large airway. (**a**) Axial nonenhanced 3D SPGR MR image (2 mm isotropic voxel, echo time 0.7 ms) has higher noise and less definition of the trachea (*white arrowhead*) and less conspicuous air trapping (*black arrow-*) heads). (**b**) Axial nonenhanced 3D SPGR MR image (3 mm isotropic voxel, echo time 0.6 ms) has lower noise and higher signal-to-noise ratio, allowing for better definition of the trachea (*white arrowhead*) and more conspicuous air trapping (*black arrowheads*)

3D GRE acquisitions are usually preferred over 2D scans, because they can provide better SNR and are less sensitive to susceptibility artifacts [2]. The 3D dataset also enables multiplanar reformats (MPR), which allows for easy review of large airway pathology [2] (Fig. 2.6). For a fixed TR, GRE sequences provide contrasts ranging from proton-density-weighted (PD-weighted, using low flip angle readouts <3°) to T1-weighted (T1-weighted at higher flip angles). The PD-weighted setting is the most appropriate to assess large airways without the use of contrast agents, while the latter is used to assess vascular structures and lung parenchymal perfusion after contrast administration.

New variants of GRE with non-Cartesian k-space acquisition (helical) schemes have been developed to reduce sensitivity to motion artifacts [10, 11]. Cartesian geometry is inherently prone to motion-induced phase distortions, even if respiratory navigation or triggering techniques are used, which results in residual ghosting artifacts. The most promising alternative is the "radial" sampling scheme, which acquires the data along rotated spokes, or "stack of stars" (StarVIBE, Siemens, Munich, Germany) [12]. Due to overs-

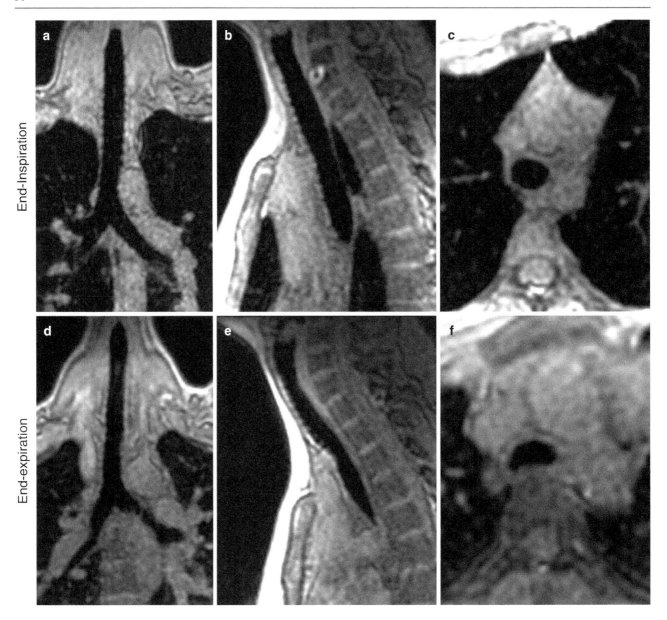

Fig. 2.6 Multiplanar reformatting (MPR) of end-inspiration and end-expiration spirometry gated 3D spoiled gradient echo (SPGR) in a 3.0 Tesla scanner on healthy subject. MR imaging acquired with a 32-channel cardiac array coil using a parallel imaging factor × 3, 12-sec acquisition time, and an isotropic voxel (2 × 2 × 2 mm). (**a**) Coronal nonenhanced 3D SPGR MR image obtained at end-inspiration. (**b**) Sagittal nonenhanced 3D SPGR MR image obtained at end-inspiration. (**c**) Axial nonenhanced 3D SPGR MR image obtained at end-inspiration. (**d**) Coronal nonenhanced 3D SPGR MR image obtained at end-expiration. (**e**) Sagittal nonenhanced 3D SPGR MR image obtained at end-expiration. (**f**) Axial nonenhanced 3D SPGR MR image obtained at end-expiration

ampling of the spokes in the center of the k-space, there is a reduction of ghosting artifacts because of a motion-averaging effect (similar to PROPELLER and BLADE scanning with FSE).

3D GRE sequences are usually combined with fat suppression techniques for large airway imaging. Fat suppression is important to cancel signal from mediastinal fat tissue, which surrounds the trachea, therefore highlighting the tracheal wall. Unfortunately fat suppression techniques may lead to signal loss in the trachea wall as well; therefore GRE two-point DIXON-based schemes are preferred to obtain homogeneous fat suppression (Fig. 2.7) [13].

Ultra-Short or Zero-TE (UTE/ZTE) Sequences UTE and ZTE are two variants of 3D GRE sequences with TE on the order of μs (microseconds) instead of ms (milliseconds). The shortening of TE allows minimization of the signal loss caused by T2* effects of air-tissue interfaces. k-space collection with UTE and ZTE can be performed both with radial or spiral trajectories achieving an oversampling of the center of the k-space [11, 14, 15]. This is desirable in large airway imaging because it reduces motion sensitivity. These sequences allow high SNR and sub-millimetric spatial resolution [11] (Fig. 2.8). UTE and ZTE are usually free-breathing acquisitions, which are combined with different respiratory triggering/gating

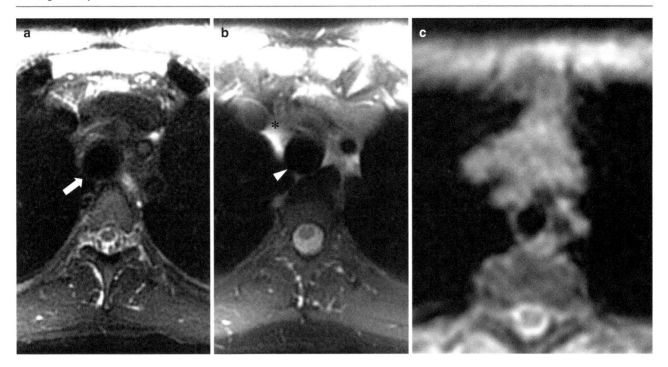

Fig. 2.7 Comparison of fat suppression techniques for large airway MR imaging. (**a**) Axial nonenhanced short tau inversion recovery (STIR) technique demonstrates generalized signal decay with reduced signal-to-noise ratio (SNR) of tracheal wall (*white arrow*). (**b**) Axial nonenhanced fat suppression technique (FATSAT) technique shows inhomogeneous fat signal cancellation with bright tissue in the anterior mediastinum (*) and low signal-to-noise ratio in the posterior tracheal wall (*arrowhead*). (**c**) Axial nonenhanced water map from two-point DIXON technique shows homogeneous SNR and fat cancellation

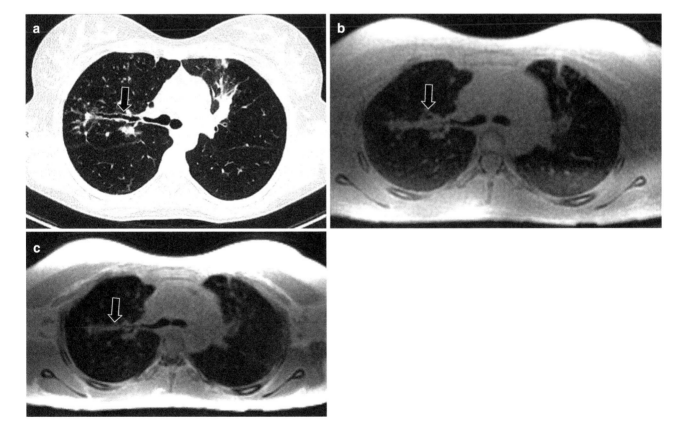

Fig. 2.8 Comparison of ultra-short echo time (UTE), zero echo time (ZTE), and CT for large airway MR imaging. (**a**) Axial nonenhanced lung window setting CT image obtained at end-expiration shows right upper lobe bronchiectasis and bronchial wall thickening (*black arrow*). (**b**) Axial nonenhanced free-breathing navigator-triggered zero echo time (ZTE) MR image obtained at end-expiration shows right upper lobe bronchiectasis and bronchial wall thickening (*black arrow*) with resolution approaching that of CT. (**c**) Axial nonenhanced pneumobelt-triggered ultra-short TE (UTE) MR image obtained at end-expiration shows right upper lobe bronchiectasis and bronchial wall thickening (*black arrow*) with resolution approaching that of CT

methods, such as prospective pneumobelt, or prospective and retrospective navigator-based echo scanning. The latter method was recently used in a group of infants to assess large airway collapse [16]. This method allows for acquisition of the images with free breathing and to retrospectively reconstruct the images in inspiration and expiration. Unfortunately respiratory gating requires long acquisition times, which can range between 6 and 15 minutes depending on the voxel size chosen (0.7–1.5 mm). Further refinements of these techniques might allow to achieve breath-hold acquisitions with spatial resolution more comparable to CT.

3D Fast Spin-Echo Sequences These are a family of 3D T2-weighted sequences that can provide isotropic resolution and allow multiplanar reformatted images with high SNR and CNR from the bronchial wall. These sequences have different acronyms according to the MR imaging vendors (CUBE, General Electric [GE], Boston, MA, USA; VISTA, or "Volume ISotropic Turbo spin echo Acquisition," Philips, Amsterdam, The Netherlands; and SPACE, or "Sampling Perfection with Application optimized Contrasts using

different flip angle Evolution," Siemens) [2]. *k*-space acquisition schemes differ between vendors but they have some similar contrast and readout characteristics, using long echo train lengths, ultra-short echo spacings, and low flip readout angles in combination with parallel and partial Fourier imaging schemes to reduce acquisition time. These sequences can achieve isotropic voxel resolutions as low as 2 mm with free breathing in a reasonable imaging time (5–10 min) (Fig. 2.9).

Dynamic MR Large Airway Imaging

The high temporal resolution and the lack of radiation have made MR imaging suitable for studying airways in true dynamic conditions (cine-MR imaging). Cine-MR imaging can be performed both with 2D and 3D acquisitions [17]. The former includes sequences, such as 2D SSFP or 2D GRE, acquiring a single thick slice in a multiphase setting. Temporal resolution ranges between 100 and 200 ms per frame with a voxel resolution of $1 \times 1 \times 5$ mm. A limitation of 2D imaging is that the trachea moves in all directions during the respiratory cycle; therefore a single slice could miss relevant airway

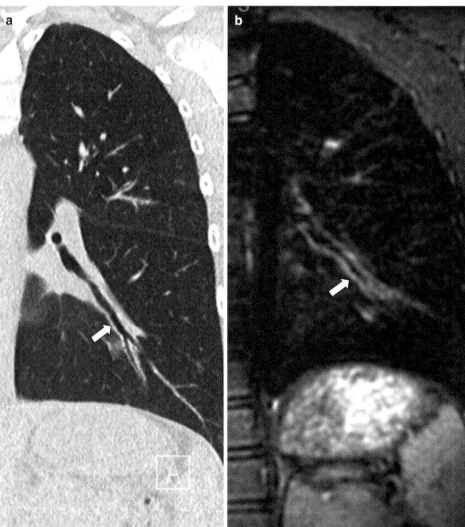

Fig. 2.9 Comparison of 3D T2-weighted MR imaging of the airway to CT in a pediatric patient with cystic fibrosis. (**a**) Coronal nonenhanced lung window setting CT image shows bronchiectasis and bronchial wall thickening (*arrow*) in left lower lobe. (**b**) Coronal nonenhanced isotropic three-dimensional (3D) CUBE (GE) T2-weighted MR image shows the bronchiectasis and bronchial wall thickening (*arrow*) resolution approaching that of CT

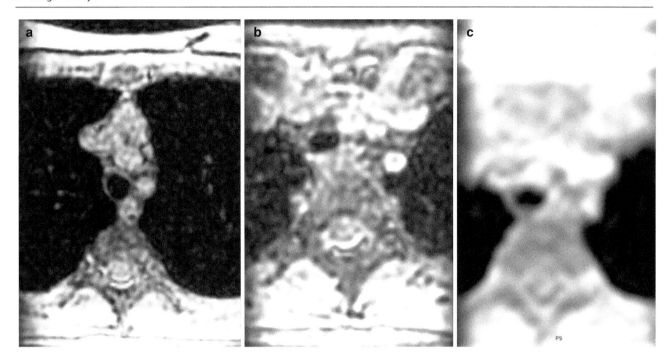

Fig. 2.10 Normal dynamic large airway MR imaging in a 12-year-old girl. (**a**) Axial nonenhanced 3D SPGR MR image obtained at end-inspiration shows a patent trachea. (**b**) Axial nonenhanced 3D SPGR MR image obtained at end-expiration shows a patent trachea which is slightly smaller than at end-inspiration, a normal finding. (**c**) Axial non- enhanced 3D SPGR MR image with *time-resolved imaging of contrast kinetics* (TRICKS) obtained during forced expiration shows a patent trachea which is slightly smaller than at end-inspiration, a normal finding

pathology during trachea movement. 3D cine-MR imaging includes 3D UTE sequence with retrospective reconstruction, previously mentioned, and 3D GRE sequences combined with keyhole imaging technique [16]. The latter includes sequences such as TRICKS, or "Time-Resolved Imaging of Contrast KineticS" (GE); DISCO, or "DIfferential Sub-sampling with Cartesian Ordering") (GE); TWIST, or "Time-resolved angiography With Interleaved Stochastic Trajectories") (Siemens); and D-TRAK, or "4D Time-Resolved Angiography using Keyhole" (Philips) [2]. These techniques allow temporal resolution in the order of 500 ms or less with isotropic voxel size between 2 and 3 mm (for a volume covering the large airways in a sagittal slab of approx. 9–12 cm). TRICKS cine-MR imaging was used to assess tracheobronchomalacia in a group of pediatric patients [18], showing that cine-MR imaging is a possible alternative to bronchoscopy and cine-CT for tracheobronchomalacia [19] (Fig. 2.10).

Anatomy

Embryology

The respiratory diverticulum starts as an outgrowth from the ventral part of the foregut around 4 weeks of gestation. The respiratory diverticulum originates from the endodermal layer, and it forms the epithelium of the larynx, trachea, and bronchi, as well as that of the lungs [20, 21]. The cartilagi- nous, muscular, and connective tissue components of the trachea and lungs are derived from the mesoderm layer of the foregut. Initially, the respiratory diverticulum is in open communication with the foregut [22]. When the diverticulum expands caudally, two longitudinal ridges, the tracheoesophageal ridges, separate it from the foregut [22]. Afterward, these ridges fuse to form the tracheoesophageal septum, which divides the foregut into a dorsal portion, the esophagus, and a ventral portion, the trachea and lung.

The lung bud then divides into right and left primary bronchial buds. Three main branches form in the right lung bud and two in the left. These initial branches correspond to the lobar bronchi of the adult lungs. The lung grows caudally and laterally, entering the pericardio-peritoneal layers [23]. At 9 weeks' gestation the pleura separates from the pericardium and peritoneum developing the visceral pleura, which covers the lung, and the parietal pleura, which covers the chest wall and diaphragm. The pattern of airway branching is complete by about the 16th week of intrauterine life [23]. Any interruption of these steps of the embryological formation (Fig. 2.11) results in tracheobronchial branching anomalies.

Normal Development and Anatomy

Although airway size changes after birth, the pattern of branching does not. Therefore, a newborn has essentially the same airway structure as an adult, but in miniature.

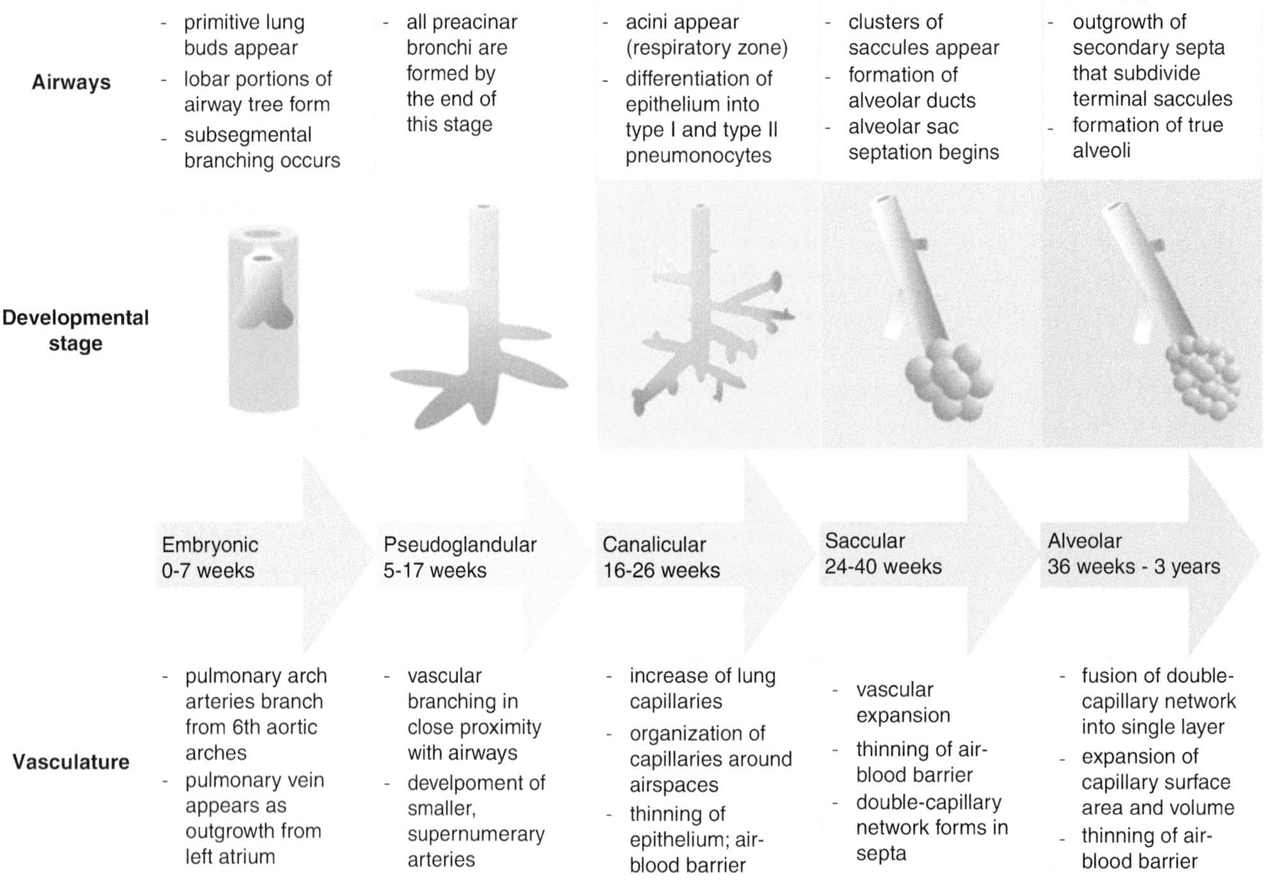

Airways	- primitive lung buds appear - lobar portions of airway tree form - subsegmental branching occurs	- all preacinar bronchi are formed by the end of this stage	- acini appear (respiratory zone) - differentiation of epithelium into type I and type II pneumonocytes	- clusters of saccules appear - formation of alveolar ducts - alveolar sac septation begins	- outgrowth of secondary septa that subdivide terminal saccules - formation of true alveoli

Developmental stage

Embryonic 0-7 weeks	Pseudoglandular 5-17 weeks	Canalicular 16-26 weeks	Saccular 24-40 weeks	Alveolar 36 weeks - 3 years

| **Vasculature** | - pulmonary arch arteries branch from 6th aortic arches
- pulmonary vein appears as outgrowth from left atrium | - vascular branching in close proximity with airways
- develpoment of smaller, supernumerary arteries | - increase of lung capillaries
- organization of capillaries around airspaces
- thinning of epithelium; air-blood barrier | - vascular expansion
- thinning of air-blood barrier
- double-capillary network forms in septa | - fusion of double-capillary network into single layer
- expansion of capillary surface area and volume
- thinning of air-blood barrier |

Fig. 2.11 Diagram illustrating normal lung development: airway structure and pulmonary vasculature

After birth, airways will keep growing until adulthood with a final diameter and length double or triple of that at birth [21, 24, 25].

In the parlance of the pathologist, the large airways include those airways extending from the mouth to the respiratory bronchiole [26]. Conversely, in the parlance of a radiologist, large airways are those airways that are visible on CT imaging, which include airways extending down to the segmental bronchi [27, 28]. Radiologists further divide large airways into upper and lower airways, where the upper airway extends from the mouth to the trachea, including the pharynx and the larynx [29].

The pharynx is a tubular structure, which connects the posterior nasal and oral cavities to the larynx and esophagus. It is divided into nasopharynx, oropharynx, and laryngopharynx. The larynx is a moving structure containing cartilage, muscles, and ligaments. The larynx performs various functions, including phonation and airway protection.

The trachea begins inferior to the cricoid cartilage of the larynx and it extends to the carina at the level of the fifth thoracic vertebra [27, 30] (Fig. 2.12). Trachea length varies between 10 and 15 cm in adults according to gender and patient length, and it contains 16–20 C-shaped cartilaginous rings open posteriorly at level of the pars membranacea, that is, the posterior wall of the trachea formed by the trachealis muscles [30]. The trachea is in the midline of the thorax and it is slightly displaced to the right by the aortic arch. The trachea bifurcates into the right and left main bronchi at the carina. The right main bronchus is more vertically positioned than the left main bronchus, resulting in a greater likelihood of foreign body aspiration or endotracheal tube entering the right bronchial lumen. Main bronchi are further divided in lobar bronchi (two on the left and three on the right), which supply each of the main lobes of the lung (upper, middle, and lower lobe on the right and upper and lower on the left side). Segmental bronchi supply each bronchopulmonary segment of the lungs [27, 30].

Anatomic Variants

Branching Anomalies

Branching anomalies depend on the embryological phase at which they occurred. A summary of the branching anomalies according to a classification based on anatomical, embryological, and functional criteria is shown in Table 2.2.

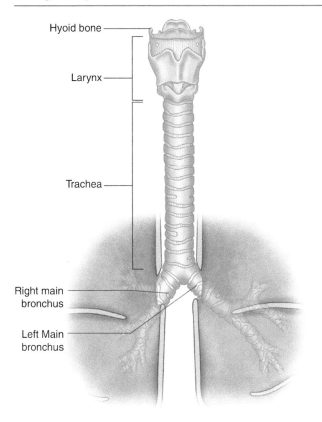

Hyoid bone

Larynx

Trachea

Right main
bronchus

Left Main
bronchus

Fig. 2.12 Anatomy of the trachea

Table 2.2 Airway branching and developmental anomalies

Developmental or anatomical defect	Resulting condition
Interruption of normal development	Agenesis-hypoplasia complex
Obstruction or compression	Tracheal stenosis
	Bronchial atresia
	Tracheal dilatation (Mounier-Kuhn syndrome)
Bronchopulmonary malformation of the foregut	Tracheoesophageal fistula
	Esophageal bronchus
	Bronchogenic cyst
Ectopic or supernumerary	Tracheal bronchus
	Accessory cardiac bronchus
	Tracheobronchial diverticulum
Malformation associated with situs anomalies	Situs inversus
	Heterotaxia

Tracheal Stenosis

Congenital tracheal stenosis is a rare condition characterized by a reduction of the tracheobronchial luminal diameter, usually greater than 50% [31]. The narrowing can be focal or generalized and may be associated with cartilaginous rings (isolated form) or compression by an extrinsic structure such as a vascular anomaly or congenital cyst [31]. Tracheal stenosis is frequently misdiagnosed as refractory asthma, causing delayed diagnosis in many cases [32]. When tracheal narrowing is diagnosed, con-

genital tracheal stenosis is a diagnosis of exclusion, when other possible etiologies such as inflammatory, traumatic, neoplastic, or iatrogenic causes of airway narrowing have been excluded.

Although CT is a current imaging modality of choice for evaluating congenital tracheal stenosis, MR imaging can be used instead and it can also demonstrate associated anomalies such as vascular malformations. On MR imaging, fixed tracheal narrowing throughout the respiratory cycle is seen in affected pediatric patients. Although axial MR imaging may be sufficient for demonstrating the degree of tracheal stenosis, the overall length of tracheal stenosis is best seen on sagittal MR imaging.

In symptomatic pediatric patients with congenital tracheal stenosis, surgical correction is currently the management of choice. While short-segment tracheal stenosis (≤5 cm) is treated with end-to-end anastomosis, patch or tracheal autograft repair is often used for long-segment tracheal stenosis. Another newer option is slide tracheoplasty, which is known to be associated with less risks of developing stricture and granulation tissue formation. Treatment result can be efficiently evaluated with MR imaging to assess postsurgical changes and residual or recurrent stenosis (Fig. 2.13).

Heterotaxy

Heterotaxies are anomalies related to the abnormal position of the organs in the thorax or abdominal cavity. Normal position of the organs (situs solitus) includes a left-sided heart and right-sided liver [33]. A mirror image of the normal organ disposition with a right-sided heart (dextrocardia) and left-sided liver is known as situs inversus. Situs inversus can be associated with congenital heart disease and primary ciliary dyskinesia (PCD). The triad of situs inversus, PCD, and chronic sinusitis (± nasal polyposis) is known as Kartagener syndrome. Situs ambiguus (heterotaxy) is an anomaly in the normal left and right distribution of the thoracic and abdominal organs which does not match the configuration of a situs inversus. A typical feature of situs ambiguus is the symmetrical and identical configuration of the bronchial tree and lung, from which derives the term isomerism [34].

In right isomerism, both lungs are trilobed with bilateral minor fissures, associated asplenia, midline positioning of the liver and stomach, intestinal malrotation, and severe cardiac anomalies. Right isomerism usually presents early due to associated congenital cyanotic heart disease and asymptomatic cases discovered in adulthood are rare (<1%) [34, 35]. In left isomerism, both lungs are bilobed, there is no minor fissure, and the main bronchi are elongated. Left isomerism is associated with midline positioning of liver and multiple small splenules, defined as polysplenia in almost half of the cases [35]. Left isomerism can be associated with intestinal malrotation and with azygos continuation of the inferior vena cava (IVC), which consist of absence of the hepatic

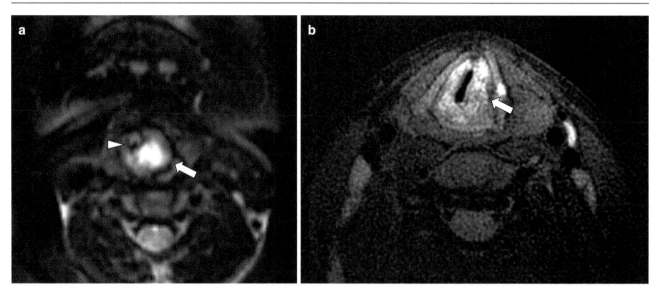

Fig. 2.13 Congenital laryngeal stenosis from a laryngeal cyst in a 1-year-old girl. (**a**) Axial nonenhanced T2-weighted fast spin-echo MR image shows a hyperintense cyst (*arrow*) in the left side of the larynx causing luminal stenosis (*arrowhead*). (**b**) Axial nonenhanced T2-weighted PROPELLER MR image obtained after resection shows thickening and deviation of the left vocal cords (*arrow*). Post operative imaging was performed when patient was 14-years-old

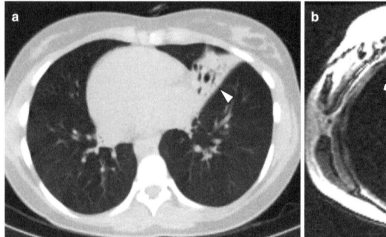

Fig. 2.14 Primary ciliary dyskinesia in a 17-year-old girl with situs inversus. (**a**) Axial nonenhanced lung window setting CT image obtained at end expiration shows dextrocardia and an area of consolidation with bronchiectasis (*arrowhead*) in the left-sided middle lobe. (**b**) Axial nonenhanced SSFP MR image shows dextrocardia with a right-sided left ventricle (*arrow*) and an area of consolidation with bronchiectasis (*arrowhead*) in the left-sided middle lobe

segment of the IVC with venous drainage of the lower half of the body via a dilated azygos vein. Cardiac abnormalities are less common in left isomerism than right isomerism, and left isomerism is more frequently asymptomatic.

Although CT is the most often used technique to assess airway pathology and associated cardiac anomalies, MR imaging can be used as an alternative, offering the benefit of cinematic assessment of large airways and cardiac physiology and pathology. In patients with situs inversus and PCD, lung pathology can be assessed with MR imaging showing typical imaging findings of dextrocardia, middle lobe consolidation, and bronchiectasis (Fig. 2.14).

In this group of patients, treatment is focused on repairing congenital heart defects (when present) and treating lung dis-

ease related to PCD. PCD treatment is mostly medical and lobectomy is not routinely suggested as therapy in PCD [36].

Spectrum of Large Airway Disorders

Congenital Large Airway Disorders

Macroglossia

Macroglossia refers to a tongue which protrudes beyond the alveolar ridge [37]. It may occur due to a focal mass or diffuse enlargement, which is associated with several genetic syndromes. Whether macroglossia is due to a focal mass or diffuse enlargement, both may lead to tongue dysfunction

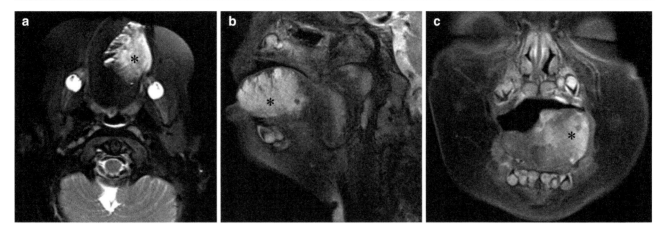

Fig. 2.15 Macroglossia due to blue rubber bleb nevus syndrome in a 5-month-old girl who presented with respiratory distress. (**a**) Axial nonenhanced T2-weighted MR image with fat suppression shows hyperintense lesion (*) in the left side of the tongue. (**b**) Sagittal nonenhanced T2-weighted MR image with fat suppression shows hyperintense lesion (*) within the tongue. (**c**) Coronal nonenhanced T2-weighted MR image with fat suppression shows hyperintense lesion (*) in the left side of the tongue

including alterations in chewing and speech and airway obstruction. Diffuse enlargement of the tongue may occur in Beckwith-Wiedemann syndrome (BWS), congenital hypothyroidism, chromosomal abnormalities, hemi-hyperplasia, and mucopolysaccharidoses (i.e., Pompe disease). Relative macroglossia is also seen in Down syndrome, micrognathia, muscular hypotonia, and angioedema. Macroglossia can also occur in cases of tissue infiltration as in case of neoplasms, neurofibromatosis, inflammatory and infectious causes, lymphatic or venous malformations (i.e., blue rubber bleb nevus syndrome), and hemangiomas. Affected pediatric patients with vascular anomalies of the tongue may present with varying symptoms depending on the size and extent of the lesion, including obstructive symptoms or recurrent bleeding.

Although CT with and without intravenous contrast is the primary imaging modality used for the evaluation of macroglossia, it has the disadvantage of requiring ionizing radiation [37]. MR imaging is an excellent alternative to CT in these cases, since it offers excellent depiction of vascular structures without the need for ionizing radiation. Angiographic MR imaging can depict the course of any abnormal vessels and provide for pre-therapeutic planning [38]. MR imaging has the added advantage of characterizing lesions in multiple sequences, often allowing for better diagnostic accuracy. For example, in a pediatric patient with macroglossia due to vascular anomalies, high-flow lesions show signal flow voids both in T1-weighted and T2-weighted images, and low-flow lesions are characterized by low signal in T1-weighted and moderately homogeneous signal in T2-weighted images (Fig. 2.15).

Whenever possible, macroglossia is managed with medical treatment, which consists of conservative measures to reduce tongue inflammation and bleeding. In cases of severe airway obstruction and/or dysphagia from macroglossia, surgical procedures are performed to reduce tongue size while maintaining tongue mobility and function [39].

Tonsillar Hypertrophy

Tonsillar hypertrophy refers to the enlargement of the lymphoid tissue located in the wall of the pharynx including the adenoids and palatine and lingual tonsils [40]. These structures are part of the immune system of the upper airways, where the first response to infectious agents takes place. In cases of repeated infection or chronic colonization (mostly by *Staphylococcus* and *Streptococcus* family organisms), these structures can become hypertrophic, limiting airflow both at the level of nasopharynx (adenoid) and oropharynx (palatine tonsils). Typical clinical findings are nasal congestion, recurrent otitis, and obstructive sleep apnea syndrome (OSAS).

Although radiographic evaluation with a lateral neck radiograph is frequently performed for assessing tonsillar hypertrophy, this technique is not a reliable method for measuring the grade of obstruction [41]. CT can demonstrate lateral or anterior-posterior narrowing of the airway with much better anatomical detail. CT is highly useful for identifying upper airway obstruction and to develop an appropriate surgical plan. For this indication, CT can be performed in supine position and in different phases of respiration to provide information about airway cross-sectional area and site of obstruction. However, CT is limited by radiation exposure risk and imaging is typically performed in a single phase of respiration. In contrast, specialized MR imaging allows both static and dynamic imaging without exposing children to increased radiation [42, 43]. MR imaging measurements of tonsillar hypertrophy show good correlation with endoscopic assessment. If lingual tonsils are greater than 10 mm in diameter and abutting both the posterior border of the tongue and the posterior pharyngeal wall, they are considered markedly enlarged (Fig. 2.16). Adenoid enlargement is diagnosed if adenoid tissue is thicker than 12 mm and if there is intermittent obstruction of the posterior nasopharynx on sagittal cine-MR imaging.

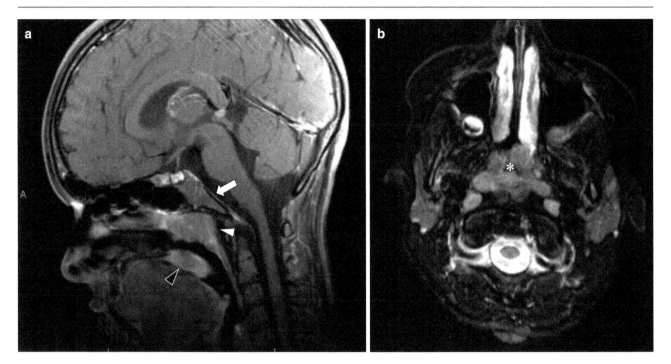

Fig. 2.16 Tonsil and adenoid hypertrophy in a 9-year-old girl who presented with breathing difficulty. (**a**) Sagittal enhanced T1-weighted MR image with fat suppression shows marked enlargement of adenoid (*arrow*), palatine tonsils (*white arrowhead*), and lingual tonsil (*black arrowhead*). (**b**) Axial enhanced T1-weighted MR image with fat suppression shows upper airway obstruction (*)

Tonsillectomy and adenoidectomy are often performed in children with chronic symptoms from tonsillar hypertrophy. Both procedures aim to improve airflow in the upper airways and to reduce recurrent infections.

Laryngeal Stenosis

Laryngeal stenosis is one of the most common causes of airway obstruction in infants and children. Laryngeal stenosis can be congenital or acquired. Acquired laryngeal stenosis is more common and is most often related to prolonged intubation. Congenital causes of laryngeal stenosis include glottic obstruction due to vocal cord thickening, congenital vocal cord paralysis due to nervous system disorders (e.g., Arnold-Chiari, hydrocephalus), laryngeal webs, congenital laryngeal cyst, and laryngomalacia [44]. Symptoms of congenital and acquired laryngeal stenosis are similar and may include stridor, dyspnea, and hypoxia [45].

Although direct visualization with endoscopy is the gold standard for diagnosis of laryngeal stenosis, radiologic evaluation plays an important role in most patients. Chest radiograph often helps to evaluate for secondary findings including atelectasis and pneumonia. CT can provide detailed anatomic information regarding the location and extension of the laryngeal stenosis; however, it often cannot differentiate between the true lumen and overlying secretions. In contrast, MR imaging can often make this differentiation due to better soft tissue characterization capability. MR imaging also has the benefit of producing cross-sectional anatomic information without the use of ionizing radiation [45].

Treatment of laryngeal stenosis usually requires surgical intervention such as laryngotracheal reconstruction with cricoid split using cartilage graft (Fig. 2.17) [45].

Congenital High Airway Obstruction Sequence

Congenital high airway obstruction sequence (CHAOS) is a rare congenital anomaly, characterized by obstruction of the fetal upper airway, including laryngeal atresia, stenosis or laryngeal cysts, and tracheal atresia or stenosis [46, 47]. The obstructed airway results in decreased clearance of the fetal lung fluid with increased intra-tracheal and lung pressure. Consequently, the lungs expand to abnormally large volumes leading to compression of mediastinal structures including the heart causing decreased venous return and hydrops [47]. CHAOS is commonly associated with genetic disorders such as Fraser's syndrome, a rare congenital syndromic anomaly characterized by tracheal/laryngeal atresia and facial and skeletal abnormalities [46].

Diagnosis is usually made prenatally by ultrasound with detection of CHAOS abnormalities around the 20th week of gestation or earlier. On prenatal ultrasound, typical signs of CHAOS are enlarged symmetrical hyper-echogenic lungs with flattening or inversion of the diaphragm [47]. The airway is dilated up to the level of the obstruction. The heart and mediastinum appear small and anteriorly displaced by the enlarged lungs. On prenatal MR imaging, the lungs are enlarged and hyperintense with flattening or inversion of the diaphragm and mediastinal displacement [48]. Compared to ultrasound, MR imaging can often better identify the level of airway obstruction due to a higher soft tissue characteriza-

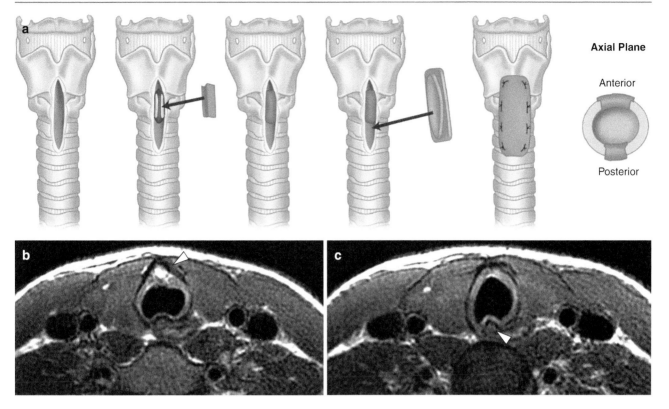

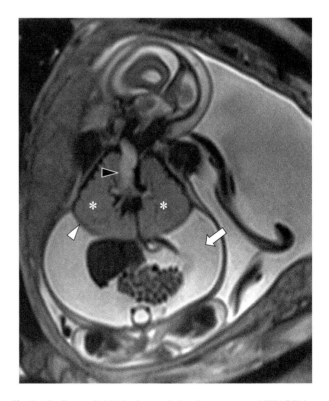

Fig. 2.17 Laryngeal stenosis treated with laryngotracheal reconstruction with cricoid split using cartilage graft in a 12-year-old boy. (**a**) Illustration of surgical procedure of anterior and posterior cricoid split with costal cartilage graft, where cricoid is opened anteriorly and pos-teriorly and two cartilage grafts are positioned to enlarge cricoid lumen. (**b**) Axial nonenhanced T2-weighted PROPELLER MR image shows the anterior graft (*arrowhead*). (**c**) Axial nonenhanced T2-weighted PROPELLER MR image shows the posterior graft (*arrowhead*)

tion and 3D capabilities [48]. Differential diagnosis of CHAOS includes causes of extrinsic compression of the airways, such as lymphatic malformation, cervical teratoma, and vascular abnormalities (Fig. 2.18).

Large series show that CHAOS is highly lethal, with occasional reports of survivors after direct postnatal surgical intervention to the upper airways [46].

Tracheoesophageal Fistula

Tracheoesophageal fistula (TEF) consists of a fistulous connection between the esophagus and trachea, often with associated esophageal atresia [49]. Congenital TEF has an incidence of 1 in 3500 births. It may be associated with other congenital abnormalities, including cardiac anomalies, VACTERL (Vertebral defects, Anal atresia, Cardiac defects, Tracheo-Esophageal fistula, Renal anomalies, and Limb abnormalities) syndrome, and gastrointestinal anomalies (e.g., malrotation, intestinal atresia) [49]. TEF and esophageal atresia are classified in five types: (1) isolated esophageal atresia without TEF (type A), (2) proximal tracheoesophageal fistula with distal esophageal atresia (type B), (3) proximal esophageal atresia with distal fistula (type C, the most frequent type), (4) double fistula with intervening esophageal atresia (type D), and (5) isolated fistula (type H) [49, 50]. Typical symptoms of TEF are coughing, choking or cyanosis during feeding, vomiting, and dyspnea.

Fig. 2.18 Congenital high airway obstruction sequence (CHAOS) in a male fetus at 27 weeks' gestation. Coronal nonenhanced T2-weighted HASTE MR image shows enlarged hyperintense lungs (*), dilated central airways (*black arrowhead*), inversion of the diaphragm (*white arrowhead*), and ascites (*arrow*)

TEF is usually first suspected based on prenatal ultrasound findings, which may include polyhydramnios, non-visualized stomach, and distended upper esophagus. Prenatal MR imaging may be subsequently performed and has been shown to have high sensitivity and specificity for the prenatal diagnosis of TEF [51, 52]. MR imaging is also an excellent tool to assess for tracheomalacia, a common complication of TEF which is described in the following sections [53] (Fig. 2.19).

TEF is treated surgically with fistula ligation and creation of a primary esophageal anastomosis. When primary anastomosis is not possible due to a long-gap esophageal atresia, a staged repair may be performed after esophageal elongation, colonic interposition graft may be utilized, or gastric pull-up may be performed [53].

Ectopic Bronchus: Tracheal Bronchus

A tracheal bronchus (TB) is an anomalous bronchus that originates directly from the trachea or the main bronchus, usually located from 6 cm above the carina up to 2 cm below [23, 54, 55]. These bronchi can be considered as normal "displaced" bronchi or supernumerary bronchi [55]. They are considered supernumerary when they coexist with a normal segmentation of the bronchial tree. In contrast, they are considered displaced when a segmental bronchus is missing from its usual normal division for a lobe. Other two possible variants are the rudimentary and anomalous TB, where the former is a blind outpouching on the right lower side of the trachea and the latter arises above the tracheal bifurcation and contains three normal bronchial segments (Fig. 2.20). TB is more frequently seen on the right side and in the upper lobes. The most common variant is the displaced TB extending to the right upper lobe [55], which is also the most frequent congenital anomaly of the tra-

cheobronchial tree overall [56]. TB is usually asymptomatic, although symptoms are more frequently present in left-sided TB and in the supernumerary form. Cough and recurrent infection are two most commonly encountered symptoms in patients with TB [55, 56].

Although the most used technique to diagnose TB remains CT, MR imaging can provide similar diagnostic capability without the need for potentially harmful ionizing radiation. On MR imaging, a TB is seen as a small tubular structure

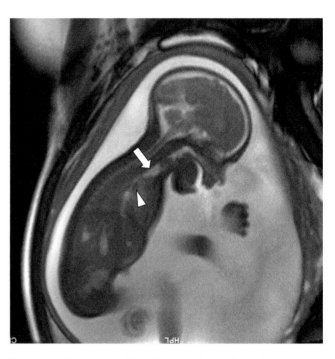

Fig. 2.19 Male fetus at 28 weeks' gestation with esophageal atresia with tracheoesophageal fistula. Sagittal T2-weighted SSFSE/HASTE MR image shows dilatation of proximal esophagus (*arrow*) with connection to the bronchial tree (*arrowhead*)

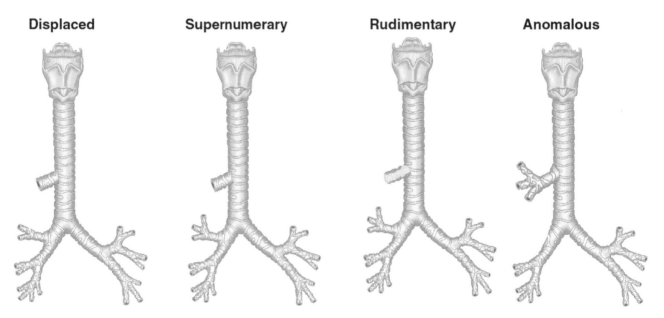

Fig. 2.20 Variation of tracheal bronchus

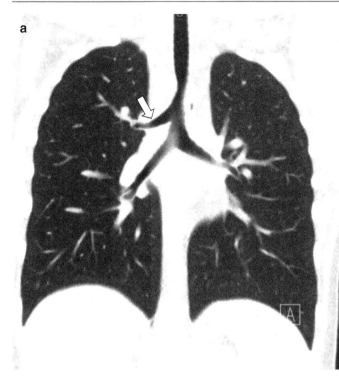
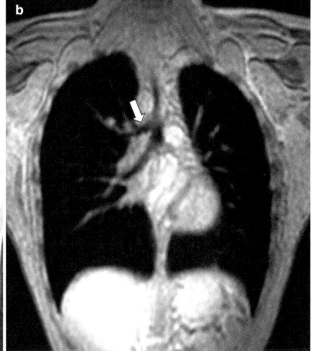

Fig. 2.21 Tracheal bronchus in a 16-year-old boy. (**a**) Coronal enhanced lung window setting CT image shows the right upper lobe bronchus (*arrow*) arising directly from the trachea. (**b**) Coronal enhanced T2-weighted HASTE MR image shows the right upper lobe bronchus (*arrow*) arising directly from the trachea

originating directly from the trachea [17]. Breath-hold acquisition at end-inspiration acquired in the coronal view enhances detection of this aberrant bronchus (Fig. 2.21).

Treatment of TB is based on the severity of the symptoms. Pediatric patients with TB and recurrent respiratory infections are treated with TB resection and lobectomy of the anomalous lobe. If the patient is asymptomatic, expectant management with bronchodilators is preferred [57].

Bronchial Atresia

Bronchial atresia is characterized by focal occlusion of a proximal segmental bronchus, with normal anatomy of the distal bronchial tree [20, 23]. The cause of bronchial atresia is still unclear, although some authors speculate that a vascular interruption during gestation may be the cause [58]. The lung parenchyma distal to the obstruction becomes isolated from the bronchial tree, but it receives collateral ventilation through the pores of Kohn, which are microscopic connections through the walls of adjacent alveoli. The atretic bronchus tends to accumulate mucus, appearing as a closed tubular structure filled with fluid and known as bronchocele [55]. Bronchial atresia is more frequently seen in the upper lobes, most often the apical-posterior segment of the left upper lobe [59]. Bronchial atresia is usually asymptomatic, although mild dyspnea, cough, and repeated infection may occur in approximately 30% of the cases [60].

On CT, bronchial atresia appears as centrally located tubular-shaped structure radiating from the airways associated with mucus impaction and hyperlucent lung parenchyma. On MR imaging, bronchial atresia is well depicted

with T2-weighted sequences, showing hyperintense signal intensity (SI) in the impacted mucus (Fig.2.22) surrounded by low SI lung parenchyma due to the chronic hyperinflation and oligemia. In order to increase detection of hyperinflation, imaging in the expiratory phase helps provide better contrast against the adjacent normal relatively hyperintense lung tissue [17]. The differential diagnosis of bronchial atresia includes all pathologies that can fill airways with mucus, such as bronchiectasis, allergic bronchopulmonary aspergillosis (ABPA), and tumor obstruction.

When asymptomatic, bronchial atresia is typically treated conservatively. When associated with symptoms, including recurrent infection, surgical resection is typically performed.

Bronchogenic Cyst

Bronchogenic cysts are remnants of the foregut (pulmonary bud), which result from anomalous ramifications arising during the development of the tracheobronchial tree [55, 61]. They have thin walls covered by columnar epithelium producing serous or mucinous material. The position of bronchogenic cysts depends on the embryological period when the defect occurs. If they develop in the early phase, they are typically located in the pericarinal region, and if they develop in a later phase, they are located within the lung parenchyma. Bronchogenic cysts are most frequently located in the subcarinal space, followed by the paratracheal regions and intra-pulmonary locations, especially the lower lobes. Rarely, bronchogenic cysts can be found in the posterior mediastinum or in an infra-diaphragmatic location [61]. Bronchogenic cysts can be asymptomatic and discovered

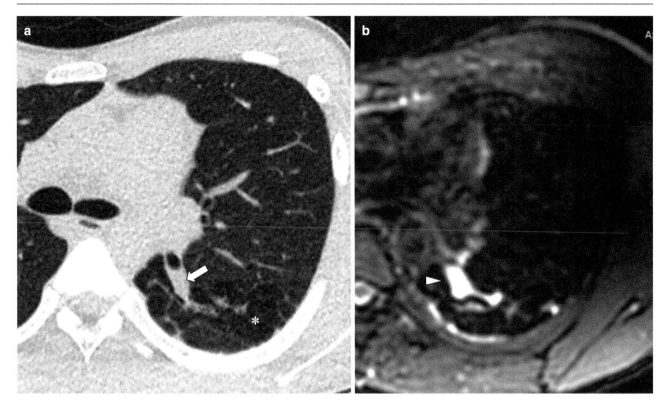

Fig. 2.22 Bronchial atresia in a 17-year-old boy. (a) Axial nonenhanced lung window setting CT image shows a tubular fluid-filled structure (*arrow*) in the left upper lobe compatible with bronchial atresia and air trapping (*) within the left upper lobe. (b) Axial nonen-

hanced T2-weighted CUBE (GE) MR image shows hyperintense signal intensity material (*arrowhead*) filling bronchial atresia. Air trapping seen on CT is not as easily seen on MR image

as incidental findings, although they can cause symptoms if superinfection occurs or if they compress surrounding structures, such as the trachea, bronchi, or esophagus.

On CXR, bronchogenic cysts appear as solitary rounded or oval opacities with well-defined contours and uniform density, which can contain an air-fluid level. On CT, they appear as solitary ovoid or rounded lesions with well-defined contours. In 50% of cases, bronchogenic cysts have a density similar to that of water, but they can be denser depending on the contents of the cyst. In cases of superinfection and communication with the airways, they can also contain blood, air, or gas [61]. Atypical features of bronchogenic cysts include thick wall, solid content, calcifications, or septa. MR imaging is an efficient alternative to CT to diagnose bronchogenic cysts. They typically demonstrate hypo- or isointense signal on T1-weighted sequences and hyperintense homogeneous signal on T2-weighted sequences, reflecting presence of water (Fig. 2.23) [17]. On post-contrast MR imaging, bronchogenic cysts show rim enhancement, typical of cystic lesions. Differential diagnosis includes esophageal duplication cyst (in the middle mediastinum) and neurogenic cyst (in the posterior mediastinum). Final diagnosis is confirmed by the presence of respiratory epithelium in the pathology specimen.

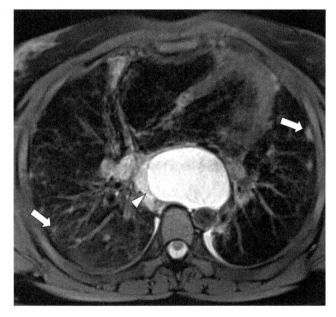

Fig. 2.23 Congenital bronchogenic cyst in a 13-year-old girl with common variable immunodeficiency (CVID). Axial nonenhanced T2-weighted PROPELLER MR image shows a hyperintense cyst (*arrowhead*) in the subcarinal region and multiple subpleural nodules (*arrows*) representing granulomas due to CVID

Typical treatment of bronchogenic cysts is surgical resection, especially when symptomatic. Some authors suggest early surgery in the post-natal period because it provides better conservation of pulmonary parenchyma, a lower incidence of inflammatory lesions, and a reduced rate of complications [62]. However, in asymptomatic patients, surgery is debated because it is associated with 20% morbidity [63, 64]. When conservative management is employed, affected patients should be informed of the 45% of risk of developing symptoms, of a 0.7% risk of developing a malignancy, and that a close long-term follow-up strategy is warranted [63, 64].

Congenital Dynamic Large Airway Disorders

Obstructive Sleep Apnea Syndrome

Obstructive sleep apnea syndrome (OSAS) is a relatively common sleep disorder, in which there is complete or partial upper airway collapse and obstruction during sleep. Typical symptoms include loud snoring or choking, frequent awakenings, disrupted sleep, excessive daytime sleepiness, fatigue, and impaired cognition [65]. Diagnosis is made by measuring the apnea-hypopnea index (AHI). AHI is considered positive for OSAS when there are five or more episodes of apnea and hypopnea per hour of sleep and associated symptoms or when there are 15 or more obstructive apnea-hypopnea events per hour of sleep regardless of symptoms.

OSAS is far more common in adult patients than children where relevant risk factors are obesity, male gender, and increasing age. In contrast, in pediatric OSAS, common risk factors are adeno-tonsillar hypertrophy, obesity, hypotonic neuromuscular diseases, and craniofacial anomalies, with a prevalence of up to 3% in children [66]. Snoring is the most common complaint in children with OSAS. Young children may present with agitated sleep and abnormal sleep positions (i.e., neck hyperextension) due to a disordered breathing. Older children often exhibit excessive daytime sleepiness with hyperactivity or inattention. When untreated, OSAS might result in cognitive deficits, attention deficit/hyperactivity disorder, poor academic achievement, and emotional instability.

Although diagnosis of pediatric OSAS is largely based on clinical history and polysomnography, imaging evaluation can be crucial to determine the cause of upper airway obstruction. Paranasal sinus radiograph and lateral neck radiograph (cephalometric analysis) are simple and highly useful methods for the detection craniofacial deformities, sinusitis, and adenoid hypertrophy [67]. With cephalometric analysis, several measurements can be performed in anatomical sites which can predispose patients to OSAS [67]. Although radiographic cephalometric analysis is often performed, both MR imaging and CT provide the advantage of multiplanar visualization [67]. MR imaging allows a better anatomical resolution of soft tissue and it does not use ionizing radiation;

therefore, it has become the major imaging method for this type of investigation [68]. MR imaging protocols for upper airways should include axial and sagittal images of the oropharyngeal and hypopharyngeal regions to assess the airway contour, the maxillomandibular relationship (e.g., retrognathia and micrognathia), the soft palate, the palate shape, the position of the hyoid bone, and the position and volume of the dorsum of the tongue. Axial reconstructions are important to assess the nasopharynx, hypopharynx, palate, dorsum of the tongue, and vocal cords [68]. Cine-MR imaging of the upper airway is particularly helpful in evaluating children with multiple sites of obstruction and to assess both static and dynamic sites of obstruction. MR images are obtained with mild sedation administered by an anesthesiologist. In these examinations, children without OSAS have minimal motion in the airway (less than 5 mm of movement), at the level of the nasopharynx, the posterior oropharynx, and the hypopharynx. However, in children with OSAS, there is typically movement greater than 5 mm at these three levels [69].

Several surgical and non-surgical treatment options for childhood OSAS are currently available, although adenotonsillectomy remains the first line therapy [70–72]. The most used nonsurgical treatment of OSAS is continuous positive airway pressure (CPAP), which is often very effective and well tolerated by many children [74, 75].

Tracheobronchomalacia

Tracheobronchomalacia (TBM) is due to a weakness of the tracheobronchial wall and/or supporting cartilage with consequent excessive collapse of the trachea and bronchi [73]. It may be congenital or secondary to trauma, infection, chronic external compression, or chronic inflammation. TBM is classified based on the etiology [74]. Type 1 lacks external compression and corresponds to "primary tracheomalacia." Type 2 is characterized by extrinsic tracheal and/or bronchial compression, which originates mainly from cardiovascular anomalies, tumors, cysts, or deformities of the chest wall (either congenital or acquired). Type 3 is an acquired malacia arising from prolonged increased ventilatory airway pressure, tracheostomy, or inflammation.

Although bronchoscopy is considered the gold standard to reach diagnosis, imaging shows similar or higher sensitivity compared to bronchoscopy [75]. End-inspiratory and end/forced -expiratory CT imaging is the most used technique to diagnose TBM, and a 50% expiratory reduction in the cross-sectional luminal area is the most often cited criteria for diagnosis of TBM in children [4]. However, this threshold might be too low, as studies in healthy adult subjects have shown that a higher threshold of 70% may be more appropriate to make the diagnosis of TBM [76]. Both bronchoscopy and CT have disadvantages when used in the pediatric population. Bronchoscopy is an invasive procedure that requires anesthesia and CT exposes children to ionizing radiation. In contrast, MR imaging can be performed in free-breathing conditions in infants with no need for anesthesia, or in older children during forced expiration to elicit better the point of airway collapse [18]. Static and dynamic MR imaging are able to demonstrate airway collapse with the same accuracy of CT without the need for ionizing radiation [19] (Fig. 2.24).

TBM is often self-limited and tends to resolve or become asymptomatic as children grow older [77, 78]. Treatment of symptomatic children with TBM includes bronchodilators, nebulized hypertonic saline to improve mucus clearance, and low-dose inhaled steroids to reduce mucosal swelling and inflammation. CPAP is also often an effective non-surgical treatment for TBM. Surgical treatment in TBM includes aortopexy, slide tracheoplasty, and stent or external splint placement [77, 78].

Infectious and Inflammatory Large Airway Disorders

Tuberculosis

Tuberculosis (TB) remains an important health issue, especially in undeveloped countries. According to the WHO, there were 234,000 deaths due to TB in children <15 years in 2018. In developed countries, TB is rare with an incidence of approximately 4% both in the United States [79] and Europe [80]. Although the primary site of infection is the lung, extrapulmonary TB can occur in children in other organs, mostly lymph nodes and the central nervous system. Typical symptoms of pulmonary TB include cough, fever, night sweats, and weight loss.

Initial screening for TB infection is usually obtained with tuberculin skin test (TST), followed by imaging. Imaging evaluation is particularly important in infants and young children, who may be asymptomatic but with a positive TST. CXR is the most frequently used screening study for TB infection because of its low cost and high availability. A common finding on CXR in a child with TB is a primary complex, which consists of a focal parenchymal opacity with hilar or subcarinal lymphadenopathy [81–83]. When disease progresses, the compression of large airways due to adenopathy often leads to development of pulmonary consolidation or atelectasis. In older pediatric patients, imaging findings of TB that are more typically seen in adults are often present on CXR, such as upper lobe airspace disease, cavitation, and pleural effusions. CT allows for better assessment of endobronchial involvement, bronchiectasis, and cavitation from TB infection [83].

The routine use of CT in TB patients is debated especially due to concern about ionizing radiation [83]. For this reason, MR imaging has been proposed as possible alternative for follow-up imaging [84]. Compared with CT, MR imaging shows similar accuracy for identifying lung lesions in non-AIDS patients with non-miliary pulmonary tuberculosis and has been shown to have a higher diagnostic performance for detecting pulmonary tissue abnormalities, mediastinal nodes, pleural abnormalities, and presence of caseation resolution [84, 85]. A combination of diffusion-weighted imaging (DWI) and subtracted contrast-enhanced (CE) MR imaging is helpful to assess disease activity in cases of mediastinal nodes/fibrosis (Fig. 2.25) [17]. Presence of diffusion restriction in the lymph nodes and peripheral enhancement suggest active TB.

Different multi-antibiotic therapy regimens are used to treat TB, such as 6–9 months of daily isoniazid, shorter two-drug regime of once-weekly isoniazid and rifapentine, or 4 months of daily rifampin [86]. Selection of the regimen depends on patient's antibiotic tolerance and treatment's adherence.

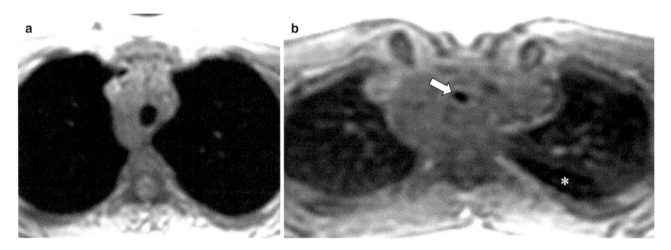

Fig. 2.24 Tracheomalacia in a 17-year-old boy with history of tracheoesophageal fistula. (**a**) Axial nonenhanced proton density-weighted 3D SPGR MR image obtained at end inspiration shows a normal caliber trachea. (**b**) Axial nonenhanced proton density-weighted 3D SPGR MR image obtained at end expiration shows 75% collapse of the trachea (*arrow*) and air trapping (*asterisk*) in the left lower lobe

Histoplasmosis

Histoplasmosis is a fungal infection caused by *Histoplasma capsulatum* frequently found worldwide but especially in North and Central America. In the United States, it is most commonly seen in the state of Ohio and the region of the Mississippi River valley [87]. Typical symptoms of pulmonary histoplasmosis include chest pain, chills, cough, fever, muscle aches and stiffness, and rash (usually small sores on the lower legs).

On CXR, pulmonary histoplasmosis can present as pneumonia with pulmonary nodules containing calcification or cavitation and mediastinal or hilar lymphadenopathy (Fig. 2.26). Because the imaging findings of pulmonary histoplasmosis are similar to TB and sarcoidosis, serology is crucial to narrow the differential diagnosis. Associated findings in histoplasmosis infection include formation of histoplasmoma (bull's-eye calcification in center of nodule), broncholithiasis, fibrosing mediastinitis, and multiple punctate splenic calcifications. Although CXR and chest CT remain the most used techniques to assess pulmonary histoplasmosis, MR imaging has been described as alternative imaging modality to assess mediastinal lymphadenopathy and response to treatment [88].

A rare complication of histoplasmosis infection is fibrosing mediastinitis (FM) [89]. FM is the deposition of collagen and fibrous tissue within the mediastinum caused by an abnormal immunologic response to histoplasmosis infection. FM is more frequently seen in young patients and it can cause compression of the superior vena cava, pulmonary veins/arteries, large airways, or esophagus. FM can be focal or diffuse.

The focal type typically appears on CT and MR imaging as localized, calcified mass in the paratracheal/subcarinal

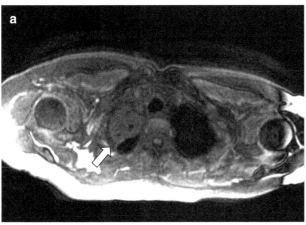
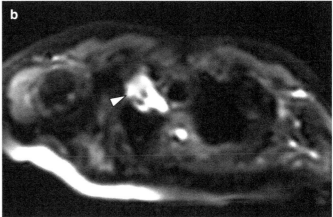

Fig. 2.25 Tuberculosis in a 16-year-old boy who presented with cough, low-grade fever, and weight loss. (Case courtesy of Vincenzo Schininà, Department of Radiology, "L. Spallanzani" National Institute for Infectious Diseases (INMI), IRCCS, Rome, Italy). (**a**) Axial nonen- hanced T1-weighted SPGR MR image shows right upper lobe consoli- dation (*arrow*). (**b**) Axial nonenhanced diffusion weighted MR image (b = 600 s/mm^2) shows restricted diffusion (*arrowhead*) within the region of consolidation

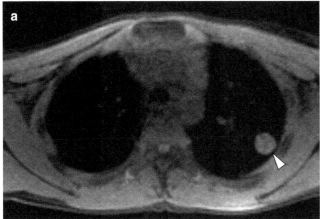
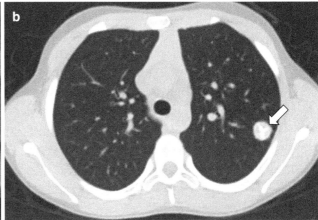

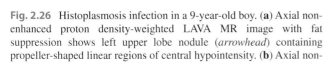

Fig. 2.26 Histoplasmosis infection in a 9-year-old boy. (**a**) Axial non- enhanced proton density-weighted LAVA MR image with fat suppression shows left upper lobe nodule (*arrowhead*) containing propeller-shaped linear regions of central hypointensity. (**b**) Axial non- enhanced lung window setting CT image shows the left upper lobe nod- ule (*arrow*), and propeller-shaped linear region is hyperdense compatible with calcification

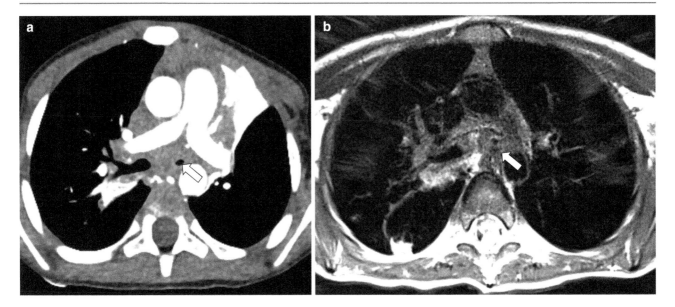

Fig. 2.27 Fibrosing mediastinitis in a 4-year-old boy who presented with progressively worsening shortness of breath and chest pain. (**a**) Axial enhanced soft tissue window setting CT image shows excessive soft tissue in the mediastinum and around the large airways with com- pression of the left main bronchus (*arrow*). (**b**) Axial nonenhanced T2-weighted PROPELLER MR image also shows the excessive soft tissue in the mediastinum and around the large airways with compres- sion of the left main bronchus (*arrow*)

regions of the mediastinum or in the pulmonary hila. The diffuse type typically appears as an infiltrating mass in mul- tiple mediastinal compartments. Contrast-enhanced imag- ing is useful to assess the extent, level, and length of stenosis of the mediastinal vessels and large airways. On MR imag- ing, FM typically appears as a heterogeneous, infiltrative mass of intermediate signal intensity on T1-weighted images and mixed areas of hypo- and hyperintensity on T2-weighted images due to areas of calcification and fibrous tissue (low SI) and areas of active inflammation (high SI) [89] (Fig. 2.27). Heterogeneous enhancement of the mass is typically seen after administration of contrast.

Treatment of pulmonary histoplasmosis includes ampho- tericin B for 2 weeks followed by itraconazole for a total of 10 weeks. Corticosteroids are given along with the antifun- gal therapy in those with severe respiratory symptoms [90]. Antifungal therapy is not typically utilized in FM. In severe cases, stents may be placed within the airways and vessels to prevent compression, and surgery may be utilized in cases of refractory disease [90].

Neoplastic Large Airway Disorders

Benign Primary Large Airway Neoplasms

Subglottic Hemangioma Infantile hemangioma is the most common pediatric tumor of head and neck [91]. It consists of a proliferation of capillaries and usually presents within the first month of life. When located in the subglottic region, infantile

hemangioma can be associated with upper airway obstruction. Affected pediatric patients typically have biphasic stridor due to upper airway narrowing. Infantile hemangioma has an initial proliferative phase with rapid growth in the first year. They tend to then grow at a slower rate until age of 5 years followed by an involution phase that occurs at 5–7 years.

Because hemangiomas have a typical appearance on visual inspection, imaging may not be necessary, although it is often employed when complications are suspected or to determine the relationship with adjacent airways and medi- astinal vessels. Initial screening is typically performed with ultrasound, typically showing a lobulated echogenic mass containing high-flow arteries and veins. On contrast- enhanced CT, infantile hemangiomas show characteristic homogeneous enhancement and rapid wash-out. On MR imaging, the appearance is usually slightly hypointense to muscle on T1-weighted images and iso- to hyperintense on T2-weighted images with flow voids and avid contrast enhancement (Fig. 2.28). In the involution phase, hemangio- mas are characterized by accumulation of fibro-fatty tissue, replacing the vascular tissue [92].

Because nearly all infantile hemangiomas eventually involute, a conservative wait-and-see approach is used for those minimally symptomatic or asymptomatic pediatric patients [93]. Symptomatic patients are often initially treated with medications that accelerate involution of the infantile hemangioma, such as propanolol. Second-line pharmaco- therapy includes corticosteroids, which are used in refractory cases. Surgical options may include intralesional injection with corticosteroids, ablation, or surgical excision [93].

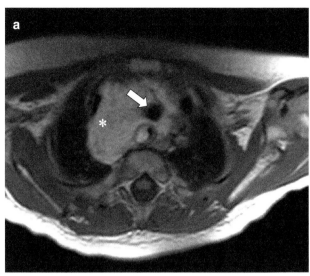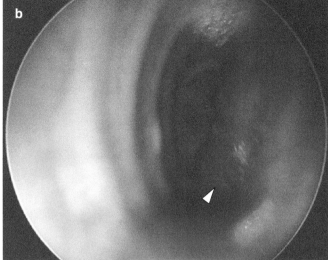

Fig. 2.28 Large airway hemangioma in a 3-month-old girl who presented with respiratory distress and subcutaneous hemangiomas. (**a**) Axial T1-weighted GRE MR image shows hyperintense lesion (*asterisk*) of the mediastinum with encasement and compression of the trachea (*arrow*). (**b**) Endoscopy image shows typical appearance of this hypervascular lesion (*arrowhead*), extending into the trachea lumen with narrowing

Respiratory Papillomatosis Respiratory papillomatosis (RP) is a condition characterized by multiple papillomas in the respiratory epithelium [94]. This occurs more commonly in the upper airways at the level of the larynx (laryngeal papillomatosis) than in the central airways (tracheobronchial papillomatosis). RP is the most common benign tumor of the trachea in children (60% of all benign tumors) [94]. RP is caused by human papilloma virus (HPV) infection, especially types 6 and 11. Human papilloma virus also causes skin and genital warts. Airway infection in children is thought to occur due to transmission to the newborn during vaginal delivery. Symptoms of chronic cough, wheezing, stridor, and hemoptysis can be present around age 2–3 years in affected patients.

The current gold standard for diagnosis is bronchoscopy, which allows direct visualization and therapeutic intervention with direct removal of the lesions. On CXR, papillomas are usually not visible, although when involving the lung parenchyma, they may appear as multiple pulmonary nodules, sometimes with cavitation. CT is the preferred method to assess the extent of disease [94]. Typical CT findings include tracheal nodules, solid or cavitated nodules in the lung parenchyma, air trapping, masses, and consolidation [94]. MR imaging can be also used as alternative to CT to visualize both airways and parenchymal changes due to RP while at the same time limiting radiation exposure. On MR imaging, papillomas typically appear as endobronchial lesions protruding into the airway lumen or as multiple lung nodules.

To date, no curative treatment for RP exists, and surgical excision of the papillomas remains the mainstay of therapy [95]. Unfortunately, lesion recurrence after surgery is common and in those patients who undergo multiple procedures, surgical complications such as larynx and glottis stenosis may occur. Coadjuvant medical treatment with agents including interferon, antiviral agents (acyclovir, ribavirin, cidofovir), retinoids, and inhibitors of the oxygenase-2 cycle may be utilized to limit HPV replication and proliferation [95].

Neurofibroma Neurofibromas are associated with neurofibromatosis type 1 (NF1) and can occur throughout the body, including the neck, thorax, and airways. NF1 is an autosomal dominant disorder and is the most common phakomatosis with an incidence 1/2000 live births [96]. In up to 50% of cases, NF1 occurs with no family history due to a sporadic spontaneous mutation.

Neurofibromas can present as a single large lesion (plexiform neurofibroma) or multiple small neurofibromas. Plexiform neurofibromas represent diffuse neural enlargement or multiple neurofibromas along the course of peripheral nerves. In the thorax, neurofibromas may involve the ribs, chest wall, lungs, and mediastinum. Mediastinal neurofibromas can cause compression of the central airway and mediastinal vessels. Furthermore, neurofibromas can directly arise from the trachea and esophagus [97]. Although diagnosis is based on clinical and genetic testing, imaging is important to assess the extension of the lesions, effect on surrounding structures and treatment planning.

On CT, neurofibromas typically have a central region of low attenuation, seen in two-thirds of the cases [96]. Sometimes, the central region of hypoattenuation tends to enhance giving a typical "target" sign appearance. On MR imaging, neurofibromas often demonstrate peripheral hyperintensity surrounding a region of central hypointensity on T2-weighted images, and enhancement may be heterogeneous if large [98] (Fig. 2.29). Plexiform neurofibromas are a more extensive form of neurofibroma that are infiltrative and have rope-like extensions along the course of the nerve with variable enhancement [98].

Asymptomatic neurofibromas are typically managed conservatively. Symptomatic mediastinal neurofibromas are usually surgically resected to decompress affected mediastinal structures [99].

Malignant Primary Large Airway Neoplasms

Tumors of the Tongue In the pediatric population, tumors of the oral cavity are more frequently benign with malignant tumors representing only 10% of oral cavity tumors. Malignant tumors include (in order of frequency) rhabdomyosarcoma, fibrosarcoma, carcinoma of the parotid, osteosarcoma, and metastatic disease [100, 101]. Among malignant tumors, rhabdomyosarcomas (RMS) are the most common. RMS is a malignant soft tissue tumor that originates from immature striated skeletal muscle cells. RMS of the head and neck region have a low tendency to cause lymph node involvement [100], but distant metastasis to other organs may occur.

Both CT and MR imaging can be used to assess the primary site of the tumor and the relationship with the surrounding structures [37]. However, MR imaging is increasingly preferred as the primary imaging method, especially for head and neck localization, because of its multiplanar capacity, ability to attenuate bone artifact, and superior soft tissue contrast. Findings on CT and MR imaging typically show an inhomogeneous solid mass with avid enhancement and variable obstruction of the oral airway (Fig. 2.30). Intratumoral necrosis, hemorrhage and adjacent bone destruction are often present. Disease staging for metastasis uses CT and/or radionuclide scans such as PET [37].

Treatment of RMS is based on a multimodal approach including surgery, chemotherapy, and/or radiation [102]. Treatment-associated sequelae may be impaired growth and function of the maxilla associated with local radiation therapy and scarring.

Nasopharyngeal Tumor Nasopharyngeal tumors are rare in children representing only 1% of malignancies in childhood [103–105]. These tumors are more frequent in Asian and Northern African children and are strongly associated with Epstein-Barr-virus infection. Peak incidence is between ages 10 and 19 years. Typical symptoms include nasal obstruction and discharge, epistaxis, hearing impairment, and neck swelling due to lymphadenopathy. Cranial

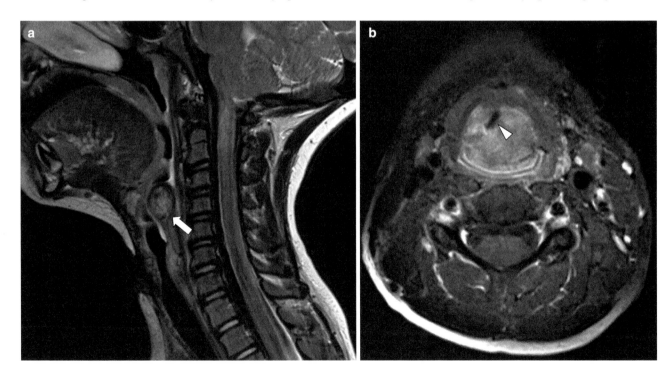

Fig. 2.29 Airway neurofibroma in a 6-year-old girl who presented with stridor. (**a**) Sagittal nonenhanced T1-weighted GRE MR image shows a nodular lesion (*arrow*) in the hypopharynx. (**b**) Axial nonen-hanced T2-weighted HASTE MR image with fat suppression shows compression of airway (*arrowhead*) at the level of the larynx

nerve palsy may be seen in advanced cases due to skull base infiltration.

On CT and MR imaging, nasopharyngeal tumors appear as large inhomogeneous masses expanding into the nasopharyngeal airway, with bone erosion and intracranial extension [105] (Fig. 2.31). The tumor usually arises in the posterolateral wall of the nasopharynx in the fossa of Rosenmüller.

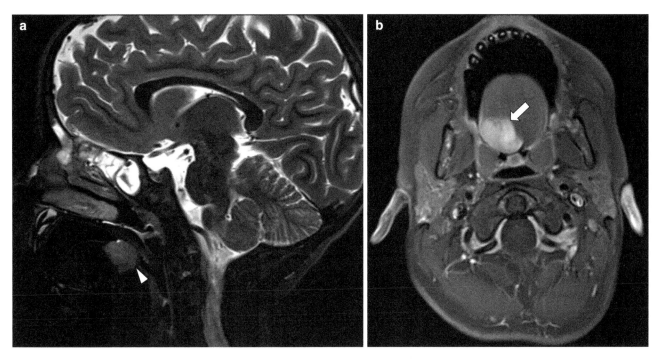

Fig. 2.30 Rhabdomyosarcoma of the tongue in a 4-year-old boy who presented with swallowing difficulty and respiratory distress. (**a**) Sagittal nonenhanced T2-weighted FSE MR image shows a hyperintense mass (*arrowhead*) arising from the right base of the tongue. (**b**) Axial enhanced T1-weighted GRE MR image with fat suppression shows avid enhancement of the mass (*arrow*)

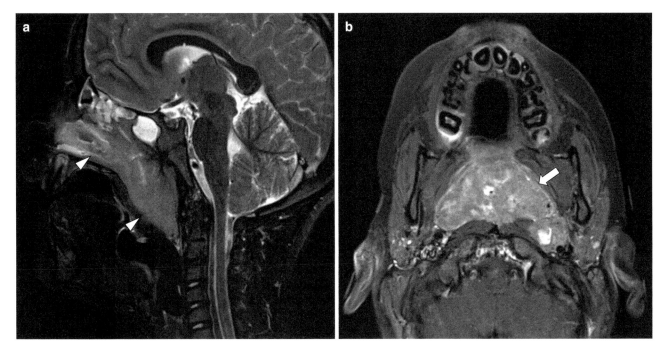

Fig. 2.31 Nasopharyngeal tumor in a 9-year-old girl who presented with respiratory distress and headaches. (**a**) Sagittal nonenhanced T2-weighted spin-echo MR image shows a mass (*arrowheads*) within the nasal cavity and nasopharynx downwardly displacing the soft palate. (**b**) Axial T1-weighted GRE MR image with fat suppression shows airway obstruction by the mass (*arrow*)

The current treatment of nasopharyngeal tumor includes surgery and/or radiation therapy and chemotherapy.

Carcinoid Tumor Although airway carcinoid tumor is rare in children, pulmonary carcinoid is the most common primary lung neoplasm in the pediatric population, typically presenting in late adolescence [106, 107]. Airway carcinoid tumors are frequently located in a main bronchus or in the proximal portion of a lobar bronchus. According to the size and location of the lesion, affected pediatric patients may present with chronic cough, hemoptysis, dyspnea, and persistent partial or total lung atelectasis. Unresolved atelectasis and pneumonia despite antibiotic treatment should suggest a possible airway carcinoid tumor. Other symptoms are related to the production of hormones such as serotonin and other bioactive amines giving cutaneous flushing, diarrhea, and bronchospasm or adrenocorticotropic hormone (ACTH) giving Cushing syndrome [108].

On CXR, carcinoid tumor typically appears as round nodule or mass in a hilar or perihilar location. When causing airway obstruction, atelectasis and mucoid impaction may be visible. Alternatively, airway carcinoid tumors may lead to hyperinflation of the affected lobe by causing a check-valve effect. If airway carcinoid tumor is small and there is no airway obstruction, CXR may be normal. CT is more sensitive than CXR for detection of airway lesions and is able to better visualize extension within and outside the large airways. On CT, carcinoid tumors typically have a lobulated contour with punctate or eccentric calcification [109]. Contrast-enhanced CT frequently shows marked enhancement due to the vascular nature of the tumors. Diagnosis is usually confirmed either by bronchoscopic biopsy (for central lesions) or by transthoracic needle biopsy (for peripheral lesions).

The use of MR imaging to assess carcinoid has been proposed, because of MR imaging's superior ability to characterize different soft tissues [109]. Using in- and out-of-phase techniques, MR imaging can provide information about the tumor fat content, which is often seen in carcinoid [110]. Moreover, MR imaging can be used as a problem-solving tool to clarify equivocal or indeterminate findings on CT. Airway carcinoid tumors show high signal intensity on T2-weighted and short-inversion-time inversion-recovery MR images, which help to distinguish them from adjacent pulmonary vessels, especially in the perihilar regions [110].

The most effective treatment for airway carcinoid tumor is complete surgical excision of the primary tumor. Surgery aims to remove the primary tumor and the involved lymph nodes [107].

Mucoepidermoid Tumor Mucoepidermoid carcinoma (MEC) is the most common malignancy of the salivary gland, accounting for about 3–15% of all salivary gland tumors [103]. Small amounts of salivary gland tissue are present in the submucosa of the trachea. Therefore, MEC can present as airway tumor [107]. Typical symptoms of airway MEC include chronic cough, dyspnea, and hemoptysis. MEC occurs more frequently in segmental bronchi than in the trachea or main bronchi and appear as sharply marginated ovoid or lobulated intraluminal nodules that adapt to the branching features of the airways [107]. MECs tend to have an indolent course characterized by local tumor invasion without metastatic disease.

Although CT is the preferred method to assess local invasion, MR imaging can be considered as alternative to limit radiation exposure in young patients. MECs are typically hypervascular tumors, which may calcify, but do not typically spread to adjacent lymph nodes. Imaging is crucial for surgical and radiation planning to achieve complete surgical resection and avoid local recurrence [111].

Long-term survival rates are excellent when complete surgical resection of MEC is achieved.

Inflammatory Myofibroblastic Tumor Inflammatory myofibroblastic tumors (IMTs) are rare entities and occur predominantly in the lung. Airway IMT is even more rare with a frequency of 0.04–0.07% of all respiratory tract tumors [112]. Initially considered as benign lesion, IMTs tend to show high recurrence rate after resection and occasionally metastasize. Cytogenetic studies have shown that approximately half of IMTs are positive for anaplastic lymphoma kinase gene rearrangements, giving them characteristics of malignant tumors [113]. IMTs consist of myofibroblastic cells and an inflammatory infiltrate of plasma cells, lymphocytes, and eosinophils. When arising in the airway, affected pediatric patients typically present with symptoms of airway obstruction and chronic cough frequently misdiagnosed as asthma or foreign body aspiration in younger children.

Imaging is important to define location and extension of the lesion. Airway IMTs may occur in the trachea or bronchi and when occurring in the trachea often demonstrate full thickness involvement of the membranous wall and the cartilaginous rings. Pulmonary IMTs present as lobulated masses with sharp distinct margins and heterogeneous contrast enhancement (Fig. 2.32). These tumors have a propensity to invade local structures, including vertebrae and thoracic vessels.

Open surgery with complete resection of IMTs is the method of choice to avoid local recurrence. When complete resection is not possible, surgery is combined with radiation therapy and/or chemotherapy.

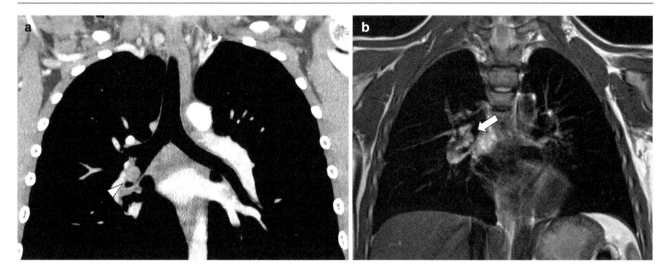

Fig. 2.32 Inflammatory myofibroblastic tumor of the airway in a 9-year-old boy who presented with respiratory distress and right-sided chest pain. (a) Coronal enhanced soft tissue window setting CT image shows endobronchial mass (*arrowhead*) within the bronchus intermedius. (b) Coronal nonenhanced T2/T1-weighted TrueFISP MR image shows the hyperintense endobronchial mass (*arrow*) within the bronchus intermedius

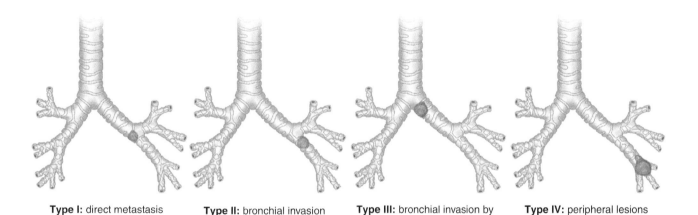

Type I: direct metastasis to the bronchus.

Type II: bronchial invasion by a parenchymal lesion.

Type III: bronchial invasion by mediastinal or hilar lymph node metastasis.

Type IV: peripheral lesions extended along the proximal bronchus.

Fig. 2.33 Four modes of endobronchial metastases. (Adapted from Kiryu et al. [116], with permission). Type I: direct metastasis to the bronchus, Type II: bronchial invasion by a parenchymal lesion, Type III: bronchial invasion by mediastinal or hilar lymph node metastasis, Type IV: peripheral lesions extended along the proximal bronchus

Metastatic Large Airway Neoplasms

Large airway metastases can occur from hematogenous tumor seeding in the airways (Type I), from large airway invasion by a nearby parenchymal lesion (Type II), from large airway invasion by mediastinal or hilar lymph node metastasis (Type III), and as peripheral lesions extended along the proximal large airway (Type IV) [114–116] (Fig. 2.33). Hematogenous spread from distant neoplasms directly to large airways (Type I) is extremely rare in pediatric patients. Airway involvement is more frequently due to invasion from an adjacent primary

tumor such as mediastinal lymphoma or metastatic lymphadenopathy (Type II) [116]. Lymphoma tends to cause extrinsic compression of the large airways and eventually obstruction. Metastatic mediastinal lymphadenopathy can occur with several other tumors as well, including Wilms tumor, neuroblastoma, testicular neoplasms, and sarcomas.

Both CT and MR imaging can be used to assess the location of an endobronchial lesion, localizing it to the trachea and main, lobar, segmental, or subsegmental bronchi. CT and MR imaging can define the shape of a lesion within the airway as polypoid, finger-in-glove, or bronchial wall thick-

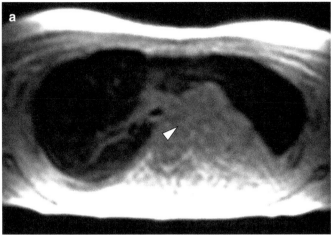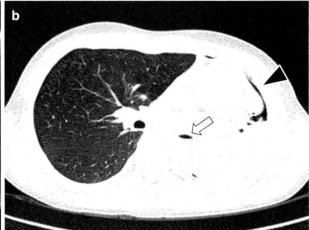

Fig. 2.34 Post-traumatic left main bronchial rupture in a 13-year-old boy who presented with respiratory distress, desaturation, and chest pain. (**a**) Axial reformat of sagittal-acquired nonenhanced proton density-weighted SPGR MR image obtained at end-expiration with nonvisualization of the left main bronchus (*white arrowhead*). (**b**) Axial nonenhanced lung window setting CT image obtained at end-expiration shows compression of the left main bronchus (*arrow*) and pneumomediastinum (*black arrowhead*)

ening. They are also excellent modalities for quantifying the number of lesions [115]. On both CT and MR imaging, metastatic lymph nodes typically appear as nodular conglomerates of enhancing soft tissue, which may develop a hypoenhancing-necrotic center. Large and aggressive tumors may cause extrinsic compression or airway invasion.

According to the type of tumor, location, and extension, a variable combination of chemotherapy and/or radiation therapy and surgery is currently used for treatment of the metastatic neoplasms of the large airways.

Acquired Large Airway Disorders

Acquired Tracheal Stenosis

Acquired tracheal stenosis in children is caused by prolonged endotracheal intubation, tracheostomy tube, or surgery. Injury of the upper airways (larynx and proximal trachea) is most often due to endotracheal intubation in newborns [117]. Infants requiring prolonged positive pressure ventilation via an endotracheal tube for a week or longer and infants requiring repeated intubations are at greatest risk for developing tracheal stenosis. Epithelial damage frequently occurs after endotracheal intubation and is accentuated when tube size does not fit patient's airway size [117]. Post-extubation stridor is the most common sign of moderate to severe subglottic stenosis or laryngeal injury.

Post-traumatic Tracheobronchial Injury

Post-traumatic tracheobronchial injuries are associated with high-energy trauma and have high associated mortality rates. Airway injury is associated with rapid symptoms of dyspnea, subcutaneous emphysema, and stridor [118]. Signs of airway injury on CXR include subcutaneous emphysema and pneumothorax [118]. CT and MR imaging are helpful for confirming the site of airway injury and identifying associated injuries (Fig. 2.34). Treatment of tracheobronchial injuries is surgical, consisting of large airway reconstruction and anastomosis or resection depending on the site of injury and extent of injury.

Postsurgical Bronchial Stenosis

Surgical treatment can also cause airway stenosis, mostly due to postsurgical complications leading to chronic inflammation and fibrosis [115]. On CT or MR imaging, bronchial stenosis appears as a focal narrowing of the airway lumen with eccentric or concentric soft tissue thickening. Causes include pressure necrosis, ischemia, and fibrosis due to the instrumentation during surgery or perianastomotic stenosis in cases of lung transplantation (Fig. 2.35). Most cases can be managed with endoscopic balloon dilation or laser treatment. However, in the most severe cases, open surgery is required.

Foreign Body Aspiration

Foreign body aspiration (FBA) is a common cause of mortality and morbidity in young children [119]. FBA occurs more frequently in the first years of life, when children tend to explore the world by putting objects into their mouths. The majority of aspirated FBs in children are found within the bronchi, especially on the right side, because of the more vertical angulation of the right main bronchus. The typical triad of symptoms in FBA is an episode of choking with severe respiratory distress and cyanosis.

On CXR, characteristic findings in FBA are unilateral hyperinflation and mediastinal shift [120]. Although affected

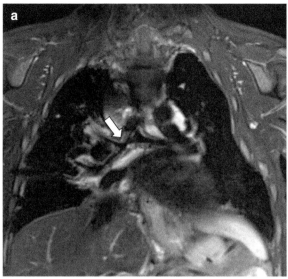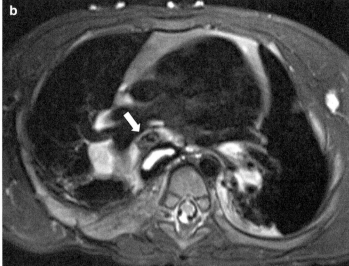

Fig. 2.35 Postsurgical bronchial stenosis in a 3-year-old boy with tracheoesophageal fistula repair. (**a**) Coronal nonenhanced T2-weighted BLADE MR image shows stenosis (*arrow*) of right main bronchus. (**b**)

Axial nonenhanced T2-weighted BLADE MR image shows stenosis (*arrow*) of right main bronchus

patients can be further investigated with bronchoscopy after CXR, cross-sectional imaging may be considered in stable pediatric patients with signs and symptoms suspicious for FBA. Findings of FBA on CT and MR imaging may include direct visualization of the foreign body, hyperinflation of a lung or lobe of the lung, and atelectasis of a lung or lobe of the lung [120] (Fig. 2.36).

Bronchoscopy is the gold-standard test for the assessment of FBA, because it allows direct visualization and removal of the FB.

Miscellaneous Large Airway Disorders

Various congenital, inflammatory, or neoplastic masses around the large airways can result in extrinsic compression of the large airway in the pediatric population. Several examples are discussed in the following section.

Lymphatic Malformation

Lymphatic malformations (LMs) are a type of vascular malformation. In general, vascular malformations are classified into low-flow lesions (lymphatic, venous, capillary, or combined) and high-flow lesions (arteriovenous malformations and arteriovenous fistulas) [91, 92, 121].

LMs are the most common low-flow vascular malformations. LMs frequently present as a cystic mass in newborns, although they may also be diagnosed later in life [91, 92, 121]. More than half of LMs are associated with genetic disorders, such as Turner syndrome, Noonan syndrome, and trisomies. LMs are most frequently located in the head and

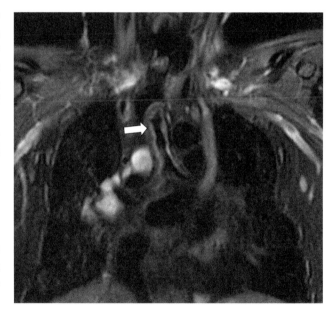

Fig. 2.36 Tracheal changes in a 16-year-old girl with prior history of battery ingestion and erosion into the trachea. Coronal nonenhanced T2-weighted FSE MR image with fat suppression shows long segment irregularity and stenosis of the trachea (*arrow*)

neck region and are the result of an embryological disorder in the development of the cervical lymphatic system. The majority of cervical LMs are diagnosed in newborns and children up to 2 years, with equal distribution between boys and girls. Lesions frequently occur posterior to the sternocleidomastoid muscle, but they can extend around the entire neck and into the mediastinum. On clinical examination, LMs appear as painless slow-growing masses with a spongy consistency. Infection or hemorrhage can lead to sudden enlargement with increased local compression, including on the airways. LMs are classified as macrocystic (>1 cm), microcystic (<1 cm), and mixed cystic forms [92]. The macrocystic is the most common type.

LMs are typically first assessed with ultrasound, which shows a uni- or multilocular cystic mass, containing fluid. Debris is often seen within the fluid, due to superimposed hemorrhage or infection. Septations of variable thickness are usually seen and may demonstrate color Doppler flow. Microcystic LMs tend to appear predominantly hyperechoic and can be confused with solid soft tissue masses. Cross-sectional imaging with CT and MR imaging are crucial for treatment planning. MR imaging is preferred over CT in order to avoid ionizing radiation exposure and because it better highlights the relationship of the lesion with the surrounding structures.

On MR imaging, LMs typically demonstrate hyperintense signal intensity on T2-weighted images (Fig. 2.37). On T1-weighted images, LMs usually demonstrate low or intermediate signal intensity. Post-contrast imaging shows septal contrast enhancement. In cases of superimposed infection or hemorrhage, the content of the cyst may be hyperintense on T1-weighted images due to the presence of proteinaceous contents and post-contrast imaging may demonstrate increased surrounding enhancement.

Treatment with surgery or intralesional sclerotherapy depends on the extent and relationship with the neighboring structures and to the type of LM. Suprahyoid microcystic LMs are more difficult to treat than macrocystic LMs in the infrahyoid and posterior cervical regions.

Castleman Disease

Castleman disease is a lymphoproliferative disorder that causes lymphadenopathy in different parts of the body [122]. Castleman disease can be unicentric, when lymphadenopathy is located in a single anatomical region (i.e., mediastinum), or multicentric, when it involves multiple regions. The latter is also associated with signs of inflammatory disease, including hepatosplenomegaly, cytopenias, and organ dysfunction due to excessive pro-inflammatory hypercytokinemia. Castleman disease can be idiopathic but is associated with infection of human herpes virus 8 (HHV-8) in immunodeficient patients (i.e., HIV-positive children). Castleman disease is also associated with malignancies such as lymphoma. Castleman disease can occur at any age, although it is more common in young adults [122]. Castleman disease is usually asymptomatic, especially in the unicentric form. If symptoms occur, they are typically related to mass effect from enlarged lymph nodes, which can cause extrinsic compression on adjacent structures including large airways. Common sites of lymphadenopathy are the chest (24%), neck (20%), abdomen (18%), and retroperitoneum (14%) [122].

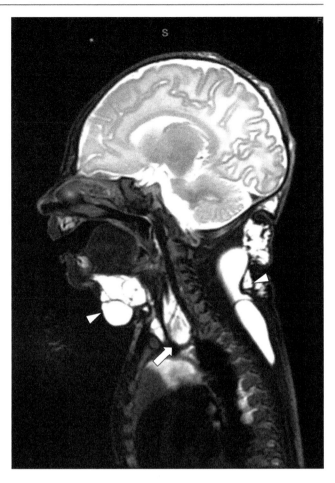

Fig. 2.37 Lymphatic malformation in a 2-day-old girl who presented with respiratory distress and palpable neck mass. Sagittal nonenhanced T2-weighted 3D CUBE (GE) MR image shows multiple hyperintense cystic lesions (*arrowheads*) in the neck, one in the anterior part of the trachea and descending in the anterior mediastinum (*arrow*)

On CXR, Castleman disease typically presents as a mediastinal or hilar mass [123]. On CT, Castleman disease typically appears as a soft tissue mass with homogeneous contrast enhancement which may cause vessel or airway compression [123]. MR imaging typically demonstrates a solid mass which is isointense to skeletal muscle on T1-weighted images, hyperintense to skeletal muscle on T2-weighted images, and avidly enhancing on post-contrast images (Fig. 2.38) [123]. PET-CT/MR imaging is also used to detect positive lymph nodes in other anatomical regions. Although the described imaging features are suggestive of Castleman disease, biopsy is necessary to confirm the diagnosis [123].

When possible, surgical resection is the method of choice to treat lymphadenopathy from Castleman disease [122]. When an enlarged lymph node from Castleman disease is close to a major structure such as large airways or major blood vessels, radiation therapy or chemotherapy is more often used for treatment.

Neuroblastoma

Neuroblastomas are tumors arising from cells in the adrenal medulla and sympathetic nervous system [124]. Neuroblastomas have variable behavior ranging from benign tumors that show spontaneous regression to aggressive malignant tumors with metastatic disease [124]. Neuroblastoma is the third most common childhood cancer, after leukemia and brain tumors,

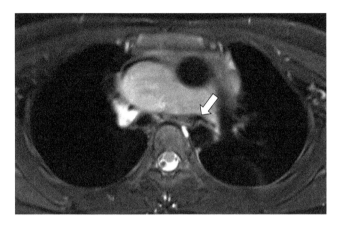

Fig. 2.38 Castleman disease in a 13-year-old girl who presented with respiratory distress. Axial nonenhanced T2-weighted HASTE MR image with fat suppression shows large hyperintense mediastinal lymph node compressing the left main bronchus (*arrow*)

and is the most common solid extracranial tumor in children [125, 126]. It is usually diagnosed in the first 2 years of life. Symptoms in children with neuroblastoma vary based on the number and location of tumors and can include both local and systemic symptoms. Approximately half of affected patients present with localized disease, with the remainder having distant metastases, especially to the bones and liver.

The most common primary site is the adrenal gland, where neuroblastomas present as asymptomatic abdominal masses or with symptoms related to local compression (abdominal pain, distension, constipation) or hypertension due to catecholamine production [125, 126]. Neuroblastoma can extend to the spinal canal and can lead to spinal cord compression and paraplegia [126, 127]. A common location in infants is the cervical and thoracic region, where they can cause compression of the symphatic trunk leading to Horner syndrome (unilateral ptosis, anhidrosis, and miosis) or compress the airways resulting in respiratory symptoms (Fig. 2.39).

Cross-sectional imaging studies such as CT and MR imaging are used to detect neuroblastoma as well as assess local extension of the tumor, lymph node involvement, and distant metastasis [125, 126]. When located in the neck and mediastinum, neuroblastoma tends to encase vascular structures and compresses large airways. On CT, neuroblastoma appears as a heterogeneous mass with contrast enhancement

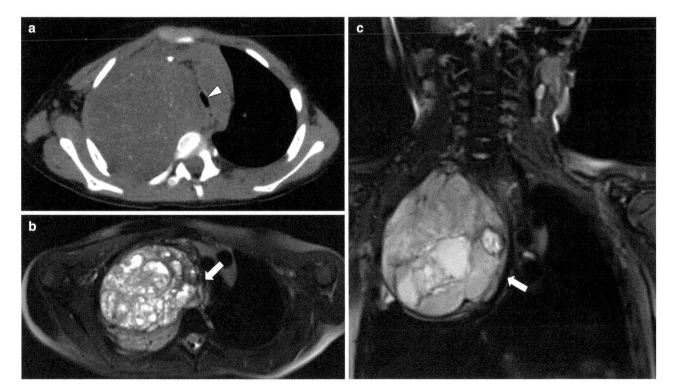

Fig. 2.39 Thoracic neuroblastoma in a 5-year-old boy who presented with respiratory distress. (**a**) Axial nonenhanced soft tissue window setting CT image shows large mass containing calcifications in the right upper thorax compressing the trachea (*arrowhead*). (**b**) Axial nonenhanced T2-weighted HASTE MR image with fat suppression shows heterogeneous hyperintense signal within the mass compressing the trachea (*arrow*). (**c**) Coronal nonenhanced T2-weighted HASTE MR image with fat suppression shows mass compressing the trachea and right main bronchus (*arrow*)

and often shows calcifications. On MR imaging, neuroblastoma appears as a heterogeneous mass that is hyperintense on T2-weighted images and restricts diffusion on diffusion-weighted images. Gadolinium contrast often improves the visualization of tumor infiltration into adjacent tissues and tumor vascularity.

The current treatment of neuroblastoma includes a combination of radiation therapy, chemotherapy, and surgical resection [125]. Prognosis depends on the location, extension, and genetics of the tumor and the age at presentation. In general, the younger the age at diagnosis, the better the survival rate.

Conclusion

The use of MR imaging for large airway evaluation in the pediatric population has three unparalleled advantages over CT. These include the absence of ionizing radiation, the ability to perform dynamic imaging, and excellent tissue characterization. Currently, various congenital and acquired pediatric large airway disorders can be evaluated using MR imaging. New sequences provide image quality comparable to CT with practical protocols that can be applied in daily clinical setting. Careful attention to patient preparation, protocol optimization, and appropriate use of sedation are the keys to obtaining diagnostic pediatric large airway MR imaging. Future developments in MR imaging and post-processing techniques (i.e., automatic MR imaging airways segmentation tools) have a great promise to further increase the use of MR imaging in pediatric patients and expand its clinical applications in various pediatric large airway disorders.

References

1. Tiddens HAWM, Kuo W, van Straten M, Ciet P. Paediatric lung imaging: the times they are a-changin. Eur Respir Rev. 2018;27(147):170097. https://doi.org/10.1183/16000617.0097-2017.
2. Ciet P, Tiddens HAWM, Wielopolski PA, et al. Magnetic resonance imaging in children: common problems and possible solutions for lung and airways imaging. Pediatr Radiol. 2015;45(13):1901–15.
3. Baez JC, Ciet P, Mulkern R, Seethamraju RT, Lee EY. Pediatric chest MR imaging: lung and airways. Magn Reson Imaging Clin N Am. 2015;23(2):337–49.
4. Lee EY, Zucker EJ, Restrepo R, Daltro P, Boiselle PM. Advanced large airway CT imaging in children: evolution from axial to 4-D assessment. Pediatr Radiol. 2013;43(3):285–97.
5. Liszewski MC, Hersman FW, Altes TA, Ohno Y, Ciet P, Warfield SK, Lee EY. Magnetic resonance imaging of pediatric lung parenchyma, airways, vasculature, ventilation, and perfusion: state of the art. Radiol Clin North Am. 2013;51(4):555–82. Review.
6. Baez JC, Seethamraju RT, Mulkern R, Ciet P, Lee EY. Pediatric chest MR imaging: sedation, techniques, and extracardiac vessels. Magn Reson Imaging Clin N Am. 2015;23(2):321–35.
7. Edwards AD, Arthurs OJ. Paediatric MRI under sedation: is it necessary? What is the evidence for the alternatives? Pediatr Radiol. 2011;41(11):1353–64.
8. Lutterbey G, Wattjes MP, Doerr D, Fischer NJ, Gieseke J, Schild HH. Atelectasis in children undergoing either propofol infusion or positive pressure ventilation anesthesia for magnetic resonance imaging. Pediatr Anesth. 2007;17(2):121–5.
9. Salamon E, Lever S, Kuo W, Ciet P, Tiddens HA. Spirometer guided chest imaging in children: it is worth the effort! Pediatr Pulmonol. 2017;52(1):48–56.
10. Gai ND, Malayeri A, Agarwal H, Evers R, Bluemke D. Evaluation of optimized breath-hold and free-breathing 3D ultrashort echo time contrast agent-free MRI of the human lung. J Magn Reson Imaging. 2016;43(5):1230–8.
11. Dournes G, Grodzki D, Macey J, Girodet PO, Fayon M, Chateil JF, et al. Quiet submillimeter MR imaging of the lung is feasible with a PETRA sequence at 1.5 T. Radiology. 2015;279(1):328.
12. Chandarana H, Block KT, Winfeld MJ, Lala SV, Mazori D, Giuffrida E, et al. Free-breathing contrast-enhanced T1-weighted gradient-echo imaging with radial k-space sampling for paediatric abdominopelvic MRI. Eur Radiol. 2014;24(2):320–6.
13. Kishida Y, Koyama H, Seki S, Yoshikawa T, Kyotani K, Okuaki T, et al. Comparison of fat suppression capability for chest MR imaging with Dixon, SPAIR and STIR techniques at 3 tesla MR system. Magn Reson Imaging. 2018;47:89–96.
14. Gibiino F, Sacolick L, Menini A, Landini L, Wiesinger F. Free-breathing, zero-TE MR lung imaging. MAGMA. 2015;28(3):207–15.
15. Kumar S, Rai R, Stemmer A, Josan S, Holloway L, Vinod S, et al. Feasibility of free breathing lung MRI for radiotherapy using non-Cartesian k-space acquisition schemes. Br J Radiol. 2017;90(1080):20170037.
16. Bates AJ, Higano NS, Hysinger EB, et al. Quantitative assessment of regional dynamic airway collapse in neonates via retrospectively respiratory-gated ^{1}H ultrashort echo time MRI. J Magn Reson Imaging. 2019;49(3):659–67.
17. Liszewski MC, Ciet P, Lee EY. MR imaging of lungs and airways in children. Magn Reson Imaging Clin N Am. 2019;27(2):201–25.
18. Ciet P, Wielopolski P, Manniesing R, Lever S, de Bruijne M, Morana G, et al. Spirometer-controlled cine magnetic resonance imaging used to diagnose tracheobronchomalacia in paediatric patients. Eur Respir J. 2014;43(1):115–24.
19. Ciet P, Boiselle PM, Heidinger B, et al. Cine MRI of tracheal dynamics in healthy volunteers and patients with tracheobronchomalacia. AJR Am J Roentgenol. 2017;209(4):757–61.
20. Berrocal T, Madrid C, Novo S, Gutiérrez J, Arjonilla A, Gómez-León N. Congenital anomalies of the tracheobronchial tree, lung, and mediastinum: embryology, radiology, and pathology. Radiographics. 2004;24:e17.
21. Holbert JM, Strollo DC. Imaging of the normal trachea. J Thorac Imaging. 1995;10(3):171–9.
22. Kotecha S. Lung growth for beginners. Paediatr Respir Rev. 2000;1(4):308–13.
23. Biyyam DR, Chapman T, Ferguson MR, Deutsch G, Dighe MK. Congenital lung abnormalities: embryologic features, prenatal diagnosis, and postnatal radiologic-pathologic correlation. Radiographics. 2010;30(6):1721–38.
24. Griscom NT, Wohl ME. Dimensions of the growing trachea related to body height. Am Rev Respir Dis. 1985;131(6):840–4.
25. Griscom NT, Wohl ME. Dimensions of the growing trachea related to age and gender. AJR Am J Roentgenol. 1986;146(2):233–7.
26. Jeffery PK. The development of large and small airways. Am J Respir Crit Care Med. 1988;157(5 Part 2):S174–80.

27. Lawrence DA, Branson B, Oliva I, Rubinowitz A. The wonderful world of the windpipe: a review of central airway anatomy and pathology. Can Assoc Radiol J. 2015;66(1):30–43.
28. Boiselle PM. Imaging of the large airways. Clin Chest Med. 2008;29(1):181–93.
29. Boiselle PM, Lee KS, Ernst A. Multidetector CT of the central airways. J Thorac Imaging. 2005;20(3):186–95.
30. Breatnach E, Abbott GC, Fraser RG. Dimensions of the normal human trachea. AJR Am J Roentgenol. 1984;142(5):903–6.
31. Hewitt RJ, Butler CR, Maughan EF, Elliott MJ. Congenital tracheo-bronchial stenosis. Semin Pediatr Surg. 2016;25(3):144–9.
32. Uchida DA, Morgan-wallace V, Richards K, Seidelman J, Muntz HR. Congenital tracheal stenosis masquerading as asthma in an adolescent: the value of spirometry. Clin Pediatr (Phila). 2009;48(4):432–4.
33. Applegate KE, Goske MJ, Pierce G, Murphy D. Situs revisited: imaging of the heterotaxy syndrome. Radiographics. 2013;19(4):837–52; discussion 853–4.
34. Yoneyama H, Kondo C, Yamasaki A, Nakanishi T, Sakai S. Comparison of situs ambiguous patterns between heterotaxy syndromes with polysplenia and asplenia. Eur J Radiol. 2015;84(11):2301–6.
35. Loomba R, Shah PH, Anderson RH, Arora Y. Radiologic considerations in heterotaxy: the need for detailed anatomic evaluation. Cureus. 2016;8(1):e470. https://doi.org/10.7759/cureus.470.
36. Shapiro AJ, Zariwala MA, Ferkol T, Davis SD, Sagel SD, Dell SD, et al.; Genetic Disorders of Mucociliary Clearance Consortium. Diagnosis, monitoring, and treatment of primary ciliary dyskinesia: PCD foundation consensus recommendations based on state of the art review. Pediatr Pulmonol. 2016;51(2):115–32. Review.
37. Donnelly LF, Jones BV, Strife JL. Imaging of pediatric tongue abnormalities. AJR Am J Roentgenol. 2000;175(2):489–93.
38. Lo Casto A, Salerno S, Cannizzaro F, Caronia A, Bencivinni F, Barbiera F, et al. MRI findings in lingual venous malformations. Dentomaxillofacial Radiol. 2003;32(5):333–6.
39. Perkins JA. Overview of macroglossia and its treatment. Curr Opin Otolaryngol Head Neck Surg. 2009;17(6):460–5.
40. Fujioka M, Young LW, Giardany BR. Radiographic evaluation of adenoidal size in children: ratio. AJR Am J Roentgenol. 1979;133(3):401–4.
41. Fernbach SK, Brouillette RT, Riggs TW, Hunt CE. Radiologic evaluation of adenoids and tonsils in children with obstructive sleep apnea: plain films and fluoroscopy. Pediatr Radiol. 1983;13(5):258–65.
42. Fricke BL, Donnelly LF, Shott SR, Kalra M, Poe SA, Chini BA, Amin RS. Comparison of lingual tonsil size as depicted on MR imaging between children with obstructive sleep apnea despite previous tonsillectomy and adenoidectomy and normal controls. Pediatr Radiol. 2006;36(6):518–23.
43. Donnelly LF, Casper KA, Chen B. Correlation on cine MR imaging of size of adenoid and palatine tonsils with degree of upper airway motion in asymptomatic sedated children. AJR Am J Roentgenol. 2002;179(2):503–8.
44. John SD, Swischuk LE. Stridor and upper airway obstruction in infants and children. Radiographics. 1992;12(4):625–43.
45. Schroeder JW, Holinger LD. Congenital laryngeal stenosis. Otolaryngol Clin North Am. 2008;41(5):865–75.
46. Sanford E, Saadai P, Lee H, Slavotinek A. Congenital high airway obstruction sequence (CHAOS): a new case and a review of phenotypic features. Am J Med Genet A. 2012;158A(12):3126–36.
47. Ryan G, Somme S, Crombleholme TM. Airway compromise in the fetus and neonate: prenatal assessment and perinatal management. Semin Fetal Neonatal Med. 2016;21(4):230–9.
48. Guimaraes CV, Linam LE, Kline-Fath BM, Donnelly LF, Calvo-Garcia MA, Rubio EI, et al. Prenatal MRI findings of fetuses with congenital high airway obstruction sequence. Korean J Radiol. 2009;10(2):129–34.
49. Goyal A, Jones MO, Couriel JM, Losty PD. Oesophageal atresia and tracheo-oesophageal fistula. Arch Dis Child Fetal Neonatal Ed. 2006;91(5):381–4. Review.
50. Garge S, Rao KL, Bawa M. The role of preoperative CT scan in patients with tracheoesophageal fistula: a review. J Pediatr Surg. 2013;48(9):1966–71.
51. Hochart V, Verpillat P, Langlois C, Garabedian C, Bigot J, Debarge VH, et al. The contribution of fetal MR imaging to the assessment of oesophageal atresia. Eur Radiol. 2015;25(2):306–14.
52. Higano NS, Bates AJ, Tkach JA, Fleck RJ, Lim FY, Woods JC, Kingma PS. Pre- and post-operative visualization of neonatal esophageal atresia / tracheoesophageal fistula via magnetic resonance imaging. J Pediatr Surg Case Rep. 2018;29:5–8.
53. Kovesi T, Rubin S. Long-term complications of congenital esophageal atresia and/or tracheoesophageal fistula. Chest. 2004;126(3):915–25.
54. Yedururi S, Guillerman RP, Chung T, Braverman RM, Dishop MK, Giannoni CM, Krishnamurthy R. Multimodality imaging of tracheobronchial disorders in children. Radiographics. 2008; 28(3):e29.
55. Desir A, Ghaye B. Congenital abnormalities of intrathoracic airways. Radiol Clin North Am. 2009;47(2):203–25.
56. Ghaye B, Szapiro D, Fanchamps J-M, Dondelinger RF. Congenital bronchial abnormalities revisited. Radiographics. 2001;21(1):105–19.
57. Doolittle AM, Mair EA. Tracheal bronchus: classification, endoscopic analysis, and airway management. Otolaryngol Neck Surg. 2002;126(3):240–3.
58. Newman B. Congenital bronchopulmonary foregut malformations: concepts and controversies. Pediatr Radiol. 2006;36(8): 773–91.
59. Kinsella BD, Sissons G, Williams MP. The radiological imaging of bronchial atresia. Br J Radiol. 1992;65(776):681–5. Review.
60. Gipson MG, Kristopher W, Hurth KM. Bronchial atresia. Radiographics. 2009;29(5):1531–5.
61. Thacker PG, Rao AG, Hill JG, Lee EY. Congenital lung anomalies in children and adults: current concepts and imaging findings. Radiol Clin North Am. 2014;52(1):155–81.
62. Fievet L, D'Journo XB, Guys JM, Thomas PA, De Lagausie P. Bronchogenic cyst: best time for surgery? Ann Thorac Surg. 2012;94(5):1695–9.
63. Kirmani B, Kirmani B, Sogliani F. Should asymptomatic bronchogenic cysts in adults be treated conservatively or with surgery? Interact Cardiovasc Thorac Surg. 2010;11(5):649–59.
64. Hall NJ, Stanton MP. Long-term outcomes of congenital lung malformations. Semin Pediatr Surg. 2017;26(5):311–6.
65. Malhotra A, White DP. Obstructive sleep apnoea. Lancet. 2002;360(9328):237–45. Review
66. Chang SJ, Chae KY. Obstructive sleep apnea syndrome in children: epidemiology, pathophysiology, diagnosis and sequelae. Korean J Pediatr. 2010;53(10):863–71.
67. Thakkar K, Yao M. Diagnostic studies in obstructive sleep apnea. Otolaryngol Clin North Am. 2007;40(4):785–805.
68. Mello Junior CF, Guimarães Filho HA, Gomes CA, Paiva CC. Radiological findings in patients with obstructive sleep apnea. J Bras Pneumol. 2013;39(1):98–101. [Article in English, Portuguese].
69. Donnelly LF. Obstructive sleep apnea in pediatric patients: evaluation with cine MR sleep studies. Radiology. 2007;236(3):768–78.
70. Brockbank JC. Update on pathophysiology and treatment of childhood obstructive sleep apnea syndrome. Paediatr Respir Rev. 2017;24:21–3.
71. Torretta S, Rosazza C, Pace ME, Iofrida E, Marchisio P. Impact of adenotonsillectomy on pediatric quality of life: review of the literature. Ital J Pediatr. 2017;43(1):107.

72. Kaditis AG, Alonso Alvarez ML, Boudewyns A, Alexopoulos EI, Ersu R, Joosten K, et al. Obstructive sleep disordered breathing in 2- to 18-year-old children: diagnosis and management. Eur Respir J. 2016;47(1):69–94.

73. Lee EY, Litmanovich D, Boiselle PM. Multidetector CT evaluation of tracheobronchomalacia. Radiol Clin North Am. 2009;47(2):261–9. Review.

74. Carden KA, Boiselle PM, Waltz DA, Ernst A. Tracheomalacia and tracheobronchomalacia in children and adults: an in-depth review. Chest. 2005;127(3):984–1005.

75. Lee KS, Sun MR, Ernst A, Feller-Kopman D, Majid A, Boiselle PM. Comparison of dynamic expiratory CT with bronchoscopy for diagnosing airway malacia: a pilot evaluation. Chest. 2007;131(3):758–64.

76. Boiselle PM, O'Donnell CR, Bankier AA, Ernst A, Millet ME, Potemkin A, Loring SH. Tracheal collapsibility in healthy volunteers during forced expiration: assessment with multidetector CT. Radiology. 2009;252(1):255–62.

77. Fraga JC, Jennings RW, Kim PC. Pediatric tracheomalacia. Semin Pediatr Surg. 2016;25(3):156–64.

78. Snijders D, Barbato A. An update on diagnosis of tracheomalacia in children. Eur J Pediatr Surg. 2015;25(4):333–5.

79. Centers for Disease Control and Prevention. Surveillance, Epidemiology, and Outbreak Investigations Branch. Division of Tuberculosis Elimination. Epidemiology of Pediatric Tuberculosis in the United States, 1993–2016. 21 Jun 2017. https://www.cdc.gov/tb/publications/slidesets/pediatrictb/PediatricTB_SlideSet_TextOnly_2016.pdf. Accessed 29 July 2019.

80. European Centre for Disease Prevention and Control/WHO Regional Office for Europe. Tuberculosis surveillance and monitoring in Europe. Report 2018. 2016 data. 2018. Sotkcholm: European Centere for Disease Prevention and Control; 2018. https://ecdc.europa.eu/sites/portal/files/documents/ecdc-tuberculosis-surveillance-monitoring-Europe-2018-rev1.pdf. Accessed 29 July 2019.

81. Fonseca-Santos J. Tuberculosis in children. Eur J Radiol. 2005;55(2):202–8.

82. Burrill J, Williams CJ, Bain G, Conder G, Hine AL, Misra RR. Tuberculosis: a radiologic review. Radiographics. 2007;27(5):1255–73.

83. Nachiappan AC, Rahbar K, Shi X, Guy ES, Mortani Barbosa EJ Jr, Shroff GS, et al. Pulmonary tuberculosis: role of radiology in diagnosis and management. Radiographics. 2017;37(1):52–72.

84. Rizzi EB, Schinina' V, Cristofaro M, Goletti D, Palmieri F, Bevilacqua N, et al. Detection of pulmonary tuberculosis: comparing MR imaging with HRCT. BMC Infect Dis. 2011;11:243. https://doi.org/10.1186/1471-2334-11-243.

85. Sodhi KS, Sharma M, Saxena AK, Mathew JL, Singh M, Khandelwal N. MRI in thoracic tuberculosis of children. Indian J Pediatr. 2017;84(9):670–6.

86. Gaensbauer J, Broadhurst R. Recent innovations in diagnosis and treatment of pediatric tuberculosis. Curr Infect Dis Rep. 2019;21(1):4. https://doi.org/10.1007/s11908-019-0662-0.

87. Chu JH, Feudtner C, Heydon K, Walsh TJ, Zaoutis TE. Hospitalizations for endemic mycoses: a population-based national study. Clin Infect Dis. 2006;42(6):822–5.

88. Kirchner SG, Hernanz-Schulman M, Stein SM, Wright PF, Heller RM. Imaging of pediatric mediastinal histoplasmosis. Radiographics. 1991;11(3):365–81.

89. Rossi SE, McAdams HP, Rosado-de-Christenson ML, Franks TJ, Galvin JR. Fibrosing mediastinitis. Radiographics. 2001;21(3):737–57. Review.

90. Wheat LJ, Freifeld AG, Kleiman MB, Baddley JW, McKinsey DS, Loyd JE, Kauffman CA. Infectious Diseases Society of America. Clinical practice guidelines for the management of patients with histoplasmosis: 2007 update by the Infectious Diseases Society of America. Clin Infect Dis. 2007;45(7):807–25.

91. Güneyli S, Ceylan N, Bayraktaroğlu S, Acar T, Savaş R. Imaging findings of vascular lesions in the head and neck. Diagn Interv Radiol. 2014;20(5):432–7.

92. Flors L, Leiva-Salinas C, Maged IM, Norton PT, Matsumoto AH, Angle JF, et al. MR imaging of soft-tissue vascular malformations: diagnosis, classification, and therapy follow-up. Radiographics. 2011;31(5):1321–40.

93. Darrow DH. Management of infantile hemangiomas of the airway. Otolaryngol Clin North Am. 2018;51(1):133–46.

94. Fortes HR, Ranke FMV, Escuissato DL, Araujo Neto CA, Zanetti G, Hochhegger B, et al. Laryngotracheobronchial papillomatosis: chest CT findings. J Bras Pneumol. 2017;43(4):259–63. [Article in English, Portuguese].

95. Fortes HR, von Ranke FM, Escuissato DL, Araujo Neto CA, Zanetti G, et al. Recurrent respiratory papillomatosis: a state-of-the-art review. Respir Med. 2017;126:116–21.

96. Fortman BJ, Kuszyk BS, Urban BA, Fishman EK. Neurofibromatosis type 1: a diagnostic mimicker at CT. Radiographics. 2001;21(3):601–12.

97. Meredith HC, Valicenti JF. Solitary neurofibroma of the trachea. Br J Radiol. 1978;51(603):218–9.

98. Kami YN, Chikui T, Okamura K, Kubota Y, Oobu K, Yabuuchi H, et al. Imaging findings of neurogenic tumours in the head and neck region. Dentomaxillofacial Radiol. 2012;41:18–23.

99. Reviron-Rabec L, Girerd B, Seferian A, Campbell K, Brosseau S, Bergot E, et al. Pulmonary complications of type 1 neurofibromatosis. Rev Mal Respir. 2016;33(6):460–73.

100. Pappo AS, Meza JL, Donaldson SS, Wharam MD, Wiener ES, Qualman SJ, et al. Treatment of localized nonorbital, nonparameningeal head and neck rhabdomyosarcoma: lessons learned from intergroup rhabdomyosarcoma studies III and IV. J Clin Oncol. 2003;21(4):638–45.

101. Weiss AR, Lyden ER, Anderson JR, Hawkins DS, Spunt SL, Walterhouse DO, et al. Histologic and clinical characteristics can guide staging evaluations for children and adolescents with rhabdomyosarcoma: a report from the Children's Oncology Group Soft Tissue Sarcoma Committee. J Clin Oncol. 2013;31(26):3226–32.

102. Tröbs RB, Mader E, Friedrich T, Bennek J. Oral tumors and tumor-like lesions in infants and children. Pediatr Surg Int. 2003;19(9–10):639–45.

103. Friedman ER, John SD. Imaging of pediatric neck masses. Radiol Clin North Am. 2011;49(4):617–32.

104. Tranvinh E, Yeom KW, Iv M. Imaging neck masses in the neonate and young infant. Semin Ultrasound CT MRI. 2015;36(2):120–37.

105. LaPlante JK, Pierson NS, Hedlund GL. Common pediatric head and neck congenital/developmental anomalies. Radiol Clin North Am. 2015;53(1):181–96.

106. Jeung M-Y, Gasser B, Gangi A, et al. Bronchial carcinoid tumors of the thorax: spectrum of radiologic findings. Radiographics. 2002;22(2):351–65.

107. Fauroux B, Aynie V, Larroquet M, Boccon-Gibod L, Ducou le Pointe H, Tamalet A, Clément A. Carcinoid and mucoepidermoid bronchial tumours in children. Eur J Pediatr. 2005;164(12):748–52.

108. Doppman JL, Pass HI, Nieman LK, Findling JW, Dwyer AJ, Feuerstein IM, et al. Detection of ACTH-producing bronchial carcinoid tumors: MR imaging vs CT. AJR Am J Roentgenol. 1991;156(1):39–43.

109. Amini B, Huang SY, Tsai J, Benveniste MF, Robledo HH, Lee EY. Primary lung and large airway neoplasms in children: current imaging evaluation with multidetector computed tomography. Radiol Clin North Am. 2013;51(4):637–57.

110. Baxi AJ, Chintapalli K, Katkar A, Restrepo CS, Betancourt SL, Sunnapwar A. Multimodality imaging findings in carcinoid tumors: a head-to-toe spectrum. Radiographics. 2017;37(2):516–36.

111. ElNayal A, Moran CA, Fox PS, Mawlawi O, Swisher SG, Marom EM. Primary salivary gland–type lung cancer: imaging and clinical predictors of outcome. AJR Am J Roentgenol. 2013;201(1):W57–63.

112. Gaissert HA, Grillo HC, Shadmehr MB, Wright CD, Gokhale M, Wain JC, Mathisen DJ. Uncommon primary tracheal tumors. Ann Thorac Surg. 2006;82(1):268–73.

113. Butrynski JE, D'Adamo DR, Hornick JL, Dal Cin P, Antonescu CR, Jhanwar SC, et al. Crizotinib in ALK-rearranged inflammatory myofibroblastic tumor. N Engl J Med. 2010;363(18):1727–33.

114. Lee EY, Greenberg SB, Boiselle PM. Multidetector computed tomography of pediatric large airway diseases: state-of-the-art. Radiol Clin North Am. 2011;49(5):869–93.

115. Semple T, Calder A, Owens CM, Padley S. Current and future approaches to large airways imaging in adults and children. Clin Radiol. 2017;72(5):356–74.

116. Kiryu T, Hoshi H, Matsui E, Iwata H, Kokubo M, Shimokawa K, Kawaguchi S. Endotracheal/endobronchial metastases : clinicopathologic study with special reference to developmental modes. Chest. 2001;119(3):768–75.

117. Downing GJ, Kilbride HW. Evaluation of airway complications in high-risk preterm infants: application of flexible fiberoptic airway endoscopy. Pediatrics. 1995;95(4):567–72.

118. Gaebler C, Mueller M, Schramm W, Eckersberger F, Vécsei V. Tracheobronchial ruptures in children. Am J Emerg Med. 1996;14(3):279–84.

119. Kiyan G, Gocmen B, Tugtepe H, Karakoc F, Dagli E, Dagli TE. Foreign body aspiration in children: the value of diagnostic criteria. Int J Pediatr Otorhinolaryngol. 2009;73(7):963–7.

120. Hunter TB, Taljanovic MS. Foreign bodies. Radiographics. 2003;23(3):731–57. Review.

121. Bhat V, Bhat V, Salins P. Imaging spectrum of hemangioma and vascular malformations of the head and neck in children and adolescents. J Clin Imaging Sci. 2014;4:31. https://doi.org/10.4103/2156-7514.135179.

122. Talat N, Belgaumkar AP, Schulte KM. Surgery in Castleman's disease: a systematic review of 404 published cases. Ann Surg. 2012;255(4):677–84.

123. Madan R, Chen J, Trotman-Dickenson B, Jacobson F, Hunsaker A. The spectrum of Castleman's disease: mimics, radiologic pathologic correlation and role of imaging in patient management. Eur J Radiol. 2012;81(1):123–31.

124. Tomolonis JA, Agarwal S, Shohet JM. Neuroblastoma pathogenesis: deregulation of embryonic neural crest development. Cell Tissue Res. 2018;372(2):245–62.

125. Brisse HJ, McCarville MB, Granata C, Krug KB, Wootton-Gorges SL, Kanegawa K, et al.; International Neuroblastoma Risk Group Project. Guidelines for imaging and staging of neuroblastic tumors: consensus report from the International Neuroblastoma Risk Group Project. Radiology. 2011;261(1):243–57.

126. Swift CC, Eklund MJ, Kraveka JM, Alazraki AL. Updates in diagnosis, management, and treatment of neuroblastoma. Radiographics. 2018;38(2):566–80.

127. Golden CB, Feusner JH. Malignant abdominal masses in children: quick guide to evaluation and diagnosis. Pediatr Clin North Am. 2002;49(6):1369–92.

Great Vessels

3

Teresa Liang, Rekha Krishnasarma, and Edward Y. Lee

Introduction

Congenital and acquired disorders of the thoracic great vessels include a broad spectrum of vascular anomalies and abnormalities. They are important causes of morbidity in the pediatric population and are associated with underlying vascular rings with respiratory and swallowing difficulties, chromosomal abnormalities, and congenital heart disease [1]. Therefore, it is essential for the radiologist to accurately recognize these thoracic vascular disorders because timely and accurate diagnosis can have important implications for prognosis and management.

Although a variety of imaging modalities have traditionally been used to evaluate thoracic great vessel disorders including chest radiograph, fluoroscopy-guided gastrointestinal studies, echocardiography, and conventional angiography, recent advances in noninvasive cross-sectional imaging studies such as multidetector computed tomography (CT) and magnetic resonance (MR) imaging have substantially enhanced evaluation of thoracic great vessel disorders in the pediatric population by taking advantage of faster acquisition times, higher spatial resolutions, and enhanced high-quality two-dimensional (2D) and three-dimensional (3D) reconstructions [2]. Due to the potentially harmful effects of ionizing radiation exposure associated with CT, MR imaging with magnetic resonance angiography (MRA) technique has become a noninvasive imaging modality of choice for a com-

plete assessment of thoracic great vessels in the pediatric population [3].

This chapter focuses on the evaluation of the congenital and acquired disorders of the thoracic great vessels in infants and children by reviewing normal anatomy including embryology and variants, up-to-date MR imaging techniques, characteristic MR imaging findings, and current management approaches.

Magnetic Resonance Imaging Techniques

MR imaging can provide anatomic detail of the thoracic great vessels in a noninvasive manner and demonstrate vessel orientation in relation to the adjacent airway and esophagus. Optimized imaging techniques are essential for achieving high-quality MR imaging studies, which are required for accurate diagnosis.

Patient Preparation

Meticulous pediatric patient preparation prior to MR imaging is crucial for the acquisition of a high-quality study. First, intravenous access for contrast administration is important to obtain first-pass MR angiography to evaluate extracardiac great vessels. For neonates, intravenous access in the arm or leg with a 22-gauge or 24-gauge needle is preferable to an umbilical venous catheter which may be associated with complications [5]. In older children, larger bore intravenous catheters such as 20-gauge or 18-gauge are typically used.

Adequate patient sedation to reduce motion artifact is imperative. Breath-holding is essential to reduce respiratory motion. However, it can require the assistance of general anesthesia if the pediatric patient is not cooperative with breath-holding instructions [6–8]. Developing a plan for sedation typically depends on patient age. For neonates, a "feed-and-wrap" technique (feeding and swaddling the child prior to being placed in the scanner) could be considered.

T. Liang (✉)
Department of Radiology, Boston Children's Hospital, Harvard Medical School, Boston, MA, USA

Department of Radiology, University of Alberta/Stollery Children's Hospital, Edmonton, AB, Canada

R. Krishnasarma
Department of Radiology, Boston Children's Hospital, Harvard Medical School, Boston, MA, USA

E. Y. Lee
Division of Thoracic Imaging, Department of Radiology, Boston Children's Hospital, Harvard Medical School, Boston, MA, USA

© Springer Nature Switzerland AG 2020
E. Y. Lee et al. (eds.), *Pediatric Body MRI*, https://doi.org/10.1007/978-3-030-31989-2_3

However, respiratory motion remains a problem when imaging the chest. Therefore, children younger than age 5 and those with cognitive delay are typically intubated and given deep sedation prior to MR imaging [9].

MR Imaging Pulse Sequences and Protocols

The main MR imaging techniques in the evaluation of thoracic great vessels include electrocardiographically (ECG)-gated black-blood imaging, bright-blood imaging, and angiographic MR imaging [5]. Table 3.1 demonstrates a suggested protocol for MR imaging of the thoracic great vessels.

Black-blood and bright-blood MR imaging sequences are both non-contrast sequences which can be employed to evaluate thoracic great vessels. Double inversion recovery imaging suppresses signal from flowing blood to create the black-blood images. By suppressing the signal from flowing blood, mural abnormalities are better defined [6]. Bright-blood imaging is performed by using a gradient refocused echo (GRE) or a balanced steady-state free precession (SSFP) sequence, both of which require relatively short acquisition times. However, they can be sensitive to field inhomogeneities that occur within the lungs and with metallic implants [5].

MRA can be obtained with or without contrast. Contrast-enhanced MRA provides excellent detail and is less prone to flow-related image artifacts than unenhanced MRA [6]. In situations that preclude the use of gadolinium, non-contrast MRA can be obtained. Due to the recent concerns regarding gadolinium deposition and with concerns of nephrogenic systemic fibrosis in patients with renal failure, non-contrast-enhanced MRA is increasingly incorporated into protocols, particularly for follow-up studies [10]. The advantage of non-contrast MR angiography is the ability to perform multiple acquisitions if the initial images prove nondiagnostic [6]. Time-of-flight MR angiography relies on the use of either 2D or 3D GRE sequences in which the constant inflow of blood into the imaging slab results in a higher signal intensity within the vessel than the surrounding soft tissues saturated by repeated radiofrequency pulses [11].

Table 3.1 Suggested pediatric thoracic great vessel MR imaging protocol

Series	Orientation	Weighting	Comments
1	Multiplanar	T2, no FS	Rapid localizer
2	Axial	T1 FSE DIR	
3	Coronal	T1 FSE DIR	
4	Axial	T1 HASTE	
5	Coronal	T2 HASTE	
6	Coronal	3D MRA	MIP and volume-rendering postprocessing

FS fat suppression, *FSE* fast spin echo, *DIR* double inversion recovery, *HASTE* half-fourier acquisition single-shot turbo spin echo, *MRA* magnetic resonance angiography, *MIP* maximum intensity projection

Anatomy

Embryology

Congenital aortic arch malformations represent a diverse spectrum of variations and anomalies arising from disordered embryogenesis of branchial arches, which result from abnormal persistence or regression of vascular segments [10]. Development of the aorta begins in utero during the 3rd week of gestation as paired dorsal and paired ventral aortic segments [12]. During the 4th and 5th gestational weeks, six paired branchial arches form, which connect the dorsal and ventral aorta as originally described by Rathke as represented in Rathke's diagram (Fig. 3.1) [10, 13, 14].

The primitive arches regress or persist in a craniocaudal fashion, to eventually form the mature aortic arch. The first and second arches regress early, with the remnant of the first arch forming maxillary arteries which contribute to the exter-

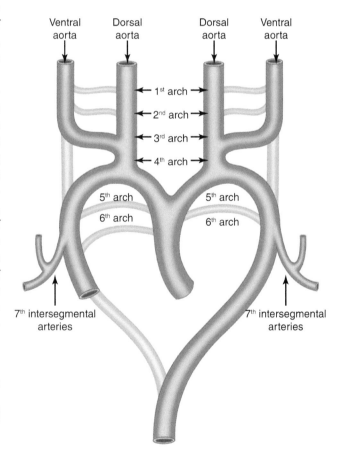

Fig. 3.1 Embryology. Rathke's diagram, a schematic representation of the development of the aortic arch and branches. The definitive aortic arch is formed from the fourth arch, while the pulmonary artery is formed from the anterior bud of the sixth arch. Parts of the third arch and anterior segments of the branchial arches contribute to the formation of left common, external, and internal carotid arteries. Areas that are shown in dark red persist, whereas those shown in pink eventually disappear

nal carotid arteries and remnants of the second arches forming the hyoid and stapedial arteries. The third arches, or the carotid arches, form the common and proximal internal carotid arteries. The fourth branchial arches contribute to the definitive mature aortic arches. The left fourth arch forms the portion of the left aortic arch between the left common carotid and left subclavian branches. The proximal right subclavian artery is formed by most of the right fourth arch. The fifth arches form rudimentary vessels that regress early. The ventral portions of the right and left sixth arches develop into the proximal right and left pulmonary arteries. The dorsal part of the right sixth arch involutes, but the dorsal part of the left sixth arch persists to form the ductus arteriosus, which connects the left pulmonary artery to the aortic arch during fetal life. After birth, the ductus arteriosus normally constricts, forming the remnant ligamentum arteriosum. On the left, the dorsal aorta persists for its entire length. On the right, the dorsal aorta involutes, except for a portion that forms the distal segment of the right subclavian artery [1, 13–17].

Most malformations of the aortic arch can be explained by Edwards' hypothetical double arch model which depicts theoretical aortic arches and ductus arteriosus on each side encircling the trachea and esophagus (Fig. 3.2). Carotid and subclavian arteries arise from their respective aortic arches. Many abnormalities of the aortic arch can be postulated by regression or persistence of segments of this hypothetical double arch system [18].

Normal Development and Anatomy

The thoracic aorta is composed of the aortic root, ascending aorta, transverse aortic arch, isthmus, and descending aorta. The normal pattern of the aorta and great vessels is a left aortic arch with a descending thoracic aorta. The three main great vessels include the brachiocephalic artery, the left common carotid artery, and the left subclavian artery (Fig. 3.3). Regression of the right dorsal aortic root (between the right subclavian artery and the descending aorta) and the right ductus arteriosus leaves the normal left aortic arch [16]. A classically configured left aortic arch and descending thoracic aorta are seen in approximately 65% of patients, and the remaining 35% of patients have anatomic variants [19–21].

Anatomic Variants

Normal variants in the anatomy of the thoracic great vessels are relatively common, asymptomatic, and typically detected incidentally by radiological examinations. When evaluating a patient for a possible congenital aortic arch or great vessel abnormality, a normal anatomic variant should be reported in order to prevent further unnecessary workup or procedures. A

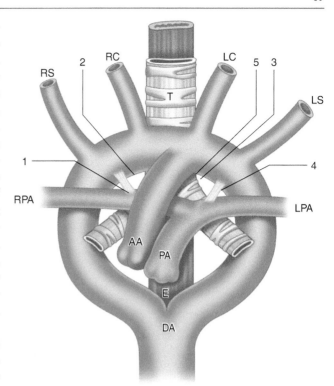

Fig. 3.2 Embryology. Edwards' hypothetical double arch model with bilateral ductus encircling the trachea and the esophagus. Breaks at 1 and 2 lead to left arch; breaks at 3 and 5 lead to right arch. A break at 1 with resorption of the right ductus results in normal anatomy. A break at 2 results in left arch with anomalous subclavian artery; typically, the right ductus resorbs and does not result in a vascular ring. A break at 4 results in right arch with mirror-image branching; the ductus courses from the innominate artery to the left pulmonary artery (not a complete ring). A break at 3 leads to right arch with aberrant subclavian artery; typically, the left ductus persists, coursing from the left subclavian to the left pulmonary artery and forming a vascular ring. A break at 5 differs in that the anomalous vessel is the innominate artery. AA ascending aorta, DA descending aorta, E esophagus, LC left carotid artery, LPA left pulmonary artery, LS left subclavian artery, PA main pulmonary artery, RC right carotid artery, RPA right pulmonary artery, RS right subclavian artery

common normal variant typically encountered on routine radiologic studies is the common origin of the brachiocephalic artery and left common carotid artery (Fig. 3.4). Another common variant which should be recognized includes origin of the left vertebral artery from the aortic arch. Both of these variants should be recognized prior to interventional and endovascular procedures such as carotid stenting or surgeries particularly in the head and neck region [20].

One of the notable exceptions of an anatomic variant that could potentially be symptomatic is the left aortic arch with aberrant right subclavian artery which can theoretically result in "dysphagia lusoria" from compression of the posterior esophagus, described later in the chapter [20]. A recent study shows that the normal three-vessel aortic arch was less common in patients with congenital heart disease [22].

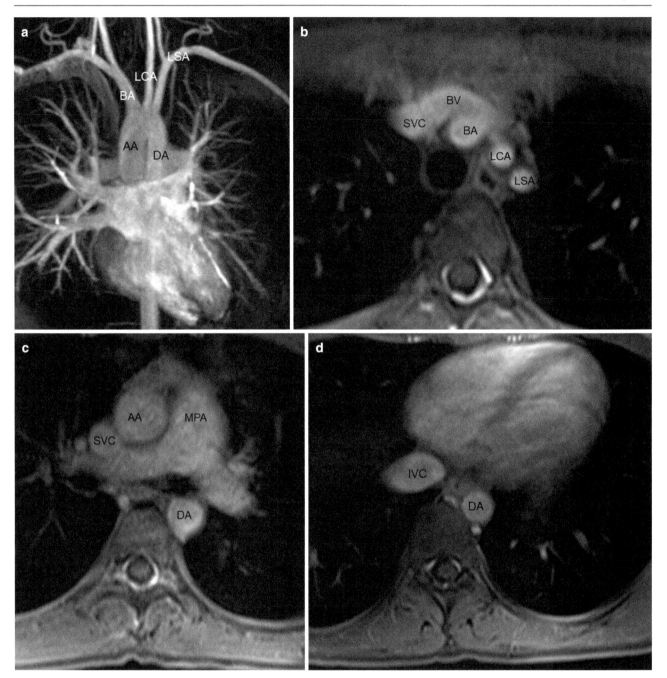

Fig. 3.3 Normal thoracic great vessel anatomy in a 16-year-old girl with recurrent hemoptysis who underwent MR imaging of the chest to evaluate for possible pulmonary arteriovenous malformations. (**a**) Coronal three-dimensional enhanced maximum intensity projection (MIP) MR image with subtraction demonstrates a normal left-sided aorta with three-vessel branching of the great vessels. AA ascending aorta, DA descending aorta, BA brachiocephalic artery, LCA left common carotid artery, LSA left subclavian artery. (**b**) Axial enhanced T1-weighted volumetric interpolated breath-hold examination (VIBE) image at the level of the great vessels demonstrates normal anatomy of the great vessels. The brachiocephalic artery (BA) is the first branch off of a left-sided aorta, the left common carotid artery (LCA) is the second branch, and the left subclavian artery (LSA) is the third branch. The brachiocephalic vein crosses anteriorly and drains into a right-sided superior vena cava (SVC). (**c**) Axial enhanced T1-weighted VIBE image at the level of the main pulmonary artery (MPA) shows normal branching of the pulmonary arteries. SVC superior vena cava, AA ascending aorta, DA descending aorta. (**d**) Axial enhanced T1-weighted VIBE image at the level of the inferior vena cava (IVC) shows that the IVC is a right-sided structure and the descending aorta (DA) is left sided

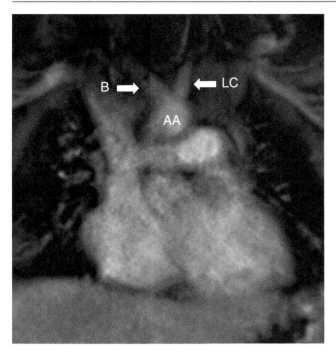

Fig. 3.4 Common origin of the brachiocephalic artery and left common carotid artery in a 2-year-old girl with anterior chest wall and mediastinal infantile hemangioma status post treatment. Coronal enhanced T1-weighted VIBE MR image at the level of the ascending aorta (AA) demonstrates common origin of the brachiocephalic artery (B) and left common carotid (LC), a normal anatomic variant

Spectrum of Great Vessel Disorders

Congenital and Developmental Great Vessel Disorders

Aortic Obstructive Lesions

Interrupted Aortic Arch Interrupted aortic arch (IAA) is a congenital great vessel anomaly in which there is total absence of a segment of the aortic arch, resulting in an interruption of luminal continuity between the ascending and descending thoracic aorta [2, 15]. Flow to the distal segment is generally supplied by a dilated patent ductus arteriosus (PDA) and is vital to maintaining survival after birth.

Among congenital cardiovascular diseases, IAA is relatively rare, comprising 1.5% of congenital mediastinal vascular anomalies [2, 23, 24]. Clinically, infants with IAA present with respiratory distress, cyanosis, or congestive heart failure during the first month of life [2, 23, 24]. A common association includes ventricular septal defect (VSD) [25]. Approximately 50% of patients with IAA exhibit chromosomal anomalies [24].

The exact embryologic etiology of IAA remains unknown. One proposed mechanism is abnormal flow during embryogenesis leading to aberrant patterns of vessel involution. Regression of the fourth arches occurs, but the site of regression varies and results in different types [14]. Three types of IAA are described based on the site of arch discontinuity (Fig. 3.5): Type A, constituting 13–42% of cases, occurs

Fig. 3.5 Interrupted aortic arch types. Type A interruption is distal to the left subclavian artery. Type B interruption is between the left common carotid artery and the left subclavian artery. Type C interruption is between the brachiocephalic trunk and the left common carotid artery. Ao aorta, PA pulmonary artery, B brachiocephalic trunk, RS right subclavian artery, RC right common carotid artery, LS left subclavian artery, LC left common carotid artery

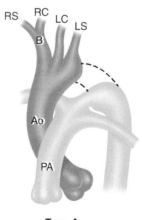

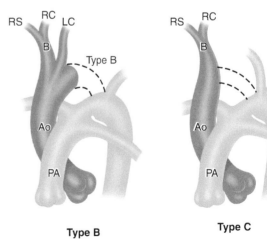

Type A   **Type B**   **Type C**

when there is interruption at the level of the distal left subclavian artery; Type B, constituting 53–84% of cases, occurs when the interruption is between the left common carotid artery and left subclavian artery and is often associated with DiGeorge syndrome (Fig. 3.6); Type C, constituting less than 5%, occurs when the interruption is between the innominate and left common carotid artery.

Cross-sectional imaging such as MRA is a valuable noninvasive imaging modality for presurgical evaluation when compared to more invasive catheter angiography. MRA has the added benefit of producing images without the need for ionizing radiation. On MRA, nonvisualization of a portion of the aortic arch can be confirmed in multiple planes, and the location, length of interruption, caliber of the thoracic aorta proximal and distal to the interruption, branching pattern, great vessel origins, patency of PDA, and presence of other cardiac abnormalities can be identified [15].

The mortality rate of patients with IAA can be as high as 90% at 1 year of age if left untreated with complications including development of a left-to-right shunt, ventricular failure, and PDA closure resulting in hypoperfusion [15]. The treatment is initially intravenous prostaglandin therapy to preserve patency of the ductus arteriosus, and this entity is definitively treated with surgical intervention in the neonatal period [14, 23, 24]. A recent study shows that as many as 40% of surviving patients eventually require reintervention on the left ventricular outflow tract by 15 years of follow-up, and echocardiography can be helpful in following these patients and identifying patients who require intervention in the future [25–27].

Aortic Stenosis Aortic stenosis is usually a congenital defect causing a fixed hemodynamically significant left ventricular outflow tract obstruction in the pediatric population [28]. Aortic stenosis encompasses multiple different pathologies depending on the location of stenosis. Valvular aortic stenosis (VAS) occurs when there is obstruction at the level of the aortic valve, often seen in the setting of a bicuspid aortic valve. Congenital stenosis of the proximal descending thoracic aorta is typical of congenital coarctation. Stenosis at the level of the thoracoabdominal aortic junction occurs in dysplastic midaortic syndrome, and stenosis of the abdominal aorta is often secondary to atherosclerosis, while iatrogenic or vasculitic processes can affect any segment of the aorta [29].

Supravalvular aortic stenosis (SVAS) is characterized by focal or diffuse narrowing at the level of the sinotubular junction (Fig. 3.7) [30]. SVAS is an elastin arteriopathy [31]. Three distinct forms of SVAS have been described, and the most common type is the "hourglass" configuration, which results in a constricting annular ridge at the superior margin of the sinuses of Valsalva [30]. Supravalvular aortic stenosis is commonly associated with Williams-Beuren syndrome, mitral valve prolapse, and pulmonary artery stenosis [32]. Affected patients typically present with angina, dyspnea, or syncope. The risk of severe endocarditis is increased in the setting of supraaortic stenosis due to altered flow mechanics [33, 34].

Cross-sectional imaging such as MR imaging is the modality of choice to demonstrate the extent of aortic stenosis prior to intervention. MR imaging can also measure the gradient across the narrowed segment. Depending on the etiology of stenosis, endovascular or surgical correction of the narrowing is often indicated. Recent studies have reported that patients with supravalvular aortic stenosis and Williams syndrome show regression of stenosis without intervention and have an overall excellent rate of survival after treatment [34, 35].

Coarctation of Aorta Aortic coarctation is a congenital condition characterized by focal constriction of the aorta near or at the level of the ductus arteriosus. The coarctation may be located proximal (preductal), at (juxtaductal), or immediately distal (postductal) to the ductus [36]. Aortic coarctations encompass 5–8% of all congenital cardiac defects [2, 37]. During development, it is proposed that this condition potentially results from abnormal migration patterns, abnormal blood flow, and/or excessive distribution of tissue around the aortic isthmus during development [36].

Aortic coarctation can be characterized based on age of presentation, which may be in infancy or adulthood. The infantile type is typically preductal, occurring at the isthmus between the left subclavian artery and the ductus. Affected infants typically present in the first 6 months of life as the ductus closes at 2 weeks. The clinical presentation can include hypoperfusion to the lower body, renal dysfunction, and acidosis. Bicuspid aortic valve is the most commonly associated congenital anomaly. Other associated anomalies include hypoplasia of the aortic arch

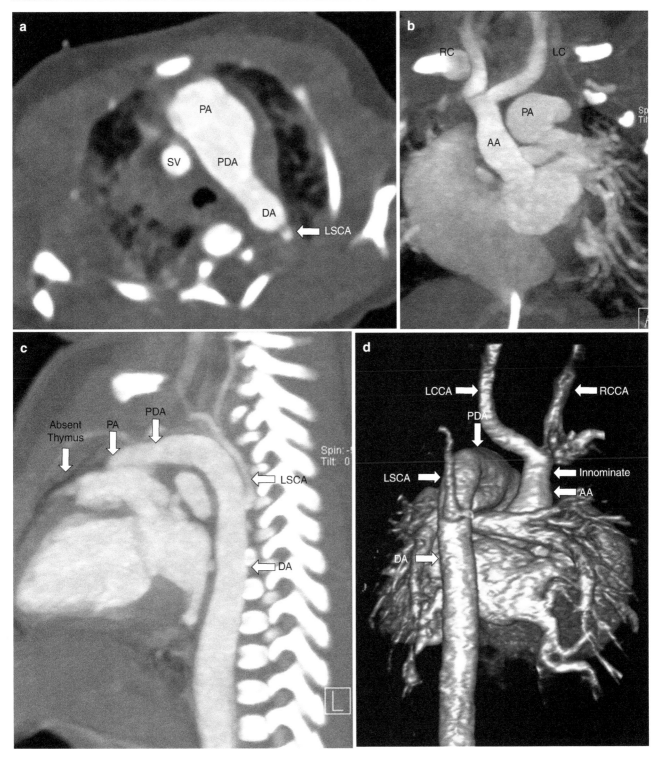

Fig. 3.6 Interrupted aortic arch in a 2-day-old full-term girl with prenatal diagnosis of a Type B interrupted aortic arch and intrauterine growth restriction (IUGR). (**a**) Axial enhanced soft tissue window setting computed tomography (CT) image shows a descending aorta (DA) with left subclavian artery (LSCA) origin (*arrow*) and a patent ductus arteriosus (PDA) between the pulmonary artery (PA) and DA. SV superior vena cava. (**b**) Coronal enhanced maximum intensity projection (MIP) soft tissue window setting CT image shows the ascending aorta (AA) giving off the innominate artery from which the right common carotid (RC) and left (LC) common carotid arteries originate. (**c**) Sagittal enhanced maximum intensity projection (MIP) soft tissue win-

dow setting CT image shows the descending aorta (DA) which gives off the left subclavian artery (LSCA). This projection also highlights the absence of the thymus, in keeping with known DiGeorge syndrome, which is commonly associated with a Type B interrupted aortic arch. PA pulmonary artery, PDA patent ductus arteriosus. (**d**) Three-dimensional CT reconstruction of the thoracic vasculature shows the right common carotid artery (RCCA) and left common carotid artery (LCCA) arising from the ascending aorta (AA). There is no communication between the AA and the descending aorta (DA). The patent ductus arteriosus (PDA) is seen in continuity with the descending aorta (DA). The left subclavian artery (LSCA) arises from the DA

(Fig. 3.8), hypoplasia of the descending aorta, and congenital heart disease such as a patent ductus arteriosus, ventricular septal defect, hypoplastic left heart, or ostial stenosis of the aortic branches. Other associated congenital or acquired diseases include Williams syndrome, Turner syndrome, giant cell arteritis, neurofibromatosis, and fibromuscular dysplasia [36]. Aortic coarctation in adults is typically juxtaductal or postductal, and affected

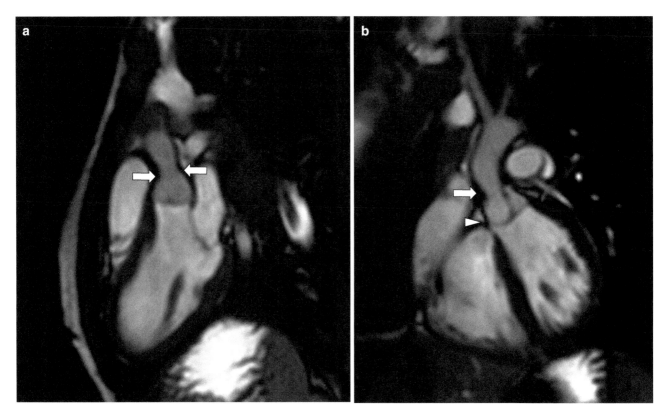

Fig. 3.7 Aortic stenosis in a 7-year-old boy with Williams syndrome and supravalvular aortic stenosis. Sagittal non-enhanced oblique balanced turbo field echo (BTFE) and coronal oblique BTFE MR images of the left ventricular outflow tract (**a, b**) show moderate supravalvular aortic stenosis with thickening of the aortic wall (*arrows*), superior to the aortic valve (*arrowhead*)

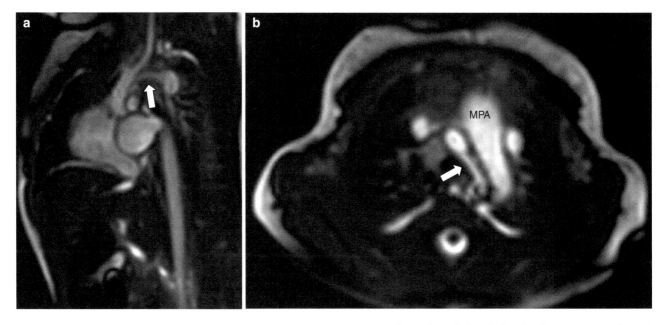

Fig. 3.8 Hypoplasia of the aortic arch in a 4-day-old girl who presented with heart failure. (**a**) Sagittal non-enhanced steady-state free precession (SSFP) and (**b**) Axial non-enhanced SSFP MR images demonstrate moderate hypoplasia of the distal transverse aortic arch (*arrows*). MPA main pulmonary artery

patients typically present later in life with arterial hypertension in the upper extremities relative to the lower extremities [2, 36].

Chest radiographs may be normal in cases of mild aortic coarctation. In more severe long-standing aortic coarctation, characteristic "figure 3" sign may be seen on chest radiograph due to enlargement of the left subclavian artery as well as pre- and post-stenotic dilatation of the descending aorta. Also seen in more prolonged courses is notching of the ribs secondary to collateral formation through the intercostal arteries, usually involving the posterior fourth to eighth ribs. Echocardiography can measure the gradient across the coarctation and demonstrate concurrent congenital heart disease. However, it is suboptimal for identifying collateral circulation, and interrupted aortic arch can mimic coarctation on echocardiogram. In current practice, catheter angiography is reserved for treatment rather than diagnosis given its invasive nature, although it can identify the pressure gradient across the coarctation and assess collateral vessels [15, 38].

Cross-sectional imaging study such as MR imaging with MRA technique with 2D and 3D volume-rendered reconstructions is a valuable noninvasive imaging modality in the diagnosis and evaluation of an aortic coarctation prior to intervention. MRA can identify the narrowed segment of the aorta (Fig. 3.9). Postoperative complications such as recurrent stenosis and aortic injury after surgical resection can also be evaluated with MRA [38].

Surgical repair with resection of the aortic coarctation with end-to-end anastomosis and subclavian flap angioplasty is the definitive management. Endovascular treatment with balloon dilation and stenting is an alternative [36, 37]. The recoarctation rate is approximately 11.5%, and a recent study shows that age of less than 15 days at repair was associated with a risk of reintervention [39].

Aortic Arch Positional Anomaly

Cervical Aortic Arch Cervical aortic arch describes an aortic arch which is unusually located high, at, or above the thoracic inlet. This vascular anomaly occurs most frequently in association with a right aortic arch, and the branching pattern is highly variable. The exact embryologic etiology is unclear, although this type of aortic arch anomaly is thought to result from persistence of the third aortic arch, rather than normal persistence of the fourth aortic arch [1, 16].

Affected patients with a cervical aortic arch are often asymptomatic [40], although symptoms can include stridor, frequent respiratory tract symptoms, and dyspnea [41]. Aneurysm formation is reported in 20% of cervical aortic arch cases due to the hemodynamic alterations resulting from kinking of the aortic arch [41, 42]. When cervical aortic arch is complicated by aneurysm formation, affected patients present with a pulsatile mass in the neck and dyspnea [41, 42].

Chest radiograph may demonstrate a superior mediastinal mass and slight deviation of the trachea to the opposite side of the aortic arch on the frontal projection. Anterior deviation of the trachea may be seen on the lateral projection [41]. Posterior indentation on the contrast-filled esophagus on the lateral projection of an esophagram may be evident [40]. MR imaging is excellent at demonstrating the high positioning of the aortic arch and other associated vascular abnormalities (Fig. 3.10).

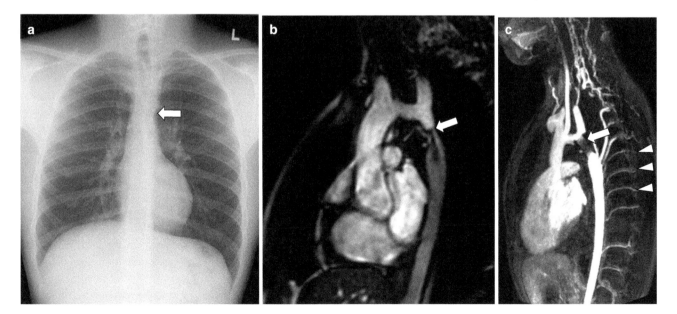

Fig. 3.9 Coarctation of the aorta in a 16-year-old boy who presented with poor exercise tolerance. (**a**) Frontal chest radiograph demonstrates an inward indentation at the level of the descending thoracic aorta, consistent with a "Figure 3" appearance (*arrow*). (**b**) Sagittal MR angiogram balanced turbo field echo image without contrast shows focal constriction (*arrow*) of the aortic arch at the level of the ductus arteriosus. (**c**) Sagittal follow-up enhanced MR angiogram maximum intensity projection (MIP) image shows improved caliber of the aorta (*arrow*) following balloon dilation and stent placement. Multiple dilated intercostal collaterals are also noted (*arrowheads*)

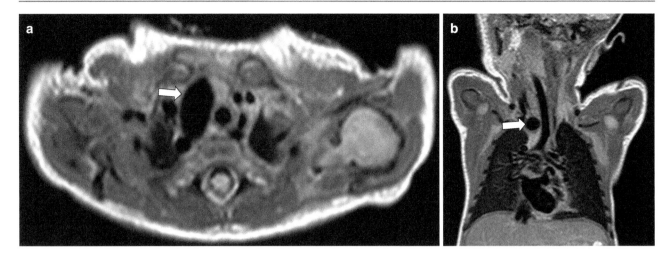

Fig. 3.10 Cervical aortic arch in a 4-day-old boy with DiGeorge syndrome, cervical right aortic arch, and Tetralogy of Fallot. (**a**) Axial non-enhanced proton density MR image and (**b**) coronal non-enhanced proton density MR image demonstrate a cervical right aortic arch (*arrows*) which is characterized by an elongated high-lying aortic arch which is at the level of the clavicles

Patients with a cervical aortic arch tend to have a benign course as the abnormality does not result in compressive symptoms, and the majority of patients do not require surgery [10, 40]. If a cervical aortic arch is complicated by aneurysm formation, endovascular repair is the primary treatment of choice [41].

Aortic Branching Anomalies

Double Aortic Arch Double aortic arch is the most common cause of vascular tracheoesophageal narrowing in symptomatic pediatric patients [2]. This type of vascular ring occurs when there is lack of regression of the ventral and dorsal aortic arches resulting in both right and left aortic arches. These right and left aortic arches arise from a single ascending aorta and encircle the trachea and esophagus. Usually one of the sixth arches persists as a ductus arteriosus or ligamentum arteriosum, most commonly on the left [1]. The double aortic arch is the most common vascular ring, and the right arch is typically dominant and more superior to the smaller left arch. Pediatric patients with a double aortic arch typically present with respiratory and gastrointestinal symptoms such as stridor, cough, wheezing, and dysphagia in the first year of life [2, 43, 44].

Imaging evaluation of clinically suspected double aortic arch initially begins with a chest radiograph, which may show a right-sided aortic arch. Fluoroscopic esophagram characteristically demonstrates lateral impression with caliber change of the esophagus at the level of the aortic arch on the frontal projection and posterior impression on the lateral projection. MRA and CTA have become the primary imaging modalities for diagnosis and presurgical planning for a double aortic arch, largely replacing catheter angiography mainly due to the noninvasive acquisition of multiplanar reformats and three-dimensional vessel imaging. MRA is often preferred over CTA due to the lack of ionizing radiation exposure.

Distinguishing an incomplete double aortic arch with distal left arch atresia from a right aortic arch with mirror-image branching can be challenging to reliably visualize on cross-sectional imaging, although the distinction is important, as a double aortic arch forms a complete vascular ring [45]. A double aortic arch demonstrates a characteristic configuration of the great vessel takeoff on cross-sectional imaging with the common carotid and subclavian arteries arising from the respective ipsilateral aortic arch, termed the "four-vessel" sign (Fig. 3.11) [46]. Multiplanar and 3D reformats also aid in deciding the surgical approach by identifying the laterality of the atretic aortic arch, which is ultimately resected to relieve compression on the trachea and esophagus. A recent study demonstrates the prevalence of tracheomalacia in patients with a double aortic arch to be 1 in 5 (20%), and, given the chronic tracheal compression and high prevalence of tracheomalacia, dynamic airway CT has been found to be useful in determining the presence and severity of tracheomalacia preoperatively or postoperatively [47, 48]. With advances in spirometer-guided MR imaging in children, tracheomalacia in pediatric patients with mediastinal vascular anomalies can also be accurately diagnosed with MR imaging [37, 49].

Definitive management for a double aortic arch includes surgical repair with video-assisted thoracoscopic surgery (VATS) division and ligation of the more atretic aortic arch to relieve the vascular ring's compression upon the trachea and esophagus, leaving the dominant aortic arch in place. VATS has been shown to be safe and effective, with a recent study demonstrating all patients following

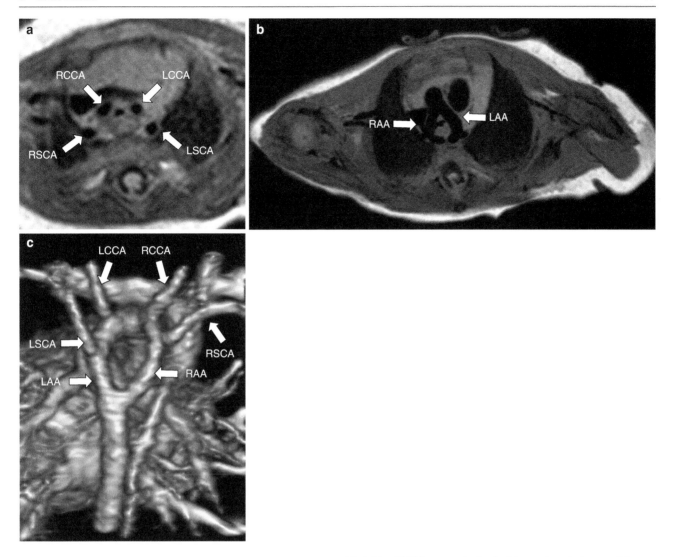

Fig. 3.11 Double aortic arch in a 37-day-old girl who presented with respiratory distress and feeding difficulty. (**a**) Axial non-enhanced proton density black-blood MR image at the level of the great vessels shows the "four-vessel" sign (RCCA right common carotid artery, RSCA right subclavian artery, LCCA left common carotid artery, LSCA left subclavian artery). (**b**) Axial non-enhanced proton density black-blood MR image at the level of the aortic arch shows a right aortic arch (RAA) and a left aortic arch (LAA) which encircle the trachea and the collapsed esophagus. (**c**) Three-dimensional reconstruction of the vascular structures from MRA in a posterior projection view demonstrates the double aortic arch with symmetric take-off of the great vessels

double aortic arch repair improved clinically at follow-up, although further studies with a larger sample of patients are required [50].

Circumflex Aortic Arch Circumflex aortic arch occurs when a portion of the arch crosses midline in a retroesophageal course above the level of the carina to the contralateral side [13, 15, 51, 52]. A circumflex aortic arch can be right or left sided. Embryologically, the circumflex aortic arch develops as the result of preservation of the proximal fourth arch [52]. In addition, it occurs when there is persistence of a segment of the contralateral sixth arch to form the ductus arteriosus and the distal portion of the right fourth arch to form the dorsal arch [52].

The ductus arteriosus extends from the descending aorta to the ipsilateral pulmonary artery, forming a complete vascular ring in patients with circumflex aortic arch [13, 53–56]. The aortic branching can be either mirror image or an aberrant right subclavian [54]. Affected pediatric patients typically present with respiratory or gastrointestinal symptoms similar to other types of vascular rings secondary to the retroesophageal compression from the transverse aortic arch. This type of vascular ring has been found to be associated with various other cardiac anomalies such as absent left pulmonary artery, ventricular septal defect, tetralogy of Fallot, and transposition of the great vessels [53, 57].

Chest radiographs may demonstrate a right aortic arch on the frontal projection and a superior mediastinal density displacing the trachea anteriorly on the lateral projection [55, 56]. Barium esophagram can demonstrate a posterior impression on the contrast-filled esophagus. Cross-sectional imaging is the best modality to evaluate a circumflex aortic arch in order to depict a transverse aortic arch crossing the midline posteriorly to descend on the contralateral side, the abnormal branching pattern, and tracheal compression (Fig. 3.12) [54].

Surgery is the definitive treatment for circumflex aortic arch. The circumflex aorta is treated with the aortic uncrossing operation, where the retroesophageal arch is mobilized anterior to the airway and anastomosed with the lateral portion of the descending aorta to relieve the posterior compression [13, 48, 58].

Right Aortic Arch—*Right Aortic Arch with Aberrant Left Subclavian Artery* Right aortic arch with an aberrant left subclavian artery consists of an aberrant origin of the left

subclavian artery with a retroesophageal course. This is the second most common type of symptomatic vascular ring after the double aortic arch in the pediatric population. Embryologically, the right aortic arch results from abnormal development of the fourth brachial arch, while the right dorsal aortic arch persists and the distal left aorta regresses [2]. The aberrant left subclavian artery arises from a Kommerell diverticulum, which is the embryonic origin of the left aberrant subclavian artery off the patent ductus arteriosus. A diverticulum of Kommerell is important to recognize on imaging because it is typically associated with the presence of an ipsilateral ligamentum arteriosum which is not visible with imaging techniques. Such ligamentum arteriosum connects the pulmonary artery to the aortic diverticulum, constituting a vascular ring [15, 44]. Affected pediatric patients present similarly to double aortic arch with respiratory distress and feeding difficulties [58].

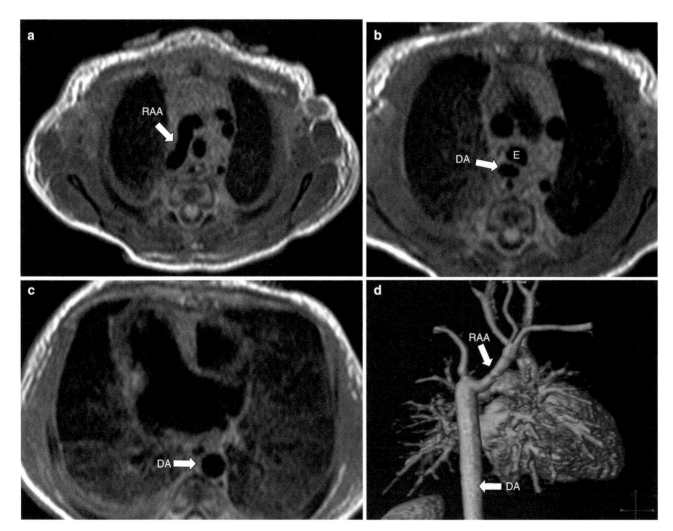

Fig. 3.12 Circumflex aortic arch in a 7-day-old girl with dextrocardia and right aortic arch found to have a circumflex right aortic arch. (**a–c**) Axial non-enhanced proton density black-blood MR images demonstrate a right-sided aortic arch (RAA) coursing horizontally from right to left, with the descending aorta (DA) compressing the esophagus (E) as it

passes posteriorly. The DA courses to the left of midline, the typical position of the descending thoracic aorta. (**d**) Three-dimensional reconstruction of the vascular structures from MRA in an oblique projection view demonstrates a right-sided aortic arch (RAA) coursing horizontally and the descending thoracic aorta (DA) coursing to the left of midline

On chest radiographs, a right-sided aortic arch with anterior tracheal bowing due to the posteriorly located aberrant retroesophageal vessel is observed. At fluoroscopy, a posterior indentation on the esophagus is identified and is indistinguishable from a double aortic arch. Definitive diagnosis is made by MRA which depicts a right-sided aortic arch with retroesophageal aberrant left subclavian artery arising from a diverticulum of Kommerell (Fig. 3.13). Dynamic airway imaging is helpful to evaluate for concomitant tracheomalacia at the level of the vascular ring [47].

Management involves surgical ligation of the vascular ring. The prognosis is generally excellent after division of the vascular ring, although symptoms may persist from tracheomalacia after repair [48].

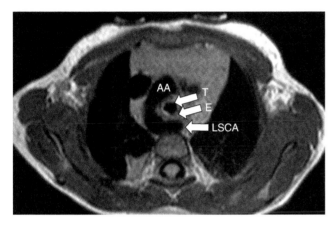

Fig. 3.13 Right aortic arch with aberrant left subclavian artery in a 16-month-old girl with velocardiofacial syndrome. Axial non-enhanced proton density black-blood turbo spin-echo MR image shows a right-sided aortic arch (AA) with a retroesophageal course of the left subclavian artery (LSCA). T trachea, E esophagus

Right Aortic Arch—*Right Aortic Arch with Mirror-Image Branching* Right aortic arch with mirror-image branching occurs if the left fourth arch regresses distal to the right subclavian artery in utero [1]. The first major vessel arising from the aortic arch is the left brachiocephalic trunk, followed by a right common carotid artery and then the right subclavian artery. This condition is not a vascular ring, since there is no connection to the ductus. Therefore, affected pediatric patients do not suffer from tracheoesophageal compression. However, it is still important for the radiologist to recognize a right aortic arch with mirror-image branching in the pediatric population because it is highly associated with congenital heart disease, which occurs in greater than 90% of cases. Tetralogy of Fallot and truncus arteriosus are the two most commonly associated congenital heart diseases. Right aortic arch with mirror-image branching is diagnosed in neonates or children as associated congenital heart disease presents in the prenatal or early postnatal period [2, 13, 17, 59]. Recent studies have also shown an association with 22q11.2 deletion and suggest that prenatal testing for karyotypes and 22q11.2 should be considered in the setting of prenatally diagnosed right aortic arch [60].

Frontal chest radiograph can demonstrate a rounded opacity in the right upper paratracheal region, potentially with leftward deviation of the trachea [17, 59]. Cross-sectional imaging studies such as contrast-enhanced MDCT and MR imaging with MRA are the best modalities to evaluate this condition, as a right aortic arch can be identified, the branching pattern can be determined, and associated congenital heart defects can be characterized (Fig. 3.14) [17, 59].

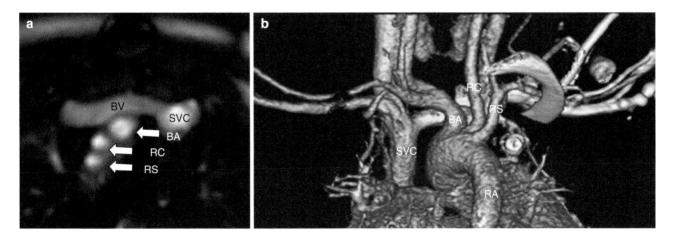

Fig. 3.14 Right aortic arch with mirror-image branching in a 12-month-old girl with tetralogy of Fallot. (**a**) Axial non-enhanced balanced turbo field echo MR image shows a right-sided aortic arch with mirror-image branching, with the left brachiocephalic artery (BA) as the first major branch, right common carotid artery (RC) as the second major branch, and right subclavian artery as the third major branch (RS). A brachiocephalic vein (BV) is seen draining in to a left-sided superior vena cava (SVC). (**b**) Posterior projection of three-dimensional reconstruction of the vascular structures from MRA shows the right-sided aortic arch (RA) and its branches: left brachiocephalic artery (BA), right common carotid artery (RC), and right subclavian artery (RS). SVC superior vena cava

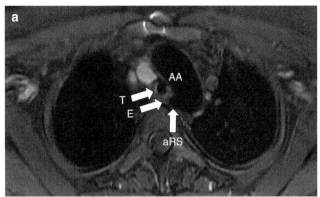
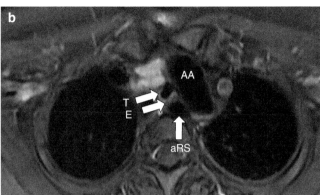
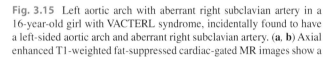

Fig. 3.15 Left aortic arch with aberrant right subclavian artery in a 16-year-old girl with VACTERL syndrome, incidentally found to have a left-sided aortic arch and aberrant right subclavian artery. (**a, b**) Axial enhanced T1-weighted fat-suppressed cardiac-gated MR images show a left-sided aortic arch (AA) giving rise to an aberrant right subclavian artery (aRS) that courses to the right, posterior to the esophagus (E) and trachea (T)

As mirror branching does not result in compressive symptoms, management of a right aortic arch with mirror-image branching focuses on identification and treatment of the associated cardiac disease.

Left Aortic Arch with Aberrant Right Subclavian Artery
A left aortic arch with aberrant right subclavian artery is generally an incidental finding and is the most common congenital aortic arch anomaly [2, 6, 13, 61, 62]. This condition arises from involution of a segment of the embryonic right fourth aortic arch between the right subclavian and right common carotid arteries [2]. The right ductus arteriosus typically regresses, and a true vascular ring does not form [61, 62]. If a right ligamentum arteriosum persists, the true vascular ring leads to subtle airway compression, and affected patients may have symptoms which are generally mild [2, 62]. The retroesophageal right subclavian can result in symptoms related to extrinsic compression on the esophagus, even in the absence of vascular ring, referred to as "dysphagia lusoria" [6, 13, 62, 63].

Barium esophagram may show oblique indentation on the posterior esophagus. MR imaging with MRA technique and 2D/3D reconstructed images can confirm the finding and can better delineate the anatomy. The branching order of the great vessels is the right common carotid artery, left common carotid artery, left subclavian artery, and aberrant right subclavian artery (Fig. 3.15) [2, 13].

A left aortic arch with aberrant right subclavian artery typically does not result in symptomatic airway or esophageal compression [61–63]. Therefore, no further management is needed once the diagnosis is made in asymptomatic pediatric patients.

Systemic Venous Anomalies

Persistent Left and Duplicated Superior Vena Cava During fetal development, the paired cardinal veins initially drain the body of the embryo, but as the fetus develops, the right cardinal vein persists to become the future right-sided superior vena cava (SVC), whereas the left cardinal vein mostly regresses with small portions forming left superior intercostal and brachiocephalic veins [15, 64]. Persistence of the left anterior cardinal vein can result in a persistent left superior vena cava (PLSVC), which is the most common congenital thoracic venous anomaly. PLSVC has an estimated prevalence of 0.3–0.5% in the general population but has an appreciably greater prevalence, estimated up to 10%, in congenital cardiac anomaly patients [15, 64–66].

The PLSVC classically drains into a dilated coronary sinus of the right atrium. However, in up to 8% of patients, the PLSVC can abnormally communicate with the left atrium, creating a small right-to-left shunt [15, 64, 67, 68]. In the setting of PLSVC, 70–90% of affected individuals have a right superior vena cava (RSVC) and a variable presence of a bridging vein communicating between the two SVCs [15, 64–66]. When both a right and left SVC are present, the anomaly is termed "mirror image" or "duplicated SVC" [15]. The RSVC may be normal, slightly smaller than the left, or absent [15, 59, 69].

Pediatric patients with PLSVC and duplicated SVC are usually asymptomatic and thus are often identified incidentally during catheter insertion or chest imaging performed for other reasons (Fig. 3.16) [15, 64]. Rarely, systemic embolization may occur, and affected pediatric patients may present with symptoms of stroke or brain abscesses [64]. Although no treatment is required, identification and descrip-

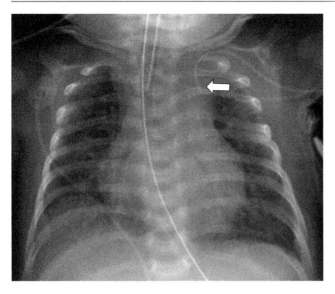

Fig. 3.16 Persistent superior vena cava in a 47-day old girl with aortic coarctation status post left arm peripherally inserted central venous catheter (PICC) placement. Frontal supine chest radiograph demonstrates the left upper extremity PICC tip (*arrow*) projecting over the upper persistent left-sided superior vena cava. Additional findings include an endotracheal tube in the mid thoracic trachea, bilateral low lung volumes with mild elevation of the right hemidiaphragm, and mild pulmonary vascular congestion

tion of its course can be valuable prior to placement of venous catheters, defibrillators, and pacemakers and for pre-operative planning [15, 69].

On frontal chest radiographs in duplicated SVC patients, there is non-specific mediastinal widening, with the presence of normal right paratracheal soft tissue opacity from the right SVC, and the PLSVC is often identified as the straight soft tissue interface in the left paratracheal region, lateral to the aortic arch (see Fig. 3.16). CT and MR imaging can confirm the presence of a PLSVC as a tubular structure originating from the junction of the left internal jugular and subclavian veins, coursing vertically to the left of the mediastinum and classically draining into the right atrium via a dilated coronary sinus (Fig. 3.17) [15, 64, 69]. While right-sided cardiac problems may result in the presence of a dilated coronary sinus, when identified, a dilated coronary sinus should raise suspicion for a PLSVC [64]. CT and MR imaging can confirm a duplicated SVC and also identify any causes of an abnormally dilated SVC [15, 59].

Single Left Superior Vena Cava Draining to Coronary Sinus An isolated PLSVC with the absence of a right SVC can rarely occur, with estimated incidences of 0.07–0.13% in patients with cardiovascular anomalies [70–73]. The incidence of cardiac anomalies is evidently increased, with estimates of up to half of patients, and the most com-

mon cardiac pathologies including atrial and ventricular septal defects (ASD and VSD), Tetralogy of Fallot, Eisenmenger syndrome, cor triatriatum, aortic coarctation, mitral atresia, and dextrocardia [15, 64, 70, 74]. Although PLSVC with absent right SVC has been frequently reported to occur in situs inversus patients (Fig. 3.18), recent studies have demonstrated many cases of the isolated PLSVC to occur in the absence of dextrocardia or heterotaxy syndrome [70, 75].

Similar to the above described pediatric patients with PLSVC/duplicated SVC, in the absence of congenital heart disease, the variation of systemic venous drainage is usually asymptomatic and often discovered incidentally [76].

Imaging findings are similar to the duplicated SVC patients; however, only a single PLSVC and no right SVC is identified. Given the increased incidence with cardiovascular anomalies, CT and MR imaging can be highly useful to identify any associated anomalies and variant anatomy (see Fig. 3.18).

Pulmonary Arterial Anomalies

Pulmonary Artery Agenesis, Aplasia, and Hypoplasia Abnormal blood flow in the dorsal aortic arch during fetal development has been postulated as the underlying pathophysiology yielding the spectrum of pulmonary agenesis, aplasia, and hypoplasia [15, 77]. The most commonly used classification proposed by Schneider and Schwalbe in 1912 [78] groups the spectrum into three categories: pulmonary agenesis corresponding to the complete absence of lung, bronchus, and vascular supply; pulmonary aplasia with absent lung and pulmonary artery but a rudimentary bronchus; and pulmonary hypoplasia with hypoplastic lung and a rudimentary bronchial tree [15, 78–80].

The clinical presentations of these pediatric patients vary, ranging from infants with respiratory distress and feeding difficulties to children with recurrent infections to asymptomatic adults [15, 77]. Morbidity and mortality are usually related to the severity of the associated cardiac, respiratory, skeletal, gastrointestinal, and genitourinary anomalies, estimated to coexist in 50–70% [79–83]. Treatment is typically symptom management, with potential surgical management for the associated anomalies [83].

Pulmonary agenesis, the most severe form, can be unilateral or bilateral, which is fatal [79, 80]. Although more common on the left [81], when it occurs on the right, there is a poorer associated prognosis with the increased mediastinal shift and distortion of the great vessels and airway [80, 81].

On radiographs, pediatric patients with pulmonary agenesis demonstrate a diffusely opacified affected hemithorax with ipsilateral mediastinal shift and compensatory hyperin-

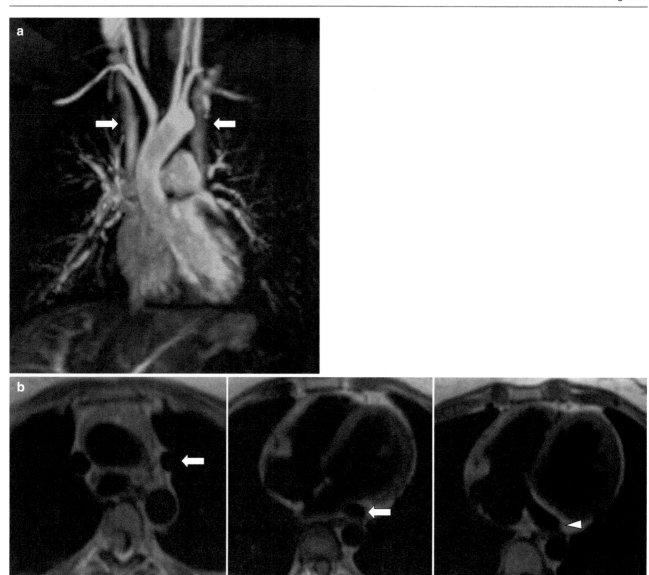

Fig. 3.17 Duplicated superior vena cava (SVC) in a 13-year-old girl who presented for further evaluation with MR imaging. (a) Coronal enhanced MR angiogram image demonstrates the duplicated SVC (*arrows*) with no bridging vein identified. (b) Axial double inversion recovery MR images demonstrate a persistent left SVC (*arrows*) draining into a dilated coronary sinus (*arrowhead*) with no bridging vein identified

flation of the contralateral lung (Fig. 3.19a) [77, 82, 83]. Cross-sectional imaging with CT or MR imaging is recommended to confirm diagnosis and identify the associated abnormalities of the involved pulmonary artery, bronchus, and lung parenchyma (Fig. 3.19b).

Depending on when the insult occurred during fetal lung development and the presence of the associated anomalies, the severity of pulmonary aplasia can vary [15, 82, 83]. On chest radiographs, the findings of pulmonary aplasia are nearly identical to the findings in pulmonary agenesis, with the involved hemithorax opacification, ipsilateral mediastinal shift, and hyperinflation of the contralateral lung [77, 82, 83]. CT or MR imaging can confirm the absence of the involved pulmonary artery and lung tissue and confirm the presence of a rudimentary bronchus arising from the carina and terminating in a blind pouch [15, 82, 83].

Congenital lung hypoplasia can occur from a primary abnormality of embryologic development or, more commonly, secondarily from compression on the developing lung and hemithorax [15]. Lung compression may result from a variety of causes including intrathoracic space-occupying lesions (such as congenital pulmonary airway malformation (CPAM), pulmonary sequestration, or congenital diaphragmatic hernias), external compression secondarily from oligohydramnios, chest wall malformations, neuromuscular or chromosomal disorders with restricted or decreased fetal breathing movements, and decreased pulmonary vascular perfusion from associated congenital cardiovascular disease [15].

Similar to its more severe counterparts, pulmonary hypoplasia shows opacification or diminished volume of the involved lung, ipsilateral mediastinal shift, and compensatory hyperinflation of the contralateral lung [77, 82, 83], and

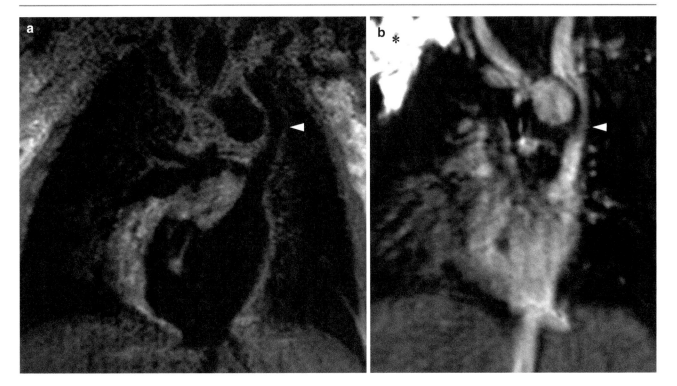

Fig. 3.18 Persistent left superior vena cava (SVC) in a 3-month-old boy with heterotaxy syndrome, right dominant atrioventricular canal, single right ventricle, pulmonary atresia, and status post right Blalock-Taussig shunt. (**a**) Coronal double inversion recovery MR image demonstrates a persistent left superior vena cava (SVC) (*arrowhead*) draining into the left common atrium. (**b**) Coronal enhanced MR angiogram image shows a persistent left SVC (*arrowhead*) draining into the left common atrium, with extravasation (*asterisk*) of contrast in the right axilla

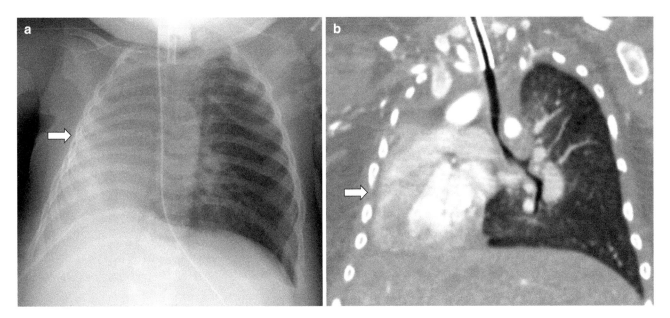

Fig. 3.19 Right pulmonary agenesis in a 58-day-old girl who presented with shortness of breath. (**a**) Frontal supine chest radiograph shows a tracheostomy in situ, with tip in proximal thoracic trachea, and diffuse opacification of the right hemithorax with ipsilateral mediastinal shift (*arrow*). (**b**) Coronal enhanced lung window setting CT image shows absence of the right pulmonary artery, right main bronchus, and right lung in keeping with right pulmonary agenesis (*arrow*)

an underlying cause such as a mass, hernia, pleural or chest wall, or diaphragmatic abnormalities may be identified (Fig. 3.20a). Although MR imaging/MRA can readily identify the pulmonary arterial and associated anomalies (Fig. 3.20b), MDCT remains superior for assessment of the bronchial tree and lung parenchyma [83].

Interruption of Proximal Pulmonary Artery / Pulmonary Artery Agenesis Proximal interruption or absence of the pulmonary artery is a rare entity estimated to occur in 1 out of 200,000 individuals, characterized by the abnormal termination of the pulmonary artery at the level of the lung hilum [15, 84–86]. This entity is thought to occur due to the failure

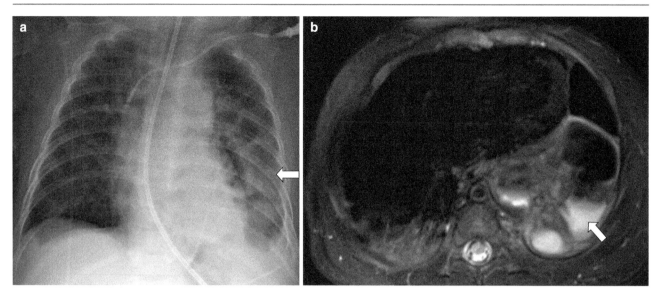

Fig. 3.20 Left pulmonary hypoplasia and left congenital diaphragmatic hernia in a 2-month-old boy who presented with shortness of breath. (**a**) Frontal supine chest radiograph shows loops of bowel (*arrow*) in the left lower hemithorax in keeping with a left-sided congenital diaphragmatic hernia and left pulmonary hypoplasia. The left

upper extremity peripherally inserted central venous catheter tip projects over the mid superior vena cava, and enteric tube tip is external to the field of view. (**b**) Axial non-enhanced T2-weighted fat-suppressed MR image demonstrates bool loops (*arrow*) herniating into the left hemithorax and left pulmonary hypoplasia

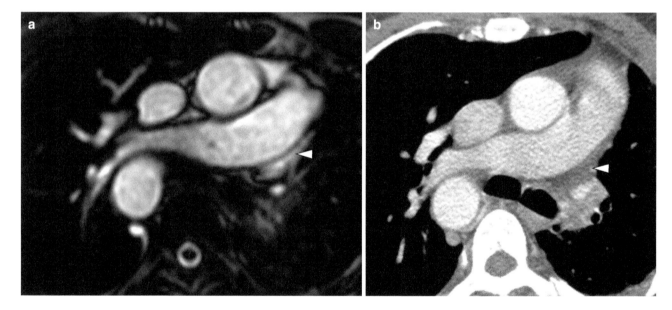

Fig. 3.21 Absent left pulmonary artery in a 54-day-old girl with tetralogy of Fallot and a right-sided aortic arch. (**a**) Axial non-enhanced T2-weighted MR image demonstrates the right-sided aortic arch and an absent left pulmonary artery (*arrowhead*). (**b**) Axial enhanced soft tissue window setting CT image shows the right-sided aortic arch and absent left pulmonary artery (*arrowhead*)

of formation of the sixth aortic arch and more commonly affects the right pulmonary artery [15, 84–86]. When it involves the left pulmonary artery, there is an association with a right-sided aortic arch and other cardiovascular anomalies including tetralogy of Fallot (Fig. 3.21) [86]. Since the embryologic origins of the hilar and distal pulmonary arteries are separate, they continue to form normally in these pediatric patients [84–86]. The affected lung receives diminished flow supplied by collaterals through the bronchial and intercostal arteries and enlargement of the contralateral pul-

monary vessels, resulting in ipsilateral pulmonary hypoplasia [84–86].

Although affected pediatric patients may remain asymptomatic, common presentations include recurrent infections, dyspnea, and pulmonary hypertension [85], and approximately 10% of affected patients present with pulmonary hemorrhage from rupture of hypertrophied collateral arteries [86]. Early treatment with surgical anastomosis or grafting of the involved pulmonary artery may improve lung and pulmonary arterial growth, whereas later presentation with

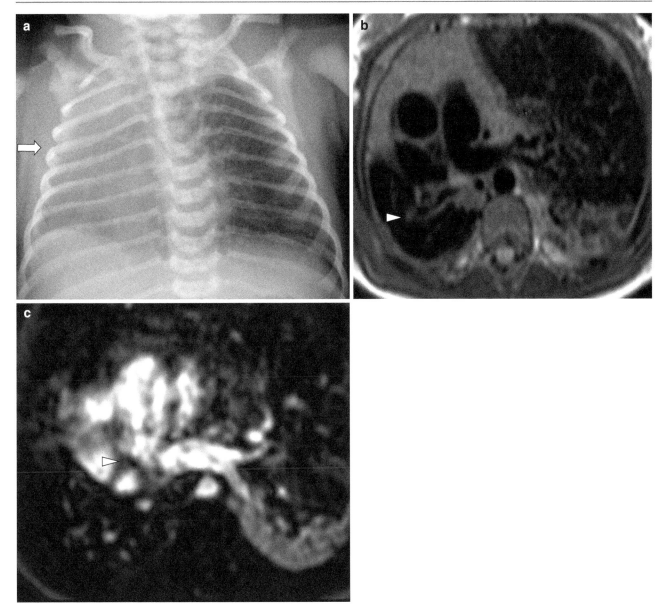

Fig. 3.22 Absent right pulmonary artery in a 59-day-old girl with complex congenital heart disease including atrial septal defect, muscular ventricular septal defect, and mildly hypoplastic tricuspid valve who presented for MR imaging for further evaluation. (**a**) Frontal supine chest radiograph shows diffuse opacification in the right hemithorax with ipsilateral midline shift (*arrow*). (**b**) Axial non-enhanced double inversion recovery MR image demonstrates an absent right pulmonary artery, hypoplastic right lung with multiple bilateral collaterals (*arrowhead*). (**c**) Axial enhanced MR angiogram image shows an absent right pulmonary artery (*arrowhead*), with multiple bilateral collaterals and hypoplastic right lung

hemoptysis or pulmonary hypertension may require embolization of collaterals [84].

On chest radiographs, affected pediatric patients have varying appearances of pulmonary hypoplasia, depending on its severity, with ipsilateral mediastinal shift and compensatory hyperinflation of the contralateral lung, a small or absent hilum, and no identifiable pulmonary artery (Fig. 3.22a) [84–86]. Findings of dilated collaterals such as rib notching and subpleural reticular opacities may also be present [15, 86]. On CT or MR imaging/MRA, the absent or interrupted pulmonary artery within 1 cm of its origin, the presence of ipsilateral pulmonary hypoplasia and multiple collateral vessels can be identified (Fig. 3.22b, c) [86]. MR imaging/MRA has the additional benefit of avoiding ionizing radiation exposure and assessing for any cardiovascular anomalies [15, 86].

Pulmonary Artery Sling The anomalous origin of the left pulmonary artery from the proximal posterior right pulmonary artery rather than from the main pulmonary artery, known as "pulmonary artery sling," is a rare mediastinal vascular anomaly resulting from complete obliteration of the primitive left sixth aortic arch during fetal development [6, 13, 84, 87]. The term sling is derived from the looping appearance of the left pulmonary artery as it passes over the right main bronchus, posterior to the trachea, and anterior to the esophagus toward the left hilum [6, 13, 84]. If the lower trachea or right main bronchus is compressed by the anomalous vessel, it can result in obstructive hyperinflation or atelectasis of the right lung, and affected pediatric patients can present during the neonatal or infancy period with stridor, respiratory distress, or hypoxia [6, 13, 15, 87].

Pulmonary artery sling is currently classified into two main types depending on the associated airway anomalies: Type I is characterized by normal airway branching with the carina at the T4 to T5 level, with compression of the trachea and right main bronchus by the anomalous pulmonary artery [13, 51, 88]. Type 1A has no associated airway abnormality, whereas Type 1B is associated with a tracheal bronchus, tracheobronchomalacia, and unilateral pulmonary hyperinflation [13, 51, 88]. In Type 2, the carina is more caudally located at the T6 level and associated with a long-segment tracheobronchial stenosis. Type 2 pulmonary slings are associated with higher morbidity and mortality during infancy, primarily related to the airway narrowing and associated anomalies including a low inverted T-shaped carina, complete tracheal rings, pulmonary hyperinflation, and congenital heart disease [51].

On chest radiographs, a variety of airway-related findings may be identified including tracheal narrowing and air trapping, and on lateral views, soft tissue between the distal esophagus and trachea with anterior deviation of the lower trachea can be seen [15, 51]. On fluoroscopic esophagram, a smooth rounded anterior esophageal indentation is typically identified [15, 51]. CT and MR imaging/MRA can readily identify the origin, course, and caliber of the anomalous left pulmonary artery (Fig. 3.23), evaluate for airway anomalies, and identify lung or cardiac anomalies [15, 51].

If patients are symptomatic, then they may undergo surgical management with ligation, division and reimplantation of the anomalous left pulmonary artery with simultaneous tracheoplasty, and repair of airway anomalies [6, 13, 15, 87].

Pulmonary Venous Anomalies

Variable Pulmonary Vein Branching During early embryological development, the lungs initially drain into the systemic veins, and the common primitive pulmonary vein forms a pouch into the primitive left atrium [69, 89]. As the lungs develop and fuse to the common pulmonary vein, the pulmonary venous connections to the cardinal and umbilicovitelline veins involute, and the common pulmonary vein incorporates into the left atrium, resulting in complete separation between the pulmonary and systemic venous systems [69, 89, 90]. The common pulmonary vein typically gives

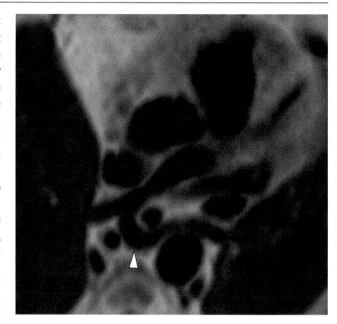

Fig. 3.23 Pulmonary artery sling in a 2-day-old girl who presented for workup of complex congenital heart disease. Axial non-enhanced double inversion recovery MR image demonstrates the pulmonary artery sling (*arrowhead*)

rise to four well-differentiated pulmonary veins, two draining each lung into the left atrium. Any disruption during the resorption pathway can result in variation in the diameter or number of pulmonary veins or abnormal drainage of the systemic veins or right atrium [69, 89, 90].

Various pulmonary vein patterns and variations have been described. However, the most common pattern, in 60–70% of the population, consists of four pulmonary veins and four well-differentiated ostia arising from the left atrium, two on the either side [89]. Variant patterns on the left typically consist of a common trunk or ostia of left superior and inferior pulmonary veins draining into the left atrium (Fig. 3.24), reported in 10–20% of people. More complex patterns usually involve one to two accessory pulmonary veins [89, 91], with the most common supernumerary pattern reported to occur in 9.0–26.6%, as a right middle lobe vein between the right superior and inferior pulmonary veins typically draining the right middle lobe [91, 92].

Contrast-enhanced ECG-gated CT and multiplanar MR imaging/MRA can be used to delineate the detailed pulmonary vein anatomy. MR imaging has the additional benefit of the lack of ionizing radiation and ability to obtain multiple sequential phases with one bolus of intravenous contrast and quantification of pulmonary venous flow volume [4, 90, 91].

Variable Pulmonary Vein Connection—Total Anomalous Pulmonary Venous Connection Total anomalous pulmonary venous connection (TAPVC) occurs when the pulmonary veins do not drain into the left atrium and form an aberrant connec-

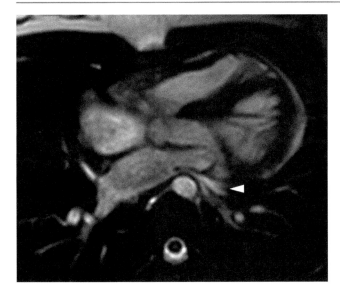

Fig. 3.24 Common left pulmonary vein in a 13-year-old girl who presented for cardiac MR imaging for evaluation of desaturation. Axial T2-weighted MR image demonstrates a common left pulmonary vein (*arrowhead*) with stenosis as it enters the left atrium. Two normal right upper and lower pulmonary veins are present

tion with another cardiovascular structure. This occurs when the common pulmonary vein fails to develop appropriately and the cardinal or umbilicovitelline vein persists during fetal development [90]. TAPVC is estimated to occur in approximately 1–5% of congenital cardiovascular anomalies [90, 93, 94]. An increased frequency of TAPVC is identified in patients with heterotaxy syndromes (Fig. 3.25) and cardiac anomalies [90, 93, 94].

Neonates with TAPVC are cyanotic with congestive heart failure, and the condition is incompatible with life if no right-to-left blood shunting is present. Shunting is typically through an atrial septal defect (ASD)/patent foramen ovale (PFO) or less commonly a patent ductus arteriosus (PDA) [90]. Advances in surgical techniques, including the use of a sutureless technique, have resulted in markedly improved 5-year survival rates, with estimates up to 97% and decreased postoperative complications of pulmonary venous obstruction [90, 94, 95].

There are four types of TAPVC characterized by pulmonary venous drainage location: supracardiac, cardiac, infracardiac, and mixed form. Supracardiac drainage or Type I is

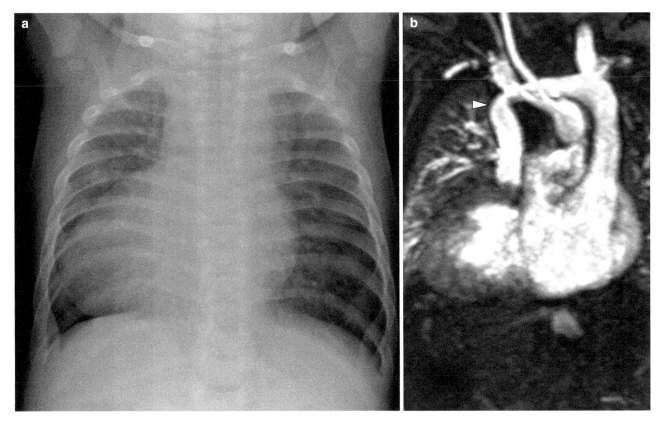

Fig. 3.25 Supracardiac total anomalous pulmonary venous connection (TAPVC) in a 4-month-old boy with heterotaxy who presented with cyanosis. (**a**) Frontal supine chest radiograph shows dextrocardia and vascular congestion. (**b**) Coronal enhanced MR angiogram image con-firms the unobstructed supracardiac total anomalous pulmonary venous connection draining to a right vertical vein (*arrowhead*). Dextrocardia and complete atrioventricular canal defect are also demonstrated

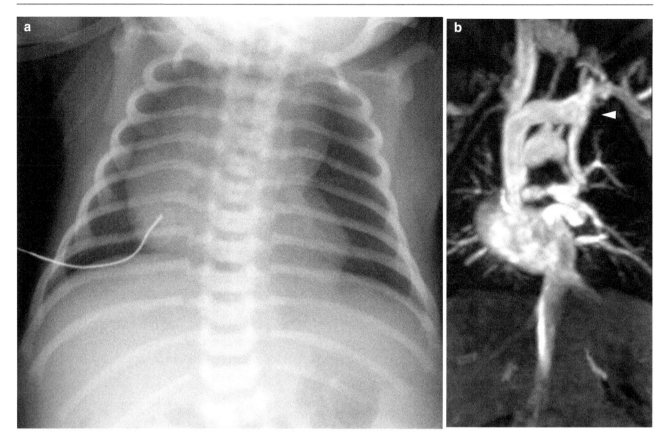

Fig. 3.26 Supracardiac total anomalous pulmonary venous connection (TAPVC) in a 0-day-old boy with heterotaxy, asplenia, bilateral morphological right bronchi, levocardia and abdominal situs, and complex cardiac disease. (a) Frontal supine chest radiograph demonstrates heterotaxy and the "snowman" sign compatible with supracardiac total anomalous pulmonary venous connection (TAPVC). (b) Coronal enhanced MR angiogram image shows TAPVC draining into the left innominate vein joining a vertical ascending confluence (*arrowhead*) joined by the right upper pulmonary vein. No left-sided superior vena cava is identified

the most common, estimated to occur in 44–55% of TAPVC [94, 96]. In this type, the most common drainage of the pulmonary veins is typically through a vertical vein to the left brachiocephalic vein and SVC, which can produce the classic "snowman" or "figure-of-eight" sign on chest radiographs (Fig. 3.26) [94, 96]. Uncommonly, these pediatric patients can have venous obstruction if the vertical vein is compressed between the pulmonary artery and left main bronchus [96]. Rarely, supracardiac TAPVC may drain directly into a right or left SVC or the azygous system [90, 94].

Cardiac TAPVC (Type II TAPVC) accounts for approximately 21–30% of TAPVC cases and is characterized by the pulmonary veins draining either into the coronary sinus (Fig. 3.27) or the right atrium [90, 94].

Type III TAPVC, accounts for approximately 13–26% of TAPVC cases, and occurs when there is an infracardiac or infradiaphragmatic connection [90, 94]. The pulmonary veins drain into a systemic infracardiac vein, such as the IVC, a hepatic or azygous vein, or the portal venous system (Fig. 3.28) [90, 94]. Because the pulmonary veins typically course below and can be compressed by the diaphragm, it is common to see obstruction in up to 78% of

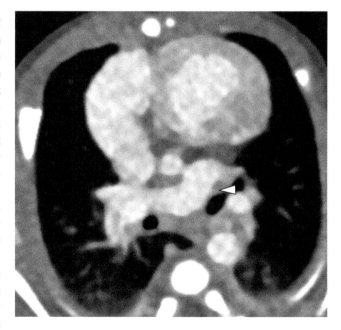

Fig. 3.27 Cardiac total anomalous pulmonary venous connection (TAPVC) in a 4-day-old boy with a hypoplastic ascending aorta who presented for evaluation of pulmonary venous drainage. Axial enhanced CT image shows three left and two right pulmonary veins draining into a large coronary sinus (*arrowhead*)

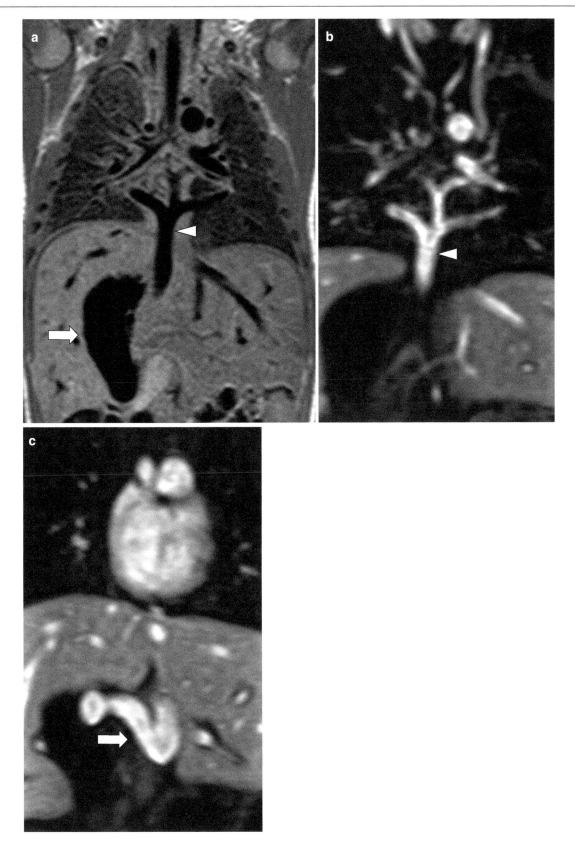

Fig. 3.28 Infracardiac TAPVC in a 2-day-old boy with heterotaxy syndrome, asplenia, and bilateral superior vena cava entering a common atrium. MR imaging was performed to further evaluate pulmonary drainage. (**a**) Coronal double inversion recovery. (**b**, **c**) Coronal enhanced MR angiogram images show an infradiaphragmatic total anomalous pulmonary venous connection (*arrowhead*) with small left and right upper pulmonary veins joining a small vertical confluence, joined inferiorly by normal-sized left and right pulmonary veins before crossing the diaphragm. The intra-hepatic portion of the confluence (*arrow*) becomes further dilated and tortuous as it joins the portal vein

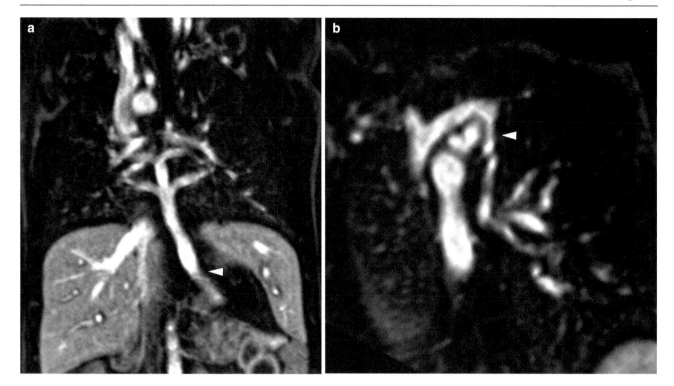

Fig. 3.29 Mixed total anomalous pulmonary venous connection (TAPVC) in a 3-day-old boy with concern for TAPVC on echocardiogram. (**a**) Coronal enhanced MR angiogram image shows a mixed-type TAPVC with bilateral upper and lower pulmonary veins draining into a vertical confluence which continues below the diaphragm into the portal vein with mild obstruction (*arrowhead*). (**b**) Oblique coronal enhanced MR angiogram image shows an accessory pulmonary vein from both the right and left lung entering into a vertical vein (*arrowhead*) draining into the left innominate vein and into the right-sided superior vena cava

these pediatric patients, which manifests as pulmonary interstitial edema with a normal-sized heart on chest radiographs [90, 94, 96].

Mixed TAPVC (Type IV TAPVC), the rarest subtype, is estimated to occur in 9% of TAPVC. It is characterized by anomalous venous connections at two or more locations (Fig. 3.29) [90, 96], with common locations including the brachiocephalic vein, SVC, azygous vein, coronary sinus, right atrium, or below the diaphragm [90, 96].

CTA and MRA are essential for preoperative planning, allowing visualization of the anomalous pulmonary veins. This is particularly valuable in the mixed forms of TAPVC as echocardiography is limited in evaluation in these cases [90]. MR imaging has the additional ability to provide hemodynamic information while measuring blood volume and flow velocities, as well as characterize effects on pulmonary arterial flow and ventricular size and function [4].

Variable Pulmonary Vein Connection—Partial Anomalous Pulmonary Venous Connection and Scimitar Syndrome
Partial anomalous pulmonary venous connection (PAPVC) is a condition in which at least one but not all the pulmonary veins drain into a location other than the left atrium, produc-

ing a left-to-right shunt [15, 89, 90]. Similar to TAPVC, this is thought to occur from abnormal persistent connections to a cardinal or umbilicovitelline vein [15, 90]. PAPVC occurs less frequently than TAPVC, with estimated rates of 0.4–0.7% [89, 90].

Depending on the number of anomalous pulmonary veins, affected pediatric patients may remain asymptomatic, and the PAPVC is discovered incidentally on imaging. However, if there is noticeably increased pulmonary flow from multiple PAPVC, affected pediatric patients may present with exercise intolerance and poor weight gain [15, 97]. Greater than 50% anomalous pulmonary blood flow has been suggested to be clinically significant [89, 90].

Although a wide variety of PAPVC patterns have been reported, the most common subtype is the drainage of the right superior pulmonary vein into the right atrium or SVC (Fig. 3.30), which can be associated with a clinically silent sinus venosus ASD [15, 89, 90]. On the left, PAPVC typically involves the left upper lobe, draining into a vertical vein joining the left brachiocephalic vein or into the coronary sinus [89, 90].

Similar to the imaging of TAPVC, contrast-enhanced ECG-gated CTA and MR imaging/MRA allow confirmation and characterization of the anomalous pulmonary venous drainage.

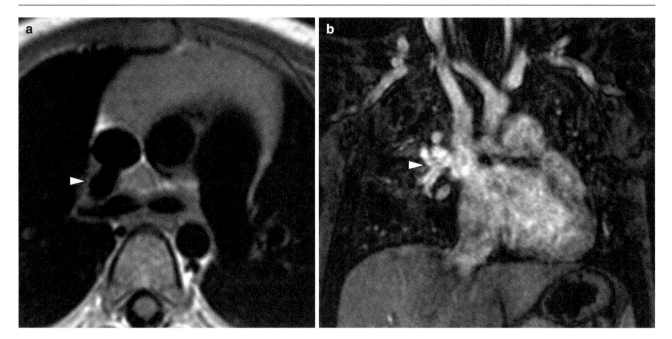

Fig. 3.30 Partial anomalous pulmonary venous return in a 4-year-old girl referred for MR imaging to evaluate pulmonary venous drainage. (a) Axial double inversion non-contrast MR image shows the right upper and middle pulmonary veins draining into the superior vena cava (SVC), just above the SVC-RA (right atrium) junction (*arrowhead*). (b) Coronal enhanced MR angiogram image demonstrates the right upper and middle pulmonary veins (*arrowhead*) draining into the SVC

In addition to the lack of ionizing radiation, velocity-encoded phase-contrast MR imaging allows the quantification of the left-to-right shunt from the PAPVC [4, 91].

Scimitar syndrome, also known as hypogenetic lung or pulmonary venolobar syndrome, is a rare form of PAPVC which almost exclusively involves the right lung, where some or all of the right pulmonary veins drain into the inferior vena cava above or below the diaphragm, azygous system, right atrium, portal venous system, or a hepatic vein [15, 89, 90, 97]. Associated anomalies include congenital heart anomalies, such as ASD in up to 25%, as well as pulmonary artery hypoplasia or aplasia, anomalous pulmonary systemic circulation, horseshoe lung, and pulmonary sequestration [15, 69, 89, 90]. Although affected pediatric patients may remain asymptomatic, in the setting of associated anomalies, they may present with dyspnea, recurrent infections, or congestive heart failure [15, 96].

Imaging findings of patients with scimitar syndrome include visualization of the anomalous crescent-shaped intrapulmonary vein adjacent to the right cardiac border, resembling the curved Turkish sword or "scimitar" (Figs. 3.31a and 3.32a). Additional imaging findings include a small ipsilateral hemithorax, ipsilateral pulmonary hypoplasia or aplasia, cardiac dextroposition, and ipsilateral systemic arterial collaterals arising from the aorta and its branch vessels (Fig. 3.31b) [89–91, 96–98]. MR imaging is fundamental for the evaluation of scimitar syndrome as it provides anatomic and hemodynamic details of the anomalous pulmonary venous drainage, lung hypoplasia, systemic arterial supply, and pulmonary blood flow distribution [4].

Although scimitar patients can be managed medically or surgically, patients presenting in infancy or with significant cardiac anomalies have suboptimal outcomes with either approach [99]. Operative repair to divert pulmonary venous blood flow away from the systemic drainage can be performed with either an intra-atrial baffle or direct reimplantation; however, post-repair stenosis or obstruction (Fig. 3.32b) or recurrent heart failure can occur [99].

Pulmonary Vein Stenosis Pulmonary vein stenosis (PVS) which can be primary (congenital) or secondary (acquired) is a rare condition characterized by luminal narrowing of the pulmonary veins and associated with high morbidity and mortality [89, 91, 100, 101]. Primary or congenital PVS is extremely rare and thought to result from abnormal embryologic incorporation of the pulmonary veins into the left atrium, with histologic features of connective tissue overgrowth, medial hypertrophy, and intimal fibrosis [89, 91, 100]. Primary PVS can involve single or multiple pulmonary veins, without a predilection for either side [15, 89, 91, 92]. PVS has been described to be associated with prematurity and severe lung disease, and 50–70% of affected patients have associated cardiac anomalies [15, 89, 100, 101]. Although dependent on the number of veins involved, the majority of affected patients present within the first 3 years of life, and an earlier symptomatic presentation has been

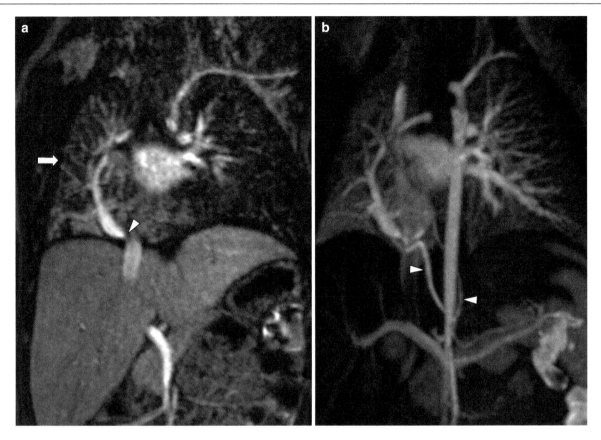

Fig. 3.31 Scimitar syndrome in a 24-day-old girl with suspicion for partial anomalous pulmonary venous connection on echocardiogram. (**a**) Coronal enhanced MR angiogram image shows partial anomalous pulmonary venous connection of all the right-sided pulmonary veins via a scimitar vein to the inferior vena cava (IVC) just below the IVC-RA (right atrium) junction, with moderate stenosis (*arrowhead*) at the entry of the scimitar vein into the IVC. The right lung is mildly hypoplastic (*arrow*), and there is dextrocardia. (**b**) Coronal maximum intensity projection (MIP) enhanced MR angiogram image demonstrates two aortopulmonary collaterals (*arrowheads*) arising from the descending aorta

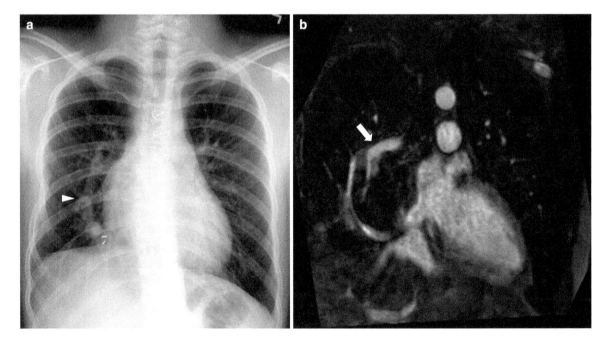

Fig. 3.32 Attempted repair of scimitar vein in a 18-year-old boy status postoperative baffle to the left atrium for scimitar syndrome, who presented for follow-up MR imaging evaluation. (**a**) Frontal chest radiograph demonstrates the anomalous crescent-shaped intrapulmonary vein (*arrowhead*) adjacent to the right cardiac border in keeping with a "scimitar" sign. (**b**) Coronary non-enhanced T2-weighted MR image shows the persistent scimitar vein (*arrow*)

reported to have increased complications and mortality [89, 100–102].

Secondary or acquired PVS, the more common type, most commonly occurs after surgery (heart or lung transplant, repair of PAPVC/TAPVC) or post-radiofrequency ablation for atrial fibrillation (in 3–8% of patients) [15, 89, 101]. Less frequently, secondary PVS can be caused by mediastinal processes resulting in extrinsic compression such as lymphadenopathy, tumor, or fibrosing mediastinitis [15, 89, 100]. Patients with PVS can present with non-specific symptoms such as cough, dyspnea, hemoptysis, and recurrent chest infections [89, 100]. However, if collateral veins develop, the symptoms can be mitigated; thus, it is important to consider PVS, in the setting of any child with pulmonary hypertension or with history of prior ablation or surgery [15, 100].

Chest radiography demonstrates the sequelae of PVS, including signs of diffuse or localized interstitial and alveolar edema [15, 84, 89]. Findings of secondary PVS, such as surgical clips, lymphadenopathy, and mediastinal calcifications, may be identified on chest radiography. MDCT with multi-planar reconstructions allows detailed assessment of the pulmonary vein narrowing and wall thickening, typically occurring near the junction with the left atrium. As PVS progresses, the abnormality can extend into the adjacent distal intraparenchymal pulmonary vein segments. CT can also assess for any associated lung parenchymal abnormalities and secondary causes of PVS [15, 84, 100]. MR imaging allows for detailed anatomic and functional assessment of the pulmonary veins using phase-contrast imaging and MRA (Fig. 3.33 and see Fig. 3.24) [4, 100]. MRI also allows for detailed assessment of associated cardiac anomalies or to identify causes of secondary PVS [100]. Pseudostenosis, apparent stenosis of the PV as it is compressed between the left atrium and the descending thoracic aorta, can be differentiated from true PVS on MR imaging as its caliber would vary throughout the cardiac cycle; alternatively, the patient can be imaged prone to eliminate any compression [91, 100].

Treatment for PVS patients depends on the severity of the stenosis and symptoms. If the patient remains asymptomatic with no significant narrowing (less than 50%), then surveillance may be performed. If patients have greater than 50%

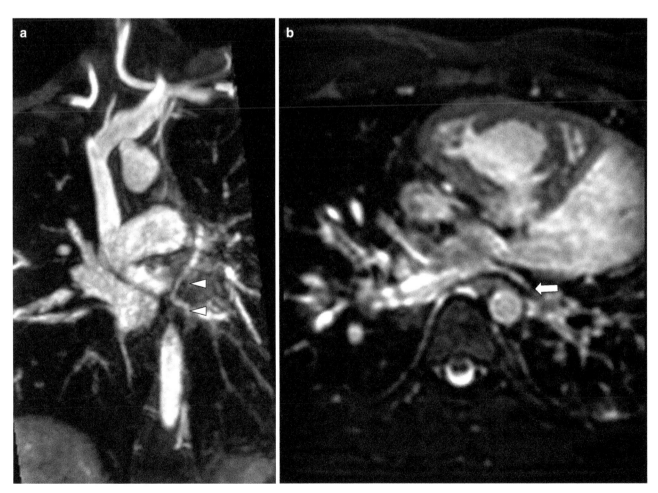

Fig. 3.33 Left pulmonary vein stenosis in a 17-year-old boy with transposition of great arteries, status post Mustard procedure with atresia of the left pulmonary vein orifice. (a) Coronal oblique enhanced MR angiogram image shows the severely hypoplastic/stenotic left upper and lower pulmonary veins (*arrowheads*). (b) Axial enhanced MR angiogram image demonstrates severely stenotic left pulmonary vein (*arrow*) and multiple tortuous venous collaterals

disease, pediatric patients are typically treated surgically [100]. Balloon angioplasty with or without stent placement has also been investigated in children but can be incredibly challenging with high rates of in-stent stenosis requiring frequent dilatations [15, 100]. However, a recent study of 93 PVS pediatric patients demonstrated no significant difference in mortality rates between the two interventions [102]. Pneumonectomy and lung transplantation are reserved for severe cases of uncontrolled hemoptysis and refractory PVS with pulmonary hypertension [15, 100].

Pulmonary Vein Atresia Pulmonary vein atresia (PVA) is thought to result from the failure of embryological incorporation of the common pulmonary vein into the left atrium [15, 89, 91, 101, 103]. Similar to PVS, the involved vein on histology demonstrates intimal thickening and fibrosis but

appears completely obstructed. PVA is the most severe manifestation of congenital PVS [15, 89, 101]. PVA can be unilateral, bilateral, or common (pulmonary veins form a confluence which does not connect to the heart or any major systemic veins) [89, 101, 103]. Depending on the distribution of involvement, clinical presentation can vary from extremely ill with severe hypoxia, respiratory distress, and metabolic acidosis in the newborn (common type) to milder presentations of recurrent pulmonary infections, hemoptysis, or pulmonary artery hypertension [15, 89, 101, 103]. Similar to patients with PVS, unilateral PVA has a high association with congenital cardiac disease and ipsilateral pulmonary hypoplasia with a diminutive pulmonary artery (Figs. 3.34 and 3.35). Whereas, common type PVA is usually an isolated cardiac anomaly but is closely associated with pulmonary lymphangiectasia [89, 101, 103].

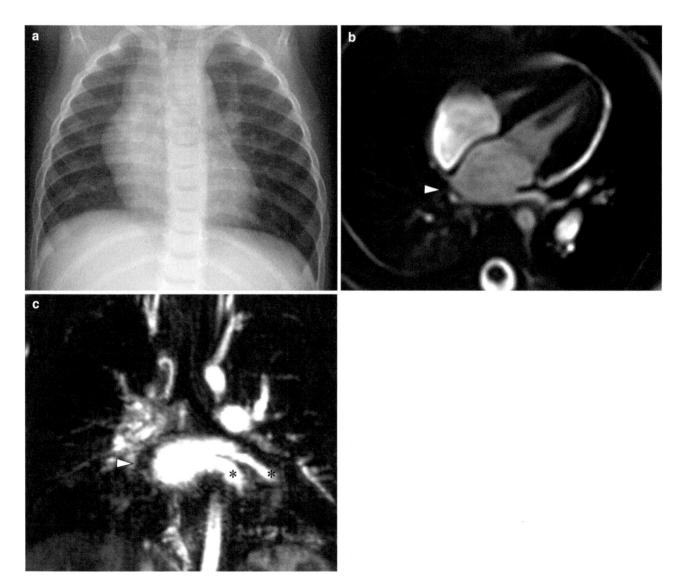

Fig. 3.34 Right pulmonary vein atresia in a 7-month-old boy with concerning echocardiogram. (**a**) Frontal chest radiograph shows a smaller right lung with decreased vascularity and mild interstitial thickening suggesting underlying mild pulmonary edema. (**b**) Axial non-enhanced

T2-weighted MR image demonstrates absence of the right upper, middle, and lower pulmonary veins (*arrowhead*). (**c**) Coronal enhanced MR angiogram image shows absence of the right pulmonary veins (*arrowhead*). The left-sided pulmonary veins are normal (*asterisks*)

In unilateral PVA, the affected lung is typically smaller with decreased vascularity, presumably related to preferential flow to the contralateral lung (see Figs. 3.34a and 3.35a) [15, 104]. Pleural thickening and findings of pulmonary venous hypertension, including septal and peribronchovascular thickening and ground glass opacities, can also be seen (see Fig. 3.35a) [15, 91, 104]. As the disease progresses, findings of pulmonary fibrosis can also be identified [15, 91]. CT and MR imaging can demonstrate the absence of pulmonary vein connections to the heart (see Figs. 3.34b, c and 3.35b, c), ipsilateral diminutive pulmonary artery, changes within the lung parenchyma and identify pulmonary to systemic venous collaterals [15, 89]. Phase-contrast MR imaging allows identification of flow reversal in the pulmonary artery, suggesting the presence of collateral vessels [104]. Unlike echocardiography, MR imaging and CT can definitively distinguish common PVA from obstructed TAPVC, which has significant prognostic implications [103].

Treatment of PVA involves surgical reformation of the pulmonary vein to left atrium connections. However, this is contingent on the size and proximity of the pulmonary venous confluence and can be very challenging with high risk of restenosis [101, 103]. If confluence reestablishment is not possible, pneumonectomy can be performed [101, 103].

Pulmonary Vein Varix Pulmonary vein varix is defined as either the focal or segmental dilation of one or more pulmonary veins, without a feeding arterial connection, as opposed to an arteriovenous fistula or malformation (AVF and AVM, respectively) [15, 89, 91, 105]. It can be congenital or acquired secondary to trauma or increased pulmonary vein pressure from mitral valve regurgitation, aortic coarctation, congenital heart disease, pulmonary vein stenosis, pulmonary hypertension, cirrhosis, or emphysema [89, 91, 105, 106]. The incidence has not been well established but most commonly occurs at the confluence of pulmonary vein and the left atrium [89, 91]. Although affected pediatric patients

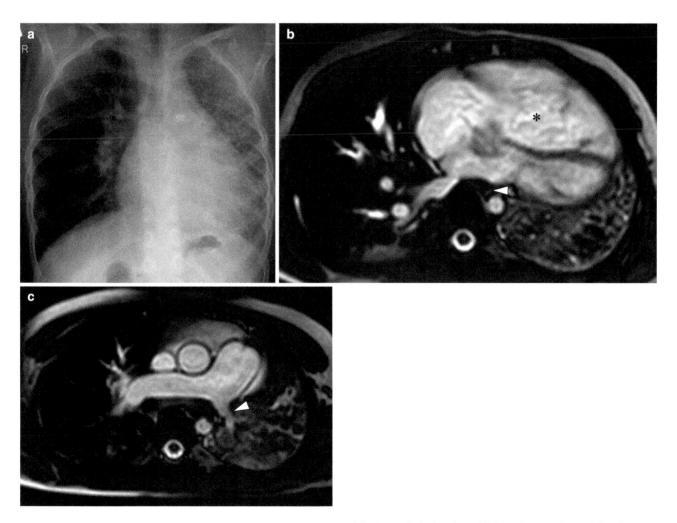

Fig. 3.35 Left pulmonary vein atresia in a 5-year-old girl with Ebstein anomaly with concerning echocardiogram. (**a**) Frontal chest radiograph shows a small left hemithorax with pulmonary edema, prominent right pulmonary artery, and a patent ductus arteriosus stent. (**b**) Axial non-enhanced T2-weighted MR image demonstrates an atrialized right ventricle (*asterisk*) in keeping with Ebstein anomaly, no left pulmonary vein (*arrowhead*), and left pulmonary hypoplasia. (**c**) Axial non-enhanced T2-weighted MR image shows a dilated right pulmonary artery, a small left pulmonary artery (*arrowhead*), and left pulmonary hypoplasia

are usually asymptomatic and discovered incidentally, they can also present with hemoptysis secondary to rupture or thromboembolic disease, recurrent lung infections, or dyspnea [15, 89, 91, 105, 106]. When symptomatic, resection is indicated, but most cases are asymptomatic, and no treatment is indicated [105].

On chest radiography and non-contrast CT, pulmonary vein varix can present as a well-defined nodule or mass near the left atrium [15, 89, 105]. Contrast-enhanced CT and MR imaging can confirm the diagnosis, with fulfillment of five angiographic criteria: normal pulmonary arterial tree, pulmonary vein draining the varix, varix drains into the left atrium, delayed drainage of varix, and tortuosity in the proximal portion of the pulmonary vein (Fig. 3.36) [91, 107]. Contrast-enhanced CT and MR imaging are essential for differentiating a varix from an AVM, based on the delayed filling and drainage of the pulmonary varix and the absence of a feeding artery [91, 105, 107].

Infectious Great Vessel Disorders

Infectious Aortitis and Mycotic Pseudoaneurysm Infectious aortitis (IA) is a rare entity seen almost exclusively in adults, partially explained by the relative lack of atherosclerosis in the pediatric population. It can occur secondarily to bacterial seeding of an existing intimal injury or atherosclerotic plaque (most common), septic emboli from endocarditis, contiguous spread from an infected site, direct bacterial inoculation from penetrating trauma, and as a complication post-angiography [108]. If the bacterial invasion results in loss of aortic wall integrity, IA may progress to form mycotic aneurysms or pseudoaneurysms and potentially rupture or form aorto-bronchial fistula (ABF) or aorto-enteric fistula (AEF), which are almost always fatal [15, 108–112].

Risk factors for IA and mycotic aneurysm include congenital aortic anomalies (such as coarctation), cardiac malformations, prior cardiac surgery, immunocompromised state, and umbilical artery catheterization [15, 109, 110]. The most common microorganisms involved include *Streptococcus pneumoniae*, *Staphylococcus*, and *Enterococcus* species, although other causative organisms include *Pneumococcus*, *Salmonella*, *Escherichia coli*, *Mycobacterium tuberculosis*, and *Treponema pallidum* [108–110]. IA symptoms are non-specific, including fever, chills, and pain at the

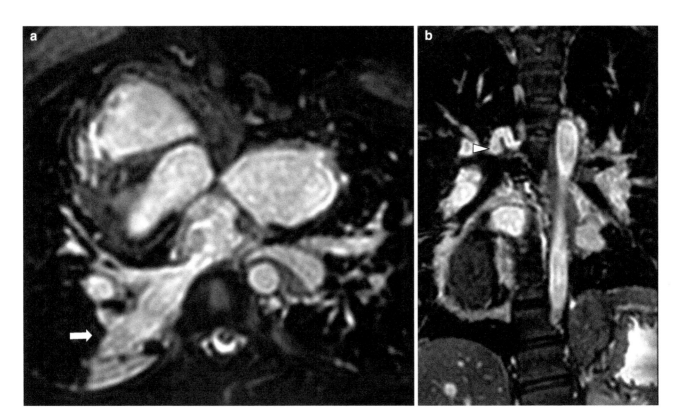

Fig. 3.36 Right pulmonary vein varix in a 12-year-old girl with heterotaxy, dextrocardia, and complex cardiac disease, status post-total anomalous pulmonary venous connection repair. (**a**) Axial enhanced MR angiogram image shows dextrocardia and a dilated and tortuous right pulmonary vein (*arrow*). (**b**) Coronal enhanced MR angiogram image demonstrates dextrocardia and the dilated tortuous right pulmonary vein (*arrowhead*) draining into the right-sided left atrium

involved location [110]. Compressive symptoms such as dysphagia, dyspnea, cough, and superior vena cava compression syndrome may occur if there is mycotic aneurysm formation [110]. If there is ABF/AEF formation, affected patients can present with hemoptysis and hematemesis, respectively [112].

Contrast-enhanced CT or MR imaging can confirm the diagnosis of infectious aortitis, with the presence of periaortic inflammation, nodularity, enhancement (Fig. 3.37), and potentially aortic intramural air and periaortic collections [15, 108]. Mycotic aneurysms/pseudoaneurysms appear saccular with irregular and thickened walls (Fig. 3.38), most commonly in the descending thoracic aorta [15, 109–111]. If present, a fistulous communication can be identified.

Treatment for AI and mycotic aneurysms/pseudoaneurysms generally consists of long-term antibiotic therapy and surgical excision with vessel reconstruction [15, 108, 110]. Endovascular repair is also a feasible option, especially in critically ill pediatric patients with fistula formation. However, the placement of foreign material at an infected site is controversial given concerns for stent infection, malpositioning with endoleak, and potential rupture [112, 113].

Vasculitic Great Vessel Disorder

Takayasu Arteritis Takayasu arteritis (TA) is a chronic autoimmune granulomatous disease of the aorta and its major branches, resulting in dilatation, stenosis, occlusion, and aneurysm formation of the affected arteries [114, 116]. Although TA most frequently affects young women in the second and third decades of life, childhood onset TA (c-TA) affects any age group, with reported ranges of 6 months to adolescence, and is the most common large vessel vasculitis in children [114, 115]. The incidence of TA has been estimated to range from 1 to 2.6 in 1 million per year [114, 116].

TA typically manifests in two phases: an acute inflammatory relapsing and remitting phase lasting weeks to months, with constitutional symptoms of anorexia, fever, night sweats, weight loss, arthralgia, and skin rash, and a chronic phase with features of distribution-specific arterial stenosis, occlusion, and ischemia [116]. In comparison to patients with adult-onset TA, patients with c-TA usually have non-specific symptoms and biomarkers, often resulting in delayed diagnosis up to four times longer than adult-onset TA [116–118]. Regardless of type, the most frequently reported symptom is hypertension [116]. Absence

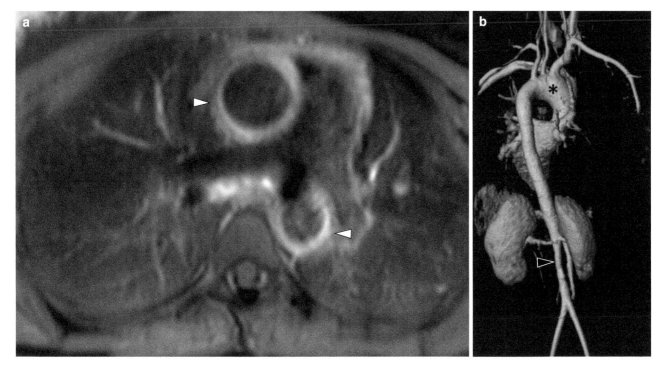

Fig. 3.37 Infectious (*Tuberculosis*) aortitis with a mycotic aneurysm in a 17-year-old girl with sepsis. (**a**) Axial non-enhanced T2-weighted fat-suppressed MR image shows circumferential aortic wall thickening (*arrowheads*) and edema at the aortic root and descending aorta in keeping with aortitis. (**b**) 3D reconstruction of enhanced MR angiogram image shows a dilated proximal aorta (*asterisk*) which becomes relatively normal in caliber after the origin of the left subclavian artery left subclavian artery. Narrowed distal aorta (*arrowhead*) is also seen

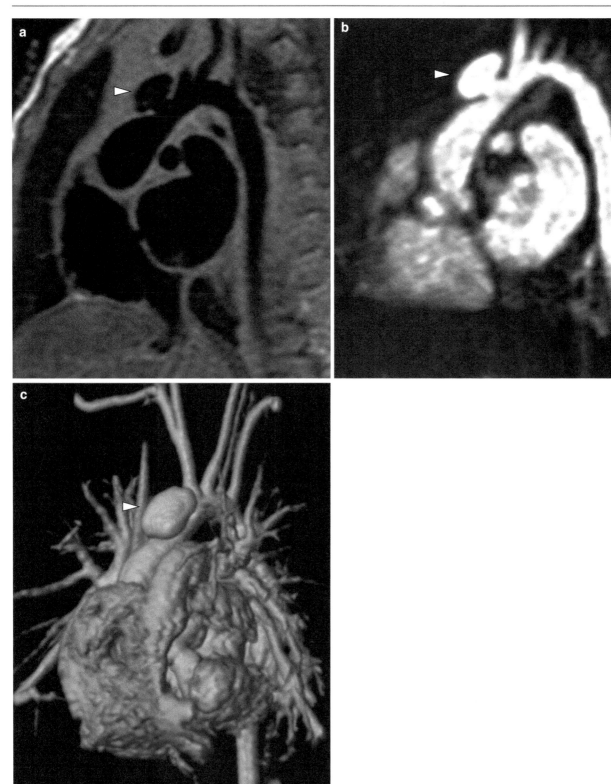

Fig. 3.38 Infectious mycotic pseudoaneurysm in a 12-day-old boy born with critical aortic stenosis, status post-balloon valvotomy with sepsis and positive methicillin-resistant *Staphylococcus aureus* (MRSA) blood cultures. (a) Sagittal non-enhanced double inversion recovery, (b) Sagittal enhanced MR angiogram, and (c) 3D reconstruction MR images show a large saccular pseudoaneurysm (*arrowheads*) in the anterior ascending aorta due to an infectious mycotic pseudoaneurysm

of extremity pulses is frequently identified in c-TA patients, whereas, unlike the typical TA patients, bruits and claudication pain are uncommon in c-TA patients [116].

Multiplanar MRA is particularly useful for identifying stenosis, dilatations, aortic wall thickening (Fig. 3.39), mural thrombi, and T2-hyperintense vessel wall edema to aid in the diagnosis of TA [114, 116]. Post-gadolinium aortic wall enhancement (Fig. 3.40 and see Fig. 3.39) is thought to correlate with disease activity [119, 120].

Treatment of TA primarily consists of first-line corticosteroids for immunosuppression and prevention of further vascular damage [119]. However, other cytotoxic agents such as methotrexate, cyclophosphamide, or azathioprine have been employed [114]. More recently, biologic therapies such as

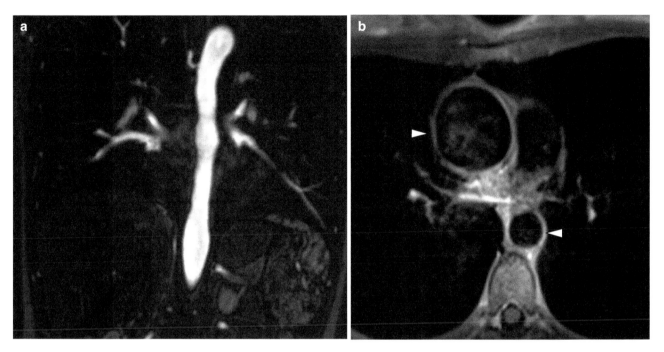

Fig. 3.39 Takayasu arteritis in an 18-year-old girl who underwent follow-up MR imaging. (**a**) Coronal enhanced MR angiogram image shows irregularity and beaded appearance of the descending thoracic aorta. (**b**) Axial enhanced T1-weighted fat-suppressed MR image shows wall thickening and enhancement (*arrowheads*) involving the thoracic aorta

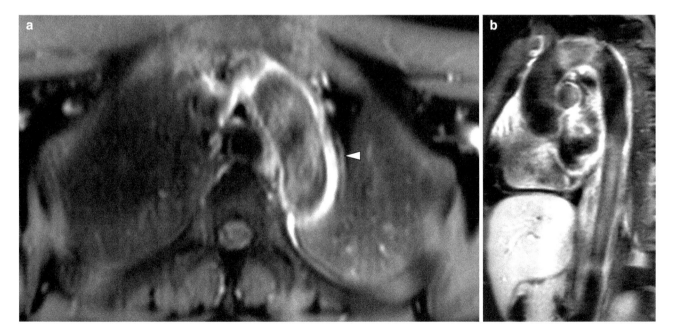

Fig. 3.40 Active Takayasu arteritis in a 15-year-old girl who presented for follow-up MR imaging. (**a**) Axial enhanced fat-suppressed MR image shows circumferential wall thickening and enhancement of aortic arch (*arrowhead*). (**b**) Sagittal enhanced fat-suppressed MR image shows diffuse circumferential wall thickening and enhancement of the thoracic aorta, just prior to the origin of the brachiocephalic artery

tocilizumab have demonstrated improved control of disease activity and may be a promising alternative treatment [115, 121]. Percutaneous or surgical revascularization techniques are reserved for critical stenotic lesions [122].

Connective Tissue Disorder

Marfan Syndrome Connective tissue diseases refer to a heterogeneous group of multi-organ heritable disorders, resulting from abnormal structure and integrity of the connective tissues. One of the relatively common disorders includes the autosomal dominant Marfan syndrome (MFS), estimated to occur in approximately 1 in 5000 individuals and most commonly associated with mutations of the fibrillin-1 gene [123, 124]. The abnormal production of fibrillin yields an extensive multiorgan phenotypic spectrum, with cardiovascular manifestations including mitral valve prolapse and regurgitation, left ventricular dilatation, cardiac failure, pulmonary artery dilatation, myocardial infarction, and, most importantly, aortic root dilation (most commonly at the sinuses of Valsalva) (Fig. 3.41) leading to aortic regurgitation, and aortic dissection, which is the main cause of MFS mortality and morbidity [123, 125]. Main pulmonary artery dilation may also occur and is associated with earlier and more severe vascular involvement [126]. Neonatal Marfan syndrome (nMFS) is a severe, rapidly progressive, and often fatal phenotypic expression of MFS, typically due to de novo mutations, with reported mortalities up to 82% before the age of 1, predominantly secondary to heart failure [125, 127, 128].

Frequent aortic surveillance is recommended to identify Marfan syndrome patients at high risk of aortic dissection. As MR imaging does not impart radiation dose and is not limited by acoustic windows, it is ideal for long-term follow-up of pediatric patients [129]. MR imaging can monitor the aortic size, precisely measure vessel diameters, and accurately characterize dissections, as it allows easy visualization of the origin and exit sites of intimal tears, dissection flap, false and true lumens, and additional vessels involved (Fig. 3.42) [129]. Additionally, MR imaging allows ventricular function, blood flow, and valvular assessment [82].

Beta-blocker therapy is the standard medical treatment for MFS patients [125]. In children, it has been suggested that a younger age of diagnosis is associated with an increased need for surgical intervention [130]. Prophylactic surgery, which has had the greatest impact on survival of MFS patients with a dilated aortic root, is recommended in children if the aortic ratio (measured aortic diameter/predicted diameter) is greater than 3 [125, 131, 132].

Acquired Great Vessel Disorders

Post-traumatic Aortic Pseudoaneurysm Pseudoaneurysm or false aneurysm, in contrast to a true aneurysm which involves all three aortic wall layers, contains less than three layers and is an extravascular hematoma contained by a fibrous capsule comminuting with the involved vessel [15].

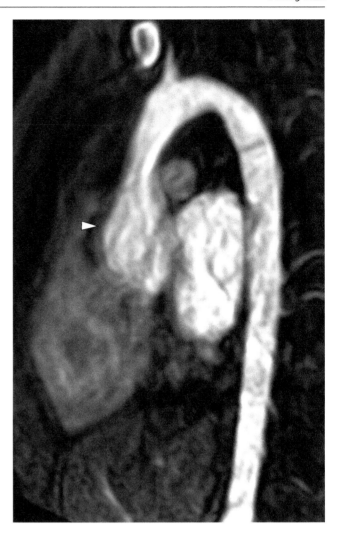

Fig. 3.41 Aortic root aneurysm in a 17-year-old boy with Marfan syndrome who underwent follow-up MR imaging. Sagittal enhanced MR angiogram image demonstrates a moderately dilated aortic root (*arrowhead*). No aortic dissection was seen

Common causes include infection (as discussed earlier), iatrogenic injury such as prior surgery, and trauma.

Thoracic vascular injuries are uncommon in the pediatric population, and although penetrating injuries can occur, blunt traumatic aortic injury is relatively more common than penetrating injuries, with estimated incidence rates of 0.1% and high mortality rates of 40–66% [133–137]. Blunt traumatic injuries are usually a result of forceful trauma such as high-speed motor vehicle collisions with multisystem injuries [133, 134, 136]. The majority of these injuries occur at the aortic isthmus, which is at the level of the ligamentum arteriosum, just distal to the left subclavian artery where the relatively mobile aortic arch becomes fixed [134, 136, 137]. Shearing injuries of the aortic intima and media layers, while the adventitia remains intact, result in pseudoaneurysm formation [134]. If unrepaired, chronic aortic pseudoaneurysms may rupture years after initial injury [15]. Additionally, a large proportion of the chronic aortic pseudoaneurysms can present as incidental findings or as apparent mediastinal masses on imaging [84].

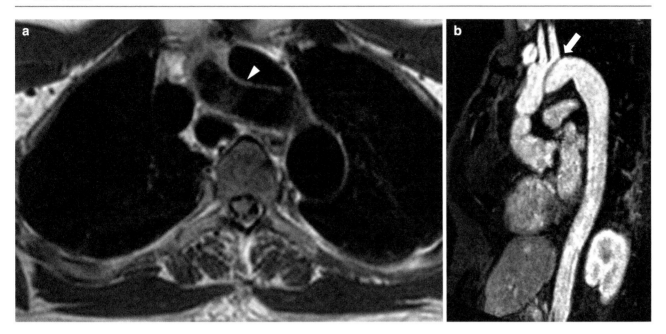

Fig. 3.42 Aortic dissection in a 22-year-old male with Marfan syndrome who underwent MR imaging for chest pain. (a) Axial non-enhanced double inversion recovery MR image shows an aortic dissection (*arrowhead*) in the mid-ascending aorta in keeping with a Type A aortic dissection. (b) Sagittal enhanced MR angiogram image shows the Type A aortic dissection (*arrow*) with the great vessels originating from the true lumen

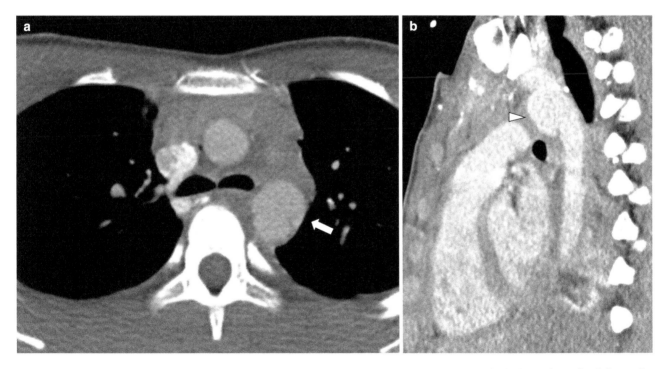

Fig. 3.43 Traumatic pseudoaneurysm in a 14-year-old boy who was involved in a motor vehicle accident. (a) Axial enhanced soft tissue window setting CT image shows an enhancing focal dilatation with luminal irregularity at the aortic isthmus in keeping with a traumatic aortic pseudoaneurysm (*arrow*). (b) Sagittal enhanced soft tissue window setting CT image shows an enhancing focal dilatation with luminal irregularity at the aortic isthmus in keeping with a traumatic aortic pseudoaneurysm (*arrowhead*)

In the setting of acute post-traumatic aortic injury, radiographs can demonstrate non-specific mediastinal widening [15, 134]. On ultrasound, a "mass" communicating with the aorta and a swirling "ying-yang" or a "to-and-fro" Doppler pattern can be visualized [15, 109]. On contrast-enhanced cross-sectional imaging (CTA or MRA), the pseudoaneurysm can be identified as an enhancing focal dilatation or diverticulum with associated luminal irregularity and an irregular outer contour (Fig. 3.43) [15]. It is important not to confuse a ductus diverticulum, a remnant of the ductus arteriosus, for a pseudoaneurysm, as they both occur at the isthmus. The ductus can be differentiated by its broader base, less vertical height, smooth margins, and obtuse angles with the aortic wall [138, 139].

Although dependent on the clinical setting, post-traumatic pseudoaneurysms are repaired semi-urgently (typically within 48 hours) [140, 141]. Although open surgical repair remains the gold standard in the pediatric population because of the smaller diameter of access vessels, with the increasing availability of smaller thoracic endografts, the popularity of endovascular aortic repair has been rapidly increasing [15, 111, 140, 141].

Aortic Dissection Thoracic aortic dissection (TAD) is defined by a tear in the intimal layer of the aortic wall with blood dissecting into the medial layer, creating a "false lumen" separated via an intimal flap from the true lumen. TAD is rare in infants and children, with incidence estimates of 0.37–3.5% of all cases [15, 142–144]. Predisposing conditions include connective tissue and inflammatory disorders (such as Marfan syndrome, as discussed earlier, and Turner syndrome), congenital cardiovascular anomalies (such as a bicuspid aortic valve or a preexisting aortic aneurysm), trauma, iatrogenic/post-surgery, hypertension, and miscellaneous activities such as cocaine use, pregnancy, and weightlifting [142–145].

The most common clinical presentation of TAD is an abrupt onset of sharp, tearing, or ripping pain, which can be migratory [142, 145]. Neurologic manifestations and signs of shock from acute heart failure, cardiac tamponade, or hypertension are also common, and extremity blood pressure differentials may also be present [142, 145]. Prompt diagnosis is crucial, with reported mortality rates of 1–2% within the first 48 hours from time of onset [142].

On radiographs, TAD can present as non-specific mediastinal widening [142]. MDCT is highly sensitive and specific for aortic dissection and identifying intrathoracic complications [142, 146]. Cross-sectional imaging with CT and MR imaging allows identification of the intimal dissection flap and characterization of the false versus true lumen (Fig. 3.44 and see Fig. 3.42) [15, 142]. A challenge with MDCT is the presence of cardiac motion artifact which can mimic acute dissection flaps. MR imaging/MRA allows multiphase acquisition which can negate this artifact; however, MR imaging/MRA is typically reserved for medically stable patients or patients with chronic dissections [142, 146].

Treatment of TAD is dependent on the corresponding Stanford classification (Fig. 3.45). Stanford Type A TAD, seen in 60–70% of cases, involves the thoracic ascending aorta and is treated as a surgical emergency [15, 146, 147]. Although surgical repair remains the gold standard, endovascular stent graft repair has become a popular alternative [143, 147]. Type B TAD only involves the descending thoracic aorta distal to the origin of the left subclavian artery (see Fig. 3.44) and is usually managed medically, unless present with complications such as a major aortic branch occlusion or renal or mesenteric ischemia [15, 143, 147].

Pulmonary Embolism Pulmonary embolism (PE) was previously thought to be a rare disease in children, with variable reported incidence rates of 0.9 up to 25 per 100,000 [148–150]. However, with the increasing use of CT pulmonary angiography (CTPA) in the evaluation of suspected PE, there is a thought that incidence rates are higher than previ-

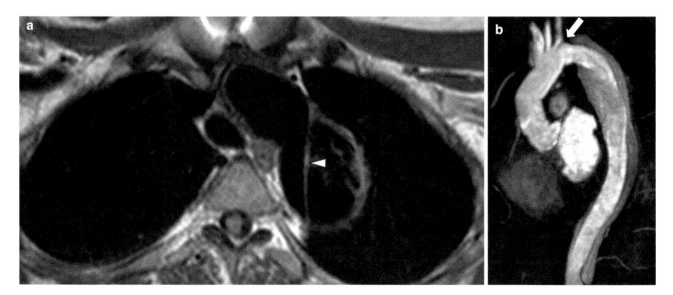

Fig. 3.44 Type B aortic dissection in a 26-year-old male with Marfan syndrome with previously repaired Type A aortic dissection who underwent follow-up MR imaging. (**a**) Axial non-enhanced double inversion recovery MR image. (**b**) Sagittal enhanced MR angiogram image shows a large Type B aortic dissection (*arrowhead* on **a** and *arrow* on **b**) originating just distal to the origin of the left subclavian artery

ously reported, with reported rates of 14–15.5% in children with clinically suspected PE who underwent a CTPA [151, 152]. Reported risk factors are variable across the pediatric age group, with dehydration, septicemia, and peripartum asphyxia as important risk factors in the neonatal period and

Stanford Classification

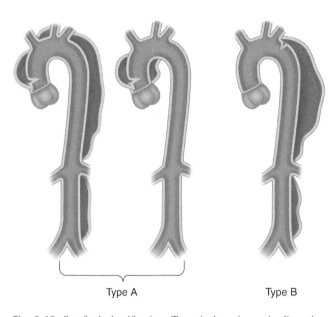

Type A   Type B

Fig. 3.45 Stanford classification. Type A thoracic aortic dissection involves the thoracic ascending aorta and requires surgical repair as the gold standard, whereas Type B only involves the descending thoracic aorta distal to the origin of the left subclavian artery and is usually managed medically, unless present with complications

malignancy, lupus erythematosus, renal disease, congenital thrombophilia, surgery, and major trauma as important risk factors in older children [151, 153–156]. However, the greatest risk factor in both age groups remains the presence of a central venous catheter [151, 153].

The classical presentation for a PE consists of pleuritic chest pain, hemoptysis, and shortness of breath; however, this usually only manifests in large PE, whereas small PE burden can often present with vague and subtle symptoms [151, 153]. Additional symptoms and signs include acute right heart failure, hypotension, dysrhythmia, syncope, and unexplained tachypnea [151, 153]. Given the variable and non-specific clinical presentation and high morbidity and mortality, especially in the setting of massive and submassive PE, it is imperative to have a high clinical suspicion in the pediatric population [157].

Chest radiographs are often normal, but when abnormal, it may show non-specific findings including cardiac enlargement, pleural effusion, atelectasis, and parenchymal opacities [151, 158]. The classically associated Westermark sign (oligemia), Hampton hump (peripheral wedge-shaped opacification), and Fleischner sign (prominent central pulmonary artery) are thought to occur in less than 20% of cases [151, 158]. CTPA is currently the gold standard, due to its high sensitivity and specificity, high spatial resolution, and availability [151]. On CTPA, the arterial filling defect is present on two or more consecutive images (Fig. 3.46), and the presence of any associated pulmonary artery enlargement, right heart dysfunction, or parenchymal changes can be readily detected [151]. The

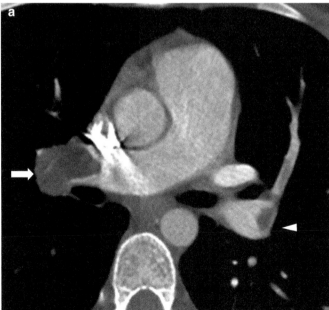

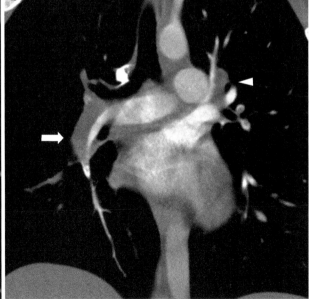

Fig. 3.46 Bilateral pulmonary embolism in a 15-year-old girl on oral contraceptive pills found to have deep vein thrombosis. (**a**) Axial enhanced CT image shows multiple filling defects in in the bilateral pulmonary arteries, including the right (*arrow*) and left (*arrowhead*)

pulmonary arteries. (**b**) Coronal enhanced CT image demonstrates multiple filling defects in in the bilateral pulmonary arteries, including the right (*arrow*) and left (*arrowhead*) pulmonary arteries

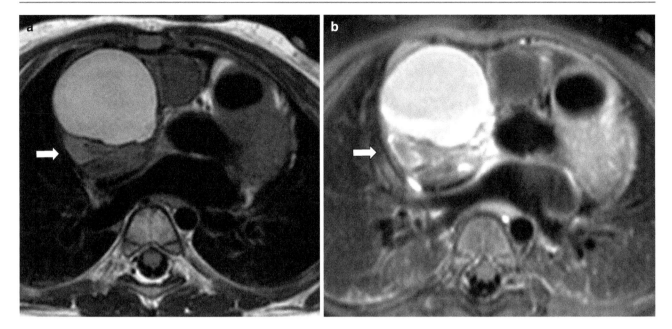

Fig. 3.47 Superior vena cava syndrome secondary to an anterior medi-astinal germ cell tumor in a 33-month-old girl who presented with neck swelling. (**a**) Axial non-enhanced double inversion recovery MR image shows a large predominantly cystic anterior mediastinal mass (*arrow*) contained within the pericardial space causing substantial mass effect on the superior vena cava (SVC) and right atrium in keeping with SVC syndrome. (**b**) Axial enhanced T1-weighted fat-suppressed MR image demonstrates the large enhancing mass (*arrow*) representing the patient's known anterior mediastinal germ cell tumor causing signifi-cant compression on the SVC and right atrium in keeping with SVC syndrome

presence of a sharply marinated and usually central filling defect with an acute margin favors an acute PE, whereas a chronic PE is eccentric and adherent to the vessel wall, sometimes with arterial wall thickening and irregularity and the presence of webs and bands [151].

Although early non-contrast MR imaging techniques were limited for assessment of PE, due to the significant motion artifacts, long acquisition times requiring sedation, and low signal-to-noise ratio (SNR), newer MRA tech-niques allow for rapid acquisition (within 20 seconds for high resolution and 4 seconds for time of flight), possibly within a single breath-hold [151]. Although prior large multicenter PIOPED III and IRM-EP studies in adults dem-onstrated limitations in the MRA for detection of PE [151, 159–161], a more recent study has demonstrated the nega-tive predictive value of MRA for assessment of PE in symptomatic patients to be comparable to CTPA [162]. Similar to CT, the presence of a pulmonary arterial filling defect on contrast-enhanced MR imaging confirms the diagnosis of a PE [151].

Treatment options for PE usually consist of anticoagu-lation therapy but are dependent on the pulmonary embo-lism size (especially in massive and submassive PE), and the patient's hemodynamic condition, thrombolysis, and surgical or interventional thrombectomy may be required [151, 157].

Superior Vena Cava Syndrome Superior vena cava syn-drome (SVCS) is a rare disease with high morbidity and mortality rates, estimated at 30% and 18%, respectively, defined by diminished venous return from the head and neck region secondary to obstruction of the SVC [163]. SVCS usually occurs secondary to external compression from oncologic pathology (most commonly lymphoma, Fig. 3.47), intrinsic thrombosis (most commonly related to central venous catheter, Fig. 3.48), or secondary to treatment of con-genital heart disease [163].

Clinical presentation can be variable, but affected patients most frequently present with head and neck edema, dis-tended neck and thoracic veins, and dyspnea [163]. Acute complications most commonly include pleural effusions and chylothorax, and long-term complications may include neu-rological conditions such as developmental delay, neurologi-cal deficits, and hydrocephalus [163].

Chest radiographs can be useful for the identification of a mediastinal or hilar mass [162]. However, cross-sectional imaging with CT or MR imaging is advantageous in identi-fying the underlying cause, characterizing the degree of obstruction or compression, recognizing the presence of col-laterals, and selecting sites for tissue sampling [164]. MR imaging has the additional benefit of being able to directly visualize blood flow and may obviate the need for intrave-nous contrast [164].

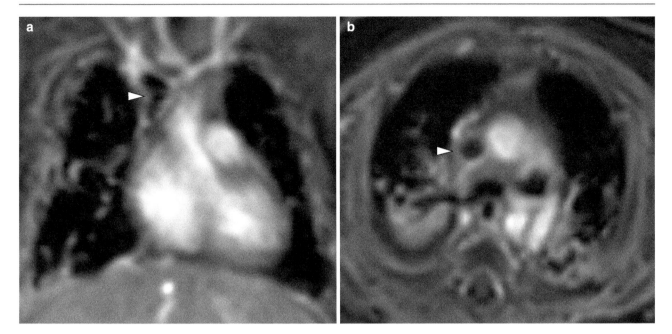

Fig. 3.48 Superior vena cava (SVC) syndrome secondary to a SVC thrombus in a 67-day-old female infant with trisomy 21, chylous effusions, and a previously placed left upper extremity central venous catheter who presented with new neck swelling. (**a**) Coronal enhanced MR angiogram image shows a large thrombus (*arrowhead*) in the superior vena cava (SVC) compatible with SVC syndrome. (**b**) Axial enhanced MR angiogram image demonstrates the large thrombus (*arrowhead*) in the SVC in keeping with SVC syndrome

Treatment for SVCS may include anticoagulation and, depending on the cause, can utilize interventional treatments such as catheterization with balloon dilatation, stenting or thrombectomy, surgical treatments such as thrombectomy, mass resection or cardiovascular correction, or oncological treatments with chemotherapy or radiation therapy depending on the scenario [161, 163].

Thoracic Outlet Syndrome The thoracic outlet is bordered by the upper mediastinum superiorly, the pectoralis minor muscle laterally, and the cervical spine posteromedially. The thoracic outlet contains the brachial plexus, subclavian vein, and artery. Thoracic outlet syndrome (TOS) occurs when there is compression on the brachial plexus, subclavian vein, and artery as they traverse the thoracic outlet [165–167]. Although TOS typically affects adolescents and young adults, it has been reported in patients as young as 4 months of age [166]. In adults, more than 90% of cases of TOS are related to nerve compression, but recent literature suggests that vascular thoracic outlet syndrome, especially venous, is much more common in the adolescent population [166–168]. One hypothesis for this discrepancy is that neurogenic TOS occurs from repetitive hyperextension or overuse injury from driving or performing jobs, which children do not commonly perform, whereas venous TOS typically occurs at the junction of the clavicle and first rib and results from strenuous hyper-abduction commonly seen in young athletes (such as pitching or weightlifting) [167]. When repetitive

venous compression results in deep venous thrombosis, this is described as Paget-Schroetter syndrome (PSS) [169]. Cervical ribs and anomalies of the first rib are the most common cause of thoracic outlet syndrome in children [166, 170].

Clinical presentation of TOS varies depending on the cause. Patients with neurogenic TOS present with pain, paresthesia, and weakness in the upper extremity, whereas patients with venous TOS present with swelling, pain, cyanosis, and distension of the upper extremity veins, and patients with arterial TOS present with weakness and signs of upper extremity ischemic insufficiency, such as claudication, pallor, and paresthesia [166, 168, 170].

Chest radiographs can demonstrate bony abnormalities in patients with suspected TOS [165]. Evaluation with contrast-enhanced MR imaging/MRA or CT, and with arms in neutral and abduction position, can confirm the diagnosis and identify any accessory muscles, compressive mass or lesion, brachial plexus signal abnormality, compression or thrombosis of the subclavian vessels, and the presence of any venous collaterals (Figs. 3.49 and 3.50) [165, 166].

TOS and PSS management is dependent on the structure involved. Vascular TOS is typically treated with physiotherapy, anticoagulation, thrombolysis, and thrombectomy, whereas neurogenic TOS can be treated symptomatically with nerve blocks [165–170]. If a structural abnormality or lesion is identified, then surgical resection or decompression is often the initial treatment [166].

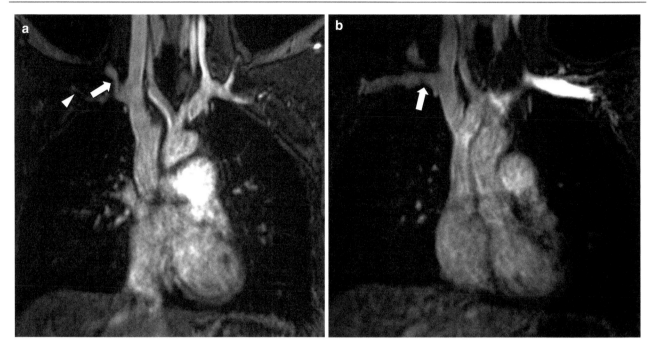

Fig. 3.49 Right thoracic outlet syndrome in a 16-year-old girl with right upper extremity pain. (**a**) Coronal enhanced MR angiogram image with the patient's arm up shows a severe narrowing (*arrow*) in the right subclavian vein between the right clavicle and anterior scalene muscle. Multiple venous collaterals (*arrowhead*) are identified in the right axil-

lary region. (**b**) Coronal enhanced MR angiogram image with the patient's arm down demonstrates resolution (*arrow*) of the external compression in the right subclavian vein and decreased prominence of the right axillary venous collaterals in keeping with venous thoracic outlet syndrome. No deep venous thrombus is identified

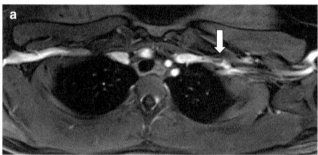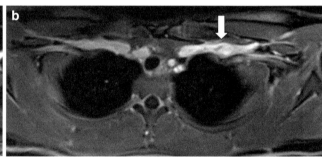

Fig. 3.50 Left Paget-Schroetter syndrome in a 14-year-old girl with left upper extremity pain and concern for venous thoracic outlet syndrome. (**a**) Axial enhanced MR angiogram image with the patient's arm up shows a focal low signal (*arrow*) within the left subclavian vein

immediately posterior to the left mid clavicle. (**b**) Axial enhanced MR angiogram image with the patient's arm down demonstrates persistent low signal within the left subclavian vein in keeping with a nonocclusive thrombus (*arrow*), compatible with Paget-Schroetter syndrome

Conclusion

Congenital and acquired thoracic vascular anomalies and abnormalities involving the thoracic aorta, pulmonary arteries and veins, and systemic veins often require cross-sectional imaging evaluation to help guide clinical diagnosis and management. In recent years, MR imaging and MRA, which can provide clinically useful anatomic and functional information, are increasingly utilized for evaluating these great vessel anomalies and abnormalities particularly in the pediatric population. For optimal patient care, it is essential for radiologists to have a clear understanding of up-to-date

MR imaging techniques, embryology and anatomy, normal development and anatomic variants, and characteristic MR imaging appearance of disorders involving the thoracic great vessels commonly encountered in daily clinical practice.

References

1. Hanneman K, Newman B, Chan F. Congenital variants and anomalies of the aortic arch. Radiographics. 2017;37(1):32–51.
2. Kondrachuk O, Yalynska T, Tammo R, Lee EY. Multidetector computed tomography evaluation of congenital mediastinal vascular anomalies in children. Semin Roentgenol. 2012;47(2):127–34.

3. Hellinger JC, Daubert M, Lee EY, Epelman M. Congenital thoracic vascular anomalies: evaluation with state-of-the-art MR imaging and MDCT. Radiol Clin North Am. 2011;49(5):96996.

4. Grosse-Wortmann L, Al-Otay A, Goo HW, Macgowan CK, Coles JG, Benson LN, et al. Anatomic and functional evaluation of pulmonary veins in children by magnetic resonance imaging. J Am Coll Cardiol. 2007;49(9):993–1002.

5. Krishnamurthy R, Lee EY. Congenital cardiovascular malformations: noninvasive imaging by MRI in neonates. Magn Reson Imaging Clin N Am. 2011;19(4):813–22; viii.

6. Baez JC, Seethamraju RT, Mulkern R, Ciet P, Lee EY. Pediatric chest MR imaging sedation, techniques, and extracardiac vessels. Magn Reson Imaging Clin N Am. 2015;23(2):321–35.

7. Boswinkel JP, Litman RS. Sedating patients for radiologic studies. Pediatr Ann. 2005;34(8):650–4, 656.

8. Manson DE. MR imaging of the chest in children. Acta Radiol. 2013;54(9):1075–85.

9. Slovis TL. Sedation and anesthesia issues in pediatric imaging. Pediatr Radiol. 2011;41(Suppl 2):514–6.

10. Priya S, Thomas R, Nagpal P, Sharma A, Steigner M. Congenital anomalies of the aortic arch. Cardiovasc Diagn Ther. 2018;8(Suppl 1):S26–44.

11. Morita S, Masukawa A, Suzuki K, Hirata M, Kojima S, Ueno E. Radiographics. 2011;31(2):E13–33.

12. Schleich JM. Images in cardiology: development of the human heart—days 15-21. Heart. 2002;87(5):487.

13. Etesami M, Ashwath R, Kanne J, et al. Computed tomography in the evaluation of vascular rings and slings. Insights Imaging. 2014;5:507–21.

14. Kellenberger CJ. Aortic arch malformations. Pediatr Radiol. 2010;40(6):976–84.

15. Laya BF, Liszewski MC, Zucker EJ, Restrepo R, Lee EY. Mediastinum. In: Lee EY, Laya BF, Liszewski MC, Retrepo R, Zucker EJ, Sarma A, editors. Pediatric thoracic imaging. Philadelphia: Wolters Kluwer; 2019. p. 189–217.

16. Kau T, Sinzig M, Gasser J, Lesnik G, Rabitsch E, Celedin S, et al. Aortic development and anomalies. Semin Intervent Radiol. 2007;24(2):141–52.

17. Oddone M, Granata C, Vercellino N, Bava E, Tomà P. Multimodality evaluation of the abnormalities of the aortic arches in children: techniques and imaging spectrum with emphasis on MRI. Pediatr Radiol. 2005;35(10):947–60.

18. Edwards JE. Anomalies of the derivatives of the aortic arch system. Med Clin North Am. 1948;32:925–49.

19. Kadir S. Regional anatomy of the thoracic aorta. In: Kadir S, editor. Atlas of normal and variant angiographic anatomy. Philadelphia; WB Saunders 1991. 19–54.

20. Karacan A, Türkvatan A, Karacan K. Anatomical variations of aortic arch branching: evaluation with computed tomographic angiography. Cardiol Young. 2014;24(3):485–93.

21. Liechty JD, Shields TW, Anson BJ. Variations pertaining to the aortic arches and their branches. Q Bull Northwest Univ Med Sch. 1957;31(2):136–43.

22. Tawfik AM, Sobh DM, Ashamallah GA, Batouty NM. Prevalence and types of aortic arch variants and anomalies in congenital heart diseases. Acad Radiol. 2019;26(7):930–6.

23. Dillman JR, Yarram SG, D'Amico AR, Hernandez RJ. Interrupted aortic arch: spectrum of MRI findings. AJR Am J Roentgenol. 2008;190(6):1467–74.

24. Lim TRU, Uy JAU. Multidetector CT scan of the thoracic aorta in the evaluation of interrupted aortic arch: a review. Asian Oceanic Forum Pediatric Radiol. 2016;2:15–23. http://edu.aospr.com/wp-content/uploads/2015/07/aofpr.pub2_.feb_.2016.pdf. Accessed 20 Aug 2019.

25. Riggs KW, Tweddell JS. How small is too small? Decision-making and management of the small aortic root in the setting of inter-rupted aortic arch. Semin Thorac Cardiovasc Surg Pediatr Card Surg Annu. 2019;22:21–6.

26. Geva T, Hornberger LK, Sanders SP, Jonas RA, Ott DA, Colan SD. Echocardiographic predictors of left ventricular outflow tract obstruction after repair of interrupted aortic arch. J Am Coll Cardiol. 1993;22(7):1953–60.

27. Jegatheeswaran A, Jacobs ML, Caldarone CA, Kirshbom PM, Williams WG, Blackstone EH, et al. Self-reported functional health status following interrupted aortic arch repair: a Congenital Heart Surgeons' Society Study. J Thorac Cardiovasc Surg. 2019;157(4):1577–87.. e10

28. Singh GK. Congenital aortic valve stenosis. Children (Basel). 2019;6:5. https://doi.org/10.3390/children6050069. Review.

29. Sebastià C, Quiroga S, Boyé R, Perez-lafuente M, Castellà E, Alvarez-castells A. Aortic stenosis: spectrum of diseases depicted at multisection CT. Radiographics. 2003;2(Spec No):S79–91.

30. Kimura-hayama ET, Meléndez G, Mendizábal AL, Meave-González A, Zambrana GF, Corona-villalobos CP. Uncommon congenital and acquired aortic diseases: role of multidetector CT angiography. Radiographics. 2010;30(1):79–98.

31. Mongé MC, Eltayeb OM, Costello JM, Johnson JT, Popescu AR, Rigsby CK, Backer CL. Brom aortoplasty for supravalvular aortic stenosis. World J Pediatr Congenit Heart Surg. 2018;9(2):139–46.

32. Aboulhosn J, Child JS. Left ventricular outflow obstruction: subaortic stenosis, bicuspid aortic valve, supravalvular aortic stenosis, and coarctation of the aorta. Circulation. 2006;114(22):2412–22.

33. Maruyoshi H, Nakatani S, Yasumura Y, Nakajima H, Niwaya K, Sasako Y, et al. Intractable infective endocarditis associated with supraaortic stenosis in Williams syndrome: a case report. J Cardiol. 2002;40(1):25–30. (Article in Japanese).

34. Cha SG, Song MK, Lee SY, Kim GB, Kwak JG, Kim WH, Bae EJ. Long-term cardiovascular outcome of Williams syndrome. Congenit Heart Dis. 2019; https://doi.org/10.1111/chd.12810. [Epub ahead of print]

35. Sharma BK, Fujiwara H, Hallman GL, Ott DA, Real GJ, Cooley DA. Supravalvar aortic stenosis: a 29-year review of surgical experience. Ann Thorac Surg. 1991;51(6):1031–9.

36. Karaosmanoglu AD, Khawaja RD, Onur MR, Kalra MK. CT and MRI of aortic coarctation: pre- and postsurgical findings. AJR Am J Roentgenol. 2015;204(3):W224–33.

37. Baez JC, Seethamraju RT, Mulken R, Ciet P, Lee EY. Pediatric chest MR imaging sedation, techniques, and extracardiac vessels. Magn Reson Imaging Clin N Am. 2015;23(2):321–35.

38. Darabian S, Zeb I, Rezaeian P, Razipour A, Budoff M. Use of noninvasive imaging in the evaluation of coarctation of aorta. J Comput Assist Tomogr. 2013;37(1):75–8.

39. Lehnert A, Villemain O, Gaudin R, Méot M, Raisky O, Bonnet D. Risk factors of mortality and recoarctation after coarctation repair in infancy. Interact Cardiovasc Thorac Surg. 2019;29:469. https://doi.org/10.1093/icvts/ivz117.

40. Kennard DR, Spigos DG, Tan WS. Cervical aortic arch: CT correlation with conventional radiologic studies. AJR Am J Roentgenol. 1983;141(2):295–7.

41. Shayan G, Shao J, Wang Y, et al. Management of cervical aortic arch complicated by multiple aneurysms. Interact Cardiovasc Thorac Surg. 2019;29:295. https://doi.org/10.1093/icvts/ivz087.

42. Pearson GD, Kan JS, Neill CA, Midgley FM, Gardner TJ, Hougen TJ. Cervical aortic arch with aneurysm formation. Am J Cardiol. 1997;79(1):112–4.

43. Kir M, Saylam GS, Karadas U, Yilmaz N, Çakmakçi H, Uzuner N, et al. Vascular rings: presentation, imaging strategies, treatment, and outcome. Pediatr Cardiol. 2012;33(4):607–17.

44. Weinberg PM. Aortic arch anomalies. J Cardiovasc Magn Reson. 2006;8(4):633–43.

45. Schlesinger AE, Krishnamurthy R, Sena LM, Guillerman RP, Chung T, DiBardino DJ, Fraser CD Jr. Incomplete double aortic

arch with atresia of the distal left arch: distinctive imaging appearance. AJR Am J Roentgenol. 2005;184(5):1634–9.

46. Gould SW, Rigsby CK, Donnelly LF, McCulloch M, Pizarro C, Epelman M. Useful signs for the assessment of vascular rings on cross-sectional imaging. Pediatr Radiol. 2015;45(13):2004–16.

47. Lee EY, Zurakowski D, Waltz DA, Mason KP, Riaz F, Ralph A, Boiselle PM. MDCT evaluation of the prevalence of tracheomalacia in children with mediastinal aortic vascular anomalies. J Thorac Imaging. 2008;23(4):258–65.

48. Ruzmetov M, Vijay P, Rodefeld MD, Turrentine MW, Brown JW. Follow-up of surgical correction of aortic arch anomalies causing tracheoesophageal compression: a 38-year single institution experience. J Pediatr Surg. 2009;44(7):1328–32.

49. Liszewski MC, Ciet P, Lee EY. MR imaging of lungs and airways in children: past and present. Magn Reson Imaging Clin N Am. 2019;27(2):201–25.

50. Koontz CS, Bhatia A, Forbess J, Wulkan ML. Video-assisted thoracoscopic division of vascular rings in pediatric patients. Am Surg. 2005;71(4):289–91.

51. Dillman JR, Attili AK, Agarwal PP, Dorfman AL, Hernandez RJ, Strouse PJ. Common and uncommon vascular rings and slings: a multi-modality review. Pediatr Radiol. 2011;41(11):1440–54.

52. Lee CH, Seo DJ, Bang JH, Goo HW, Park JJ. Translocation of the aortic arch with Norwood procedure for hypoplastic left heart syndrome variant with circumflex retroesophageal aortic arch. Korean J Thorac Cardiovasc Surg. 2014;47(4):389–93.

53. Mcleary MS, Frye LL, Young LW. Magnetic resonance imaging of a left circumflex aortic arch and aberrant right subclavian artery: the other vascular ring. Pediatr Radiol. 1998;28(4):263–5.

54. Hernanz-Schulman M. Vascular rings: a practical approach to imaging diagnosis. Pediatr Radiol. 2005;35(10):961–79.

55. Blieden LC, Schneeweiss A, Deutsch V, Neufeld HN. Right aortic arch with left descending aorta (circumflex aorta). Pediatr Radiol. 1978;6(4):208–10.

56. Schuford WH, Sybers RG, Gordon IJ, Baron MG, Caron GC. Circumflex retroesophageal right aortic arch simulating a mediastinal tumor or dissecting aneurysm. AJR Am J Roentgenol. 1986;146(3):491–6.

57. Watanabe M, Kawasaki S, Sato H, Minami K, Shimazaki S, Akimoto K, et al. Left aortic arch with right descending aorta and right ligamentum arteriosum associated with d-TGA and large VSD: surgical treatment of a rare form of vascular ring. J Pediatr Surg. 1995;30(9):1363–5.

58. Backer CL, Mavroudis C. Congenital Heart Surgery Nomenclature and Database Project: patent ductus arteriosus, coarctation of the aorta, interrupted aortic arch. Ann Thorac Surg. 2000;69(Suppl 4):S298–307.

59. Carter BW, de Groot PM, Godoy MC, Marom EM, Wu CC. Imaging of the mediastinum: vascular lesions as a potential pitfall. Semin Roetgenol. 2015;50(3):241–50.

60. Velipasaoglu M, Sentürk M, Ayaz R, Atesli B, Tanir HM. Characteristics of prenatally detected right aortic arch cases in a single institution. J Obstet Gynaecol. 2018;38(7):895–8.

61. Ramos-Duran L, Nance JW, Schoepf UJ, Henzlelr T, Apfaltrer P, Hlalvacek AM. Developmental aortic arch anomalies in infants and children assessed with CT angiography. AJR Am J Roentgenol. 2012;198(5):W466–74.

62. Donnelly LF, Fleck RJ, Parcharn P, Ziegler MA, Fricke BL, Cotton RT. Aberrant subclavian arteries: cross sectional imaging in infants and children referred for evaluation of extrinsic airway compression. AJR Am J Roentgenol. 2002;178(5):1269–74.

63. Ranganath SH, Lee EY, Restrepo R, Eisenberg RL. Mediastinal masses in children. AJR Am J Roengenol. 2012;198(3):W197–216.

64. Sonavane SK, Milner DM, Singh SP, Aal AKA, Shahir KS, Chaturvedi A. Comprehensive imaging review of the superior vena cava. Radiographics. 2015;35(7):1873–92.

65. Ratliff HL, Yousufuddin M, Lieving WR, Watson BE, Malas A, Rosencrance G, McCowan RJ. Persistent left superior vena cava: case reports and clinical implications. Int J Cardiol. 2006;113(2):242–6.

66. Fares WH, Birchard KR, Yankaskas JR. Persistent left superior vena cava identified during central line placement: a case report. Respir Med CME. 2011;4(3):141–3.

67. Dillman JR, Hernandez RJ. Role of CT in evaluation of congenital cardiovascular diseases. AJR Am J Roentgenol. 2009;192(5):1219–31.

68. Biffi M, Boriani G, Frabetti L, Bronzetti G, Branzi A. Left superior vena cava persistence in patients undergoing pacemaker or cardioverter-defibrillator implantation: a 10-year experience. Chest. 2001;120(1):139–44.

69. Demos TC, Posniak HV, Pierce KL, Olson MC, Muscato M. Venous anomalies of the thorax. AJR Am J Roentgenol. 2004;182(5):1139–50.

70. Ari ME, Doğan V, Özgür S, Ceylan Ö, Ertuğrul İ, Kayalı Ş, et al. Persistent left superior vena cava accompanying congenital heart disease in children: experience of a tertiary care center. Echocardiography. 2017;34(3):436–40.

71. Waikar HD, Lahie YK, De Zoysa L, Chand P, Kamalanesan RP. Systemic venous anomalies: absent right superior vena cava with persistent left superior vena cava. J Cardiothorac Vasc Anesth. 2004;18(3):332–5.

72. Guarnieri GF, Romano F, Clericò L, Balducci G. Absent right and persistent left superior vena cava: fetal and neonatal echocardiographic diagnosis. Pediatr Cardiol. 2006;27(5):646–8.

73. Pugliese P, Murzi B, Aliboni M, Eufrate S. Absent right superior vena cava and persistent left superior vena cava: clinical and surgical considerations. J Cardiovasc Surg (Torino). 1984;25(2):134–7.

74. Sheikh AS, Mazhar S. Persistent left superior vena cava with absent right superior vena cava: review of the literature and clinical implications. Echocardiography. 2014;31(5):674–9.

75. Winter FS. Persistent left superior vena cava. Survey of the world literature and report of thirty additional cases. Angiology. 1954;5(2):90–132.

76. Bartram U, Van Praagh SV, Levine JC, Hines M, Bensky A, Van Praagh R. Absent right superior vena cava in visceroatrial situs solitus. Am J Cardiol. 1997;80(2):175–83. Review.

77. Abbey P, Narula MK, Anand R. Congenital malformations and developmental anomalies of the lung. Curr Radiol Rep. 2014;2:71.

78. Schneider P, Schwalbe E. Die Morphologic der Missbildungen des Menschen und der Tiere, vol. 3. Jena: G Fischer; 1912. p. 812–22.

79. Wasileska E, Lee EY, Eisenberg RL. Unilateral hyperlucent lung in children. AJR Am J Roentgenol. 2012;198(5):W400–14.

80. Newman B, Gondor M. MR evaluation of right pulmonary agenesis and vascular airway compression in pediatric patients. AJR Am J Roentgenol. 1997;168(1):55–8.

81. Kayemba-Kay's S, Couvrat-Carcauzon V, Goua V, Podevin G, Marteau M, Sapin E, Levard G. Unilateral pulmonary agenesis: a report of four cases, two diagnosed antenatally and literature review. Pediatr Pulmonol. 2014;49(3):E96–102.

82. Daltro P, Fricke BL, Kuroki I, Domingues R, Donnelly LF. CT of congenital lung lesions in pediatric patients. AJR Am J Reontgenol. 2004;183(5):1497–506.

83. Mutlu H, Basekim C, Silit E, Pekkafali Z, Ozturk E, Karaman B, et al. Gadolinium-enhanced 3d MR angiography of pulmonary hypoplasia and aplasia. AJR Am J Roentgenol. 2006;187(2):398–403.

84. Thacker PG, Schooler GR, Caplan MJ, Lee EY. Developmental lung malformations in children: recent advances in imaging techniques, classification system, and imaging findings. J Thorac Imaging. 2015;30(1):29–43; quiz 44–5.

85. Ellis K. Fleischner lecture. Developmental abnormalities in the systemic blood supply to the lungs. AJR Am J Roentgenol. 1991;156(4):669–79.

86. Carter BW, Lichtenberger JP, Wu CC. Congenital abnormalities of the pulmonary arteries in adults. AJR Am J Roentgenol. 2014;202(4):W308–13.

87. Smith BM, Lu JC, Dorfman AL, Mahani MG, Agarwal PP. Rings and slings revisited. Magn Reson Imaging Clin N Am. 2015;23(1):127–35.

88. Wells TR, Gwinn JL, Landing BH. Reconsideration of the anatomy of sling left pulmonary artery: the association of one form with bridging bronchus and imperforate anus: anatomic and diagnostic aspects. J Pediatr Surg. 1988;23(10):892–8.

89. Varona Porres D, Morenza OP, Pallisa E, Rogue A, Andreu J, Martinez M. Learning from the pulmonary veins. Radiographics. 2013;33(4):999–1022.

90. Dillman JR, Yarram SG, Hernandez RJ. Imaging of pulmonary venous developmental anomalies. AJR Am J Roentgenol. 2009;192(5):1272–85.

91. Hassani C, Saremi F. Comprehensive cross-sectional imaging of the pulmonary veins. Radiographics. 2017;37(1):1928–54.

92. Marom EM, Herndon JE, Kim YH, McAdams HP. Variations in pulmonary venous drainage to the left atrium: implications for radiofrequency ablation. Radiology. 2004;230(3):824–9.

93. White CS, Baffa JM, Haney PJ, Pace ME, Campbell AB. MR imaging of congenital anomalies of the thoracic veins. Radiographics. 1997;17(3):595–608.

94. Karamlou T, Gurofsky R, Al Sukhni E, Coles JG, Williams WG, Caldarone CA, et al. Factors associated with mortality and reoperation in 377 children with total anomalous pulmonary venous connection. Circulation. 2007;115(12):1591–8.

95. Wu Y, Wu Z, Zheng J, Li Y, Zhou Y, Kuang H, et al. Sutureless technique versus conventional surgery in the primary treatment of total anomalous pulmonary venous connection: a systematic review and meta-analysis. J Cardiothorac Surg. 2018;13(1):69.

96. Ferguson E, Krishnamurthy R, Oldham SA. Classic imaging signs of congenital cardiovascular abnormalities. Radiographics. 2007;27(5):1323–34.

97. Dyer KT, Hlavacek AM, Meinel FG, De Cecco CN, McQuiston AD, Schoepf UJ, Pietris NP. Imaging in congenital pulmonary vein anomalies: the role of computed tomography. Pediatr Radiol. 2014;44(9):1158–68.

98. Haramati LB, Moche IE, Rivera VT, Patel PV, Heyneman L, McAdams HP, et al. Computed tomography of partial anomalous pulmonary venous connection in adults. J Comput Assist Tomogr. 2003;27(5):743–9.

99. Wang H, Kalfa D, Rosenbaum MS, Ginns JN, Lewis MJ, Glickstein JS, et al. Scimitar syndrome in children and adults: natural history, outcomes, and risk analysis. Ann Thorac Surg. 2018;105(2):592–8.

100. Pazos-Lopez P, Garcia-Rodriguez C, Guitian-Gonzalez A, Paredes-Galan E, Alvarez-Moure MA, Rodriguez-Albarez M, et al. Pulmonary vein stenosis: etiology, diagnosis and management. World J Cardiol. 2016;8(1):81–8.

101. Song MK, Bae EJ, Jeong SI, Kang IS, Kim NK, Choi JY, et al. Clinical characteristics and prognostic factors of primary pulmonary vein stenosis or atresia in children. Ann Thorac Surg. 2013;95(1):229–34.

102. DiLorenzo MP, Santo A, Rome JJ, Zhang H, Faerber JA, Mercer-Rosa L, Hopper RK. Pulmonary vein stenosis: outcomes in children with congenital heart disease and prematurity. Semin Thoracic Surg. 2019;31(2):266–73.

103. Perez M, Kumar TK, Briceno-Medina M, Alsheikh-Ali M, Sathanandam S, Knott-Craig CJ. Common pulmonary vein atresia: report of three cases and review of the literature. Cardiol Young. 2016;26(4):629–35.

104. Heyneman LE, Nolan RL, Harrison K, McAdams P. Congenital unilateral pulmonary vein atresia radiology findings in three adults. AJR Am J Roentgenol. 2001;177(3):681–5.

105. Lee EY, Boiselle PM, Cleveland RH. Multidetector CT evaluation of congenital lung anomalies. Radiology. 2008;47(3):632–48.

106. Onteddu NK, Palumbo A, Kalva SP. Pulmonary vein varix with pulmonary vein stenosis. J Vasc Interv Radiol. 2017;28(1):147.

107. Berecova Z, Neuschl V, Boruta P, Masura J, Ghersin E. A complex pulmonary vein varix: diagnosis with ECG gated MDCT, MRI and invasive pulmonary angiography. J Radiol Case Rep. 2012;6(12):9–16.

108. Schwartz SB, Fisher D, Reinus C, Shahroor S. Infectious aortitis: a rare cause of chest pain in a child. Pediatr Emerg Care. 2011;27(7):654–6.

109. Restrepo R, Ranson M, Chait PG, Connolly BL, Temple MJ, Amaral J, John P. Extracranial aneurysms in children: practical classification and correlative imaging. AJR Am J Roentgenol. 2003;181(3):867–78.

110. Lopes RJ, Almeida J, Dias PJ, Pinho P, Marciel MJ. Infectious thoracic aortitis: a literature review. Clin Cardiol. 2009;32(9):488–90.

111. Voitle E, Hofmann W, Cejna M. Aortic emergencies – diagnosis and treatment: a pictorial review. Insights Imaging. 2015;6(1):7–32.

112. Kan C, Lee H, Yang Y. Role of endovascular aortic repair in the treatment of infected aortic aneurysms complicated by aortoenteric or aortobronchial fistulae. Thorac Cardiovasc Surg. 2018;66(3):240–7.

113. Deipolyi AR, Czaplicki CD, Oklu R. Inflammatory and infectious aortic diseases. Cardiovasc Diagn Ther. 2018;8(Suppl 1):S61–70.

114. Ranieri D. Great vessels of children: Takayasu's arteritis. Pediatr Ann. 2015;44(6):e148–52.

115. Aeschlimann FA, Eng SW, Sheikh S, Laxer RM, Hebert D, Noone D, et al. Childhood Takayasu arteritis: disease course and response to therapy. Arthritis Res Ther. 2017;19(1):255.

116. Mathew AJ, Goel R, Kumar S, Danda D. Childhood-onset Takayasu arteritis: an update. Int J Rheum Dis. 2016;19(2):112–26.

117. Kerr GS, Hallahan CW, Giordana J, Leavitt RY, Fauci AS, Rottem M, et al. Takayasu arteritis. Ann Intern Med. 1994;120(11):919–29.

118. Lupi-Herrara E, Sanchez-Torres G, Marcushamer J, Mispireta J, Horwitz S, Vela JE. Takayasu's arteritis. Clinical study of 107 cases. Am Heart J. 1977;93(1):94–103.

119. Nastri MV, Baptista LP, Baroni RH, Blasbalg R, de Avila LF, Leite CC, et al. Gadolinum-enhanced three-dimensional MR angiography of Takayasu arteritis. Radiographics. 2004;24(3):773–86.

120. Papa M, De Cobelli F, Baldissera E, Dagna L, Schiani E, Sabbadini M, et al. Takayasu arteritis: intravascular contrast medium for MR angiography in the evaluation of disease activity. AJR Am J Roentgenol. 2012;198(3):W279–84.

121. Batu ED, Sonmez HE, Hazirolan T, Ozaltin F, Bilginer Y, Ozen S. Tocilizumab treatment in childhood Takayasu arteritis: case series of four patients and systematic review of the literature. Semin Arthritis Rheum. 2017;46(4):529–35.

122. Johnston SL, Lock RJ, Gompels MM. Takayasu arteritis: a review. J Clin Pathol. 2002;55(7):481–6.

123. Tinkle BT, Seal HM. Committee on genetics. Health supervision for children with Marfan syndrome. Pediatrics. 2013;132(4):e1059–72.

124. Dietz HC, Loeys B, Carta L, Ramirez F. Recent progress towards a molecular understanding of Marfan syndrome. Am J Med Genet C Semin Med Genet. 2005;139C(1):4–9.
125. Ekhomu O, Naheed Z. Aortic involvement in pediatric Marfan syndrome: a review. Pediatr Cardiol. 2015;36(5):887–95.
126. Stark VC, Huemmer M, Olfe J, Mueller GC, Kozlik-Feldmann F, Mir TS. The pulmonary artery in pediatric patients with Marfan syndrome: an underestimated aspect of the disease. Pediatr Cardiol. 2018;39(6):1194–9.
127. Bresters D, Nikkels PG, Meijboom EJ, Hoorntje TM, Pals G, Beemers FA. Clinical, pathological and molecular genetic findings in a case of neonatal Marfan syndrome. Acta Paediatr. 1999;88(1):98–101.
128. Bucchorn R, Kertess-Szlaninka T, Dippacher S, Hulpke-Wette M. Neonatal Marfan syndrome: improving the bad prognosis with a strict conservative treatment with carvedilol? Open J Thorac Surg. 2014;4(2):44–7.
129. Dormand H, Mohiaddin RH. Cardiovascular magnetic resonance in Marfan syndrome. J Cardiovasc Magn Reson. 2013;15:33.
130. Yetman AT, Huang P, Bornemeier RA, McCrindle BW. Comparison of outcome of the Marfan syndrome in patients diagnosed at ≤age 6 years versus those diagnosed at >6 years of age. Am J Cardiol. 2003;91(1):102–3.
131. Pyeritz RE. Marfan syndrome: 30 years of research equals 30 years of additional life expectancy. Heart. 2009;95(3):173–5.
132. Keane MG, Pyeritz RE. Medical management of Marfan syndrome. Circulation. 2008;117(21):2802–13.
133. Pabon-Ramos WM, Williams DM, Strouse PJ. Radiologic evaluation of blunt thoracic aortic injury in pediatric patients. AJR Am J Roentgenol. 2010;194(5):1197–203.
134. Moore MA, Wallae C, Westra SJ. The imaging of paediatric thoracic trauma. Pediatr Radiol. 2009;39(5):485–96.
135. Sinclair DS. Traumatic aortic injury: an imaging review. Emerg Radiol. 2002;9(1):13–20.
136. Hammer MR, Dillman JR, Chong ST, Strouse PJ. Imaging of pediatric thoracic trauma. Semin Roentgenol. 2012;47(2):135–46.
137. Westra SJ, Wallace EC. Imaging evaluation of pediatric chest trauma. Radiol Clin North Am. 2005;43(2):267–81.
138. Agrawa PP, Chughtai A, Matzinger FR, Kazerooni EA. Multidetector CT of thoracic aortic aneurysms. Radiographics. 2009;29(2):537–52.
139. Ann JH, Kim EY, Jeong YM, Kim JH, Kim HS, Choi HY. Morphologic evaluation of ductus diverticulum using multi-detector computed tomography: comparison with traumatic pseudoaneurysm of the aortic isthmus. Iran J Radiol. 2016;13(4):e38016.
140. Keyhani K, Estera AL, Safi HJ, Azizzadeh A. Endovascular repair of traumatic aortic injury in a pediatric patient. J Vasc Surg. 2009;50(3):562–4.
141. Hosn MA, Nicholson R, Turek J, Sharp WJ, Pascarella L. Endovascular treatment of a traumatic thoracic aortic injury in an eight-year old patient: case report and review of literature. Ann Vasc Surg. 2017;39:292.e1–4.
142. Fikar CR, Koch S. Etiologic factors of acute aortic dissection in children and young adults. Clin Pediatr (Phila). 2000;39(2):71–80.
143. Hua HU, Tashiro J, Allen CJ, Rey J, Perez EA, Sola JE. Hospital survival of aortic dissection in children. J Surg Res. 2015;196(2):399–403.
144. Fikar CR, Fikar R. Aortic dissection in childhood and adolescence: an analysis of occurrences over a 10-year interval in New York state. Clin Cardiol. 2009;32(6):E23–6.
145. Zalstein E, Hamilton R, Zucker N, Diamant S, Webb G. Aortic dissection in children and young adults: diagnosis, patients at risk, and outcomes. Cardiol Young. 2003;13(4):341–4.
146. Johnson PT, Horton KM, Fishman EK. Aortic valve and ascending thoracic aorta: evaluation with isotropic MDCT. AJR Am J Roentgenol. 2010;195(5):1072–81.
147. Nienaber CA, Powell JT. Management of acute aortic syndromes. Eur Heart J. 2012;33(1):26–35.
148. Agha BS, Sturm JJ, Simon HK, Hirsh DA. Pulmonary embolism in the pediatric emergency department. Pediatrics. 2013;132(4):663–7.
149. Stein PD, Kayali F, Olson RE. Incidence of venous thromboembolism in infants and children: data from National Hospital Discharge Survey. J Pediatr. 2004;145(5):563–5.
150. Andrew M, David M, Adams M, Ali K, Anderson R, Barnard D, et al. Venous thromboembolic complications (VTE) in children: first analyses of the Canadian Registry of VTE. Blood. 1994;83(5):1251–7.
151. Thacker PG, Lee EY. Pulmonary embolism in children. AJR Am J Roentgenol. 2015;204(6):1278–88.
152. Kritsaneepaiboon S, Lee EY, Zurakowski D, Strauss KJ, Boiselle PM. MDCT pulmonary angiography evaluation of pulmonary embolism in children. AJR Am J Roentgenol. 2009;192(5):1246–52.
153. Patocka C, Nemeth J. Pulmonary embolism in pediatrics. J Emerg Med. 2012;42(1):105–16.
154. Babyn PS, Gahunia HK, Massicotte P. Pulmonary thromboembolism in children. Pediatr Radiol. 2005;35(3):258–74.
155. Schmidt B, Andrew M. Neonatal thrombosis: report of a prospective Canadian and international registry. Pediatrics. 1995;96(5 Pt 1):939–43.
156. van Ommen CH, Heijboer H, Buller HR, Hirasing RA, Heijmans HS, Peters M. Venous thromboembolism in childhood: a prospective two-year registry in the Netherlands. J Pediatr. 2001;139(5):676–81.
157. Pelland-Marcotte MC, Tucker C, Klaassen A, Avila ML, Amid A, Amiri N, et al. Outcomes and risk factors of massive and submassive pulmonary embolism in children: a retrospective cohort study. Lancet Haematol. 2019;6(3):e144–53.
158. Elliott CG, Goldhaber SZ, Visani L, DeRosa M. Chest radiographs in acute pulmonary embolism: results from the International Cooperative Pulmonary Embolism Registry. Chest. 2000;118(1):33–8.
159. Stein PD, Chenevert TL, Fowler SE, Goodman LR, Gottschalk A, Hales CA, et al. Gadolinum-enhanced magnetic resonance angiography for pulmonary embolism: a multicenter prospective study (PIOPED III). Ann Intern Med. 2010;152(7):434–43.
160. Revel MP, Sanchez O, Couchon S, Planquette B, Hernigou A, Niarra R, et al. Diagnostic accuracy of magnetic resonance imaging for an acute pulmonary embolism: results of the 'IRM-EP' study. J Thromb Haemost. 2012;10(5):743–50.
161. Benson DG, Schiebler ML, Nagle SK, François CJ. Magnetic resonance imaging for the evaluation of pulmonary embolism. Top Magn Reson Imaging. 2017;26(4):145–51.
162. Schiebler ML, Nagle SK, Francois CJ, Repplinger MD, Hamedani AG, Vigen KK, et al. Effectiveness of MR angiography for the primary diagnosis of acute pulmonary embolism: clinical outcomes at 3 months and 1 year. J Magn Reson Imaging. 2013;8(4):914–25.
163. Nossair F, Schoettler P, Starr J, Chan AKC, Kirov I, Paes B, et al. Pediatric superior vena cava syndrome: an evidence-based systematic review of literature. Pediatr Blood Cancer. 2018;65(9):e27225.
164. Abner A. Approach to the patient who presents with superior vena cava obstruction. Chest. 1993;104(4 Suppl):394S–7S.
165. Raptis CA, Sridhar S, Thompson RW, Fowler KJ, Bhalla S. Imaging of the patient with thoracic outlet syndrome. Radiographics. 2016;36(4):984–1000.

166. Chavhan GB, Batmanabane V, Muthusami P, Towbin AJ, Borschel GH. MRI of thoracic outlet syndrome in children. Pediatr Radiol. 2017;47(10):1222–34.
167. Arthur LG, Teich S, Hogan M, Caniano DA, Smead W. Pediatric thoracic outlet syndrome: a disorder with serious vascular complications. J Pediatr Surg. 2008;43(6):1089–94.
168. Chang K, Graf E, Davis K, Demos J, Roethle T, Freischlag JA. Spectrum of thoracic outlet syndrome presentation in adolescents. Arch Surg. 2011;146(12):1383–7.
169. Trenor CC, Fisher JG, Khan FA, Sparks EA, Duzan J, Harney K, et al. Paget-Schroetter syndrome in 21 children: outcomes after multidisciplinary care. J Pediatr. 2015;166(6):1493–7.
170. Vu AT, Patel PA, Elhadi H, Schwentker AR, Yakuboff KP. Thoracic outlet syndrome in the pediatric population: case series. J Hand Surg Am. 2014;39(3):484–7.

Lymphatics

4

Kyung Rae Kim, Edward Y. Lee, and Raja Shaikh

Introduction

The lymphatic system plays an essential role in the transport of metabolites, fluid balance, and immune regulation, which can be affected by various disease processes [1, 2]. The two traditional lymphatic imaging techniques are direct cannulation of the lymphatic vessels (pedal lymphangiography) and interstitial injection of contrast agents that migrate into the lymphatic vessels (lymphoscintigraphy and lower extremity magnetic resonance (MR) lymphangiography). However, these imaging techniques cannot be reliably used to image the central conducting lymphatic system due to dilution of contrast and prolonged image duration [3–5].

A novel technique, in which contrast is injected directly into inguinal lymph nodes combined with improved MR imaging technology, has greatly improved the imaging evaluation of central lymphatic vessels. Central lymphatic imaging is most commonly indicated for pediatric patients with clinical manifestations related to abnormal lymphatic flow or leak. MR lymphangiography can be utilized for planning various medical, interventional, and surgical treatments in lymphatic diseases and be used to evaluate treatment response. This has traditionally been achieved with conventional fluoroscopic intranodal lymphangiography with oil contrast; however, MR lymphangiography is becoming a preferred modality because it provides additional advantages of obtaining high-quality cross-sectional anatomical information and real-time dynamic imaging with no exposure to ionizing radiation. Additional risks of conventional fluoroscopic intranodal lymphangiography in patients with a right-to-left cardiac shunt, severe pulmonary insufficiency, and thyroid dysfunction are also avoided by utilizing MR lymphangiography [6–8].

This chapter reviews up-to-date imaging techniques and clinical applications of MR lymphangiography for assessing central conducting lymphatic ducts and their abnormalities in the pediatric population.

K. R. Kim
Division of Interventional Radiology,
Department of Radiology, UNC Medical Center/University of North Carolina School of Medicine,
Chapel Hill, NC, USA
e-mail: kyung_kim@med.unc.edu

E. Y. Lee
Division of Thoracic Imaging,
Department of Radiology,
Boston Children's Hospital, Harvard Medical School,
Boston, MA, USA
e-mail: Edward.Lee@childrens.harvard.edu

R. Shaikh (✉)
Division of Interventional Radiology,
Department of Radiology,
Boston Children's Hospital, Harvard Medical School,
Boston, MA, USA
e-mail: Raja.Shikh@childrens.harvard.edu

Magnetic Resonance Imaging Techniques

Patient Preparation

In order to perform MR lymphangiography, pediatric patients are first placed supine on a detachable MR imaging table in the preparation room over the posterior element of the torso receiver coil. Infants and young children (<10 years old) are usually placed under general anesthesia for the procedure. Light sedation can be used in older children if necessary in order to reduce anxiety. Most children older than 15 years of age can tolerate MR lymphangiography with only local anesthetic at the site of groin accesses. A controlled ventilation technique (breath-hold) is required to obtain motion artifact-free imaging, and communication

© Springer Nature Switzerland AG 2020
E. Y. Lee et al. (eds.), *Pediatric Body MRI*, https://doi.org/10.1007/978-3-030-31989-2_4

with the anesthesiology team prior to the procedure is crucial.

The inguinal lymph nodes are then identified with ultrasound. In small pediatric patients with severe lymphatic flow anomalies, detecting the lymph nodes can be challenging. A careful exploration with ultrasound extending above the inguinal crease should be performed to search for accessible lymph nodes. After sterilely preparing both groins, 22- to 25-gauge needles or angiocatheters connected to low-volume connecting tubes are used to access the lymph nodes [3, 9]. The placement of long connecting tubes allows the contrast to be injected from outside the bore of the magnet without moving the patient. The tip of the needle is positioned in the medulla, and few drops of sterile water or saline can be gently injected to confirm optimal access without evidence of extravasation. The connecting tubing is then secured to the patient's thigh. It is crucial to minimize the patient's movement during transfer to the MR suite to prevent needle dislodgment. A hybrid MR and fluoroscopy unit can be used to confirm intranodal needle position with injection of iodinated contrast agent under fluoroscopy followed by transfer of the patient to the MR scanner [9].

MR Imaging Pulse Sequences and Protocols

Currently, MR lymphangiography is predominantly performed utilizing 1.5-Tesla systems, although there are efforts to utilize the higher-resolution properties of 3-Tesla systems [10]. A torso coil is typically used to provide imaging coverage from the neck to the upper one-third of the thigh. Adequate right-to-left coverage to image the central channels during volumetric imaging should be planned. Time to scan (and length of breath-holds) increases with larger coverage volumes, so selection of an appropriate field of view is essential. These trade-offs should be carefully considered to appropriately plan optimal imaging.

The commonly employed MR imaging sequences during MR lymphangiography include (1) T2-weighted imaging; (2) pre- and post-contrast T1-weighted dynamic MR imaging; (3) pre- and post-contrast steady-state free precession (SSFP); and (4) three-dimensional balanced steady-state gradient echo, which provides excellent visualization of the vessels in relation to the lymphatic channels. T2-weighted imaging is obtained in axial or coronal plane to evaluate the overall anatomy and any suspected abnormalities or vascular anomalies. Prior to any contrast injection, a 3D SSFP sequence with fat suppression is acquired in a sagittal plane. Following this, pre-contrast coronal 3D spoiled gradient-recalled echo T1-weighted imaging with fat suppression is acquired. These images are then evaluated at the work station and repeated if necessary for optimization. It is crucial to obtain good coverage and resolution of the T1-weighted pre-contrast images to be used as masks for subtraction after subsequent post-contrast imaging [9]. The contrast is then injected through the preplaced groin lymph node access at a slow and well-controlled rate (0.5–1.0 ml/min).

Post-contrast 3D spoiled gradient-recalled echo T1-weighted imaging with fat suppression is intermittently repeated at approximately 30–45 seconds or longer based on the transit rate of the contrast. The contrast first opacifies the iliac and lumbar lymphatic channels ascending cranially along the central lymphatics, cisterna chyli, and thoracic duct, which crosses the midline at the mid-thoracic level to reach the neck where it makes a posterior to anterior turn to terminate at the venous angle at the junction of the left subclavian and internal jugular veins (Figs. 4.1 and 4.2). Usually, gadolinium appears in the iliac and lumbar lymphatics within 1–2 min of injection, into the midline trunk by 2–3 min, and within the cisterna chyli in 3–6 min, and it opacifies the thoracic duct and the terminal segment at the venous angle in less than 10 min. When optimal visualization of the central lymphatic channels (cisterna chyli and thoracic duct) is noted, a 3D SSFP post-contrast sequence can be obtained.

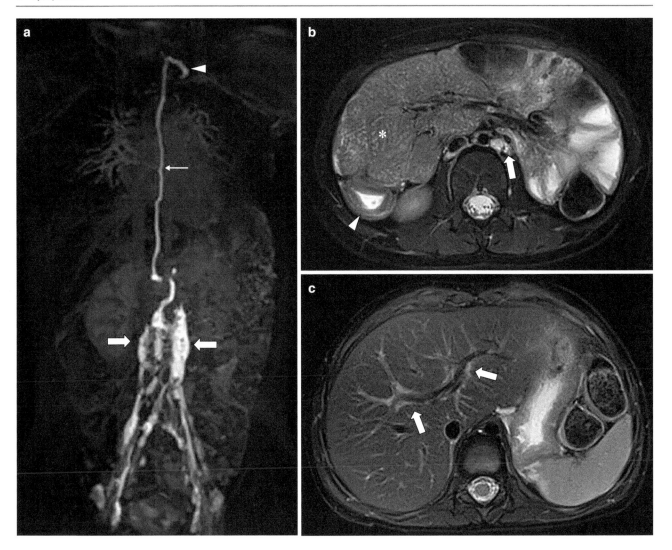

Fig. 4.1 Protein-losing enteropathy in a 4-year-old girl who presented for the evaluation of central lymphatic system. (**a**) Coronal maximum intensity projection image of T1-weighted fat-suppressed dynamic contrast-enhanced MR lymphangiogram shows increased filling of lymphatic contrast in the lumbar lymphatic channels (*large arrows*) secondary to lymphatic reflux. The normal course of the thoracic duct (*small arrow*) in the mediastinum and its termination at the venous angle (*arrowhead*) are noted. (**b**) Axial non-enhanced T2-weighted fat-suppressed MR image shows extensive diffuse wall thickening of the small bowel (*) and ascending colon (*arrowhead*) as well as dilated periaortic lymphatic channels (*arrow*). (**c**) Axial non-enhanced T2-weighted fat-suppressed MR image shows diffuse periportal high signal intensity (*arrows*) secondary to lymphatic congestion and reflux

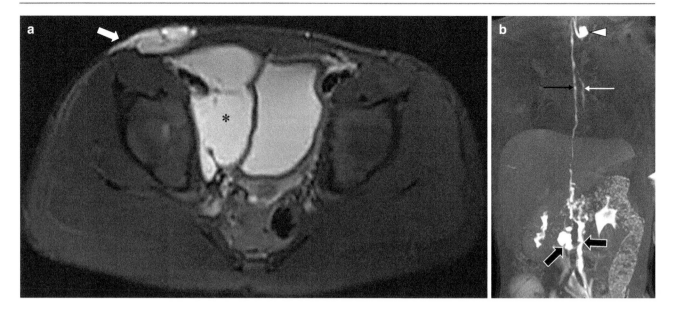

Fig. 4.2 Lymphatic malformation in a 12-year-old girl who presented with swelling and discomfort in the right groin. (**a**) Axial non-enhanced T2-weighted fat-suppressed MR image demonstrates extensive lymphatic macrocysts in the right groin (*arrow*) and pelvis (∗) which represent dilated central lymphatic channels. (**b**) Coronal maximum intensity projection MR image of T1-weighted fat-suppressed dynamic contrast-

enhanced MR lymphangiogram shows increased filling of lymphatic contrast in the lumbar lymphatic channels (*large black arrows*) secondary to lymphatic reflux. Also noted are parallel accessory thoracic duct (*small white arrow*) as well as orthotopic thoracic duct (*small black arrow*) and its termination (*arrowhead*)

Table 4.1 Dynamic magnetic resonance lymphangiography protocol

Sequence	TR	TE	TI	FA (degrees)	Matrix	ST (mm)	NEX	Bandwidth (Hz)	Plane
3D SSFP	4.0	1.9	90	90	160 × 320	1.2	0.5	434	Sagittal
3D spoiled gradient-recalled echo	4.0	1.9	16	25	190 × 280	1.8	1	244	Coronal
SSFSE T2-weighted	4500	97	0	90	384 × 256	4	0.5	400	Axial or coronal

Adapted from Shaikh et al. [1], with permission
SSFP steady-state free precession, *SSFSE* single shot fast spin echo, *TR* repetition time, *TE* echo time, *TI* inversion time, *FA* flip angle, *ST* slice thickness, *NEX* number of excitations

All contrast is washed out of the lymphatic channels in 15–20 min with the appearance of enhancement of renal parenchyma [3]. Delayed imaging can be performed if needed. The complete image data set is reviewed before concluding the study. The parameters used for these sequences are detailed in Table 4.1 [1].

Multiplanar reconstruction (MPR) and post-contrast subtraction images are obtained from a 3D volumetric image data set. Maximum intensity projection (MIP) volume-rendering images are reconstructed by selecting the highest signal voxels to improve the visibility of the lymphatic channels and are typically reformatted in a coronal plane. Customized off-axis MIP images which are tailored to the specific anatomy at the time of the exam are especially helpful in delineating the course of the thoracic duct [11].

Contrast Agents

For dynamic contrast-enhanced MR imaging, any routinely used macrocyclic nonionic gadolinium agent can be used.

Currently, the contrast dose is the same standard dose of 0.1 mmol/kg of body weight used for routine intravenous injection. The calculated volume can be further diluted with saline to increase the final volume.

Anatomy

Embryology

In humans, the lymphatic system starts to develop at the end of the 5th week of gestation [12]. The lymphatic vessels arise by the budding of primary lymph sacs from the veins that form initially in the jugular-axillary area and then in the retroperitoneum, mediastinum, and pelvis. All of the primordial lymph sacs fuse at different stages of development and lose their connections with veins, except for 2–3 connections between jugular-axillary lymph sacs and venous angles. The thoracic duct system is formed by the union of a duct or ducts growing caudad from the jugular sacs and a plexus arising from the cisterna chyli and extending cephalad (Fig. 4.3) [13–15].

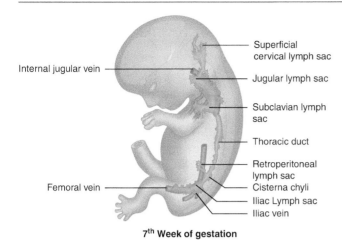

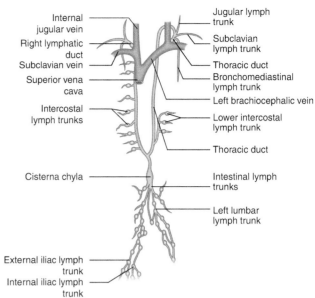

Fig. 4.3 Embryology of the lymphatic system. The lymphatic vessels arise by the budding of primary lymph sacs from the veins that form initially in the jugular-axillary area and then in the retroperitoneum, mediastinum, and pelvis. All of the primordial lymph sacs fuse at different stages of development and lose their connections with veins, except for 2–3 connections between jugular-axillary lymph sacs and venous angles. The thoracic duct system is formed by the union of a duct or ducts growing caudad from the jugular sacs and a plexus arising from the cisterna chyli and extending cephalad

Fig. 4.4 Normal anatomy of the lymphatic system. The thoracic duct usually starts with the cisterna chyli and crosses from the retroperitoneum into the mediastinum in the space between the aorta and azygous vein, through the aortic hiatus. As it ascends through the mediastinum, it accepts paired intercostal lymphatic ducts from the lower 6–7 intercostal spaces as well as lymphatic ducts from multiple mediastinal structures. The thoracic duct ascends in the posterior mediastinum to the right of the midline, and the duct crosses midline at the level of T5 and ascends toward the thoracic inlet along the left edge of the esophagus

Normal Development and Anatomy

Lymph vessels absorb excess interstitial fluid and proteins and transport them into the venous circulation [16]. The lymphatic system regulates tissue pressure and fluid status and provides a conduit for immune surveillance. About 4 to 5 L of lymph circulates per day and an average of 100 ml per hour flow in the thoracic duct. Depending on diet, approximately 1.5 to 2 L of chyle (intestinal lymph) is transported through the thoracic duct per day [17]. Similar to the veins, lymphatic vessels have valves and intermittently contract, which aid lymph flow. Alpha adrenoreceptors and histamine and bradykinin receptors located on lymphatic vessels may help these contractions. Lymph flow is also facilitated by movement of adjacent tissues and pulsations of nearby arteries to propel the lymph against gravity [18].

The lymphatic channels are generally small, tortuous, beaded, and can have an interrupted course. For example, the iliac and lumbar lymphatics may be comprised of multiple channels coursing in parallel toward the midline. These channels tend to become fewer in number and larger in caliber as they reach the midline and drain into the cisterna chyli, which is located behind the lower part of the right crural pillar between the aorta and inferior vena cava. The cisterna chyli is often formed by the confluence of the left lumbar trunk, the intestinal trunk, and, rarely, the right lumbar trunk, although these relationships are inconsistent [11, 14, 19].

The thoracic duct is the largest and longest lymphatic duct in the body. It represents the terminal part of the lymphatic system and drains lymph from 80–90% of the body. The remaining 10–20% of the body, including the right side of the head and neck, right upper extremity, right side of the chest, right lung, and heart, are drained by the right lymphatic duct. The thoracic duct drains into the left venous angle, and the right lymphatic duct drains into the right venous angle. The thoracic duct usually starts with the cisterna chyli and crosses from the retroperitoneum into the mediastinum in the space between the aorta and azygous vein, through the aortic hiatus. As it ascends through the mediastinum, it accepts paired intercostal lymphatic ducts from the lower 6–7 intercostal spaces as well as lymphatic ducts from multiple mediastinal structures. The thoracic duct ascends in the posterior mediastinum to the right of the midline, and the duct crosses midline at the level of T5 and ascends toward the thoracic inlet along the left edge of the esophagus (Fig. 4.4) [9, 14, 19–22].

In the intestines, the lymphatic system also transports nutrients and other substances absorbed from the bowel lumen. Most lymph from the gastrointestinal tract comes from the small intestine, where fluids, extravascular protein, and fat pass into the lymphatics. The increased flow during digestion is mostly from the absorbed water and fat, as protein and carbohydrate ingestion has been found to cause little or no increase in lymph flow. This intestinal lymph, known as chyle, is rich in triglycerides and chylomicrons. The initial lymphatic networks are noncontractile blind-ended vessels lacking smooth muscles and valves [14, 23, 24]. There are two collecting systems in the bowel: the

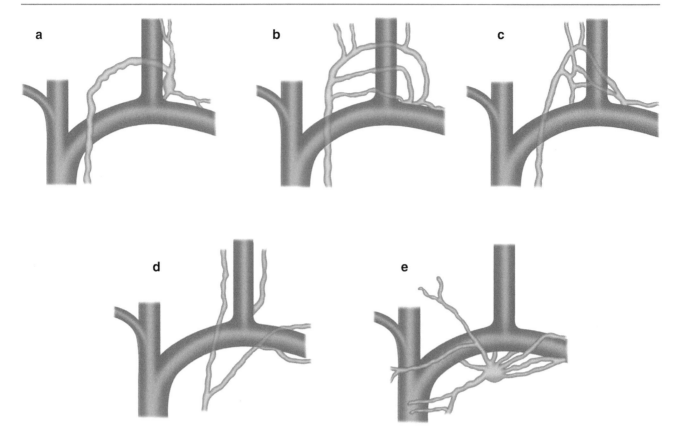

Fig. 4.5 Variations of the entry of the thoracic duct into the venous system. (**a**) Single thoracic duct and a simple junction. (**b**) Plexiform ramification of the final segment of a thoracic duct with a simple junc-

tion. (**c**) Delta-like entry of the thoracic duct. (**d**) Duplication of the final segment of the thoracic duct and two separate junctions. (**e**) Ampullary enlargement of the thoracic duct with multiple terminal branches

intestinal villi with its submucosal network of lymphatics and the muscle layer lymphatic network. These two networks do not form a continuous draining system but intercommunicate extensively. The lymphatics in the villi and the submucosal layer network do not have smooth muscle and rely on intestinal peristalsis to transport chyle upstream. These networks drain into the collecting lymphatics near the mesenteric border of the intestine [25]. These then drain via the intestinal lymphatic trunks to the para-aortic lymph nodes.

The pulmonary lymphatic network is distributed in the connective tissue of the subpleural layer, interlobular septa, intersegmental septa, perivascular space, and peribronchial region. The subpleural, interlobular, and intersegmental septal lymphatics drain along the pulmonary vein into the hilar lymph nodes. Perivascular and peribronchial lymphatics transport lymph to the hila via collecting lymphatics in the bronchial adventitia and by those related to the branches of the pulmonary artery. The right lymphatic duct mainly drains lymph from both lungs, and the thoracic duct predominantly drains the apical portion of the left lung. A chylothorax is formed if there is disruption of this network and chyle collects within the pleural space [26].

Any disruption or disorder in the interconnected chain of this complex collecting system can give rise to diseases of the lymphatic system.

Anatomic Variants

The cisterna chyli is highly inconsistent in appearance and shape. It is most commonly located at the level of L1–L2 in the right paramedian region but may be located midline or left paramedian. It may appear as a fusiform dilated lymphatic channel or a network of several smaller channels. It may be completely absent in 30% of patients [10].

In general, the thoracic duct is more consistent in appearance and is most often seen as a single duct coursing through the chest toward the neck. However, variations are more common in the neck. It may branch into multiple channels in 40–60% of cases, where it may bifurcate or trifurcate prior to draining into the venous angle (Fig. 4.5) [11, 14, 19–22].

Spectrum of Lymphatic Disorders

Abnormal drainage of lymphatic fluid can be due to incompetent or poorly formed lymphatic channels, elevated central venous pressures, or anatomical interruption of the lymphatic channels. The patterns that are commonly seen on MR lymphangiography in the presence of any lymphatic drainage abnormality include (1) non-filling or retarded antegrade flow of contrast from peripheral to central lymphatics; (2) dilated

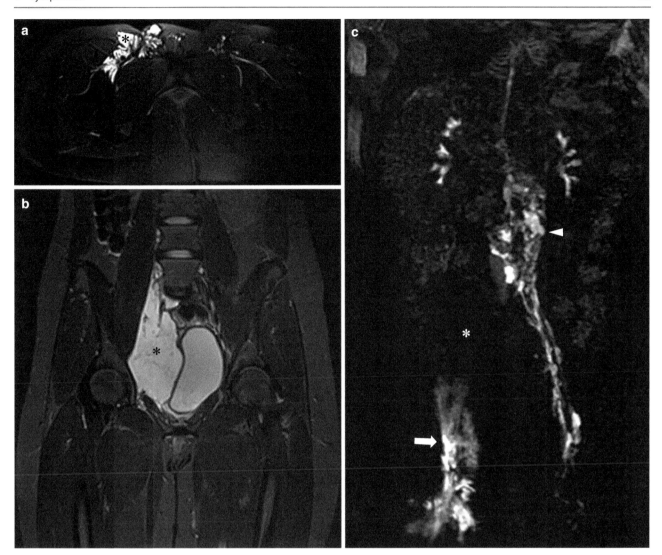

Fig. 4.6 Lymphatic malformation in a 14-year-old girl who presented with swelling and discomfort in the right groin. (**a**) Axial non-enhanced T2-weighted fat-suppressed MR image shows lymphatic macrocysts (∗) in the right inguinal region which represent dilated lymphatic channels. (**b**) Coronal non-enhanced T2-weighted fat-suppressed MR image demonstrates extensive lymphatic macrocysts (∗) in the pelvis which represent dilated central lymphatic channels. (**c**) Coronal maximum intensity projection image of T1-weighted fat-suppressed dynamic contrast-enhanced MR lymphangiogram shows contrast pooling in the right inguinal and pelvic macrocysts (*arrow*) with non-opacification of right iliac lymphatic channels (∗). Also noted are abnormally dilated central lymphatic channels (*arrowhead*)

lymphatic channels; (3) rerouting or anomalous filling of lymphatic channels, typically away from the midline; (4) retrograde filling of lymphatics; and (5) leaks in the retroperitoneal space, peritoneal, pleural, or pericardial cavities.

Congenital Disorders of Central Conducting Lymphatic Anomaly

Central conducting lymphatic anomaly (CCLA) is a broad entity involving several conditions resulting from central conducting lymphatic dysfunction. Affected pediatric patients typically present with chylous ascites, pericardial or pleural effusion, protein-losing enteropathy, plastic bronchitis, and, less frequently, peripheral edema.

When occurring early in life, CCLA may be related to an immature lymphatic system or congenital dysfunctional lymphatic drainage. Resulting dilation of normal lymphatic channels is referred to as primary lymphangiectasia, which is most often secondary to more proximal obstruction, lymphatic valvular incompetence, or aplasia/hypoplasia of the central lymphatic system (Figs. 4.6 and 4.7 and see Figs. 4.1 and 4.2). Primary lymphangiectasia can also involve the pulmonary, intestinal, and hepatic lymphatic vasculature (see Fig. 4.1) [27].

Neonates affected with CCLA often present with chylothorax, chylous ascites, hydrops fetalis, protein-losing enteropathy, or lung disease. In older pediatric patients, these may occur in isolation (e.g., isolated idiopathic chylothorax) or in association with other lymphatic diseases such as generalized lymphatic anomaly (GLA), Gorham disease, Noonan syndrome, and kaposiform lymphangiomatosis (KLA) (Fig. 4.8). The main cause of morbidity and mortality in these patients is deterioration of pulmonary function due to interstitial lung disease and chylothorax.

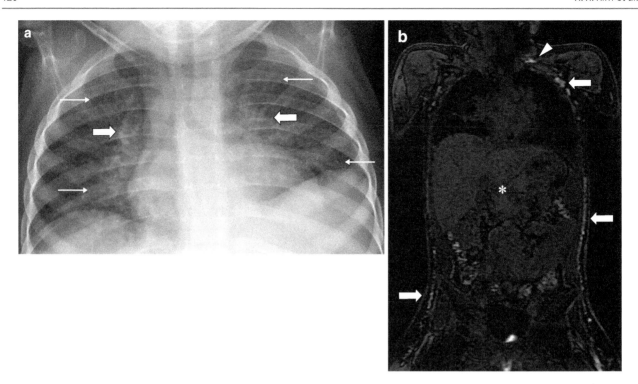

Fig. 4.7 Generalized hereditary lymphedema in a 2-year-old girl who presented with recurrent pulmonary infections and chylous pleural effusions. (**a**) Frontal chest radiograph shows hilar fullness (*large arrows*) and increased interstitial markings (*small arrows*) within the lung parenchyma. (**b**) Coronal T1-weighted fat-suppressed dynamic contrast-enhanced image from MR lymphangiogram shows non-opacification of the central lymphatic channels (*) due to congenital aplasia. There is rerouting of lymphatic flow via the truncal body wall lymphatic channels (*arrows*) to the neck lymphatics at the expected location of the terminal segment of the thoracic duct at the venous angle (*arrowhead*)

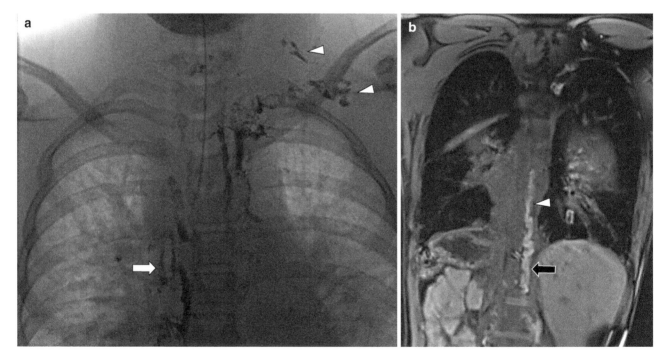

Fig. 4.8 Kaposiform lymphangiomatosis with mediastinal and pulmonary involvement in a 12-year-old girl who presented for the evaluation of central lymphatic system and received sirolimus treatment. (**a**) Frontal chest radiograph obtained during fluoroscopic intranodal lymphangiography demonstrates lymphatic oil contrast reflux to the right peribronchovascular lymphatic channels (*arrow*) and left jugular and subclavian lymphatic channels (*arrowheads*). (**b**) Coronal T1-weighted fat-suppressed dynamic contrast-enhanced image from MR lymphangiogram shows dilated cisterna chyli (*arrow*) and thoracic duct (*arrowhead*). (**c**) Coronal non-enhanced T2-weighted fat-suppressed MR image shows abnormal high signal intensities in the mediastinum (*) extending along the peribronchovascular lymphatic channels (*arrows*) and left supraclavicular region (*arrowhead*) due to lymphatic reflux

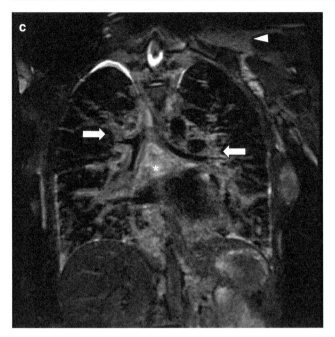

Fig. 4.8 (continued)

MR lymphangiography imaging typically shows anomalous or hypoplastic lymphatic channels, presence of dermal lymphatic flow, dilated incompetent central channels, diminished or absent cranial transition of lymphatic flow, lymphatic reflux, and fluid accumulation. Secondary signs of mesenteric edema, bowel wall edema, or peribronchial interstitial thickening with opacification and formation of collateral lymphatic vessels may be seen. The specific location of the possible chylous leak may not always be detected. Occasionally, the terminal segment of the thoracic duct at the venous angle is dysfunctional, and it may remain unopacified on MR lymphangiography or exhibit aberrant anatomy with reflux of contrast into the cervical lymphatics (Fig. 4.9). If the thoracic duct is occluded at the level of the neck, a microsurgical thoracic duct-to-vein connection can be considered. Percutaneous embolization is contraindicated in these cases [9, 28].

The finding of abnormal pulmonary lymphatic flow away from the thoracic duct toward the lung parenchyma and mediastinum and through aberrant lymphatics is known as pulmonary lymphatic perfusion syndrome (PLPS) which can cause chylous effusions and plastic bronchitis [9]. Plastic bronchitis is a rare condition characterized by a branching bronchial cast, which is formed by exudation of protein-rich

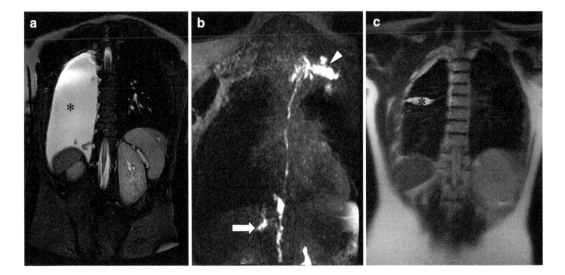

Fig. 4.9 Recurrent chylous pleural effusion and bony abnormalities of the right clavicle, lower cervical vertebral bodies, and right ribs in a 13-year-old girl who presented for the evaluation of central lymphatic system. (a) Coronal non-enhanced T2-weighted MR image shows a large right pleural effusion (∗). (b) Coronal maximum intensity projection (MIP) image of T1-weighted, fat-suppressed dynamic contrast-enhanced MR lymphangiogram shows abnormal lymphatic contrast reflux into a right lower intercostal lymphatic channel (*arrow*) and into the left jugular and subclavian lymphatic channels (*arrowhead*). (c) Coronal non-enhanced T2-weighted MR image following sirolimus treatment shows significant treatment response compared to pretreatment imaging, with only a small right pleural effusion (∗)

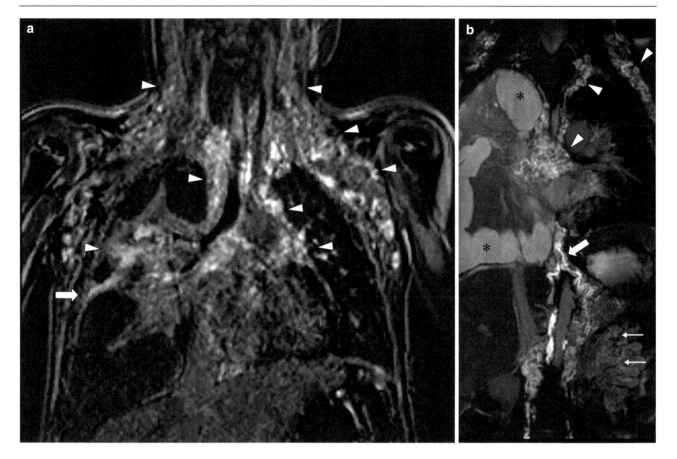

Fig. 4.10 Chylous pleural effusion due to elevated central venous pressure in a 5-year-old boy status post-fenestrated Fontan procedure for treatment of hypoplastic left heart syndrome. (**a**) Coronal T1-weighted fat-suppressed dynamic contrast-enhanced image from MR lymphangiogram shows extensive infiltrative lymphatics in the mediastinal, peribronchovascular, jugular, subclavian, and axillary regions (*arrowheads*). There is contrast extravasation and pooling in the right pleural space (*arrow*). (**b**) Coronal maximum intensity projection (MIP) image of T1-weighted fat-suppressed dynamic contrast-enhanced MR lymphangiogram shows congestion and lymphatic reflux in the mediastinal, cervical, and axillary lymphatic channels (*arrowheads*) and the right-sided chylous pleural effusion (∗). Also noted are the dilated intestinal lymphatic trunk (*large arrow*) and the mesenteric lymphatic channels (*small arrows*) secondary to lymphatic reflux

chyle into the airway. The cast may obstruct the airway and can lead to respiratory insufficiency or even asphyxia. These conditions may be treated with venolymphatic anastomosis, although the long-term benefit of this procedure has not been thoroughly evaluated [29, 30]. MR lymphangiography is also useful for the evaluation of response following medical or surgical treatment (see Figs. 4.8 and 4.9).

Iatrogenic Disorders of Central Conducting Lymphatic Anomaly

Surgical procedures near the central lymphatic ducts can be complicated by inadvertent injury. Most commonly, this occurs following surgery for congenital cardiac disease, with an incidence of 2.8–3.9% [31, 32]. Additionally, procedures that result in elevated right heart pressures such as Fontan and Glenn procedures may result in postoperative chylothorax and chronic plastic bronchitis (Fig. 4.10) [32, 33].

Surgical procedures to treat cysts arising from the lymphatic system in the abdomen and pelvis can result in significant chylous ascites. Dynamic MR lymphangiography can reveal the leak and underlying dysfunctional central lymphatic system (Fig. 4.11).

Pediatric patients with long-term central lines in the left-sided central veins may develop central venous stenosis at the venous angle resulting in occlusion of the thoracic duct or lymphatic reflux due to elevated central pressure. These

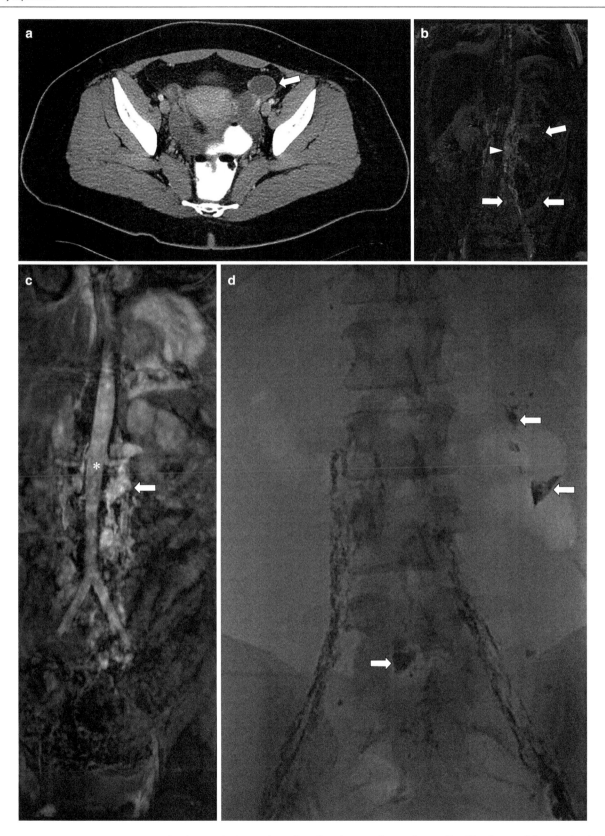

Fig. 4.11 Recurrent chylous ascites following surgical resection of adnexal pelvic cysts in a 23-year-old female who presented for the evaluation of central lymphatic system. The cysts were reported as lymphatic cysts on surgical pathology. (**a**) Axial enhanced CT image of the pelvis before surgical resection shows non-enhancing adnexal lymphatic macrocysts (*arrow*). (**b**) Coronal maximum intensity projection image of T1-weighted fat-suppressed dynamic contrast-enhanced MR lym- phangiogram shows abnormally dilated central lymphatic channels (*arrowhead*) and droplets of free contrast into the peritoneal cavity (*arrows*). (**c**) Coronal enhanced SSFP image shows the lymphatic channels (*arrow*) in relation to the vessels (∗). (**d**) Frontal radiograph of the abdomen obtained during fluoroscopic intranodal lymphangiography confirms the extravasation (*arrows*) of oil contrast into the peritoneal cavity

patients present with abnormal central lymphatic flow, pericardial or pleural chylous effusion, and pulmonary parenchymal lymphatic reflux and infrequently with features of plastic bronchitis.

Conclusion

MR lymphangiography is an excellent and noninvasive imaging modality to identify specific areas of lymphatic obstruction, leak, or abnormal perfusion. It is an invaluable tool to evaluate the outcome of a medical or surgical treatment of a central conducting lymphatic anomaly in the pediatric population. MR imaging has emerged as an essential tool in the evaluation of lymphatic disorders and continues to evolve and advance with the emergence of newer imaging sequences and higher-strength magnetic fields.

References

1. Shaikh R, Biko DM, Lee EY. MR imaging evaluation of pediatric lymphatics: overview of techniques and imaging findings. Magn Reson Imaging Clin. 2019;27(2):373–85.
2. Dori Y. Novel lymphatic imaging techniques. Tech Vasc Interv Radiol. 2016;19(4):255–61.
3. Krishnamurthy R, Hernandez A, Kavuk S, Annam A, Pimpalwar S. Imaging the central conducting lymphatics: initial experience with dynamic MR lymphangiography. Radiology. 2015;274(3):871–8.
4. Weiss M, Baumeister RG, Tatsch K, Hahn K. Lymphoscintigraphy for non-invasive long term follow-up of functional outcome in patients with autologous lymph vessel transplantation. Nuklearmedizin. 1996;35(6):236–42.. [Article in German]
5. Weissleder H, Weissleder R. Lymphedema: evaluation of qualitative and quantitative lymphoscintigraphy in 238 patients. Radiology. 1988;167(3):729–35.
6. Sheybani A, Gaba RC, Minocha J. Cerebral embolization of ethiodized oil following intranodal lymphangiography. Semin Intervent Radiol. 2015;32(1):10–3.
7. Alomari MH, Lillis A, Kerr C, Newburger JW, Quinonez L, Alomari AI. The use of non-ionic contrast agent for lymphangiography and embolization of the thoracic duct. Cardiovasc Intervent Radiol. 2019;42(3):481–3.
8. Cherella CE, Breault DT, Thaker V, Levine B-S, Smith JR. Early identification of primary hypothyroidism in neonates exposed to intralymphatic iodinated contrast: a case series. J Clin Endocrinol Metab. 2018;103(10):3585–8.
9. Chavhan GB, Amaral JG, Temple M, Itkin M. MR lymphangiography in children: technique and potential applications. Radiographics. 2017;37(6):1775–90.
10. Notohamiprodjo M, Baumeister RG, Jakobs TF, Bauner KU, Boehm HF, Horng A, et al. MR-lymphangiography at 3.0 T—a feasibility study. Eur Radiol. 2009;19(11):2771–8.
11. Pamarthi V, Pabon-Ramos WM, Marnell V, Hurwitz LM. MRI of the central lymphatic system: indications, imaging technique, and pre-procedural planning. Top Magn Reson Imaging. 2017;26(4):175–80.
12. Louveau A, Smirnov I, Keyes TJ, Eccles JD, Rouhani SJ, Peske JD, et al. Structural and functional features of central nervous system lymphatic vessels. Nature. 2015;523(7560):337–41.
13. Williams KR, Burford TH. The management of chylothorax. Ann Surg. 1964;160:131–40.
14. Hsu MC, Itkin M. Lymphatic anatomy. Tech Vasc Interv Radiol. 2016;19(4):247–54.
15. Van der Putte S, Van Limborgh J. The embryonic development of the main lymphatics in man. Acta Morphol Neerl Scand. 1980;18(4):323–35.
16. Földi M, Földi E, Strößenreuther R, Kubik S. Földi's textbook of lymphology: for physicians and lymphedema therapists. Philadelphia: Elsevier; 2012.
17. El-Chemaly S, Levine SJ, Moss J. Lymphatics in lung disease. Ann N Y Acad Sci. 2008;1131:195–202.
18. Levick J, McHale N. The physiology of lymph production and propulsion. In: Browse N, Burnand K, Mortimer PS, editors. Diseases of the lymphatics. London: Arnold (Hodder); 2003. p. 44–64.
19. Loukas M, Wartmann CT, Louis RG Jr, Tubbs RS, Salter EG, Gupta AA, et al. Cisterna chyli: a detailed anatomic investigation. Clin Anat. 2007;20(6):683–8.
20. Hematti H, Mehran RJ. Anatomy of the thoracic duct. Thorac Surg Clin. 2011;21(2):229–38.
21. Riquet M, Barthes FLP, Souilamas R, Hidden G. Thoracic duct tributaries from intrathoracic organs. Ann Thorac Surg. 2002;73(3):892–8.
22. Skandalakis JE, Skandalakis LJ, Skandalakis PN. Anatomy of the lymphatics. Surg Oncol Clin N Am. 2007;16(1):1–16.
23. Schmid-Schonbein GW. Microlymphatics and lymph flow. Physiol Rev. 1990;70(4):987–1028.
24. Loukas M, Bellary SS, Kuklinski M, Ferrauiola J, Yadav A, Shoja MM, et al. The lymphatic system: a historical perspective. Clin Anat. 2011;24(7):807–16.
25. Unthank JL, Bohlen HG. Lymphatic pathways and role of valves in lymph propulsion from small intestine. Am J Physiol. 1988;254(3. Pt 1):G389–98.
26. McGrath EE, Blades Z, Anderson PB. Chylothorax: aetiology, diagnosis and therapeutic options. Respir Med. 2010;104(1):1–8.
27. Esther CR Jr, Barker PM. Pulmonary lymphangiectasia: diagnosis and clinical course. Pediatr Pulmonol. 2004;38(4):308–13.
28. Taghinia AH, Upton J, Trenor CC III, Alomari AI, Lillis AP, Shaikh R, et al. Lymphaticovenous bypass of the thoracic duct for the treatment of chylous leak in central conducting lymphatic anomalies. J Pediatr Surg. 2019;54(3):562–8.
29. Melduni RM, Oh JK, Bunch TJ, Sinak LJ, Gloviczki P. Reconstruction of occluded thoracic duct for treatment of chylopericardium: a novel surgical therapy. J Vasc Surg. 2008;48(6):1600–2.
30. Schild HH, Strassburg CP, Welz A, Kalff J. Treatment options in patients with chylothorax. Dtsch Arztebl Int. 2013;110(48):819–26.
31. Bauman ME, Moher C, Bruce AK, Kuhle S, Kaur S, Massicotte MP. Chylothorax in children with congenital heart disease: incidence of thrombosis. Thromb Res. 2013;132(2):e83–5.
32. Mery CM, Moffett BS, Khan MS, Zhang W, Guzman-Pruneda FA, Fraser CD Jr, et al. Incidence and treatment of chylothorax after cardiac surgery in children: analysis of a large multi-institution database. J Thorac Cardiovasc Surg. 2014;147(2):678–86.e1; discussion 85–6.
33. Dori Y, Keller MS, Rome JJ, Gillespie MJ, Glatz AC, Dodds K, et al. Percutaneous lymphatic embolization of abnormal pulmonary lymphatic flow as treatment of plastic bronchitis in patients with congenital heart disease. Circulation. 2016;133(12):1160–70.

Mediastinum

Alison R. Hart and Edward Y. Lee

Introduction

The mediastinum is the most common location of chest masses in the pediatric patient. The large number of structures contained within the mediastinum and the numerous pathologies which originate in the mediastinum complicates diagnosis and highlights the importance of imaging. While traditionally utilized as problem-solving tool for other modalities such as radiography, ultrasound, and computed tomography (CT), the use of MR imaging in the workup, treatment planning, and evaluation of response in mediastinal pathology is increasing, particularly in the pediatric population.

This chapter discusses up-to-date MR imaging techniques including pediatric patient preparation as well as MR imaging pulse sequences and protocols. In addition, mediastinal anatomy including embryology, normal development, and anatomic variants are reviewed. Furthermore, selected pediatric mediastinal disorders that are encountered in daily clinical practice are discussed based on a practical three mediastinal compartmental imaging approach.

Magnetic Resonance Imaging Techniques

Patient Preparation

MR imaging provides superior soft tissue characterization capability and precise anatomic detail making it an ideal imaging modality to evaluate the pediatric mediastinum. Specific MR imaging sequences can be utilized in imaging the mediastinum to highlight inherent differences in tissue characteristics. For example, MR imaging is capable of differentiating cystic from solid lesions and can demonstrate intralesional fat [1]. Unlike CT where image generation requires the use of potentially harmful ionizing radiation, MR imaging is acquired without ionizing radiation. This is an important advantage in the imaging of pediatric patients who are more susceptible to the potentially harmful effects of radiation [2].

Chest MR imaging is specifically challenging in children as image quality is directly linked to patient cooperation [3]. Motion in chest MR imaging may be secondary to physiologic cardiac and respiratory motion or due to body movement. Patient motion in MR imaging can successfully be reduced in children over the age of 6 years through the use of simulation, distraction techniques, coaching, explanation, and reassurance [1]. Despite these measures, sedation is frequently required in children less than 6 years of age, those with cognitive disability, or children with hearing problems, claustrophobia, or anxiety [3]. Cardiac motion artifacts may be reduced through the use of cardiac gating in which the cardiac cycle is monitored and images acquired only during diastole [4]. Respiratory motion may be minimized by breath holding, although this may be difficult to accomplish in young pediatric patients. Rapid pulse sequences or respiratory gating may be utilized to limit respiratory motion with the caveat that respiratory gating requires longer sequence time, thereby increasing examination length [4].

MR Imaging Pulse Sequences and Protocols

MR imaging of the chest can be performed at 1.5 Tesla (T) or 3.0 T MRI scanners (Table 5.1). Imaging at higher field strength increases both signal-to-noise ratio and contrast-to-noise ratio improving both the spatial and temporal resolution of acquired images [1]. Phased array receiver coils are generally preferred because they are closer in proximity to the intrathoracic structures. This shorter distance increases

A. R. Hart
Diagnostic Imaging, Rhode Island Hospital, Brown University, Providence, RI, USA

E. Y. Lee (✉)
Division of Thoracic Imaging, Department of Radiology, Boston Children's Hospital, Harvard Medical School, Boston, MA, USA
e-mail: Edward.Lee@childrens.harvard.edu

Table 5.1 Pediatric Mediastinal Mass MR Imaging Protocols

Mediastinal mass screening protocol	Mediastinal mass characterization protocol
3 PLANE LOC	3 PLANE LOC
AX T1 VIBE DIXON	AX T1 VIBE DIXON
COR T2 FS	AX T2 FS
AX T2 FS	COR T2 FS
	AX FSE DIR T2

LOC localizer, *AX* axial, *VIBE* volumetric interpolated breath-hold sequence, *COR* coronal, *FS* fat suppression, *FSE* fast spin echo, *DIR* double inversion recovery

signal-to-noise ratio while decreasing imaging time through the use of parallel imaging [3].

MR sequences utilized in the evaluation of the mediastinum should be selected based on the clinical question. T1-weighted, T2-weighted, pre-, and post-contrast fat-suppressed sequences are the mainstays of MR imaging evaluation. Fat suppression techniques are utilized to minimize the signal from the adipose tissue and improve contrast. Gradient echo in- and out-of-phase imaging can allow for the detection of microscopic fat via chemical shift [3]. Dynamic contrast imaging with chelated extracellular gadolinium agents can also provide detailed information as to the degree of vascularity, pattern of enhancement, and proximity to adjacent mediastinal structures such as vessels [1].

Anatomy

Embryology

Because of the myriad of anatomic structures contained within the mediastinum, its development results from the complex interplay of numerous primordial structures. The primordium of the body cavities arises during the fourth week from the partitioning of the intraembryonic coelom into three well-defined spaces: the pericardial, paired pericardioperitoneal canals, and peritoneal cavities [5]. The septum transversum is the first partition to form, later to become the central tendon of the diaphragm, thereby separating the pericardial and peritoneal cavities. Arranged lateral to the proximal foregut, the coronally oriented, paired pericardioperitoneal canals later partition to become the pleural and pericardial cavities.

Simultaneously within the fourth week, the tracheoesophageal septum arises at the caudal foregut partitioning the ventral laryngotracheal tube (the origin of the larynx, trachea, bronchi, and lungs) from a dorsal component later destined to become the oropharynx and esophagus [5]. From the laryngotracheal tube, a ventral diverticulum forms from which the respiratory bud is derived [6]. Further division of the respiratory bud produces left and right bronchial buds, the future lungs, which grow into the pericardioperitoneal canals [6].

Growth of the primordial bronchial buds into the pericardioperitoneal canals stimulates the development of a membranous ridge at the lateral wall of each canal, the pleuropericardial

and pleuroperitoneal folds. The pleuroperitoneal folds extend ventromedially from the dorsolateral abdominal wall fusing with the dorsal mesentery of the esophagus and septum transversum in the sixth week of gestation, an action through which the pleural and peritoneal cavities are defined [6]. The pleuropericardial folds grow medially to surround the heart ultimately fusing with one another and the ventral foregut during the seventh week of gestation, thus defining pleural and pericardial cavities [6] (Fig. 5.1). This combined fusion of the pleuropericardial and pleuroperitoneal folds thus creates the mediastinum and the diaphragm [7].

The nervous system arises during the third week of gestation. The neural plate folds to become the neural tube. Neural crest cells, a specialized cell population which arise from the dorsal neural tube, then become precursors to spinal and autonomic ganglia and Schwann cells [5]. Myelin sheaths, which form around nerve fibers in the spinal cord, originate from oligodendrocytes derived from neuroepithelium through a process which begins during the late fetal period and continues during the first postnatal year [6]. The osseous structures of the thorax originate from thickening of the intraembryonic mesoderm. This mesoderm arises lateral to the neural tube and ultimately differentiates into somites and then sclerotomes from which the vertebral bodies and ribs are derived [6].

The heart arises from cardiogenic precursors within the mesoderm which form the primary heart tube within the fourth week of gestational life. The heart tube then loops, remodels, realigns, and septates to form the embryonic heart [5]. The dominant venous structures in the thorax stem from the common cardinal veins which are initially contained within the pleuropericardial membranes [6]. The great arterial vessels arise from paired aortic arches which then attach to the primitive heart tube [5].

Arising from the anterior endodermal foregut, the pharyngeal organs, including the thyroid, thymus, and parathyroid glands, originate from paired branchial pouches. The thymus typically arises from the third ventral pharyngeal pouch. It

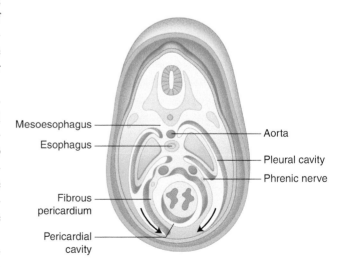

Fig. 5.1 Primordial mediastinum during the seventh week of gestation

then elongates and descends to fuse at the midline, anterior to the aortic arch, by the eighth gestational week [7]. During this process, the thymopharyngeal duct contained within the thymic buds obliterates [8]. During the tenth week of gestation, lymphoid cells migrate into the thymus [9].

Normal Development and Anatomy

The mediastinum can be compartmentalized in an attempt to better localize mediastinal abnormalities and aid in the formulation of an appropriate differential diagnosis (Fig. 5.2)

Fig. 5.2 Mediastinal compartment. (**a**) Coronal view of the anatomic definition. (**b**) Sagittal view of the anatomic definitions

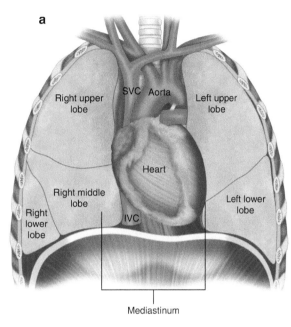

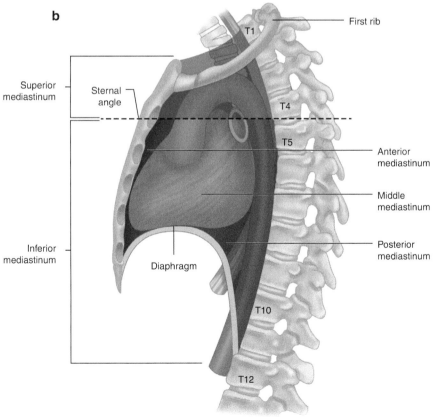

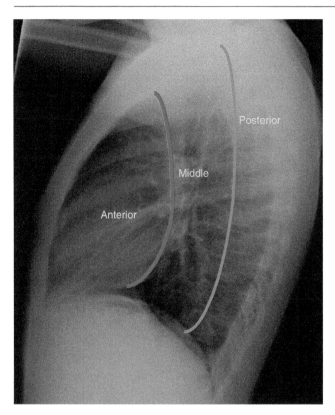

Fig. 5.3 Annotated sagittal chest radiograph demonstrating the traditional anatomic imaging delineation of the anterior, middle, and posterior mediastinal compartments

This compartmentalization was historically accomplished via the nonanatomic division of the lateral chest radiograph [10] (Fig. 5.3). While invaluable for the identification of mediastinal lesions on radiography, the availability of multiple classification models limited the localization of some mediastinal lesions and was a source of confusion among providers of different specialties [11]. More recently, a new system of division has been adopted to standardize the classification of mediastinal lesions based upon specific anatomy which can be readily identified on cross-sectional imaging [11].

The three compartments of the International Thymic Malignancy Interest Group (ITMIG) model (prevascular, visceral, and paravertebral) can be thought of similarly to the classic anterior, middle, and posterior compartments defined radiographically (Fig. 5.4) (Table 5.2). Each compartment is bordered superiorly by the thoracic inlet and inferiorly by the diaphragm. The thoracic inlet is defined by the osseous structures at the superior aspect of the thorax including the superior cortex of the manubrium, the bilateral first ribs, and the superior endplate of the first thoracic vertebral body [11].

The prevascular compartment (anterior mediastinum) is bound anteriorly by the sternum, posteriorly by the pericardium, and laterally by the parietal pleura [11]. The

structures in the prevascular compartment thus include the thymus, lymph nodes, adipose tissue, internal mammary vessels, and left brachiocephalic vein. The visceral compartment (middle mediastinum) is bordered anteriorly by the pericardium and posteriorly by a vertical line positioned 1 cm posterior to the anterior margin of the thoracic vertebral bodies [11]. Thus, the visceral compartment can be further subdivided into vascular (the heart, great vessels, and thoracic duct) and nonvascular structures (the tracheobronchial tree, the esophagus, and the lymph nodes). The paravertebral compartment (posterior mediastinum) begins at the posterior margin of the visceral compartment, 1 cm posterior to the anterior margin of the thoracic vertebral bodies, and extends posteriorly to the chest wall and laterally to the transverse processes of the thoracic vertebral bodies [11]. The structures contained within this compartment thus include the thoracic spine and paravertebral soft tissues including the thoracic nerve roots.

While the classification of mediastinal structures to a respective compartment is helpful to guide diagnosis, intervention, and treatment, large lesions which span multiple compartments are inherently difficult to categorize. Two methods, first described on CT but which can be readily extrapolated for use on MR imaging, can thus be helpful to the radiologist tasked with the localization of mediastinal lesions. The first, the "center method," defines the center of the mediastinal abnormality and thus its appropriate compartment on the basis of the axial image at the site of greatest axial dimension [12]. The second, the "structure displacement tool," further helps to define a lesion's mediastinal compartment through careful examination of the structures with which it displaces. For example, a large lesion centered in the prevascular (anterior) mediastinum may exert local mass effect on anterior mediastinal structures as well as posterior mass effect on visceral (middle) compartment structures [12].

Anatomic Variants

Ectopic Thymus

The thymus is a bilobed, H-shaped, homogeneous organ which drapes over the structures within prevascular/anterior mediastinum. Critical to the maturation and differentiation of T cells, the thymus plays a central role in cellular immunity [13]. In pediatric patients less than 5 years of age, the thymus is prominent with a quadrilateral shape and convex margins. After the age of 5 years, the thymus gradually decreases in size, becomes less prominent, and has a triangular morphology. With age, the thymic margins continue to straighten. The thymus reaches its maximum weight in adolescence undergoing progressive replacement

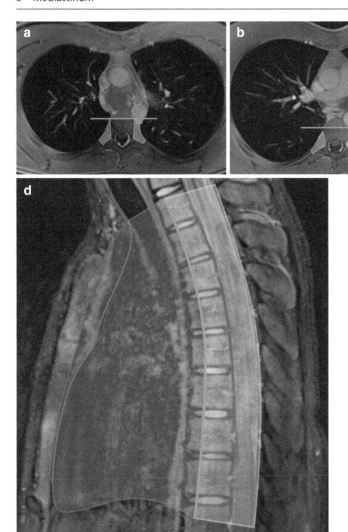

Fig. 5.4 MRI adaptation of the CT-based mediastinal compartment scheme developed by the International Thymic Malignancy Interest Group (ITMIG). Axial T2-weighted fat-suppressed MR images just below the level of the aortic arch (**a**), at the level of the main pulmonary artery (**b**), and at the level of the heart (**c**) show the prevascular/anterior (*red*), visceral/middle (*green*), and paravertebral/posterior (*yellow*) mediastinal compartments. (**d**) Sagittal T2-weighted fat-suppressed MR image demonstrates the three compartments in the sagittal plane

Table 5.2 MR imaging characteristics and locations of mediastinal masses in the pediatric population

	Soft tissue component	Fat component	Fluid component
Anterior (prevascular) mediastinal masses	Ectopic thymus	Thymolipoma	Thymic cyst
	Thymic herniation	Germ cell tumor	Lymphatic malformation
	Thymoma		
	Thymic carcinoma		
	Lymphoma		
	Midline NUT cell tumor		
Middle (visceral) mediastinal masses	Infectious lymphadenopathy		Foregut duplication cyst
	Neoplastic lymphadenopathy		
	Sarcoidosis		
	Castleman disease		
Posterior (paravertebral) mediastinal masses	Sympathetic chain ganglion origin tumors	Extramedullary hematopoiesis	Neurogenic cyst
	Nerve root origin tumors		

by fibrofatty tissue thereafter. In adults, the residual thymus weighs less than half its weight at infancy and is not readily identifiable [13].

The thymus demonstrates homogenous intermediate T2 signal intensity and mild T1 hyperintensity with respect to muscle. Given the changing composition of the thymus with age, it is not surprising that the MR imaging signal characteristics of the thymus shift. As a child grows, there is increasing thymic T1 hyperintensity to reflect the increasing percentage of intracellular fat. Similarly, the out-of-phase gradient echo sequence can be compared to in-phase gradient sequences; fatty thymic tissue drops in signal intensity on out-of-phase images reflective of the degree of fat infiltration.

Accessory thymic tissue results due to rests of normal thymic tissue along the path of thymic descent. Accordingly, accessory thymic tissue can occur anywhere along the course of the thymopharyngeal duct from the mandible to the superior mediastinum [7]. One such variant, the retrocaval thymus, is the result of posterior extension of accessory thymic tissue interposed between the superior vena cava and great arteries. Although retrocaval thymus can mimic a mediastinal mass or right upper lobe mass on chest radiography, cross-sectional MR imaging evaluation demonstrates continuity with the normally positioned thymus and homogenous signal characteristics. Ectopic thymic tissue, conversely, is

presumably the result of an aberrant migration pathway leading to the presence of thymic tissue in abnormal locations, including the base of the skull [13] (Fig. 5.5).

Thymic Herniation

Suprasternal extension of the thymus is a commonly documented phenomenon in infants [13]. In these cases, no luminal tracheal narrowing or respiratory symptoms result although the abnormality may be alarming to caregivers and providers as a palpable mass is frequently present [14]. More rarely, cases of intermittent herniation of the mediastinal thymus into the neck with Valsalva maneuver have been reported in older children presumably on the basis of loose mediastinal connective tissue [15]. Demonstration of homogenous tissue in continuity with the normal mediastinal thymic tissue is diagnostic on both neck ultrasound and MR imaging (Fig. 5.6). Dynamic MR imaging performed with and without Valsalva maneuver can be performed to isolate the abnormality if it occurs intermittently [15].

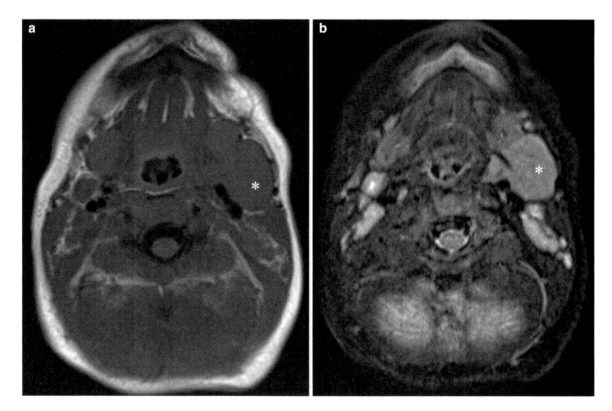

Fig. 5.5 Ectopic thymic tissue (histologically proven) in a 5-month-old boy with seizures and incidentally found left submandibular mass. (a) Axial T1-weighted fat-suppressed MR image demonstrates a circumscribed mass (*asterisk*) which is isointense to skeletal muscle and located in the left neck posterior to the left submandibular gland. (b) Axial T2-weighted fat-suppressed MR image shows that the mass (*asterisk*) is

hyperintense to skeletal muscle. (c) Coronal T2-weighted fat-suppressed MR images demonstrate the inferior extension of the mass (*asterisk*) into the infrahyoid neck. The normal thymus is observed within the superior mediastinum (*arrowhead*). (d) Axial T1-weighted post-contrast MR image demonstrates mild enhancement with tissue architecture suggestive of glandular ectopic thymus (*asterisk*)

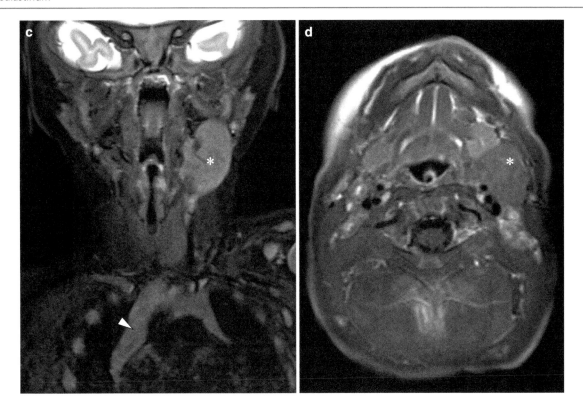

Fig. 5.5 (continued)

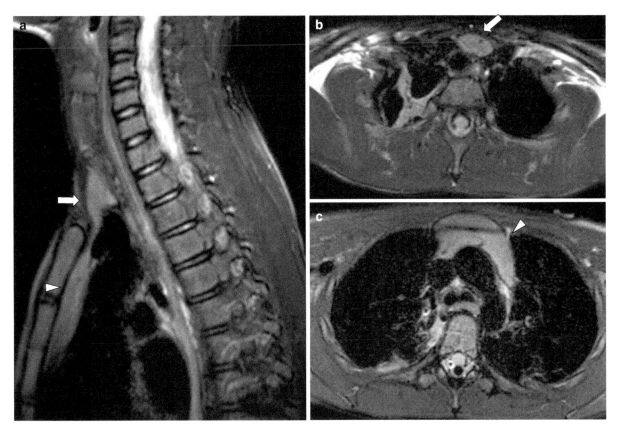

Fig. 5.6 Herniation of thymic tissue into the neck in a 10-year-old boy who presented with palpable neck mass. (**a**) Sagittal T2-weighted fat-suppressed MR image demonstrates extension of homogenous signal intensity tissue (*arrow*) above the sternal notch into the neck in continuity with the normal retrosternal thymus (*arrowhead*). (**b**) Axial T2-weighted fat-suppressed MR image at the thoracic inlet level shows thymus (*arrow*) herniating into the neck. (**c**) Axial T2-weighted fat-suppressed MR image at the level of the aortic arch shows the normal thymus (*arrowhead*), which is identical in signal and contiguous with the herniated thymus

Spectrum of Mediastinal Disorders

Anterior (Prevascular) Mediastinal Lesions

Congenital Disorders

Aplasia or Hypoplasia of the Thymus Rarely, thymic hypoplasia or complete aplasia may occur, most frequently in the setting of a global immunodeficiency syndrome such as DiGeorge syndrome or severe combined immunodeficiency (SCID) (Fig. 5.7). DiGeorge syndrome is caused by a chromosomal 22 deletion. This deletion leads to abnormal formation of the third and fourth pharyngeal pouches during embryologic development from which the thymus and the parathyroid glands are formed [13]. Varying severity of primary T-cell deficiency may result. Lack of T cells predisposes patients to disseminated viral, fungal, and parasitic infections and abnormal antibody response [16]. Affected pediatric patients also may suffer from hypoparathyroidism and cardiovascular anomalies. Additionally, characteristic facial features are associated with DiGeorge syndrome which include micrognathia, low-set ears, and hypertelorism [16].

Severe combined immunodeficiency (SCID) syndromes are a group of disorders characterized by the absence of T and B cells. Inherited in either X-linked or recessive fashion, SCID is universally fatal without immune reconstitution due to the development of severe opportunistic infections early in life. As T cells are absent and therefore do not migrate into the thymus, there is abnormal thymic development. This manifests in aplasia or severe thymic hypoplasia [13].

Lastly, relative absence of the thymus on imaging may result from prior cardiothoracic surgery. A median sternotomy for anterior approach to the heart routinely requires removal of the thymus [17]. Thus, pediatric patients who

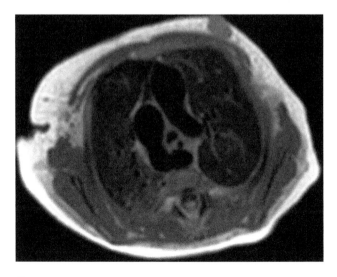

Fig. 5.7 Aplasia of the thymus in a 3-week-old girl with DiGeorge syndrome. Axial proton-density black blood turbo spin echo MR image shows a complete aplasia of the thymus. A right-sided aortic arch is also seen

have undergone median sternotomy may appear to lack a thymus on subsequent imaging. As a result, these patients may demonstrate decreased peripheral T-cell count and impaired T-cell maturation though the implications between this and future infection or malignancy is unknown [17].

Benign Neoplastic Disorders

Thymic Cyst A thymic cyst is a remnant of the embryonic thymopharyngeal duct and thus can occur anywhere along the course of the thymopharyngeal duct from the piriform sinus to the mediastinum. Most, however, are associated with the carotid sheath and lateral infrahyoid neck. In some cases, a fibrous connection with the thymus may persist. Although usually asymptomatic, symptoms such as respiratory distress or dysphagia can result from mass effect upon adjacent structures if lesions become large. Rare in adults, thymic cysts are most commonly diagnosed before the second decade of life. Complete surgical resection is the treatment of choice once such lesions are diagnosed with excellent prognosis.

While visualization of Hassall's corpuscles confirms the diagnosis histologically, prior to surgical resection, cross-sectional imaging plays an important role in determining the presence, location, and extent of such lesions [18]. Due to superior soft tissue contrast resolution as compared with CT and especially useful in cases where attenuation characteristics are indeterminate, MR imaging evaluation can better differentiate cystic versus solid lesions. Thymic cysts are typically uniformly hyperintense on T2-weighted images and may show variable signal intensity on T1-weighted images (Fig. 5.8). Lesions containing serous fluid are hypointense on T1-weighted images, whereas lesions complicated by hemorrhage or infection may be hyperintense on T1-weighted images [19]. Lesions may be comprised of a large, dominant cyst or multiloculated. Following contrast administration, there is no internal enhancement. Thin mural and septal enhancement may occur. Occasionally, mural nodularity and thickening may be present, usually secondary to prior infection or hemorrhage.

Many differential possibilities exist for simple or multiloculated cystic lesions in the mediastinum including lymphatic malformation, brachial cleft cyst, thyroglossal duct cyst, foregut duplication cyst, and germ cell tumor. Cystic changes may be seen within a mediastinal mass, including Hodgkin lymphoma or other neoplastic processes [20].

Thymolipoma Thymolipomas are rare, benign lesions comprised of thymic tissue and fibrous septae interwoven with macroscopic fat [18]. The amount of fat within the lesion is commonly 50–85%, although lesions with up to 95% fat have been reported [11]. Given their slow growth and pliability due to the predominance of fat, thymolipomas can easily conform to adjacent mediastinal structures oftentimes growing quite large prior to their discovery. Thus, most are incidentally discovered on chest radiograph, where

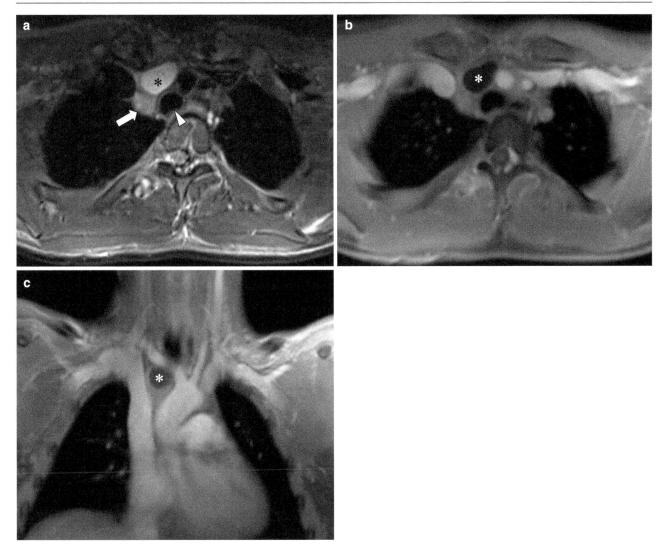

Fig. 5.8 Incidentally found thymic cyst in a 16-year-old boy who presented for evaluation of right scapular pain following a sports injury (confirmed upon surgical resection). (**a**) Axial T2-weighted fat-suppressed MR image demonstrates a well-circumscribed, unilocular hyperintense lesion (*asterisk*) in the anterior mediastinum located anterolateral to the trachea (*arrowhead*) on the right surrounded by normal thymus (*arrow*). (**b**) Axial T1-weighted fat-suppressed post-contrast MR image shows no contrast enhancement within the thymic cyst (*asterisk*). (**c**) Coronal T1-weighted fat-suppressed post-contrast MR image shows no contrast enhancement within the thymic cyst (*asterisk*)

they can easily be confused for more common causes of mediastinal enlargement such as cardiomegaly or a pericardial tumor. Symptoms may result due to mass effect on adjacent mediastinal structures and include dyspnea, cough, arrhythmia, and chest pain. Rare associations with myasthenia gravis, aplastic anemia, thyrotoxicosis, and Graves' disease has been reported [21]. Unless symptomatic, no treatment is required for thymolipomas.

Due to the combination of fat and thymic tissue, thymolipomas characteristically demonstrate a whorled appearance on cross-sectional imaging [21]. The lesion is well-defined and contained by a capsule without invasion into adjacent mediastinal structures. On MR imaging, lesions demonstrate mixed signal on T1-weighted images. On T1-weighted images, linear bands of hyperintense fat are interspersed with hypointense bands of thymic and fibrous tissue which are similar in intensity to adjacent skeletal muscle (Fig. 5.9).

Germ Cell Tumor Prior to the sixth week of development, germ cells traverse the mediastinum as they descend caudally from the yolk sac. As germ cells give rise to gametes in both sexes, they migrate to the gut tube and then via the gut mesentery to the genital ridge [5]. Premature arrest therefore may result in rests of germ cells at extragonadal locations. Germ cell tumors are the third most common mediastinal mass in children, accounting for 6–15% of all mediastinal tumors [22]. Germ cell tumors frequently appear as fat-containing masses within the mediastinum. Teratoma, a tumor derived from tissues of all three germ cells layers, is the most common subtype of extragonadal germ cell tumor within the mediastinum [20].

Germ cell tumors can be broadly divided into three subtypes: teratoma (including mature, immature, and teratoma with malignant transformation), seminoma, and nonseminomatous malignant germ cell tumor. Seminomatous germ cell tumors are the most likely to be malignant [23]. Approximately

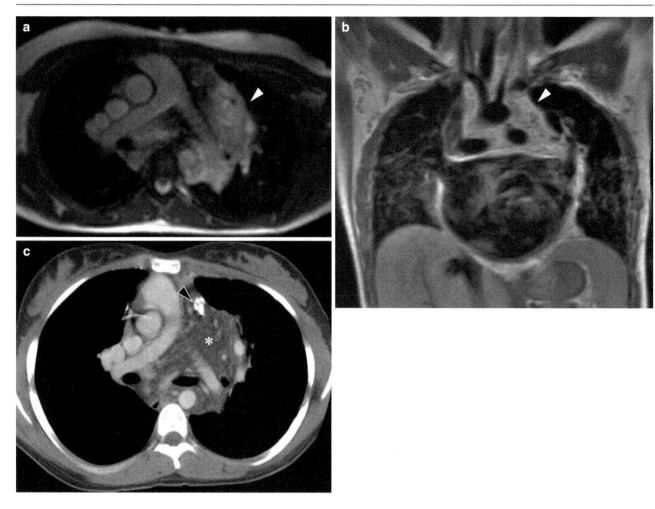

Fig. 5.9 Incidentally discovered thymolipoma in a 15-year-old girl with history of restrictive cardiomyopathy and congenital mitral prolapse resulting in severe left atrial enlargement (histologically proven). (**a**) Axial T1-weighted MR image demonstrates a large mass (*white arrowhead*) insinuating around the mediastinal vessels with areas of hyperintensity, representing fat, interspersed with regions of hypointensity, representing bands of thymic and fibrous tissue. (**b**) Coronal T1-weighted MR image demonstrates a large mass (*white arrowhead*) insinuating around the mediastinal vessels with areas of hyperintensity, representing fat, interspersed with regions of hypointensity, representing bands of thymic and fibrous tissue. (**c**) Axial contrast-enhanced CT of the chest shows the mass (*asterisk*) to be heterogeneous and hypodense with associated calcification (*black arrowhead*)

4% of all malignant germ cell tumors occur within the mediastinum [24]. When this is the case, imaging of the gonads must be performed as primary malignant germ cell tumors of the mediastinum are indistinguishable on imaging from primary gonadal tumor metastasis [18]. Mediastinal metastases from primary gonadal germ cell tumors, however, almost universally also demonstrate retroperitoneal lymph node metastases [23].

Complete surgical resection is the treatment of choice for mature benign germ cell tumors with excellent prognosis. Although most mediastinal malignant germ cell tumors can also be successfully resected following adjuvant chemotherapy, the overall prognosis is worse compared with those of primary gonadal or other extragonadal origin [20, 24].

While the presence of an anterior mediastinal germ cell tumor may be suspected radiologically, cross-sectional evaluation is required to confirm diagnosis and evaluate disease extent.

Traditionally, CT was the preferred imaging technique due to its improved spatial resolution over radiography. Because teratomas are the most common germ cell tumor within the mediastinum and are comprised of all three germ cells layers, most characteristically contain fat. Additionally, soft tissue, calcification, cystic, and solid components are generally present [21]. As a result, MR imaging has emerged as a useful modality to differentiate soft tissue components and confirm the presence of fat without requiring the use of ionizing radiation.

On MR imaging, teratomas are well circumscribed with heterogeneous internal signal on both T1- and T2-weighted images due to the varying characteristics of its comprised tissues. Macroscopic fat is hyperintense on T1-weighted images and shows signal loss on fat-suppressed sequences (Fig. 5.10). Cystic elements demonstrate intrinsic hyperintensity on T2-weighted images and hypointensity on

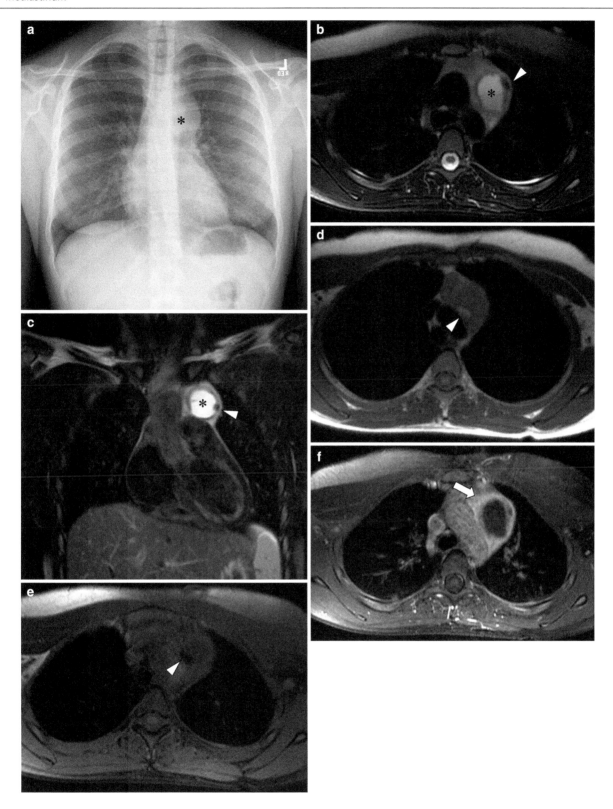

Fig. 5.10 Anterior mediastinal mature teratoma in a 17-year-old girl who presented with left-sided chest pain (histologically proven). (**a**) Frontal chest radiograph demonstrates a mass (*asterisk*) at the superior mediastinum on the left. (**b**) Axial T2-weighted fat-suppressed MR image demonstrates a well-circumscribed, centrally hyperintense lesion (*asterisk*) within the left anterior superior mediastinum containing a hypointense calcification (*arrowhead*). (**c**) Coronal T2-weighted fat-suppressed MR image demonstrates a well-circumscribed, centrally hyperintense lesion (*asterisk*) within the left anterior superior mediastinum containing a hypointense calcification (*arrowhead*). (**d**) Axial T1-weighted MR image demonstrates a focus of hyperintensity (*arrowhead*) at the medial margin of the lesion compatible with macroscopic fat. (**e**) Axial T1-weighted fat-suppressed MR image shows loss of signal (*arrowhead*) within this region, confirming the presence of macroscopic fat. (**f**) Axial T1-weighted fat-suppressed contrast-enhanced MR image demonstrates peripheral enhancement (*white arrow*)

T1-weighted images. Soft tissue components are isointense to muscle [23]. The presence of microscopic fat can be confirmed by signal loss on out-of-phase gradient sequences due to chemical shift artifact. The extent and associated complications of these tumors can also be evaluated with MR imaging [25]. Rupture of mature teratomas has been reported, and spilled contents may result in pneumonitis, pleural effusion, or pericardial effusion depending upon location [7, 20].

Unlike teratomas, seminomatous and nonseminomatous malignant germ cell tumors have a less characteristic MR imaging appearance. Both demonstrate heterogeneous signal intensity on T1- and T2-weighted images and variable enhancement on post-contrast imaging. While both may demonstrate high signal intensity on T2-weighted MR images suggestive of cystic necrosis, this MR imaging appearance is more common in nonseminomatous malignant germ cell tumors [23]. Additionally, like other malignant entities, both seminomas and nonseminomatous malignant germ cell tumors may obliterate fat planes and extend into adjacent mediastinal compartments. MR imaging is the most sensitive modality to evaluate the degree of anatomic infiltration due to its excellent contrast resolution [25].

Lymphatic Malformation Lymphatic malformations can occur anywhere throughout the body and are comprised of a variable number of endothelial-lined channels without muscular walls [26]. Histologically, these lesions stain positive for lymphatic markers. The incidence of lymphatic malformation at birth is 1 in 5000 [27]. While common in the anterior cervical region, due to its large volume of lymphatic tissue, primary mediastinal lymphatic malformations are rare [28]. Extension of cervical lymphatic malformations into the mediastinum, however, can be seen with large lesions [26]. When small, such lesions are generally asymptomatic. If there is superimposed infection or hemorrhage, symptoms may result. Larger lesions can also produce symptoms due to mass effect such as airway compression or vascular compromise [28].

Offering superior soft tissue resolution as compared with CT, MR imaging is vital in the evaluation of lymphatic malformations. Deeper involvement occurs in 6% of palpable, superficial lymphatic malformations, and MR imaging provides superior characterization of involved tissue planes [28]. Large lesions are frequently composed of both microcystic and macrocystic components. Microcystic components measure smaller than 1 cm, whereas macrocystic elements are those which measure larger than 1–2 cm. Lesions may be mass-like and well-defined or infiltrative. On T2-weighted images, lymphatic malformations are hyperintense lesions surrounded by a thin wall with thin internal septa (Fig. 5.11). Whereas peripheral and septal enhancement of macrocystic components is common, microcystic components enhance more homogenously and therefore frequently appear solid at imaging [26]. Lesions containing proteinaceous material or hemorrhage may be hyperintense on T1-weighted images or may contain fluid-fluid levels.

Because lymphatic malformations can vary substantially in their size, shape, extent of deeper involvement, and involvement of adjacent structures, accurate MR imaging characterization is required to guide management. While macrocystic regions may be amenable to percutaneous sclerotherapy, microcystic components may require surgical excision with or without concomitant medical therapy [26]. The complexity of lymphatic malformations highlights the importance of a multidisciplinary approach in their management.

Malignant Neoplastic Disorders

Thymoma Thymomas are epithelial neoplasms which contain a variable amount of lymphoid tissue. Rare in the pediatric population, thymomas account for less than 1% all of mediastinal tumors in children. Thymomas are typically diagnosed as an anterior mediastinal neoplasm in adults, usually within the fifth and sixth decades of life without sex predilection [9]. While oftentimes asymptomatic, symptoms can result from compression or invasion of adjacent structures. Notably, when thymomas occur in children, they are usually aggressive with poor prognosis [29]. While thymoma-associated paraneoplastic syndromes have been documented in children, including immunodeficiency and red cell aplasia, the common association between myasthenia gravis and thymoma in adults is rarely observed in the pediatric population [30]. Thymomas may be staged as invasive or noninvasive on the basis of capsular extension on imaging [18]. Complete surgical resection improves long-term survival. Chemotherapy and/or radiation may be required in advanced stages or cases where complete surgical resection cannot be achieved [30].

Up to 25% of thymomas may be radiographically occult [29]. Thus, cross-sectional imaging is invaluable for the diag-

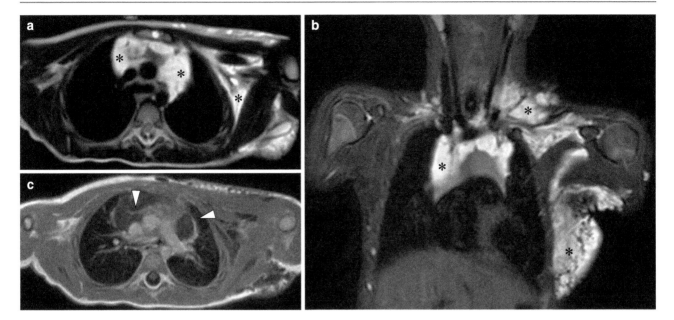

Fig. 5.11 Lymphatic malformation of the anterior mediastinum and left chest wall in a 3-year-old boy with prenatal diagnosis of lymphatic malformation. (a) Axial T2-weighted fat-suppressed MR image demonstrates hyperintense, infiltrative lesion *(asterisks)* within the anterior mediastinum and left axilla comprised of both macro- and microcystic components with thin intervening septa. (b) Coronal T2-weighted fat-suppressed MR image shows the lesion *(asterisks)* extending through the anterior mediastinum, left supraclavicular region, and left axilla. (c) Axial T1-weighted fat-suppressed contrast-enhanced MR image demonstrates peripheral and septal enhancement *(arrowheads)*

nosis, characterization, staging, and treatment of thymomas. On MR imaging, noninvasive thymomas are typically oval or lobulated, located off of the midline, and homogenous and hyperintense on T2-weighted images [19] (Fig. 5.12). The lack of signal dropout on out-of-phase gradient echo sequences helps confirm the lack of microscopic fat thus differentiating thymomas from thymic hyperplasia [1]. Invasive thymomas, conversely, demonstrate irregular contour, disruption of mediastinal boundaries, heterogeneous signal intensity, and often areas of necrosis [1]. Recently, diffusion characteristics and time to peak enhancement have been studied as a means of differentiating high-risk from low-risk lesions with promising result [19].

Thymic Carcinoma Exceedingly rare in children, thymic carcinomas are aggressive, epithelial neoplasms which may arise from malignant transformation of an existing thymoma [31]. Histologically, thymic carcinomas demonstrate hallmark features of invasive malignancies including increased mitoses, nuclear atypia, and necrosis [18]. Symptoms due to local invasion may be present at diagnosis and include chest pain, weight loss, respiratory distress, superior vena cava syndrome, fatigue, and night sweats [31]. Surgical resection remains the gold standard for treatment of thymic carcinoma with neoadjuvant chemotherapy and adjuvant radiation as required.

On MR imaging, thymic carcinomas are frequently large and irregular. The degree of local invasion, especially vascular, and metastatic involvement is best categorized by MR imaging [18] (Fig. 5.13). Contrary to the homogenous appearance of thymomas, thymic carcinomas typically demonstrate heterogeneous hyperintensity on both T1- and T2-weighted sequences due to hemorrhage and necrosis [7]. Calcification is common, occurring in greater than 60% of patients with thymic carcinoma [31]. Following contrast administration, there is heterogeneous enhancement.

Lymphoma Lymphoma is the most common mass in the anterior mediastinum in the pediatric population [20]. Arising from constituent cells of the immune system or their precursors, mediastinal lymphoma may be subclassified as

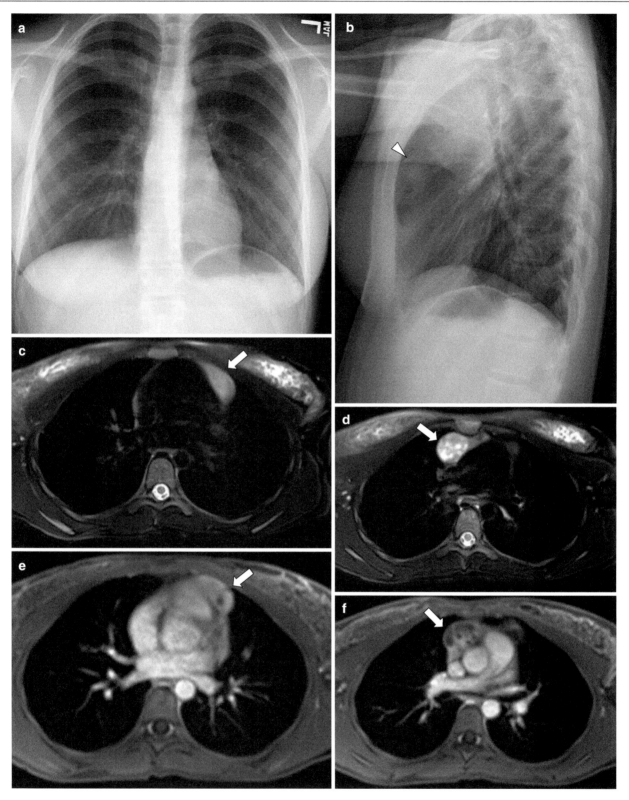

Fig. 5.12 Anterior mediastinal thymoma in a 16-year-old girl who presented with persistent cough. (**a**) Frontal chest radiograph shows subtle widening of the superior mediastinum. (**b**) Lateral chest radiograph demonstrates a well-circumscribed opacity (*arrowhead*) in the retrosternal clear space. (**c**) Axial T2-weighted fat-suppressed MR image demonstrates an ovoid heterogeneous hyperintense well-defined mass (*arrow*) in the left anterior mediastinum. (**d**) Axial T2-weighted fat-suppressed MR image demonstrates an additional ovoid heterogeneous hyperintense well-defined mass (*arrow*) in the right anterior mediastinum. (**e**) Axial T1-weighted fat-suppressed contrast-enhanced MR image of the left-sided mass (*arrow*) demonstrates heterogeneous enhancement in areas of relative hypointensity on T2-weighted image. (**f**) Axial T1-weighted fat-suppressed contrast-enhanced MR image of the right-sided mass (*arrow*) demonstrates heterogeneous enhancement in areas of relative hypointensity on T2-weighted image

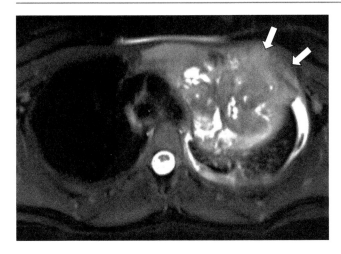

Fig. 5.13 Thymic carcinoma in a 13-year-old girl who presented with chest pain and weight loss. Axial T2-weighted MR image shows a large heterogeneous mass with local invasion (*arrows*) into adjacent chest wall

Hodgkin or non-Hodgkin. Hodgkin lymphoma is characterized histologically by the presence of Reed-Sternberg cells, large abnormal lymphocytes that may contain more than one nucleus. Non-Hodgkin lymphoma, alternately, is characterized histologically as the abnormal clonal proliferation of immature immunologic B or T cells.

Hodgkin lymphoma represents 40–50% of cases of pediatric lymphoma. Thoracic involvement is demonstrated in 85% of cases [32]. Hodgkin lymphoma more commonly affects young adults over the age of 20 without specific gender predilection. Four main histologic subtypes of Hodgkin lymphoma are described. The nodular sclerosing subtype accounts for 65% of cases in the pediatric population [33]. Affected pediatric patients typically present with painless adenopathy, most frequently in the neck. Two-thirds of affected patients demonstrate mediastinal involvement at initial presentation, which may cause symptoms related to mass effect [33]. Hodgkin lymphoma is staged according to the Ann Arbor staging system, which classifies the disease on the basis of anatomic lymph node involvement, presence of B symptoms, and extranodal involvement [13]. The 5-year survival rate for Hodgkin lymphoma is greater than 90% [7].

Non-Hodgkin lymphoma is more common in patients less than 10 years of age and more frequently affects boys [13]. Thoracic involvement is present in 45% of cases of non-Hodgkin lymphoma [32]. As compared with adults, children with non-Hodgkin lymphoma more commonly demonstrate extranodal thoracic or abdominal involvement which may manifest with acute symptoms such as pain, compressive symptoms, and biliary or urinary tract obstruction [33]. Non-Hodgkin lymphoma is staged according to the St. Jude staging system, which divides patients into "limited" (stage 1 and

2) and "extensive" (stage 3 and 4) disease [13]. The histologic subtype and tumor bulk are the most important prognostic factors [32].

On cross-sectional imaging, lymphoma of either subtype presents as a lobulated, multinodular, infiltrative mass which tends to encase adjacent structures rather than invade them [11]. While imaging is imperative for accurate staging, histologic sampling is required for definitive diagnosis [1]. Masses in lymphoma are typically homogenously hypointense on T1-weighted images, hyperintense on T2-weighted images, and show variable enhancement after the administration of contrast (Fig. 5.14). Central necrosis may also occur which produces a heterogeneous appearance on T2-weighted and post-contrast MR images. MR imaging can also assess pericardial or CNS involvement. Recently, diffusion-weighted MR imaging has been utilized to aid in differentiating lymphoma from other common mediastinal masses such as thymomas or thymic rebound [1, 19]. As a result of increased cellular density and cellular atypia, lymphoma demonstrates a low ADC value on diffusion-weighted MR imaging which can help differentiate it from other benign processes such as thymic rebound [1].

Midline NUT Cell Tumor NUT midline carcinoma is recently described, rare, aggressive, and malignant epithelial neoplasm. It is characterized by chromosomal rearrangement of the gene encoding nuclear protein of the testis (NUT) on chromosome 15 [34]. Variably, fusion with BRD4 on chromosome 19 results in a novel BRD4-NUT oncogene which may block cellular differentiation and contribute to carcinogenesis [35]. Although initially described in children and young adults, the tumor has now been described in older adults [36]. Approximately 90% of cases arise from midline anatomic sites, most commonly the thorax, head, and neck [37]. Affected patients present with symptoms referable to the site of malignancy. Definitive diagnosis of a NUT midline carcinoma is based solely upon histology and immunochemistry demonstration of monoclonal antibody nuclear reactivity for NUT [34]. Prognosis is poor with patients surviving an average of 6.7 months, and there is only one known case of curative treatment to date [37].

Imaging characteristics of NUT midline carcinoma are nonspecific as the majority of affected patients present with advanced disease [37]. On MR imaging, the tumor is generally large, heterogeneous, hypointense on T1-weighted images, and hyperintense on T2-weighted images. Following contrast administration, there is heterogeneous enhancement, often with central necrosis [36] (Fig. 5.15). MR imaging can serve as an adjunct to CT to assess for vascular or cardiac invasion and can aid in the detection of osseous metastatic disease [37].

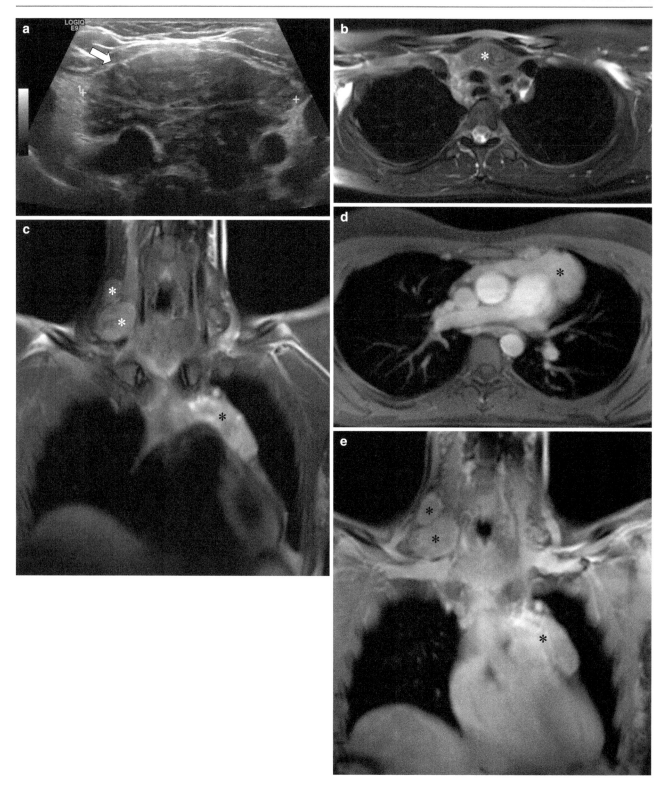

Fig. 5.14 Hodgkin lymphoma in an 18-year-old girl who presented with sore throat and pressure sensation in the anterior neck and chest leading to thyroid ultrasound and subsequent MR imaging evaluation (histologically proven). (**a**) Transverse grayscale ultrasound image demonstrates a heterogeneous anterior mediastinal mass (*arrow*). (**b**) Axial T2-weighted fat-suppressed MR image demonstrates an anterior mediastinal mass (*asterisk*) abutting the mediastinal vessels. (**c**) Coronal T2-weighted fat-suppressed MR image shows the mass (*asterisks*) extending into the neck and draping over the heart. (**d**) Axial T1-weighted fat-suppressed contrast-enhanced MR image shows homogenous enhancement of the large, multilobulated, anterior mediastinal mass (*asterisk*). (**e**) Coronal T1-weighted fat-suppressed contrast-enhanced MR image shows homogenous enhancement of the large, multilobulated, anterior mediastinal and right sided neck masses (*asterisks*)

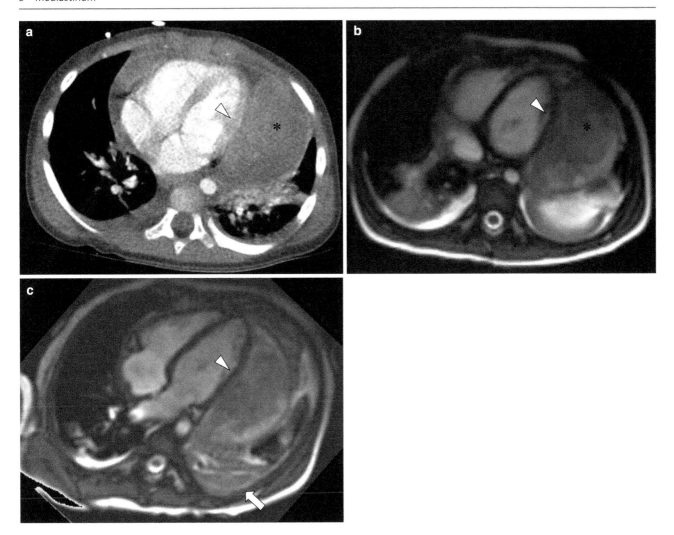

Fig. 5.15 Midline NUT cell tumor in a 2-year-old girl who presented with chest pain, fatigue, and fever (histologically proven). (**a**) Axial contrast-enhanced soft tissue window setting CT image demonstrates a heterogeneous mass (*asterisk*) adjacent to the free wall of the left ventricle (*arrowhead*). (**b**) Axial T2-weighted MR image shows the large heterogeneous mass (*asterisk*) adjacent to the left ventricle (*arrowhead*) with soft tissue and fluid components. (**c**) Axial balanced steady-state gradient echo sequence MR image demonstrates a separate left ventricular wall (*arrowhead*) without direct invasion. There is associated collapse of the left lower lobe (*arrow*)

Middle (Visceral) Mediastinal Lesions

Lymphadenopathy

Infectious Lymphadenopathy Infection is a common cause of mediastinal adenopathy in the pediatric population. Granulomatous infections such as tuberculosis and histoplasmosis classically cause significant mediastinal adenopathy in children [38]. Tuberculosis is caused by the acid-fast bacillus *Mycobacterium tuberculosis* and is a leading infectious cause of death and disability worldwide [7]. While most commonly manifesting with pulmonary involvement, concurrent mediastinal adenopathy is common and more prevalent in younger children [7]. Histoplasmosis infection occurs secondary to the dimorphic fungi *Histoplasma cap-sulatum* which is found in the soil of endemic areas [20]. After germination within the alveoli, the fungus disseminates via the reticuloendothelial system to mediastinal and hilar lymph nodes. In some cases, enlarged mediastinal lymph nodes with central caseation may result, which later calcify [39].

The MR imaging appearance of infectious mediastinal lymphadenopathy may be nonspecific. Homogenous or heterogeneous soft tissues masses within the mediastinum due to conglomerates of enlarged lymph nodes are most common [1] (Fig. 5.16). Mediastinal lymph nodes due to tuberculosis may demonstrate hypointensity on T2-weighted images and peripheral enhancement on contrast-enhanced images [7]. Calcified lymph nodes from histoplasmosis demonstrate hypointense signal intensity on all sequences.

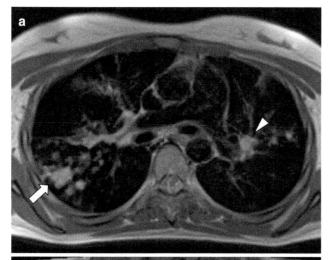

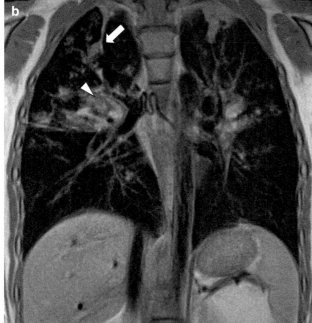

Fig. 5.16 Mycobacterial lung infection in a 17-year-old girl with cystic fibrosis. (**a**) Axial T2-weighted MR image demonstrates nodular airspace disease most prominent in the right upper lobe (*arrow*) and left hilar adenopathy (*arrowhead*). (**b**) Coronal T1-weighted MR image shows nodular airspace disease most prominent in the right upper lobe (*arrow*) and right hilar adenopathy (*arrowhead*)

Neoplastic Lymphadenopathy

Primary Neoplasm Lymphoma is the most common primary neoplasm in children to cause middle mediastinal adenopathy [22]. As with lymphoma in the prevascular/anterior compartment, lymphoma in the visceral/middle mediastinum typically manifests as a large, lobulated, infiltrative soft tissue mass which insinuates around adjacent structures. Although usually homogenous at presentation, as lesions increase in size, there may be hemorrhage, or they may undergo central necrosis [13]. These features may result in a heterogeneous imaging appearance. Following

treatment, calcification may occur due to treatment-induced necrosis, which manifests as foci of low signal intensity on all MR imaging sequences [40].

Metastatic Disease Metastatic disease is an uncommon cause of mediastinal adenopathy in the pediatric population [22]. Sarcomas, testicular neoplasms, Wilms tumor, and other malignancies of the abdomen and pelvis are the most common primary malignancies which result in mediastinal involvement [18]. MR imaging appearance of mediastinal adenopathy is usually nonspecific, resulting in a conglomerate mass of enlarged homogenous or heterogeneous lymph nodes with variable degrees of contrast enhancement (Fig. 5.17). Rarely, metastatic mediastinal lymph nodes may ossify prior to the initiation of therapy, as is the case with metastatic osteosarcoma, thus providing a clue to their primary origin [41].

Other Causes of Mediastinal Adenopathy

While less common than infectious or neoplastic etiologies, other processes may result in mediastinal adenopathy.

Sarcoidosis Sarcoidosis is a rare systemic disorder characterized by the formation of noncaseating granulomas [42]. While younger children are more likely to manifest with a triad of skin, joint, and eye involvement, older children generally present similar to adults with pulmonary and mediastinal involvement [42]. Intrathoracic lymphadenopathy is the most commonly observed sign of sarcoidosis typically involving the hilar and right paratracheal stations (Fig. 5.18) [43]. Previous study has demonstrated high levels of agreement between CT and MR imaging for the thoracic manifestations of sarcoidosis, including perilymphatic nodularity and hilar and mediastinal lymphadenopathy [44]. In addition, recently, contrast-enhanced lung MRI with fast imaging sequences has been shown to be highly sensitive imaging modality and compatible with CT in the evaluation of both lung and cardiac abnormalities in pediatric sarcoidosis [45].

Castleman Disease Castleman disease is a non-neoplastic, nonclonal, lymphoproliferative disorder characterized by lymph node hyperplasia which results in middle mediastinal adenopathy [7, 20]. Rare in children, adenopathy typically involves the hilar or right paratracheal stations [20]. Castleman disease can be present in isolation (unicentric disease) or can result in association with concurrent disease processes such as infection and malignancy [46]. Because of similarities in appearance and its ability to mimic both benign and malignant pathologies, Castleman disease should be included on the differential for mediastinal adenopathy. Unlike other manifestations of mediastinal adenopathy, Castleman disease lesions demonstrate heterogeneous hyperintensity on both

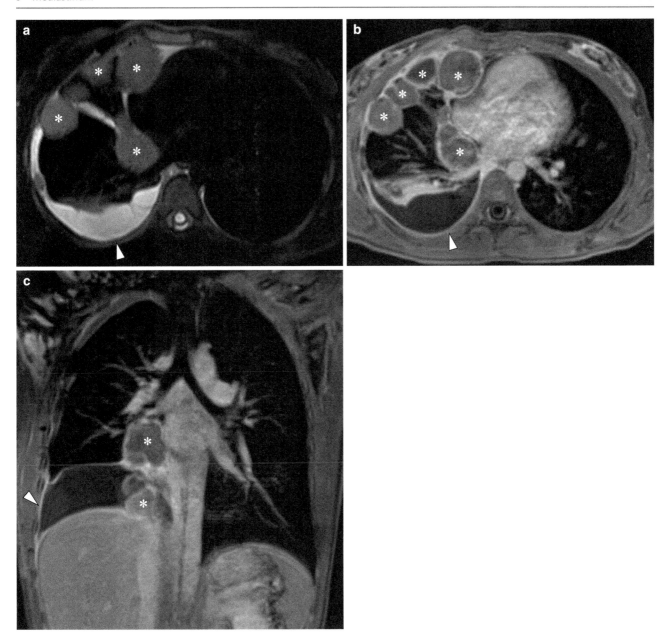

Fig. 5.17 Metastatic synovial sarcoma in a 14-year-old girl who presented with chest pain. (**a**) Axial T2-weighted fat-suppressed MR image demonstrates multiple T2-weighted mildly hyperintense masses (*asterisks*) within the right hilum and right anterior thorax and an associated right pleural effusion (*arrowhead*). (**b**) Axial T1-weighted fat-suppressed contrast-enhanced MR image demonstrates heterogeneous contrast enhancement of the masses (*asterisks*) and peripheral enhancement of the right pleural effusion (*arrowhead*). (**c**) Coronal T1-weighted fat-suppressed contrast-enhanced MR image demonstrates heterogeneous contrast enhancement of the masses (*asterisks*) and peripheral enhancement of the right pleural effusion (*arrowhead*)

T1- and T2-weighted images and, characteristically, homogenous intense enhancement following contrast administration [46] (Fig. 5.19).

Foregut Duplication Cysts

Foregut duplication cysts, including bronchogenic cyst, esophageal duplication cyst, and neuroenteric cyst, result from developmental malformations of the embryonic foregut. Unable to be differentiated on imaging on the basis of their cystic portion alone, foregut duplication cysts are classified histologically on the basis of their cellular composition into bronchogenic, esophageal, and neuroenteric subtypes. Foregut duplication cysts are the most common primary lesion in the vascular/middle mediastinal compartment and account for 11% of mediastinal masses [22].

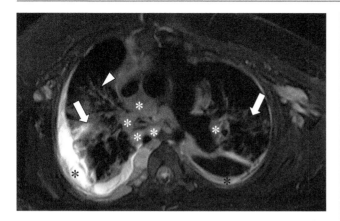

Fig. 5.18 Sarcoidosis in a 12-year-old girl who presented with respiratory distress. Axial T2-weighted fat-suppressed MR image demonstrates multiple enlarged paratracheal and bilateral hilar lymph nodes (*white asterisks*). Lymphangitic spread characterized by underlying septal thickening (*arrowhead*) and fibrotic changes (*arrows*) including bronchiectasis, volume loss, and architectural distortion are also seen. In addition, bilateral pleural effusions (*black asterisks*) are also present

Bronchogenic Cyst Bronchogenic cyst results from abnormal budding of the ventral foregut in embryological lung development [47]. Although bronchogenic cysts may occur anywhere along the tracheobronchial tree, most commonly, they are found at the carina or paratracheal regions [7]. Dyspnea may result from localized mass effect on the airway. Infection may also produce symptoms or result in a connection to the tracheobronchial tree through which the cyst may become air-filled [48].

Esophageal Duplication Cyst Esophageal duplication cysts arise from abnormal division of the posterior foregut. Most frequently occurring along the upper third of the esophagus, esophageal duplication cysts may produce dysphagia due to localized mass effect [18]. Less commonly, esophageal duplication cysts may detach from the esophagus and migrate into the lung during development [18]. Esophageal duplication cysts may also contain gastric mucosa which can ulcerate and bleed [49].

Neuroenteric Cyst Neuroenteric cysts result from a failure in the division of the primitive neural crest from the gastrointestinal tract. Most frequently located in the paravertebral compartment adjacent to the spine, neuroenteric cysts may extend into or communicate with the spinal column and result in pain. Communication with the spinal column may be associated with an osseous defect, a unique secondary characteristic through which neuroenteric cysts may be differentiated from bronchogenic and esophageal duplication cysts on imaging.

On MR imaging, foregut duplication cysts of all subtypes are well circumscribed, ovoid, or round with T2 hyperintensity. T1 signal is variable depending upon the cyst contents. If the cyst contains protein, as with superimposed hemorrhage, hyperintensity on T1-weighted images may result. Following contrast administration, an enhancing wall may

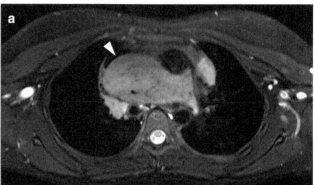

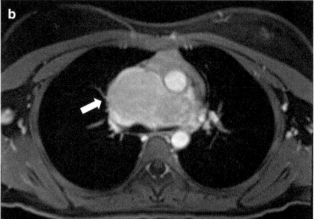

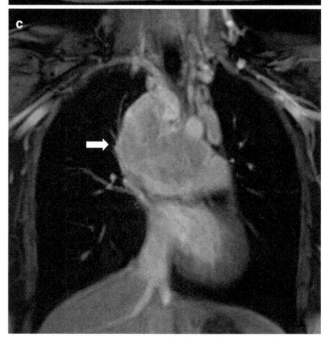

Fig. 5.19 Castleman disease in a 13-year-old girl who presented with shortness of breath, fatigue, and cough who found to have a mediastinal mass on echocardiogram prompting MR imaging. Biopsy confirmed histologic characteristics of Castleman disease. (**a**) Axial T2-weighted fat-suppressed MR image demonstrates homogenous, hyperintense mediastinal mass (*arrowhead*). (**b**) Axial T1-weighted fat-suppressed contrast-enhanced MR image demonstrates homogenous enhancement of the mass (*arrow*). (**c**) Coronal T1-weighted fat-suppressed contrast-enhanced MR image demonstrates homogenous enhancement of the mass (*arrow*)

be visualized especially in the setting of superimposed infection. In all cases, MR imaging can be helpful in cases where CT characteristics are indeterminate to further differentiate cystic from solid lesions [19] (Figs. 5.20, 5.21, and 5.22). Complete surgical resection is the currently accepted definitive treatment particularly in symptomatic pediatric patients with foregut duplication cysts.

Posterior (Paravertebral) Mediastinal Lesions

Neoplastic Disorders

Sympathetic Chain Ganglion Origin Tumors

Ganglioneuroma, Ganglioneuroblastoma, and Neuroblastoma Up to 90% of posterior mediastinal masses are

neuroblastic in origin [20]. Those tumors that arise from the autonomic ganglion cells (ganglioneuromas, ganglioneuroblastomas, and neuroblastomas) constitute a spectrum of benign to malignant lesions with varying degrees of cellular differentiation [50]. Approximately 2/3 occur in patients less than 20 years of age, grow parallel to the spine in a craniocaudal orientation, and are malignant [50].

Ganglioneuromas are benign, fully differentiated neuronal tumors comprised of primordial neural crest cells in combination with mature ganglion cells and other mature tissue [51]. Most tumors occur in children greater than 10 years of age and are attached to a sympathetic nerve or an intercostal nerve trunk [50]. Because these tumors are slow growing, they may result in mass effect with associated symptoms including painless, progressive scoliosis [52]. Complete surgical resection is curative with excellent prognosis.

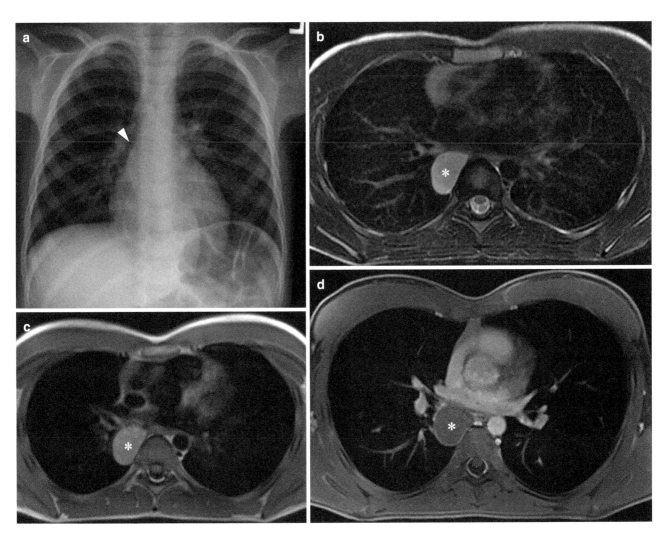

Fig. 5.20 Bronchogenic cyst in a 16-year-old boy who presented with chest pain (histologically proven). (**a**) Frontal chest radiograph demonstrates a right hilar mass (*arrowhead*). (**b**) Axial T2-weighted fat-suppressed MR image demonstrates a well-circumscribed, hyperintense, oval lesion (*asterisk*) at the border of the middle and posterior medias-

tinum to the right of midline. (**c**) Axial T1-weighted fat-suppressed MR image demonstrates increased T1 signal intensity within the lesion (*asterisk*) compatible with proteinaceous fluid content. (**d**) Axial T1-weighted fat-suppressed contrast-enhanced MR image demonstrates a thin enhancing wall surrounding the lesion (*asterisk*)

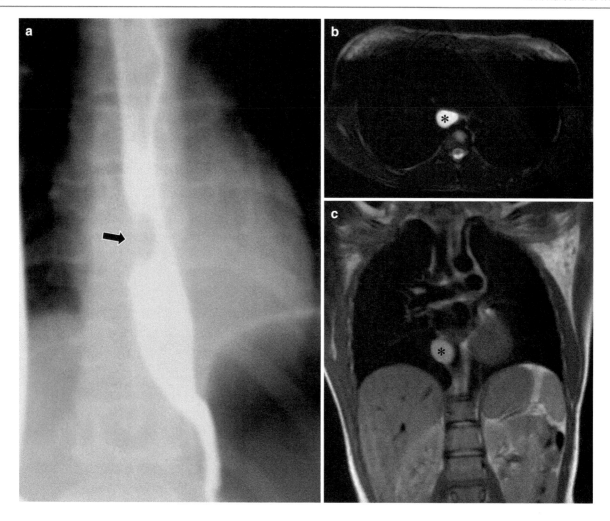

Fig. 5.21 Esophageal duplication cyst in a 17-year-old girl who presented with epigastric abdominal pain occurring after meals. (a) Frontal spot fluoroscopic image from an esophagram demonstrates a smoothly marginated soft tissue mass (*arrow*) causing a scalloped impression on the esophageal lumen. (b) Axial T2-weighted MR image demonstrates an oval-shaped, fluid intensity cyst (*asterisk*) within the middle mediastinum at the right lateral aspect of the esophagus. (c) Coronal double IR FSE proton density weighted MR image demonstrates hyperintense signal within the cyst (*asterisk*) compatible with proteinaceous fluid content

Ganglioneuroblastomas are the fourth most common tumor in childhood [50]. Representing transitional tumors between ganglioneuromas and neuroblastomas, ganglioneuroblastomas contain both benign and malignant elements. Histologically, ganglioneuroblastomas are comprised of undifferentiated neuroblasts and mature ganglion cells [50]. These tumors occur most frequently in children between 2 and 4 years of age without gender predilection [53].

Neuroblastoma is the third most common cause of malignancy in the pediatric population with a reported incidence of 1/8000–1/10,000 [54]. Thoracic neuroblastoma accounts for the minority of neuroblastoma cases, although prognosis is better as compared with primary abdominal neuroblastoma [55]. Neuroblastoma more commonly affects boys under the age of 8 with 50% of cases diagnosed before the age of 2 years [53]. Histologically, neuroblastomas are comprised of small, blue, round, neuroepithelial cells of glial or ganglionic differentiation with little intervening stroma [50]. Staging is based upon the presence of metastatic dis-

ease and image-defined risk factors including tumor encasement or invasion of adjacent vessels and organs [8].

The histologic type of neuroblastic tumor cannot be reliably distinguished by imaging alone, and histologic correlation is required for diagnosis [20]. On MR imaging, ganglioneuromas generally demonstrate homogenous signal characteristics with intermediate signal intensity on all sequences (Fig. 5.23). Occasionally, a whorled appearance may be demonstrated with linear areas of low signal intensity [50]. Ganglioneuroblastomas vary in appearance on MR imaging. They may be well circumscribed and mimic ganglioneuroma, be locally invasive, or demonstrate metastatic disease (Fig. 5.24). Similarly, neuroblastomas demonstrate variable imaging characteristics and may be homogenous or heterogeneous [55]. Cystic change or hemorrhage may occur. MR imaging is generally preferred over CT for staging of the neuroblastic tumors due to its ability to demonstrate intraspinal extension, marrow replacement, and hepatic metastases [50] (Fig. 5.25).

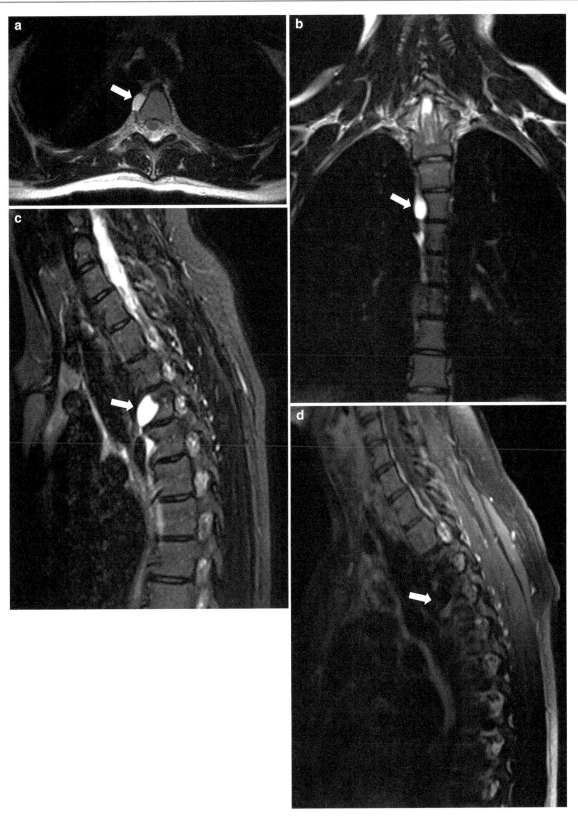

Fig. 5.22 Neuroenteric cyst in a 16-year-old girl who presented with back pain. (**a**) Axial T2-weighted MR image demonstrates a well-defined, ovoid, cystic structure (*arrow*) abutting the anterior aspect of the right T3 vertebral body with mild osseous remodeling of the vertebral body. (**b**) Coronal T2-weighted MR image shows the cystic lesion (*arrow*) adjacent to the T3 vertebral body and extending inferiorly to the level of T4. (**c**) Sagittal inversion-recovery MR image demonstrates intrinsic hyperintensity of the cyst (*arrow*). (**d**) Sagittal T1-weighted fat-suppressed contrast-enhanced MR images show no enhancement within the cyst (*arrow*)

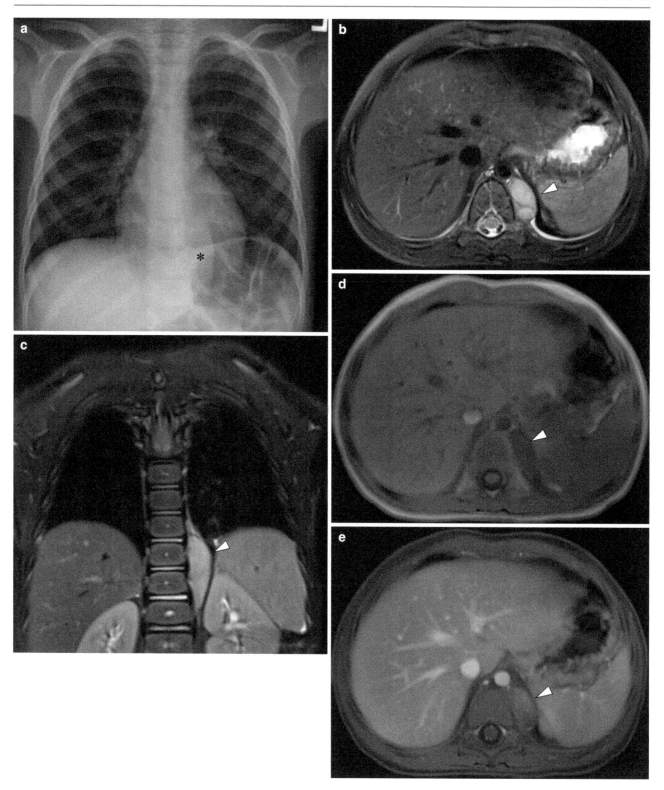

Fig. 5.23 Ganglioneuroma in a 4-year-old boy who presented with cough and fever. A left paraspinal mass due to ganglioneuroma was incidentally found (histologically proven). (**a**) Frontal chest radiograph demonstrates a left paraspinal mass (*asterisk*). (**b**) Axial T2-weighted fat-suppressed MR image shows a left paravertebral, hyperintense, well-circumscribed mass (*arrowhead*). (**c**) Coronal T2-weighted fat-suppressed MR image shows the mass (*arrowhead*) vertically oriented and fusiform. (**d**) Axial T1-weighted fat-suppressed MR image demonstrates intrinsic T1 hypointensity of the mass (*arrowhead*). (**e**) Axial T1-weighted fat-suppressed contrast-enhanced MR image demonstrates heterogeneous contrast enhancement within the mass (*arrowhead*)

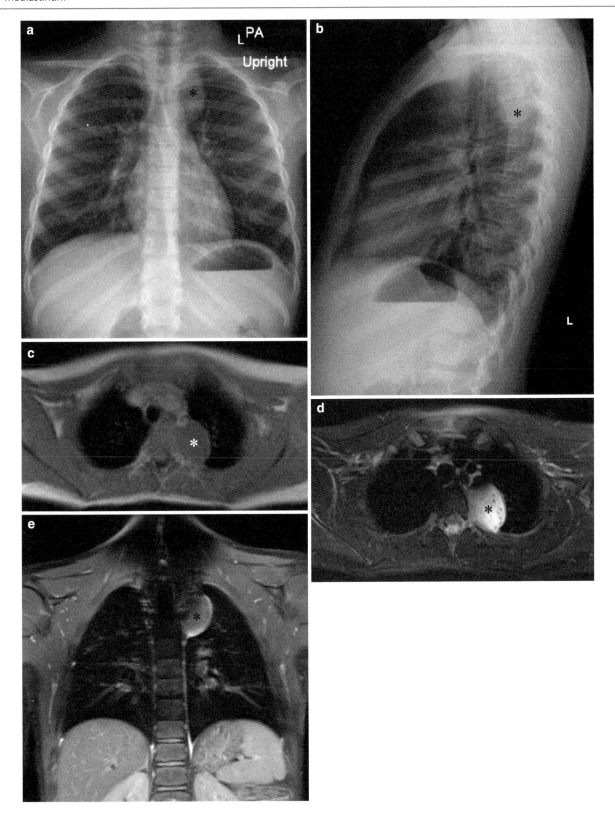

Fig. 5.24 Ganglioneuroblastoma in a 7-year-old girl who presented with cough and fever. (**a**) Frontal chest radiograph demonstrates a smoothly marginated mass (*asterisk*) which projects over the left lung apex. (**b**) Lateral chest radiograph demonstrates posterior mediastinal location of the mass (*asterisk*). (**c**) Axial T1-weighted MR image shows hypointense mass (*asterisk*) within the left posterior mediastinum. (**d**) Axial T2-weighted MRI image shows hyperintensity within the mass (*asterisk*). (**e**) Coronal T1-weighted fat-suppressed contrast-enhanced MR image demonstrates homogenous enhancement within the mass (*asterisk*)

A. R. Hart and E. Y. Lee

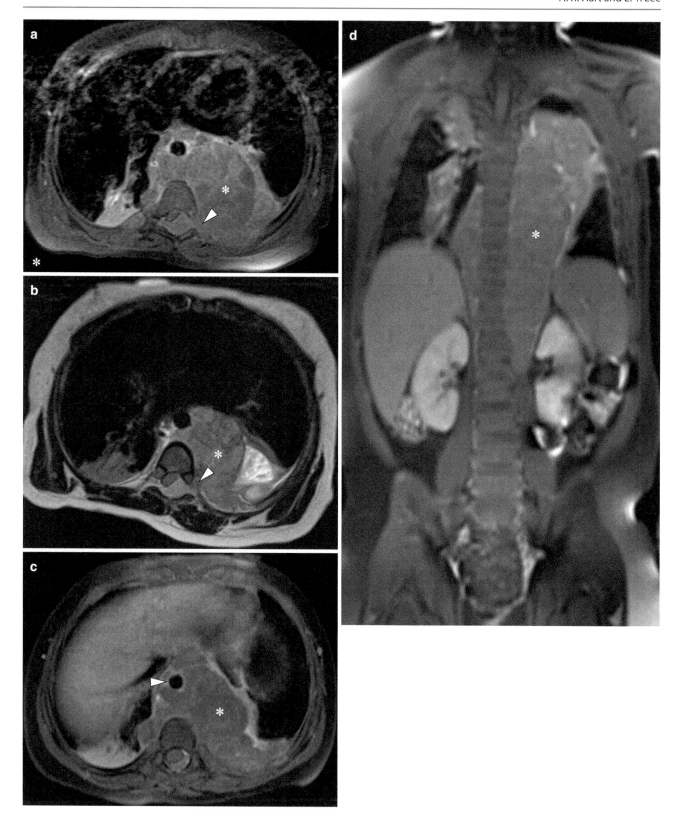

Fig. 5.25 Neuroblastoma in a 16-month-old girl who presented with lower extremity flaccid paralysis (histologically proven). (**a**) Axial T1-weighted fat-suppressed MR image demonstrates a large, left paraspinal mass (*asterisk*) at the posterior mediastinum extending across the midline from left to right with mixed signal intensity and neuroforaminal invasion (*arrowhead*). (**b**) Axial T2-weighted MR image demonstrates a large, left paraspinal mass (*asterisk*) at the posterior mediastinum extending across the midline from left to right with mixed signal intensity and neuroforaminal invasion (*arrowhead*). (**c**) Axial T1-weighted fat-suppressed contrast-enhanced MR image demonstrates heterogeneous enhancement of the mass (*asterisk*) and lifting of the thoracic aorta (*arrowhead*) off of the spine. (**d**) Coronal T1-weighted fat-suppressed contrast-enhanced MR image demonstrates the longitudinal extent of the mass (*asterisk*) along the thoracic spine

Nerve Root Origin Tumors

Neurofibroma Neurofibromas may occur in isolation or in association with neurofibromatosis type I (NF1), the most common neurocutaneous syndrome [56]. Neurofibromas associated with NF1 tend to more frequently undergo malignant degeneration and be larger than those occurring spontaneously though the rate of malignant transformation remains low [57]. Pathologically, neurofibromas are unencapsulated, soft tissue tumors composed of Schwann cells, fibroblasts, and perineural cells which grow in a disorganized manner [58]. Because they grow in a longitudinal, fusiform manner, they are unable to be surgically separated from the parent nerve with which they are associated [57]. This requires that the parent nerve be sacrificed at time of surgical resection.

On MR imaging, neurofibromas are classically hypointense on T1-weighted images and hyperintense on T2-weighted images, with avid contrast enhancement. A characteristic target sign may also be identified with a hypointense cen-

tral region and a periphery of hyperintensity on T2-weighted sequences [57]. Plexiform neurofibromas are a subtype of neurofibroma that is often described as having the appearance of a "bag of worms" and is the result of fusiform enlargement of nerve roots and peripheral nerve fibers [58] (Fig. 5.26). Both neurofibromas and plexiform neurofibromas may be associated with neuroforaminal enlargement and demonstrate a dumbbell shape.

Schwannoma Schwannomas are encapsulated neoplasms composed primarily of Schwann cells which grow eccentrically along the involved nerve. This eccentric growth pattern allows for complete separation of the lesion from the parent nerve at time of surgical resection [57]. The propensity of malignant degeneration of schwannomas is very low and is less than that of neurofibromas. Like neurofibromas, schwannomas may be singular or multiple. Schwannomas are multiple in neurofibromatosis type II which is defined by the presence of bilateral vestibular schwannomas with or without meningiomas, ependymomas, neurofibromas, and spinal

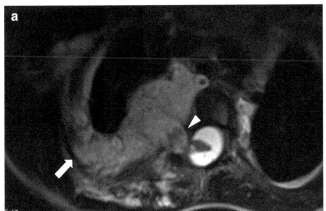

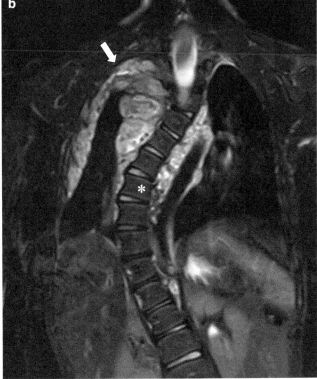

Fig. 5.26 Multiple plexiform neurofibromas in a 5-year-old boy with history of neurofibromatosis type 1. (**a**) Axial T2-weighted fat-suppressed MR image demonstrates lobulated T2 hyperintense lesions (*arrow*) throughout the right paraspinal region. There is associated neu-

roforaminal enlargement (*arrowhead*). (**b**) Coronal T2-weighted fat-suppressed MR image demonstrates lobulated T2 hyperintense lesions (*arrow*) throughout the right paraspinal region and scoliotic curvature (*asterisk*)

and peripheral nerve schwannomas [59]. Neurofibromatosis type II is inherited in an autosomal dominant fashion due to germ line mutation of the NF gene on chromosome 22 [59].

In most cases, schwannomas cannot be differentiated from neurofibromas on MR imaging because they demonstrate similar imaging characteristics of low signal intensity on T1-weighted sequences, high signal intensity on T2-weighted sequences, and avid contrast enhancement [57] (Fig. 5.27). Eccentric location with respect to its parent nerve may suggest schwannoma, as neurofibromas tend to be more centrally located. Schwannomas also tend to more frequently undergo cystic degeneration, hyalinization, and calcification as compared to neurofibromas resulting in a more heterogeneous appearance on imaging [59].

Other Posterior Mediastinal Lesions

Extramedullary Hematopoiesis Another important differential consideration for a paravertebral mass, extramedullary hematopoiesis occurs when there are too few blood cells to satisfy the body's demand [60]. Most frequently demonstrated with myelodysplasia and severe anemia, failure of hematopoietic marrow results in the proliferation of hematopoietic cells outside of the bone marrow [61]. In fetal development, the spleen and the liver are responsible for hematopoiesis. Before birth, the site of hematopoiesis shifts to the bone marrow [62]. Although the exact pathophysiology is unknown, sites of hematopoiesis can again shift in response to need [61]. Mass-like paraspinal involvement is a common site of extramedullary hematopoiesis and can mimic a soft tissue neoplasm.

Characteristic MR imaging features can help establish a diagnosis of extramedullary hematopoiesis, especially in the setting of a predisposing medical condition, and can obviate the need for biopsy and histologic correlation. Paraspinal hematopoietic masses are generally bilateral, well-defined, and lobulated. Lesions may extend into the central spinal canal resulting in compression [63]. Active hematopoietic masses demonstrate intermediate signal intensity on T1- and T2-weighted images with mild enhancement on post-contrast images (Fig. 5.28). Older, inactive lesions demonstrate diffusely increased signal on T1- and T2-weighted images, due

to fatty replacement, or diffusely decreased signal on T1- and T2-weighted images, due to iron deposition in the setting of frequent blood transfusions [64].

Posterior Diaphragmatic Hernia Derived from the complex interplay of four major embryologic structures (the septum transversum, pleuroperitoneal membranes, dorsal mesentery of the esophagus, and body wall), the diaphragm separates the thoracic from abdominal cavities. The diaphragm is also the major muscle responsible for quiet breathing [65]. Congenital diaphragmatic hernia is often a life-threatening condition presenting at birth and is often associated with additional anatomic abnormalities including cardiac, extremity, and CNS [66]. Occasionally, diaphragmatic hernia may present as an incidental finding in an older child or adult.

A Bochdalek hernia is a congenital diaphragmatic hernia believed to be caused by an embryonic defect in the fusion of the pleuroperitoneal fold with the septum transversum and intercostal muscles [65]. Due to herniation of intra-abdominal contents into the chest, congenital diaphragmatic hernia may substantially impact pulmonary development. The most common cause of morbidity and mortality associated with congenital diaphragmatic hernia is pulmonary hypoplasia. Decreased fetal lung volumes in congenital diaphragmatic hernia are associated with lower survival rates and increased probability of developing chronic lung disease [67].

Fetal MR imaging has been shown to provide additional information over ultrasound and guide treatment [66]. Low in signal on all MR imaging sequences, the diaphragm can be easily identified on fetal MR imaging separating the thoracic and abdominal cavities [65]. In the setting of congenital diaphragmatic hernia, the diaphragm on the side of abnormality is more difficult to identify. MR imaging can assess for herniation of the bowel, liver, and other abdominal structures into the thorax and identify associated abnormalities [66]. Fetal MR imaging can also be used to calculate fetal lung volume, with lower lung volumes associated with increased morbidity and the need for postnatal ECMO therapy [67]. Postnatally, MR imaging can also be utilized to characterize the diaphragmatic defect, define affected structures, and guide surgical management [66] (Fig. 5.29).

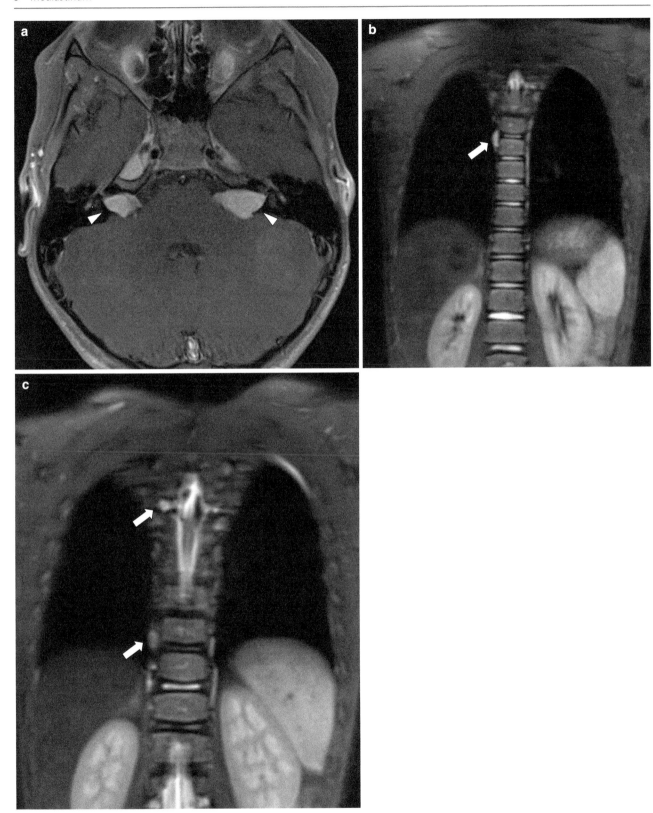

Fig. 5.27 Bilateral vestibular schwannomas and multiple spinal schwannomas in a 10-year-old boy with history of neurofibromatosis type 2. (**a**) Axial T1-weighted fat-suppressed contrast-enhanced MR image demonstrates homogenously enhancing masses (*arrowheads*) within bilateral internal auditory canals. (**b**) Coronal T2-weighted fat-suppressed MR image demonstrates T2 hyperintense, homogenous lesion (*arrow*) of the spinal nerve root. (**c**) Coronal T2-weighted fat-suppressed MR image demonstrates additional T2 hyperintense, homogenous lesions (*arrows*) of the spinal nerve root

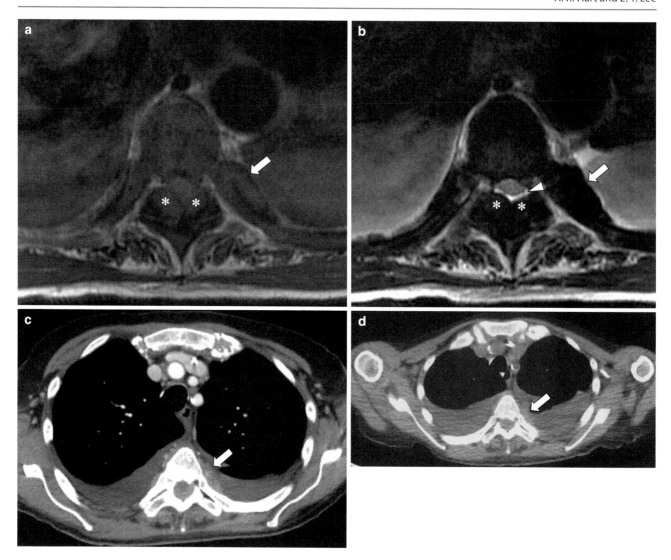

Fig. 5.28 Extramedullary hematopoiesis in a 17-year-old girl with myelodysplastic syndrome. (**a**) Axial T2-weighted MR image demonstrates lobulated intermediate signal intensity masses (*arrow*) along the inner cortex of the left fourth rib and at the posterior elements of the vertebra (*asterisks*). (**b**) Axial T1-weighted MR image demonstrates lobulated hypointense lesions (*arrow*) along the inner cortex of the left fourth rib and at the posterior elements of the vertebra (asterisks) with mass effect on the posterior thecal sac (*arrowhead*). (**c**) Axial enhanced soft tissue window setting CT image at the level of the T4 vertebral body demonstrates mild contrast enhancement of the lobulated lesion (*arrow*) along the inner cortex of the left fourth rib. (**d**) FDG-PET/CT image at the T4 vertebral body level demonstrates mild corresponding FDG avidity (*arrow*)

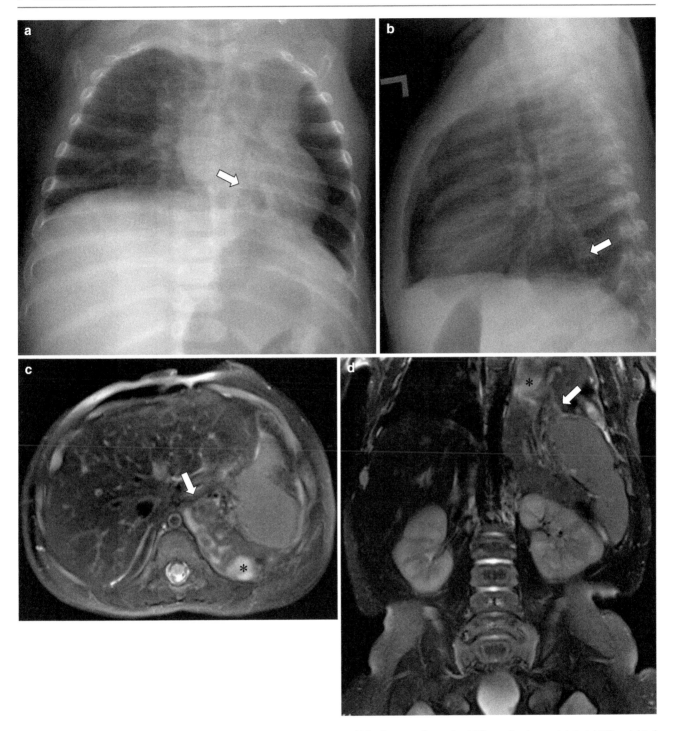

Fig. 5.29 Recurrent diaphragmatic defect containing herniated stomach and bowel in a 5-month-old boy with history of congenital diaphragmatic hernia status post neonatal repair who presented with increased work of breathing. (**a**) Frontal chest radiographs demonstrate retrocardiac lucency (*arrow*) representing herniated bowel. (**b**) Lateral chest radiographs show that the herniated bowel (*arrow*) is located within the posterior and middle mediastinum. (**c**) Axial T2-weighted fat-suppressed MR image demonstrates bowel (*arrow*) and stomach (*asterisk*) herniating into the left hemithorax. (**d**) Coronal T2-weighted fat-suppressed MR image shows bowel (*arrow*) and stomach (*asterisk*) herniating into the left hemithorax

Conclusion

The excellent soft tissue characterization capability and exceptional anatomic detail that MR imaging can provide allow for superior assessment of pediatric mediastinal lesions as compared with other imaging modalities. Individualized and tailored MR imaging techniques may be utilized to characterize mediastinal abnormalities based upon their unique features in the pediatric population. MR imaging also concurrently allows for the evaluation of disease extent and anatomic relationship to other mediastinal structures. Unlike CT, MR imaging does not require the use of potentially harmful ionizing radiation and is thus particularly attractive for pediatric patients who are more susceptible to these potentially harmful effects. Clear knowledge of the characteristic MR appearance of various pediatric mediastinal masses and a practical use of the three mediastinal compartmental imaging approach can often help narrow the differential diagnosis and thus optimize pediatric patient management.

References

1. Acharya PT, Ali S, Stanescu AL, Phillips GS, Lee EY. Pediatric mediastinal masses. Magn Reson Imaging Clin N Am. 2019;27(2):227–42.
2. Kleinerman RA. Radiation-sensitive genetically susceptible pediatric sub-populations. Pediatr Radiol. 2008;39(S1):27–31.
3. Ciet P, Tiddens HAWM, Wielopolski PA, Wild JM, Lee EY, Morana G, et al. Magnetic imaging in children: common problems and possible solutions for lung and airways imaging. Pediatr Radiol. 2015;45(13):1901–15.
4. Baez JC, Seethamraju RT, Mulkern R, Ciet P, Lee EY. Pediatric chest MR imaging. Magn Reson Imaging Clin N Am. 2015;23(2):321–35.
5. Schoenwolf GC, Bleyl SB, Brauer PR, Francis-West PH. Development of the respiratory system and body cavities. In: Larsen WJ, Schoenwolf GC, Bleyl SB, Brauer PR, editors. Larsen's human embryology. 5th ed. Edinburgh: Churchill Livingstone; 2015. p. 251–66.
6. Moore KL, Persaud TVN, Torchia MG. Body cavities, mesenteries, and diaphragm. In: Moore KL, Persaud TVN, Torchia MG, editors. The developing human: clinically oriented embryology. Philadelphia: Elsevier; 2020. p. 131–42.
7. Laya B, Lee EY, Liszewski MC, Zucker EJ, Restrepo R, Zucker EJ, Lee EY. Mediastinum. In: Lee EY, editor. Pediatric thoracic imaging. Philadelphia: Wolters Kluwer; 2019. p. 150–217.
8. Adzick NS, Farmer DL. Cysts of the lungs and mediastinum. In: Coran AG, Adzick NS, Krummel TM, Laberge JM, Shamberger RC, Caldamone AA, editors. Pediatric surgery. 7th ed. Philadelphia: Elsevier; 2012. p. 825–35.
9. Nasseri F, Eftekhari F. Clinical and radiologic review of the normal and abnormal thymus: pearls and pitfalls. Radiographics. 2010;30(2):413–28.
10. Whitten CR, Khan S, Munneke GJ, Grubnic S. A diagnostic approach to mediastinal abnormalities. Radiographics. 2007;27(3):657–71.
11. Carter BW, Benveniste MF, Madan R, Godoy MC, de Groot PM, Truong MT, et al. ITMIG classification of mediastinal compartments and multidisciplinary approach to mediastinal masses. Radiographics. 2017;37(2):413–36.
12. Carter BW, Tomiyama N, Bhora FY, Rosado de Christenson ML, Nakajima J, Boiselle PM, et al. A modern definition of mediastinal compartments. J Thorac Oncol. 2014;9(9):S97–S101.
13. Sams CM, Voss SD. Imaging of the pediatric thymus and thymic disorders. In: Garcia-Peña P, Guillerman RP, editors. Pediatric chest imaging. 3rd ed. Berlin/Heidelberg: Springer; 2014. p. 327–48.
14. Mandell GA, Bellah RD, Boulden ME, Sherman NH, Harcke HT, Padman RJ, et al. Cervical trachea: dynamics in response to herniation of the normal thymus. Radiology. 1993;186(2):383–6.
15. Wong KT, Lee DLY, Chan MSM, Tsang RKY, Yuen EHY, Ahuja AT. Unusual anterior neck mass visible only during valsalva's maneuver in a child. AJR Am J Roentgenol. 2005;185(5):1355–7.
16. Zi Yin E, Frush DP, Donnelly LF, Buckley RH. Primary immunodeficiency disorders in pediatric patients. AJR Am J Roentgenol. 2001;176(6):1541–52.
17. MacDonald K, Mackenzie S. What happens to the thymus in children who have undergone a median sternotomy? Pediatr Radiol. 2009;39(6):616–21.
18. Ranganath SH, Lee EY, Restrepo R, Eisenberg RL. Mediastinal masses in children. AJR Am J Roentgenol. 2012;198(3):W197–216.
19. Daye D, Ackman JB. Characterization of mediastinal masses by MRI: techniques and applications. Appl Radiol. 2017:10–32.
20. Thacker PG, Sodi KS, Gooneratne NA, Fonda C, Ciet P, Lee EY. Mediastinum. In: Lee EY, editor. Pediatric radiology: practical imaging evaluation of infants and children. Philadelphia: Wolters Kluwer; 2018. p. 609–39.
21. Gaerte SC, Meyer CA, Winer-Muram HT, Tarver RD, Conces DJ. Fat-containing lesions of the chest. Radiographics. 2002;22(Suppl 1):S61–78.
22. Lee EY. Evaluation of non-vascular mediastinal masses in infants and children: an evidence-based practical approach. Pediatr Radiol. 2009;39(S2):184–90.
23. Takahashi K, Al-Janabi NJ. Computed tomography and magnetic resonance imaging of mediastinal tumors. J Magn Reson Imaging. 2010;32(6):1325–39.
24. Billmire DF. Malignant germ cell tumors in childhood. Semin Pediatr Surg. 2006;15(1):30–6.
25. Drevelegas A, Palladas P, Scordalaki A. Mediastinal germ cell tumors: a radiologic–pathologic review. Eur Radiol. 2001;11(10):1925–32.
26. Merrow AC, Gupta A, Patel MN, Adams DM. 2014 Revised classification of vascular lesions from the international society for the study of vascular anomalies: radiologic-pathologic update. Radiographics. 2016;36(5):1494–516.
27. Xu Y, Xu D, Chen Z. Giant lymphatic malformations of the mediastinum in children: report of three cases. Clin Imaging. 2012;36(5):606–8.
28. Ghaffarpour N, Burgos CM, Wester T. Surgical excision is the treatment of choice for cervical lymphatic malformations with mediastinal expansion. J Pediatr Surg. 2018;53(9):1820–4.
29. Rothstein DH, Voss SD, Isakoff M, Puder M. Thymoma in a child: case report and review of the literature. Pediatr Surg Int. 2005;21(7):548–51.
30. Petroze R, McGahren ED. Pediatric chest II. Benign tumors and cysts. Surg Clin North Am. 2012;92(3):645–58.
31. Stachowicz-Stencel T, Orbach D, Brecht I, Schneider D, Bien E, Synakiewicz A, et al. Thymoma and thymic carcinoma in children and adolescents: a report from the European Cooperative Study Group for Pediatric Rare Tumors (EXPeRT). Eur J Cancer. 2015;51(16):2444–52.
32. Bae YA, Lee KS. Cross-sectional evaluation of thoracic lymphoma. Thorac Surg Clin. 2010;20(1):175–86.
33. Toma P, Granata C, Rossi A, Garaventa A. Multimodality imaging of Hodgkin disease and non-Hodgkin lymphomas in children. Radiographics. 2007;27(5):1335–54.

34. Stelow EB. A review of NUT midline carcinoma. Head Neck Pathol. 2011;5(1):31–5.

35. Nelson BA, Lee EY, French CA, Bauer DE, Vargas SO. BRD4-NUT carcinoma of the mediastinum in a pediatric patient. J Thorac Imaging. 2010;25(3):W93–W6.

36. Polsani A, Braithwaite KA, Alazraki AL, Abramowsky C, Shehata BM. NUT midline carcinoma: an imaging case series and review of literature. Pediatr Radiol. 2011;42(2):205–10.

37. Bair RJ, Chick JF, Chauhan NR, French C, Madan R. Demystifying NUT midline carcinoma: radiologic and pathologic correlations of an aggressive malignancy. AJR Am J Roentgenol. 2014;203(4):W391–W9.

38. Thacker PG, Mahani MG, Heider A, Lee EY. Imaging evaluation of mediastinal masses in children and adults. J Thorac Imaging. 2015;30(4):247–67.

39. Kirchner SG, Hernanz-Schulman M, Stein SM, Wright PF, Heller RM. Imaging of pediatric mediastinal histoplasmosis. Radiographics. 1991;11(3):365–81.

40. Keraliya AR, Tirumani SH, Shinagare AB, Ramaiya NH. Beyond PET/CT in Hodgkin lymphoma: a comprehensive review of the role of imaging at initial presentation, during follow-up and for assessment of treatment-related complications. Insights Imaging. 2015;6(3):381–92.

41. Rastogi R, Garg R, Thulkar S, Bakhshi S, Gupta A. Unusual thoracic CT manifestations of osteosarcoma: review of 16 cases. Pediatr Radiol. 2008;38(5):551–8.

42. Shetty AK, Gedalia A. Childhood sarcoidosis: a rare but fascinating disorder. Pediatr Rheumatol. 2008;6(1):16.

43. Koyama T, Ueda H, Togashi K, Umeoka S, Kataoka M, Nagai S. Radiologic manifestations of sarcoidosis in various organs. Radiographics. 2004;24(1):87–104.

44. Chung JH, Little BP, Forssen AV, Yong J, Nambu A, Kazlouski D, et al. Proton MRI in the evaluation of pulmonary sarcoidosis: comparison to chest CT. Eur J Radiol. 2013;82(12):2378–85.

45. Gorkem SB, Kose S, Lee EY, Doganay S, Coskun AS, Kose M. Thoracic MRI evaluation of sarcoidosis in children. Pediatr Pulmonol. 2017;52(4):494–9.

46. Bonekamp D, Horton KM, Hruban RH, Fishman EK. Castleman disease: the great mimic. Radiographics. 2011;31(6):1793–807.

47. Son JK, Lee EY, Eisenberg RL. Focal nonvascular thoracic masses in children. AJR Am J Roentgenol. 2011;196(3):W224–W39.

48. Juanpere S, Cañete N, Ortuño P, Martínez S, Sanchez G, Bernado L. A diagnostic approach to the mediastinal masses. Insights Imaging. 2012;4(1):29–52.

49. Hryhorczuk AL, Lee EY, Eisenberg RL. Esophageal abnormalities in pediatric patients. AJR Am J Roentgenol. 2013;201(4):W519–W32.

50. Pavlus JD, Carter BW, Tolley MD, Keung ES, Khorashadi L, Lichtenberger JP. Imaging of thoracic neurogenic tumors. AJR Am J Roentgenol. 2016;207(3):552–61.

51. Ozawa Y, Kobayashi S, Hara M, Shibamoto Y. Morphological differences between schwannomas and ganglioneuromas in the mediastinum: utility of the craniocaudal length to major axis ratio. Br J Radiol. 2014;87(1036):20130777.

52. Wang X, Yang L, Shi M, Liu X, Liu Y, Wang J. Retroperitoneal ganglioneuroma combined with scoliosis. Medicine. 2018;97(37):e12328.

53. Lee JY, Lee KS, Han J, Yoon H-K, Kim TS, Han BK, et al. Spectrum of neurogenic tumors in the thorax: CT and pathologic findings. J Comput Assist Tomogr. 1999;23(3):399–406.

54. Demirag F, Yazicioglu A, Aydogdu K, Kaya S, Karaoglanoglu N, Bicakcioglu P. Intrathoracic neurogenic tumors. Thorac Cardiovasc Surg. 2013;62(02):147–52.

55. Lyons K, Paul Guillerman R, McHugh K. Pulmonary and extrathymic mediastinal tumors. In: Garcia-Peña P, Guillerman RP, editors. Pediatric chest imaging. 3rd ed. Berlin/Heidelberg: Springer; 2014. p. 349–71.

56. Khong P-L, Goh WHS, Wong VCN, Fung C-W, Ooi G-C. MR imaging of spinal tumors in children with neurofibromatosis 1. AJR Am J Roentgenol. 2003;180(2):413–7.

57. Lin J, Martel W. Cross-sectional imaging of peripheral nerve sheath tumors. AJR Am J Roentgenol. 2001;176(1):75–82.

58. Hrehorovich PA, Franke HR, Maximin S, Caracta P. Malignant peripheral nerve sheath tumor. Radiographics. 2003;23(3):790–4.

59. Koontz NA, Wiens AL, Agarwal A, Hingtgen CM, Emerson RE, Mosier KM. Schwannomatosis: the overlooked neurofibromatosis? AJR Am J Roentgenol. 2013;200(6):W646–W53.

60. Berkmen YM, Zalta BA. Case 126: extramedullary hematopoiesis. Radiology. 2007;245(3):905–8.

61. Bowling MR, Cauthen CG, Perry CD, Patel NP, Bergman S, Link KM, et al. Pulmonary extramedullary hematopoiesis. J Thorac Imaging. 2008;23(2):138–41.

62. Ginzel AW, Kransdorf MJ, Peterson JJ, Garner HW, Murphey MD. Mass-like extramedullary hematopoiesis: imaging features. Skeletal Radiol. 2011;41(8):911–6.

63. Georgiades CS, Neyman EG, Francis IR, Sneider MB, Fishman EK. Typical and atypical presentations of extramedullary hemopoiesis. AJR Am J Roentgenol. 2002;179(5):1239–43.

64. Tsitouridis J, Stamos S, Hassapopoulou E, Tsitouridis K, Nikolopoulos P. Extramedullary paraspinal hematopoiesis in thalassemia: CT and MRI evaluation. Eur J Radiol. 1999;30(1):33–8.

65. Chavhan GB, Babyn PS, Cohen RA, Langer JC. Multimodality imaging of the pediatric diaphragm: anatomy and pathologic conditions. Radiographics. 2010;30(7):1797–817.

66. Liszewski MC, Zucker EJ, Laya BF, Restrepo R, Lee EY. Diaphragm. In: Lee EY, editor. Pediatric thoracic imaging. Philadelphia: Wolters Kluwer; 2019. p. 327–44.

67. Debus A, Hagelstein C, Kilian AK, Weiss C, Schönberg SO, Schaible T, et al. Fetal lung volume in congenital diaphragmatic hernia: association of prenatal mr imaging findings with postnatal chronic lung disease. Radiology. 2013;266(3):887–95.

Chest Wall and Diaphragm

Jessica Kurian

Introduction

The chest wall protects and supports the lungs and thoracic vascular structures. It contributes to physiologic motion of the thorax during respiration, as well as stabilization of shoulder and arm movements. The chest wall is comprised of numerous structures including bones (sternum, ribs, and spine), skin and subcutaneous tissue, muscle, nerves, and vessels. In infants and children, the chest wall is more cartilaginous than in adults and therefore less rigid.

The diaphragm is the primary muscle responsible for active breathing. The diaphragm contracts during inspiration, in conjunction with the accessory muscles of respiration, enlarging the thoracic cavity and drawing air into the lungs [1]. In addition to respiration, the diaphragm also plays a role in esophageal function (emesis, reflux barrier), regulation of intraabdominal pressure (aiding in urination and defecation), and stabilization of the spine [1, 2].

In this chapter, up-to-date techniques for MR imaging of the pediatric chest wall and diaphragm are discussed. Embryology, normal development and anatomy, anatomic variants, and clinical and MR imaging features of various clinically important congenital and acquired disorders involving the chest wall and diaphragm in infants and children are also reviewed.

Magnetic Resonance Imaging Techniques

Patient Preparation

To prepare a pediatric patient for MR imaging of the chest wall or diaphragm, the child's age and ability to hold still, follow instructions, and perform breath-holding must be

carefully considered. Additionally, the clinical indication for the study and the potential effects of patient motion on the area of interest should be considered. The non-sedated "feed and wrap" technique can be attempted for young infants, usually less than 3 months of age but sometimes as old as 6 months [3, 4]. Approximately 3–4 hours after the last feed, the baby is fed in a room near the MR imaging suite and then swaddled using multiple blankets to induce natural sleep, before transfer onto the scan table. The blankets also serve to restrain the infant, although some institutions choose to use a dedicated infant immobilization device.

After the newborn period, the majority of infants and young children require moderate sedation or general anesthesia. To scan children awake, behavioral techniques (familiarity with the scanner, practice of breathing techniques, etc.), radiology child life specialists, and MR imaging video goggles can help decrease motion artifact and improve patient tolerance of extended scan times. These methods can be attempted in patients as young as 5 years old, depending on the child's ability to cooperate. As some motion may be inevitable even in cooperative children, motion-resistant sequences and motion-correction techniques are helpful, particularly in patients between 5 and 10 years old [5]. For patients who are being assessed for chest wall lesions, an MRI-specific adhesive marker should be placed on the skin at the site of concern.

MR Imaging Pulse Sequences and Protocols

Chest Wall Evaluation

When performing MR imaging of the chest wall, it is best to tailor each case to the size and location of the suspected lesion with regard to pulse sequences, imaging plane, field of view, and coil type [6]. Chest wall examinations should begin with a large field of view, using a cardiac coil for infants and small children under 5 years of age and a phased array torso coil in older children and adolescents [7]. If needed, smaller field of view images can be obtained using a surface coil.

J. Kurian (✉)
Department of Radiology, Montefiore Medical Center,
Albert Einstein College of Medicine, Bronx, NY, USA
e-mail: jkurian@montefiore.org

© Springer Nature Switzerland AG 2020
E. Y. Lee et al. (eds.), *Pediatric Body MRI*, https://doi.org/10.1007/978-3-030-31989-2_6

Table 6.1 Practical chest wall MR imaging protocol

Sequence	Acronym (GE/Philips/Siemens)	Plane	FS	Slice thickness/gap (mm)	FOV	Mode	Notes
T2 single shot	SSFSE/SSTSE/HASTE	Cor	None	4/1	Entire chest	FB or BH	
STIR	STIR	Cor or Sag	Yes	3–4/1	Fit to patient – may include the entire chest or target to area of concern	BH or RT	
T1	FSE/TSE/TSE	Ax or Cor	None	3–4/1		BH or RT	
T2	FSE/TSE/TSE	Ax	SPAIR	5/0		RT	
3D SPGR	LAVA/THRIVE/VIBE	Ax	Yes	4/0		BH	Pre-contrast
3D SPGR	LAVA/THRIVE/VIBE	Ax, Cor, and Sag	Yes	4/0		BH	Post-contrast
T1	FSE/TSE/TSE		SPAIR	3–4/1		BH or RT	Optional – may substitute for pre- and post-contrast imaging
DWI	DWI	Ax	–	4/1		BH	Optional
bSSFP	FIESTA/bFFE/TruFISP	Ax	None	5/1	Entire chest	FB or BH	Optional, may use as single sequence exam for Haller index

Notes: Slice thickness can be increased for larger patients and to reduce scan time. Respiratory triggering can be substituted for breath-hold in patients who are sedated or unable to breath-hold

FS fat suppression, *FOV* field of view, *Ax* axial, *Cor* coronal, *Sag* sagittal, *STIR* short tau inversion recovery, *SPAIR* spectral adiabatic inversion recovery, *SPGR* spoiled gradient recalled, *DWI* diffusion-weighted imaging, *bSSFP* balanced steady-state free precession, *FB* free breathing, *BH* breath-hold, *RT* respiratory triggered

To limit breathing artifacts, breath-hold and/or respiratory triggering should be used, and prone imaging can also be considered to minimize anterior chest wall motion [7, 8]. Cardiac gating is only necessary if the mediastinal structures are also being assessed. For dedicated MR imaging of the sternum, coronal views can be obtained obliquely along the sternum, prescribed from the sagittal images. Although pulse sequences and slice orientation should be geared to the suspected disease, a typical examination should include axial, sagittal, and coronal images with T1 and T2 weighting, as well as a fat-suppressed sequence and contrast-enhanced images. A suggested practical chest wall MR imaging protocol is provided in Table 6.1.

Diaphragm Evaluation

MR imaging of the diaphragm is still an evolving field. Existing work in this area has primarily dealt with diaphragmatic motion and lung volumes in adults, particularly in patients with neuromuscular disorders [9].

For assessment of diaphragmatic masses, standard pulse sequences as used for other anatomic body MR imaging exams are sufficient, and examinations can be performed with breath-hold or quiet breathing. For demonstration of diaphragmatic motion, fast gradient recalled echo (GRE) pulse sequences are reliable; however other rapid pulse sequences such as single-shot fast spin echo, spoiled gradient echo, and balanced steady-state free precession may be used [1, 10–12]. To assess motion, MR imaging is obtained with deep breathing to approximate vital capacity, by instructing the patient to inhale and exhale slowly and maximally [10]. Sagittal and/or coronal images should be included for measurement of diaphragmatic excursion [10, 11]. During the examination, respiration is monitored with a pressure belt.

Anatomy

Embryology

Chest Wall

The chest wall begins developing in the third week of gestation from paraxial and lateral plate mesoderm, and some of its components continue to develop even after birth [13]. The paraxial mesoderm segments into somites, which differentiate into three different types: sclerotomes, myotomes, and dermatomes (Fig. 6.1). Sclerotomes are arranged segmentally and migrate toward the neural tube to form the vertebrae. Small regions of mesenchyme that develop along the lateral aspects of the vertebral arches subsequently lengthen to form the ribs. The cartilaginous ribs undergo endochondral ossification, with the primary ossification center forming near the angle of the ribs. During adolescence, secondary ossification centers form at the heads and tubercles of the ribs.

After the sclerotomes migrate to form the vertebrae, the remaining mesoderm (dermomyotome) separates into dermatomes and myotomes. The dermatomes form the skin and connective tissue of the chest wall. The myotomes are comprised of two subcomponents: epimeres and hypomeres. The epimeres form the deep muscles of the back, and the hypomeres form the muscles of the ventrolateral body wall, including the intercostal muscles.

The sternum forms independently from lateral plate mesoderm (Fig. 6.2). A longitudinal pair of mesenchymal structures called sternal bars fuse in the midline in a craniocaudal fashion, terminating with the xiphoid process. As with the ribs, the cartilaginous sternum subsequently ossifies; however, the xiphoid process does not ossify until after birth [14].

Diaphragm

The diaphragm is formed between the 4th and 12th weeks of gestation from four components: the transverse septum, pleuroperitoneal folds, esophageal mesentery, and muscular body wall (Fig. 6.3) [1, 15]. The transverse septum is located anteriorly and centrally and fuses laterally with the body wall and posteriorly with the pleuroperitoneal folds and esophageal mesentery. The transverse septum becomes the central muscular tendon of the diaphragm and is the origin of the myoblasts that migrate to form the rest of the muscular diaphragm [2].

The esophageal mesentery forms the median portion of the diaphragm, and the "crura" of the diaphragm are created when muscle fibers grow into the mesentery. The transverse

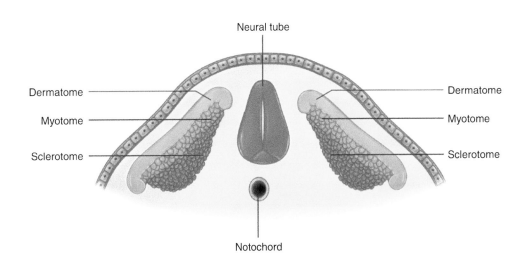

Fig. 6.1 Embryology of the chest wall. Diagram shows the developing components of the chest wall. The somites differentiate into three components: sclerotomes, which migrate toward the neural tube to form the vertebrae; dermatomes, which form the skin and connective tissue; and myotomes, which form the muscles of the back and body wall

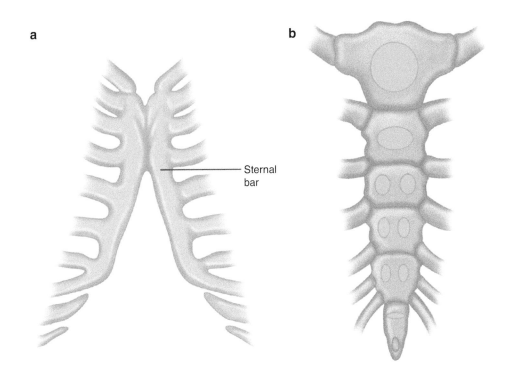

Fig. 6.2 Development of the sternum. (**a**) Diagram depicts the appearance of the sternum at the 9th week of gestation, consisting of longitudinal sternal bars, which fuse in a craniocaudal fashion. (**b**) The fully developed sternum, with the blue regions indicating the original ossification centers

Fig. 6.3 Embryology of the
diaphragm. Diagram depicts
the four major structures that
form the diaphragm: the
transverse septum,
pleuroperitoneal folds,
esophageal mesentery, and
muscular body wall

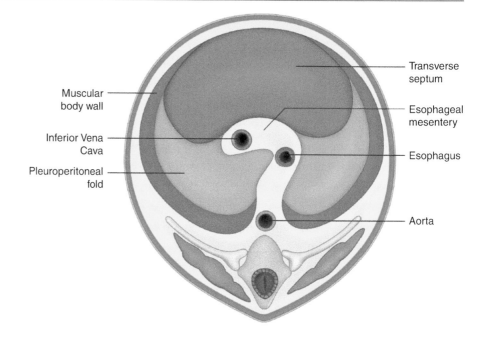

Fig. 6.4 Chest wall
anatomy—skeletal. Diagram
shows the bony structures that
comprise the skeleton of the
chest wall

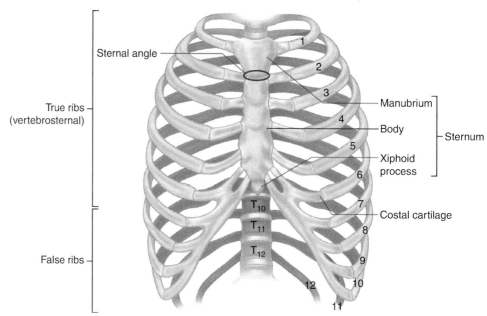

septum initially lies opposite the upper cervical somites. The
ventral rami from the C3, C4, and C5 spinal nerves subsequently grow through the pleuropericardial membrane into
the transverse septum to form the phrenic nerve.

Normal Development and Anatomy

Chest Wall

The thoracic skeleton is comprised of the sternum, the 12
thoracic vertebrae, and the 12 paired ribs and costal cartilages (Fig. 6.4) [16]. The ribs are anchored to the T1–T12
vertebrae. The first through seventh ribs connect to the
sternum through the costal cartilages ("true" ribs). The

8th through 12th ribs do not articulate with the sternum
("false" ribs). The sternum consists of the manubrium,
sternal body, and xiphoid process. The sternal angle or
angle of Louis is a bony ridge between the manubrium
and sternal body, which is continuous with the second rib
and typically the landmark for the level of the tracheal
bifurcation.

The anterior chest wall muscles include the pectoralis
major, a large fan-shaped muscle, and deep to this the pectoralis minor (Fig. 6.5) [17]. The extrinsic or superficial back
muscles include the latissimus dorsi (a large muscle which
has extensive attachments to the spine), the serratus anterior
posterolaterally, and the trapezius and rhomboids posteromedially. The oblique muscles, though considered part of the

Fig. 6.5 Chest wall anatomy—muscular. Diagram shows the (*top*) anterior and (*bottom*) posterior muscles of the chest wall

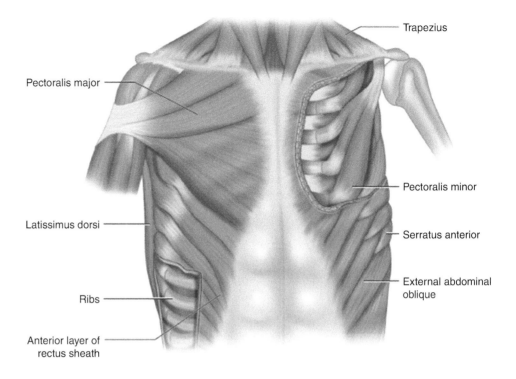

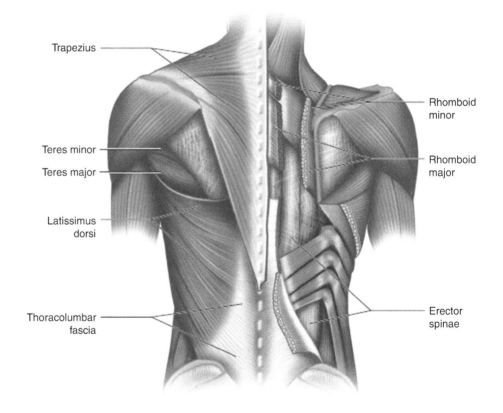

abdominal wall, attach to the lower seventh to eighth ribs. The intrinsic or deep back muscles include numerous muscles that maintain posture and control of vertebral movement (erector spinae and transversospinalis groups). The deepest

muscles of the chest wall are the three layers of intercostal muscles.

The blood supply and innervation of the chest wall are primarily via the intercostal vessels and nerves and the brachial plexus [17]. The intercostal nerves are formed from the anterior rami of the spinal nerves. The paraspinal muscles are innervated by the posterior rami of the spinal nerves. The blood supply to the sternum is from the paired internal mammary arteries, which are branches of the subclavian arteries. The ventral chest wall is also supplied by numerous collaterals between the subclavian artery branches and the deep epigastric artery branches.

The high contrast resolution of MR imaging allows the chest wall structures to be easily depicted (Fig. 6.6). The intercostal vessels and nerves cannot be visualized on routine imaging unless involved in a pathologic process.

Diaphragm

The diaphragm is a dome-shaped skeletal muscle that denotes the anatomical separation between the thoracic and abdominal cavities (Fig. 6.7) [2, 18]. The right diaphragm is usually slightly higher than the left [19]. The diaphragm extends from the fifth–sixth ribs anteriorly to the tenth rib posteriorly and has multiple attachments to the body wall

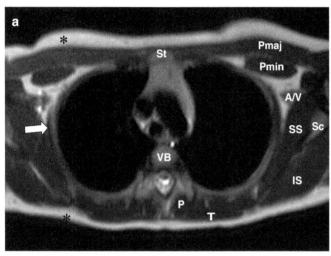
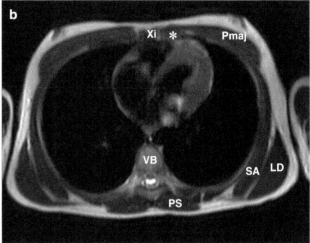

Fig. 6.6 Normal chest wall in an 8-year-old girl. (**a**) Axial non-enhanced T2-weighted MR image at the level of the sternal notch (St) depicts normal chest wall anatomy, including the subcutaneous fat (∗), pectoralis major (Pmaj), pectoralis minor (Pmin), scapula (Sc), subscapularis (SS), infraspinatus (IS), trapezius (T), paraspinal muscles (P), axillary artery and vein (A/V), vertebral body (VB), and ribs *(arrow)*. (**b**) Axial non-enhanced T2-weighted MR image at the level of the xiphoid process (Xi) depicts normal chest wall anatomy, including the pectoralis major (Pmaj), serratus anterior (SA), latissimus dorsi (LD), paraspinal muscles (PS), vertebral body (VB), and costal cartilage (∗)

Fig. 6.7 Diaphragm anatomy. Diagram shows the muscles and ligaments that comprise the diaphragm, as well as the three diaphragmatic hiatuses

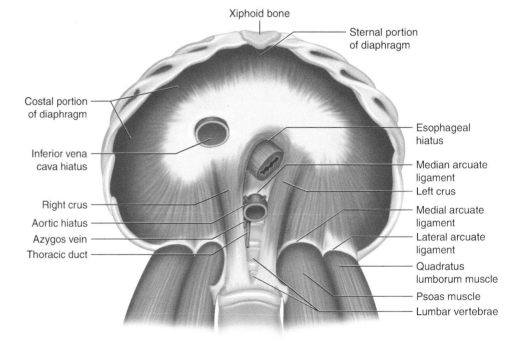

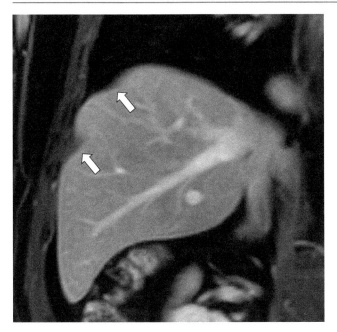

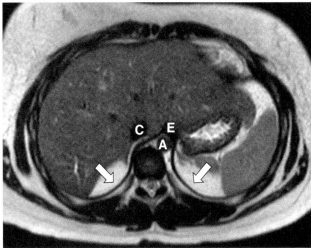

Fig. 6.10 Normal diaphragm in a 16-year-old girl. Axial non-enhanced T2-weighted MR image through the lower chest shows the diaphragm as a low-signal band (*arrows*). The esophageal hiatus (E), aorta (A), and inferior vena cava (C) are visible

Fig. 6.8 Diaphragmatic slips in a 16-year-old boy. Coronal enhanced T1-weighted fat-suppressed MR image demonstrates hypointense muscular slips (*arrows*) indenting the liver contour

the condition known as median arcuate ligament syndrome, thickening or low positioning of the median arcuate ligament can compress the celiac artery and/or celiac plexus leading to chronic abdominal pain [21, 22].

The diaphragm contains three openings: the caval hiatus at the T8 level containing the IVC and right phrenic nerve branches; the esophageal hiatus at the T10 level containing the esophagus, vagal nerves, and small esophageal arteries; and the aortic hiatus at the T12 level containing the aorta, azygos and hemiazygos veins, and thoracic duct [1, 2, 15].

The paired phrenic nerves provide innervation to the diaphragm [23]. These are formed from the C3–C5 nerve roots and course from the posterolateral neck into the anterior thorax and along the surface of the pericardium, before arborizing on the diaphragm surface [23, 24]. The pericardiophrenic and musculophrenic arteries (branches of the internal thoracic and inferior phrenic arteries) supply the diaphragm [21].

On MR imaging, the diaphragm appears as a thin sheet of muscle, with signal intensity typically lower than other skeletal muscle [21] (Fig. 6.10).

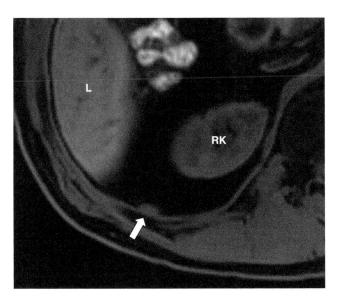

Fig. 6.9 Prominent lateral arcuate ligament of the diaphragm in a 17-year-old boy. Axial non-enhanced T1-weighted fat-suppressed MR image shows a nodular structure (*arrow*) in the right posterior pararenal space, consistent with a lateral arcuate ligament. L liver, RK right kidney

Anatomic Variants

Chest Wall

Minor variations in morphology of the anterior chest wall are common, occurring in one-third of children [25, 26]. These include tilted sternum, prominent convexity of the rib or costal cartilage, asymmetry of the costal cartilage, and bifid ribs [25–27] (Figs. 6.11 and 6.12). Small paracostal subcutaneous nodules may also be seen, thought to represent islands of cartilage [25, 26]. These variations generally carry no clinical significance; however, they are frequently the cause of imaging referrals for palpable chest lumps.

including the sternum, ribs, and vertebrae. The diaphragmatic "slips" of the muscle which attach to the anterior ribs, as well as the medial and lateral arcuate ligaments which attach to the psoas, quadratus lumborum, and vertebrae, may be visible on imaging and should not be mistaken for nodules (Figs. 6.8 and 6.9). The diaphragmatic crura at the median portion of the diaphragm attach posteriorly to the upper lumbar vertebrae and discs. The right and left crus are connected by the fibrous median arcuate ligament [20]. In

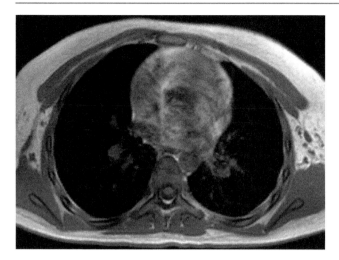

Fig. 6.11 Tilted sternum in a 16-year-old girl who presented with chest wall asymmetry. Axial non-enhanced T1-weighted MR image demonstrates oblique rather than horizontal orientation of the sternum, resulting in asymmetry of the chest wall

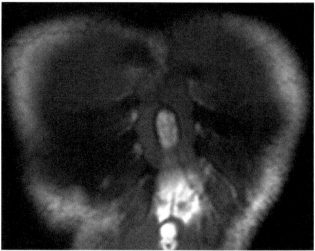

Fig. 6.13 Sternal foramen in a 17-year-old boy. Coronal non-enhanced T1-weighted MR image shows an ovoid defect in the midline sternal body

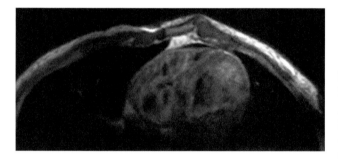

Fig. 6.12 Anatomic variant of the chest wall in a 16-year-old boy who presented with palpable chest lump. Axial T1-weighted non-enhanced MR image demonstrates focal anterior protrusion of the chest wall to the left of midline, due to prominent convexity of the costal cartilage and tilting of the sternum

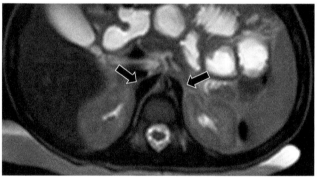

Fig. 6.14 Prominent diaphragmatic crura in a 21-month-old boy. Axial non-enhanced T2-weighted MR image shows a thickened or nodular appearance of the crura (*arrows*), which is a normal finding in small children

There are several minor developmental variants of the sternum, the most common of which is the sternal foramen, found in 5% of the population [28]. It consists of a 3–18 mm smooth round- or oval-shaped defect in the midline sternal body, caused by incomplete fusion of the sternal bars [29] (Fig. 6.13). The finding is asymptomatic but may need precautions during sternal punctures and acupuncture. In contrast, cleft sternum is a rare abnormality with a larger defect between the sternal halves, which may be seen with other disorders such as pentalogy of Cantrell [29].

The sternalis muscle is a variant of chest wall musculature found in 1–18% of the population and is more often unilateral than bilateral [30]. It courses perpendicular to the medial edge of the pectoralis major, and there is wide variation in its size. It has no known clinical significance and should not be mistaken for a chest wall lesion [31].

Diaphragm

In small children, particularly under the age of 5 years, the crura are relatively larger in size and may have a nodular appearance, mimicking adenopathy [21] (Fig. 6.14).

There are three variations in imaging appearance of the anterior portion of the diaphragm, based on the cephalo-caudad relationship of the xiphoid to the central tendon [32]. These are described on CT but are sometimes visible on MR imaging as well. In type 1, the most frequent type (48%), the central tendon is cephalic to the xiphoid resulting in a smooth contour of the anterior diaphragm on axial images. In type 2 (28%), the central tendon is caudal to the xiphoid, resulting in a divergent appearance of the diaphragm in the midline on axial images. In type 3 (11%), the central tendon is at the same level of the xiphoid, resulting in a thick and irregular appearance of the anterior diaphragm on axial images.

Spectrum of Chest Wall Disorders

Congenital and Developmental Chest Wall Disorders

Congenital and developmental disorders of the chest wall can be recognized on MR imaging in pediatric patients referred for workup of focal lesions or chest wall deformities. The following sections describe the spectrum of these disorders with attention to anomalies of the ribs, sternum, clavicles, and chest wall musculature.

Rib Anomalies

Numerical Rib Anomalies

Supernumerary ribs may be present as a normal variant but are also associated with trisomy 21 and VATER (vertebral, anus, tracheoesophageal, and renal anomalies) [33, 34]. Eleven paired ribs are commonly seen in normal patients (5–8%), as well as in one-third of trisomy 21 patients.

Morphological Rib Anomalies

There is a wide spectrum of morphological deformities of the ribs. Some examples include developmental fusion between ribs, articulation or bony bridging between ribs, and bifid or forked configuration of ribs [27, 35, 36] (Fig. 6.15). These may be considered anatomic variants as they are typically of no clinical significance. Shortening of a mid-thoracic (sixth, seventh, or eighth) rib is a common incidental finding seen in up to 16% of the population [36, 37]. More severe shortening of numerous ribs, such that they do not reach the sternum, is a finding in the short-rib polydactyly syndromes. Intrathoracic ribs are rare supernumerary ribs most commonly found on the right side within the mid-thorax [35].

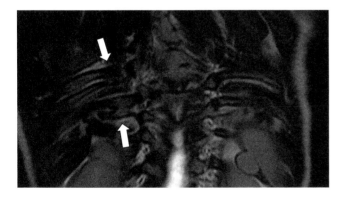

Fig. 6.15 Rib anomalies in a 2-year-old girl with scoliosis. Coronal non-enhanced T2-weighted MR image through the posterior chest demonstrates multiple fusion anomalies (*arrows*) of the right-sided ribs

Cervical Rib

Cervical ribs are seen in 0.2–8% of the population and may be unilateral or bilateral [35]. Cervical ribs are supernumerary ribs arising from the seventh cervical vertebrae and may terminate blindly or fuse distally to the first rib [38] (Fig. 6.16). While typically incidental, cervical ribs are also associated with Klippel-Feil anomaly [34]. In older children and adults, cervical ribs can contribute to thoracic outlet syndrome by compression of the subclavian vessels or brachial plexus [38, 39].

Pectus Excavatum

Pectus excavatum is the most common congenital deformity of the chest wall with a range of incidence of 1 in 400–1000 and a male-to-female ratio of 5:1 [40]. In this deformity, the inferior aspect of the sternum is depressed inward resulting in concavity of the chest wall. The depression is often asymmetric with right-sided predominance due to rotation of the sternum [41]. Pectus excavatum is familial in 45% of patients

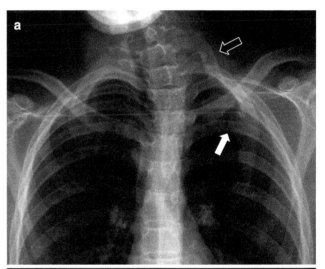

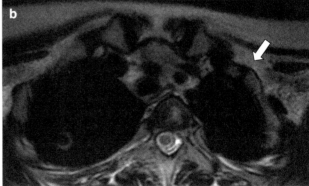

Fig. 6.16 Large cervical rib in a 10-year-old girl who presented with thoracic outlet syndrome. (**a**) Frontal chest radiograph shows a large left cervical rib (*black arrow*) which articulates with the second rib (*white arrow*). The left first rib is absent. (**b**) Axial non-enhanced T2-weighted MR image shows the left cervical rib articulating (*arrow*) with the second rib

[7]. Associated anomalies include scoliosis and connective tissue diseases (Marfan and Ehlers-Danlos syndromes) [41]. The etiology of pectus deformities is thought to be due to misdirected growth of the lower costal cartilages, rather than abnormal growth of the sternum itself [41].

The Haller index is a measure of severity of pectus excavatum deformity [42]. It is calculated from an axial image by dividing the maximum transverse dimension of the thorax (from the inner margin of the ribs) by the minimum anteroposterior dimension of the thorax [42]. An index less than 2.56 is normal. An index greater than 3.25 is an indication for surgery, along with compromised pulmonary or cardiac function [42]. While the Haller index was initially described on CT, a single MR acquisition in the axial plane can easily serve the same purpose while avoiding ionizing radiation [43–45] (Fig. 6.17). Balanced steady-state free precession is a good choice of pulse sequence because it is rapid and produces high signal-to-noise ratio images [44, 45]. Short acquisition times can minimize respiratory artifact. Pectus protocols vary across institutions as to use of breath-hold versus free breathing, although it should be noted that inspiratory breath-hold images usually underestimate the Haller index [46]. Cardiac gating is not required.

Pectus Carinatum

Pectus carinatum is the second most common chest wall deformity, occurring in 1 in 1500 live births [40]. In this deformity, the sternum protrudes outward. Three types of carinatum deformity are recognized [29]. In classic carinatum, known as "keel chest" or "pyramidal chest," the lower third of the sternum protrudes outward. In lateral pectus cari-

natum, there is unilateral protrusion of the costal cartilages with contralateral rotation of the sternum. In "pouter pigeon breast," the protrusion is at the sterno-manubrial junction, and the sternal body may be depressed resulting in a mixed defect [29, 47].

Pectus carinatum is associated with the same disorders as listed above for pectus excavatum; however, cardiopulmonary symptoms are less common. MR imaging may be used for surgical planning, particularly in patients with mixed defects (Fig. 6.18).

Poland Syndrome

Poland syndrome is defined by absence of the pectoralis muscle. It is typically unilateral and occurs on the right side more than the left. This disorder is sporadic with incidence of 1 in 30,000 and has male predominance [41]. Three categories of Poland syndrome are recognized. In the mild or partial type, there is only absence of the pectoralis muscle. In the moderate or classic type, there is also costochondral hypoplasia and unilateral hand deformity (syndactyly). In the severe type, there are multiple deficits including rib defects, latissimus and deltoid hypoplasia, and sometimes dextrocardia, ectrodactyly, and unilateral renal agenesis [29, 48]. Hypoplasia of the breast, nipple, and subcutaneous tissue, as well as axillary alopecia, may be seen in Poland syndrome. The most accepted theory for pathogenesis of this

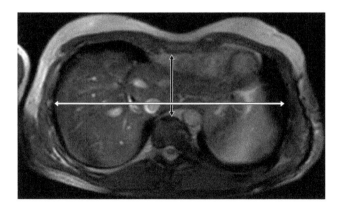

Fig. 6.17 Pectus excavatum in a 14-year-old boy who presented with chest wall deformity. Axial non-enhanced balanced FFE MR image demonstrates inward depression of the sternum consistent with pectus excavatum. The Haller index is obtained by dividing the transverse dimension of the chest (*white line*) by the narrowest anteroposterior dimension of the chest (*black line*). In this patient, the Haller index measured 3.9

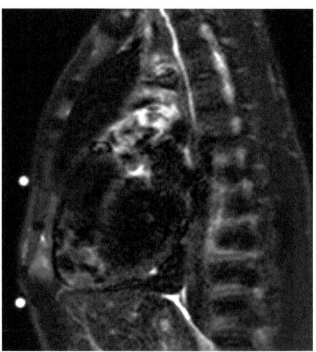

Fig. 6.18 Pectus carinatum in a 19-year-old boy who presented with chest wall deformity. Sagittal non-enhanced STIR MR image demonstrates outward protrusion of the lower third of the sternum (*denoted by skin markers*) consistent with pectus carinatum

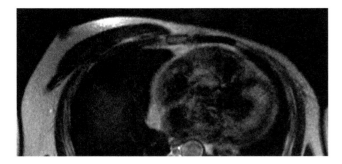

Fig. 6.19 Poland syndrome in an 18-year-old boy. Axial non-enhanced T2-weighted MR image demonstrates absence of the left pectoral muscles and thinning of the left chest wall soft tissues, consistent with Poland syndrome

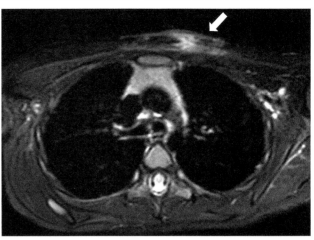

Fig. 6.20 Cellulitis in a 4-year-old boy who presented with chest wall pain and fever. Axial non-enhanced T2-weighted fat-suppressed MR image demonstrates ill-defined edema (*arrow*) of the subcutaneous tissue of the left upper chest wall, with associated skin thickening, consistent with cellulitis

disorder is in disruption of subclavian blood supply during limb bud development [29, 49].

MR imaging is useful for diagnostic purposes and to delineate the extent of muscle, soft tissue, and bone involvement [50] (Fig. 6.19). MR imaging can be used to assess the size of the latissimus dorsi and the anterior abdominal wall muscles, to plan for muscle flap reconstruction [16, 50, 51].

Cleidocranial Dysplasia

Cleidocranial dysplasia is a rare autosomal dominant skeletal dysplasia affecting bones that form through intramembranous ossification, including the clavicles, skull, and pelvis [52]. The typical findings include the following triad: partial or complete absence of the clavicles, supernumerary or impacted teeth, and delayed fontanel closure [16, 53]. There is a broad spectrum of additional skeletal findings, some of which include short stature, midface hypoplasia, kyphoscoliosis, pelvic bone hypoplasia with pseudo-widening of the symphysis pubis, and brachydactyly.

In addition to clavicular hypoplasia, the thoracic deformities seen on imaging include shortened ribs with a bell-shaped thorax, as well as vertebral anomalies. When a congenital clavicular abnormality is identified, affected pediatric patients should undergo genetic workup for this syndrome; however, once the diagnosis has been established, no specific imaging follow-up is needed [16, 53]. Radiologists may encounter thoracic findings of this syndrome on MR imaging in patients referred for workup of spinal deformities [54].

Infectious Chest Wall Disorders

Infections of the chest wall in children are uncommon and may occur by direct extension or hematogenous spread [16, 47]. Soft tissue and/or bone can be affected. An overview of the spectrum of chest wall infections is described in the sections below.

Cellulitis

Cellulitis is a bacterial infection of the skin, subcutaneous tissue, and superficial fascia, with sparing of the muscle and deep fascia [55]. It is most commonly caused by *Staphylococcus aureus* or *Streptococcus pyogenes* and presents with erythema, swelling, warmth, pain, fever, and chills. While cellulitis is a clinical diagnosis, imaging may be requested to investigate complications such as soft tissue abscess and muscle or bone involvement. Cellulitis of the chest wall follows the same imaging pattern as it does for other areas of the body.

On MR imaging, findings include soft tissue thickening, edema signal on fluid-sensitive sequences, and post-contrast enhancement (Fig. 6.20). These findings are more apparent on MR imaging compared to other imaging modalities because of its high contrast resolution and sensitivity for edema [8].

Cellulitis must be distinguished from necrotizing fasciitis, which involves the deep soft tissues, progresses much more rapidly, and has significant morbidity and mortality if untreated. Necrotizing fasciitis is exceedingly rare in children and is unusual to present in the chest wall [56]. Predisposing factors include immunosuppression and skin wounds [56, 57]. Affected pediatric patients may present with sepsis and multiorgan failure, and the degree of pain is disproportionately higher than skin involvement [55]. When involving the chest wall, hemorrhagic changes can be seen [56]. The presence of T2 hyperintensity and thickening of the deep peripheral and intermuscular fascia are sensitive but nonspecific on MR imaging [8, 55]. The rare finding of soft tissue gas characterized by low-signal foci with blooming artifact on gradient echo is highly specific [55, 58].

Abscess

Chest wall abscess is an unusual manifestation of primary chest wall infection in the pediatric population. Soft tissue abscess can be seen after an open wound or thoracic surgery, and bony abscess may result from osteomyelitis, costochondritis, or sternoclavicular joint infection [59]. The presence of a primary chest wall abscess should prompt a workup for tuberculosis (discussed in a subsequent section) [48, 60].

Similar to abscess in other body parts, on MR imaging, a chest wall abscess presents as an inflammatory mass, with a central fluid portion with high signal on T2-weighted and STIR sequences, and peripheral enhancement (Fig. 6.21). The central signal may vary if there is blood or high protein content in the abscess cavity [61]. The differential diagnosis is a centrally necrotic tumor [8].

Osteomyelitis

Osteomyelitis of the chest wall is exceedingly rare and can affect the ribs, sternum, or vertebrae. Bacterial infections are more common than fungal infections, which can be seen in immunocompromised pediatric patients [7]. Causative organisms include *Staphylococcus aureus*, *Mycobacterium tuberculosis*, *Actinomyces*, *Aspergillus*, and *Candida* [7, 62]. Symptoms are similar to those of other chest wall infections including fever, leukocytosis, erythema, swelling, and pain.

MR imaging is useful in identifying the presence of osteomyelitis, delineating its extent, and identifying osseous or peri-osseous abscesses. The hallmark finding on MR imaging is bone marrow edema, which can occur with or without frank bone destruction, and is associated with adjacent soft tissue inflammation [8] (Fig. 6.22). Use of intravenous contrast assists with detection of abscesses.

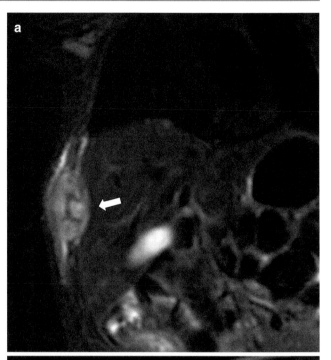

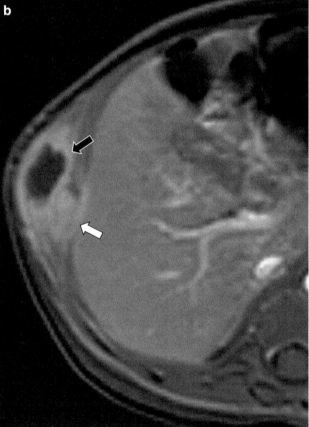

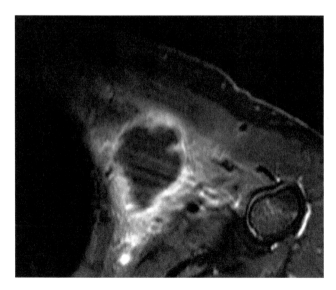

Fig. 6.21 Abscess in a 7-year-old girl who presented with chest wall pain, swelling, and fever. Axial enhanced T1-weighted fat-suppressed MR image demonstrates a large subpectoral fluid collection with a thick enhancing rim, consistent with an abscess

Fig. 6.22 Osteomyelitis in a 3-month-old boy who presented with fever and chest wall swelling. (**a**) Coronal non-enhanced STIR MR image demonstrates expansion and marrow edema of a right-sided rib (*arrow*), with surrounding high-signal inflammatory tissue and soft tissue edema, consistent with osteomyelitis. (**b**) Axial enhanced T1-weighted fat-suppressed MR image demonstrates enhancement of the affected rib (*white arrow*), with an adjacent thick-walled fluid collection (*black arrow*) consistent with abscess

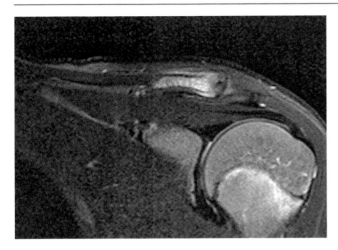

Fig. 6.23 Chronic nonbacterial osteomyelitis (CNO) in a 15-year-old boy who presented with shoulder pain. Coronal non-enhanced STIR MR image demonstrates edema and periosteal reaction of the left clavicle

The differential diagnosis for osteomyelitis of the chest wall includes chronic nonbacterial osteomyelitis (CNO). This is a chronic relapsing-remitting disorder of unknown etiology which may be autoimmune in nature. Its first presentation is often in childhood, with symptoms of osteomyelitis but with no organism on biopsy cultures [63]. The usual chest wall sites of CNO include the clavicles, ribs, and sternum. In the acute and healing phases, MR imaging findings can be essentially identical to those of infectious osteomyelitis (Fig. 6.23).

Tuberculosis

Mycobacterium tuberculosis (TB) infection of the chest wall may result from hematogenous seeding after pulmonary infection or less commonly as a primary infection [48, 64, 65]. Intrathoracic TB involving lymph nodes or pleura can burrow into the chest wall and present as a lump or mass [66]. Chest wall abscess has also been reported as a complication of BCG vaccination in children [60, 67]. TB infections of the chest wall can affect the ribs and sternum and less commonly the soft tissues [62, 66, 67]. Imaging findings include osseous and cartilaginous erosion with adjacent soft tissue abscesses [62, 68].

On MR imaging, TB osteomyelitis demonstrates irregular alteration of marrow signal, cortical destruction, and ill-defined soft tissue, sometimes with formation of sinus or fistula tracts [69]. As with other chest wall abscesses, TB abscesses can mimic a centrally necrotic tumor.

Actinomycosis

Actinomycosis is a bacterial infection associated with dental caries, which can rarely involve the lungs, pleura, and chest wall [48, 70]. Actinomycosis is known to cross anatomic boundaries and can breach pulmonary fissures, spread through the pleura to the diaphragm, chest wall soft tissues,

or bones, and form fistulas and sinus tracts [16, 48]. Suggestive findings on imaging are a lower lobe pulmonary consolidation with empyema and erosion or periostitis of ribs [70]. While CT can demonstrate these findings, MR imaging is more helpful to delineate soft tissue extension and identify fistulas and abscesses [16, 71].

Empyema Necessitans

Empyema necessitans (EN) is a complication of empyema in which pus from the pleural space ruptures into the chest wall, most commonly at the anterolateral aspect through an intercostal space [72]. EN is rare in children and is classically caused by actinomyces or tuberculosis, although other bacterial and fungal agents can be responsible [73, 74]. Regardless of the organism, MR imaging findings are similar to those described in the section on actinomycosis, with an inflammatory pleural collection extending to the soft tissues of the chest wall (Fig. 6.24). The process can mimic a tumor and may require biopsy, although lack of rib changes favors infection over malignancy [74].

Neoplastic Chest Wall Disorders

MR imaging is useful in depicting the tissue composition and anatomic extent of chest wall masses. Many soft tissue masses cannot be distinguished as benign or malignant solely based on imaging. However, MR imaging characteristics in conjunction with patient age, presentation, and location of the mass can help to narrow the differential diagnosis. Additionally, MR imaging assessment of osseous chest wall lesions should be correlated with radiographic and/or CT findings. MR imaging features of pediatric primary chest wall neoplasms are described in the following sections.

Benign Primary Soft Tissue Neoplasms of the Chest Wall

Brown Fat/Hibernoma

Brown adipose tissue or brown fat (BF) consists of small adipocytes that are metabolically active and involved in thermogenesis, in contrast to white or yellow adipose tissue which consists of larger adipocytes that store triglycerides [75]. BF is normally present in neonates and is thought to gradually decrease after infancy, although metabolically active BF can be seen on FDG-PET studies in older children and adults, and may represent a mixture of brown and white adipocyte tissue [75–77]. BF activity correlates inversely with obesity [77].

In infants, thoracic BF is bilateral and symmetric, seen most commonly around the scapula, axilla, intercostal spaces, base of neck, and supraclavicular regions [78] (Fig. 6.25). MR imaging can characterize differences between brown and white fat. Because of its greater meta-

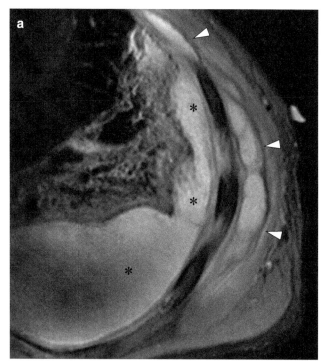

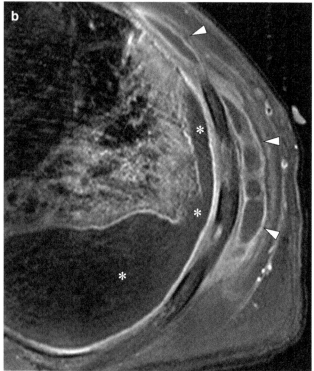

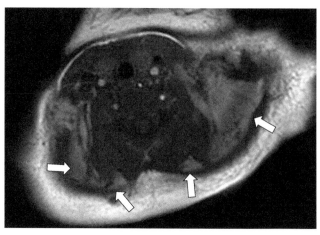

Fig. 6.25 Prominent brown adipose tissue in a 1-month-old boy. Axial non-enhanced T1-weighted MR image demonstrates symmetric distribution of brown adipose tissue (*arrows*) in the supraclavicular and paraspinal regions at the base of the neck. The signal is hyperintense to the muscle but slightly hypointense to subcutaneous fat

Fig. 6.24 Empyema necessitans in an 18-year-old boy who presented with chest wall pain and fever. (**a**) Axial non-enhanced T2-weighted fat-suppressed MR image demonstrates a loculated pleural effusion (*) consistent with empyema, adjacent to abnormal heterogeneous signal in the lung due to pneumonia. There are lobulated fluid collections (*arrowheads*) in the chest wall representing transpleural rupture of the empyema. (**b**) Axial enhanced T1-weighted fat-suppressed MR image demonstrates thick rim enhancement of the empyema (*), as well as of the chest wall fluid collections (*arrowheads*) which are consistent with empyema necessitans

bolic activity and lower amount of triglycerides, BF demonstrates lower fat-signal fraction on chemical shift Dixon MR imaging [75]. Due to greater oxygen consumption, greater blood perfusion, and larger amount of mitochondria with intracellular iron, BF also demonstrates lower $T2^*$ relaxation times [75, 76].

Hibernoma is a rare benign tumor of BF that presents as a painless slow-growing mass, usually arising in sites corresponding to the fetal distribution of BF, but also found in other sites such as the thigh [79–81]. The specific diagnosis is usually not made on imaging alone because the appearance overlaps with other neoplasms [79]. Although hibernomas contain fat, on T1-weighted MR images, they are hyperintense to the muscle but hypointense relative to subcutaneous fat, with minimal chemical shift artifact and lack of complete signal suppression on STIR [78–81] (Fig. 6.26). These tumors are well circumscribed and highly vascular with avid enhancement and may contain thin septal bands [78–81].

Lipoma and Lipoblastoma

Adipocytic tumors in children include benign lesions (lipoma and lipoblastoma) and malignant lesions (liposarcoma). Other chest wall masses may also demonstrate internal fat, including hibernoma, fibrous hamartoma, and involuting hemangiomas, as described in other sections of this chapter.

The chest wall and trunk is a relatively common site for benign lipomas, especially the upper back [61]. Most lipomas are superficial (subcutaneous); however, deep lipomas can affect the inter- or intramuscular compartments of the chest wall [82]. Because they are composed of mature adipocytes (i.e., macroscopic fat), lipomas follow the same MR imaging characteristics as subcutaneous fat on all sequences,

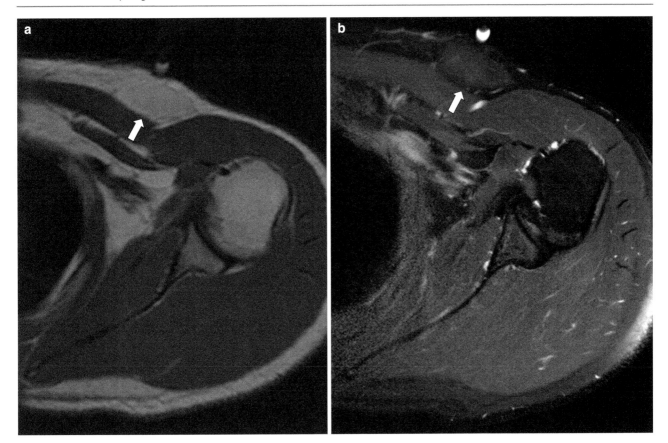

Fig. 6.26 Hibernoma in a 17-year-old boy who presented with chest wall mass. (a) Axial non-enhanced T1-weighted MR image demonstrates a mass (*arrow*) in the subcutaneous tissue of the left anterior chest wall, which is isointense to slightly hypointense to the subcutaneous fat. (b) Axial non-enhanced T2-weighted fat-suppressed MR image demonstrates that the mass (*arrow*) is minimally hyperintense to the subcutaneous fat, due to lack of complete fat signal suppression

including high signal on T1- and T2-weighted MR images, and fat suppression on STIR [61] (Fig. 6.27). Lesions do not enhance aside from minimal enhancement of a few thin septa (<2 mm) [61, 82, 83].

Lipoblastoma is an uncommon rapidly growing benign tumor, which lacks metastatic potential but can be locally invasive. It arises from immature adipocytes (embryonal fat tissue) and presents in infants and young children under the age of 3 years. On MR imaging, lipoblastomas demonstrate fat signal but are more heterogeneous than simple lipomas due to the presence of stromal tissue [61, 82]. The differential diagnosis for this MR imaging appearance is liposarcoma; however, liposarcoma is exceedingly rare in the pediatric age group [61].

The terms lipomatosis and lipoblastomatosis refer to non-encapsulated versions of the above lesions, which can be diffusely proliferative and sometimes infiltrate deep into the musculature [61] (Fig. 6.28).

Desmoid Fibromatosis

Desmoid-type fibromatosis (DF) is a benign myofibroblastic tumor which is slow growing and does not metastasize

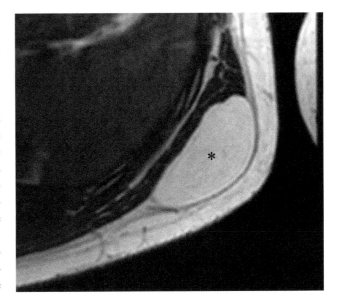

Fig. 6.27 Lipoma in a 16-year-old boy who presented with palpable chest wall mass. Axial non-enhanced T1-weighted MR image demonstrates a homogeneous encapsulated mass (*) in the left chest wall overlying the latissimus dorsi, which was isointense to the subcutaneous fat on all sequences

but can be locally aggressive with a high tendency for recurrence [84, 85]. It is also known as aggressive fibromatosis or desmoid tumor and is seen with greater incidence in APC gene mutations such as familial adenomatous polyposis (Gardner syndrome). DF is a rare lesion that can occur in any location, but when involving the chest wall, sites include the intercostal muscles, axilla, and shoulder or supraclavicular region [8, 85].

MR imaging is important for defining regional extent of DF for therapeutic planning and post-treatment monitoring [86,

87]. Chest wall DF is isointense to the muscle on T1-weighted MR images, hyperintense or intermediate on T2-weighted MR images and has heterogeneous but usually strong enhancement [85–87] (Fig. 6.29). Non-enhancing low-signal bands may be present [84, 85, 88]. DF may be well-defined or infiltrative [88]. "Fascial tails" may be seen, with linear extension of signal abnormality along fascial planes [84, 89].

Myofibroma and Infantile Myofibromatosis

Myofibroma (MF; solitary) and infantile myofibromatosis (IM; multicentric) are additional entities within the benign category of pediatric fibroblastic-myofibroblastic lesions. These are the most common fibrous tumors of infancy, with the majority of cases presenting at birth or within the first 2 years of life, although older patients can be affected [84, 90]. Solitary MF most commonly affects the skin and subcutaneous tissue, whereas multicentric IM can also involve the muscle, bone, and viscera [84, 90, 91]. The most common sites of involvement are the head, neck, and trunk [84].

MR imaging is the most important imaging technique for assessing the extent of MF/IM; however, the appearance is nonspecific. Signal intensity is variable on T1 and mixed but predominantly hyperintense on T2, and enhancement is typically peripheral due to central necrosis [84, 90, 91] (Fig. 6.30). Lesions may be well-defined or infiltrative and may contain hemorrhagic components, calcification, or cystic change [47, 84]. Affected bones can demonstrate erosion, sclerotic margins, cortical expansion, scalloping, or pathologic fracture [47, 84, 90]. Although MF/IM is a benign lesion and usually spontaneously regresses in 1–2 years, visceral involvement

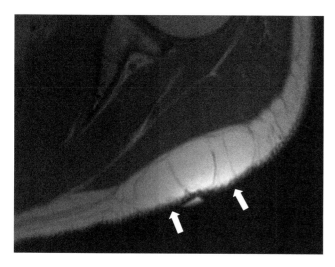

Fig. 6.28 Lipomatosis in a 17-year-old girl who presented with palpable chest wall mass. Axial non-enhanced T1-weighted MR image demonstrates a mass-like region (*arrows*) in the left shoulder posterior to the deltoid, which was isointense to the subcutaneous fat on all sequences but is nonencapsulated

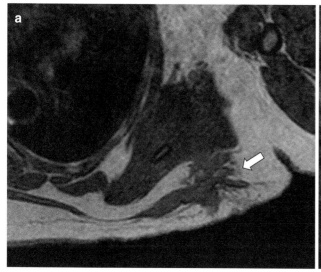 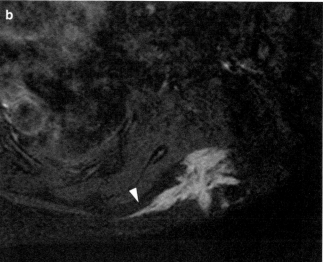

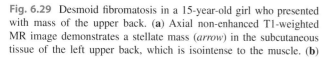

Fig. 6.29 Desmoid fibromatosis in a 15-year-old girl who presented with mass of the upper back. (**a**) Axial non-enhanced T1-weighted MR image demonstrates a stellate mass (*arrow*) in the subcutaneous tissue of the left upper back, which is isointense to the muscle. (**b**)

Axial enhanced T1-weighted fat-suppressed MR image shows strong enhancement of the mass, with a "fascial tail" (*arrowhead*) extending medially along the superficial fascia

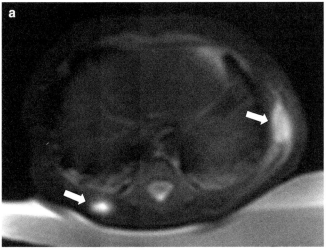

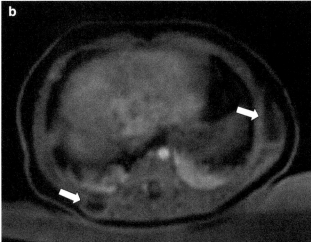

Fig. 6.30 Infantile myofibromatosis in a 7-week-old boy who presented with multiple palpable chest wall nodules. (**a**) Axial non-enhanced T2-weighted fat-suppressed MR image shows well-defined hyperintense nodules (*arrows*) in the right posterior and left lateral chest wall. (**b**) Axial enhanced T1-weighted fat-suppressed MR image shows that the nodules (*arrows*) demonstrate peripheral enhancement, typical of myofibromas

requires aggressive therapy due to high mortality. Whole-body MR imaging can be helpful for diagnosis and follow-up of visceral and/or multicentric disease [92–94].

Fibrous Hamartoma

Fibrous hamartoma of infancy (FH) is a benign subcutaneous fibrous tumor, presenting as a rapidly growing mass in the first 2 years of life, and may be present at birth [84]. Common locations of FH include the trunk, upper extremities, and inguinal regions [92]. Lesions demonstrate three histological components: bundles of fibrocollagenous tissue, islands of primitive mesenchyma, and mature fat [84, 92]. The MR imaging appearance of FH is reflective of this histology, usually demonstrating an infiltrative or nonencapsulated mass with a serpentine pattern of T1 and T2 hypointense fibrous strands, interspersed with hyperintense fat [92, 95]. This MR imaging appearance, in the appropriate clinical setting, is highly suggestive of the diagnosis [95].

Neurofibroma

Neurofibroma is the most common peripheral neurogenic tumor in the pediatric population [92]. Neurofibroma is a benign nerve sheath tumor arising from Schwann cells and takes one of three forms: localized or solitary (90%), diffuse, and plexiform [96]. Plexiform neurofibroma is a pathognomonic finding of neurofibromatosis type 1. Chest wall neurogenic tumors may arise from intercostal nerves or a spinal nerve root [97].

On MR imaging, localized neurofibroma is a well-defined fusiform mass that is isointense to the muscle on T1-weighted MR images, hyperintense on T2-weighted MR images and has avid or heterogeneous enhancement [8, 92, 98] (Fig. 6.31). Also on T2-weighted MR images, a target sign is typical, seen as central hypointensity with a hyperintense rim; this finding

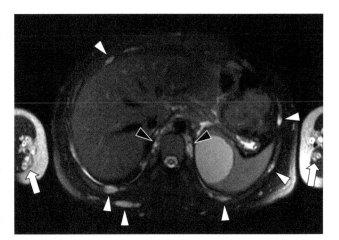

Fig. 6.31 Neurofibromatosis type 1 and multiple chest wall neurofibromas in a 15-year-old boy. Axial non-enhanced T2-weighted fat-suppressed MR image demonstrates multiple ovoid T2 hyperintense lesions (*white arrowheads*) through the chest wall soft tissues and intercostal regions consistent with neurofibromas. There are plexiform neurofibromas in the paraspinal region (*black arrowheads*). Plexiform neurofibromas are also seen in both arms (*arrows*), which demonstrate the "target" sign of neurofibroma

helps differentiate neurofibromas from malignant peripheral nerve sheath tumors [98]. Other findings associated with solitary neurofibromas, such as the major nerve/tail sign and split fat sign, are seen in extremity lesions but have not been commonly described for chest wall lesions [96]. Pressure erosion of adjacent osseous structures may be seen [97]. Plexiform neurofibromas are larger and multinodular, extending along a nerve trunk with a "bag of worms" appearance [92, 97]. Diffuse neurofibroma and superficial plexiform neurofibroma affect the skin and subcutaneous tissue with an infiltrating morphology and lack of target sign [96, 99].

Schwannoma

Schwannoma is another benign tumor of Schwann cells, rarely found in the pediatric population, which are usually solitary but can be multiple in schwannomatosis and neurofibromatosis type 2 [96]. Unlike neurofibromas, schwannomas are eccentric and at surgical excision are separable from the nerve [92]. In the paraspinal location, these lesions may acquire a dumbbell shape by growing into the spinal canal through the neural foramen [97]. Schwannomas share many of the same MR imaging signal characteristics described above for neurofibromas [92, 96]. However, some schwannomas can be large and undergo internal necrosis or hemorrhage, leading to loss of the target sign and mimicking the appearance of a sarcoma [8, 92, 96, 97].

Benign Primary Osseous Neoplasms of the Chest Wall

Osteoid Osteoma and Osteoblastoma

Osteoid osteoma (OO) is a benign osteoblastic tumor with a central osteoid-rich nidus surrounded by vascular connective tissue and reactive sclerotic bone [100, 101]. It invariably presents with pain, which is classically nocturnal and relieved with aspirin or non-steroidal anti-inflammatory drugs. Most are seen in the lower extremities, although they can occur in any part of the skeleton; 10–20% occur in the spine with predilection for the posterior elements [100]. OO of the ribs can occur but is rare [102, 103]. OO of the spine or rib can cause painful scoliosis in children [102].

On MR imaging, calcification of the nidus as well as the surrounding osteosclerosis may be seen as low signal on both T1- and T2-weighted MR imaging [100] (Fig. 6.32). However, the nidus can be difficult to recognize on MR imaging, and CT is usually required. MR imaging demonstrates perilesional and soft tissue edema, which may mimic a more aggressive tumor. Location in the lamina or pedicle of the vertebrae should raise suspicion for OO [101].

Osteoblastoma is histologically similar to OO, but is larger (>2.0 cm), and can be locally aggressive [101]. Osteoblastomas also have predilection for the posterior elements of the spine and can rarely affect the ribs and sternum [102, 104, 105]. Osteoblastoma may resemble a large OO, but some aggressive lesions are also characterized by lytic expansion and/or a soft tissue component [106]. The signal on T2-weighted MR imaging can be variable or mixed, depending on the degree of internal matrix mineralization. As with osteoid osteoma, the perilesional edema and enhancement can be striking on MR imaging, making it difficult to distinguish the lesion boundaries from the inflammatory response or "flare phenomenon" [101, 106].

Osteochondroma

Osteochondroma or exostosis is the most common benign bone tumor, although it is rare in the chest wall unless part of the multiple hereditary exostoses syndrome [107]. These lesions can arise from any bone with an epiphysis or apophysis, including the ribs and scapula. In the ribs, they are often seen at the costochondral junction [16, 108]. They consist of an osseous protuberance continuous with the cortex and medulla of the parent bone, with an overlying cap of hyaline cartilage. Chest wall osteochondromas can present with cosmetic deformity or pain and sometimes intrathoracic complications such as pleural effusion or pneumothorax [107]. Thickness of the cartilage cap greater than 2 cm raises suspicion for malignant degeneration to chondrosarcoma [109].

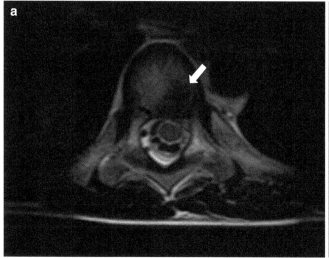
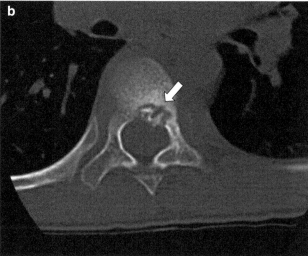

Fig. 6.32 Osteoid osteoma in an 8-year-old boy who presented with painful scoliosis. (a) Axial non-enhanced T2-weighted MR image demonstrates edema surrounding a low-signal region (*arrow*) in the posterior vertebral body. There is edema of the posterior elements, ribs, and paraspinal soft tissue. (b) Axial non-enhanced CT image at the same level demonstrates the calcified nidus of osteoid osteoma (*arrow*), with surrounding osteosclerosis

MR imaging is useful for demonstrating corticomedullary continuity, the thickness of the cartilage cap which is hyperintense on fluid-sensitive sequences, and the presence of bursa formation or compression of neurovascular structures [16, 107] (Fig. 6.33).

Mesenchymal Hamartoma

Mesenchymal hamartoma of the chest wall is a rare lesion arising from the rib in newborns and infants and may be detected prenatally [110]. These are not true neoplasms but rather a benign proliferation of skeletal tissue with a large cartilaginous component, as well as hemorrhagic cavities in the form of secondary aneurysmal bone cyst (ABC) [111]. Mesenchymal hamartoma manifests as a large partially calcified chest wall mass, involving one or more ribs, with intrathoracic projection of an extrapleural soft tissue component [110, 111].

MR imaging demonstrates heterogeneous signal intensity, enhancement of solid portions, and foci of high signal intensity on T1-weighted MR images and/or fluid-fluid levels representing the hemorrhagic cavities [111]. Although the imaging appearance can mimic a malignancy, the newborn age, rib origin, and presence of secondary ABC formation are highly suggestive of this diagnosis [111].

Fibrous Dysplasia

Fibrous dysplasia (FD) is the most common primary bone lesion of the chest wall. It is a fibro-osseous lesion thought to represent primitive bone-forming mesenchyme that fails to

remodel into mature bone [8, 108]. Seventy to 80% are monostotic, and 20–30% are polyostotic; polyostotic FD may be seen as part of McCune-Albright syndrome. Affected pediatric patients may present with chest wall deformity or pathologic fracture.

On MR imaging, FD is a sharply defined sometimes expansile medullary lesion, with a low-signal-intensity (sclerotic) rim (Fig. 6.34). It does not always follow the signal characteristics of pure fibrous tissue [112]. Internal signal intensity can be variable on T2-weighted MR images (low, intermedi-

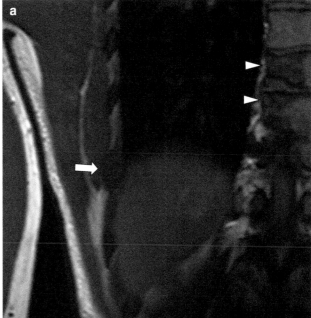

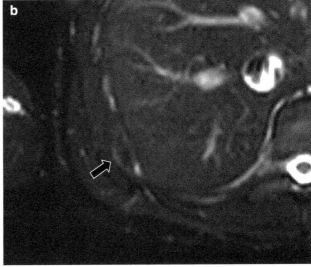

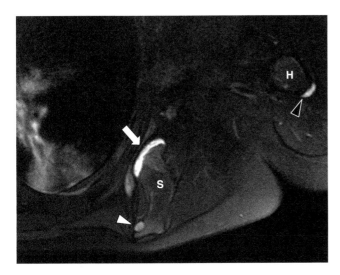

Fig. 6.33 Multiple hereditary exostoses in a 6-year-old boy with chest wall deformity. Axial non-enhanced T2-weighted fat-suppressed MR image demonstrates a protuberant lesion arising from the medial aspect of the body of the scapula (S), which is continuous with the medullary cavity and has a thin hyperintense cartilage cap (*arrow*), consistent with osteochondroma. There is mild edema adjacent to the cap which may represent early adventitial bursa formation. Additional smaller osteochondromas are seen arising from the posterior scapula (*white arrowhead*) and humerus (H; *black arrowhead*)

Fig. 6.34 Polyostotic fibrous dysplasia in a 17-year-old girl. (**a**) Coronal non-enhanced T1-weighted MR image shows an expansile hypointense rib lesion (*white arrow*). Additional hypointense lesions (*arrowheads*) with low-signal rims are present in the thoracic vertebrae. (**b**) Axial enhanced T1-weighted fat-suppressed MR image shows hypointensity of the lesion with minimal peripheral enhancement (*black arrow*), consistent with fibrous dysplasia

ate, or high) depending on the degree of calcification, fat, and cystic degeneration and low on T1-weighted MR images [108, 112]. Most lesions demonstrate enhancement, but the pattern may vary from peripheral to patchy to homogeneous [112].

Aneurysmal Bone Cyst

Aneurysmal bone cysts (ABCs) are benign osteolytic lesions that cause bone expansion and cortical thinning and contain multiple blood-filled cavities lined by osteoclastic giant cells [16]. ABC may arise as a primary lesion or secondary as a reaction to another lesion. In the chest wall, ABCs are found in the posterior elements of the spine and less commonly the ribs [16, 108]. Suggestive MR imaging features are a thin-walled septated lesion with a low-signal rim and fluid-fluid levels corresponding to the hemorrhagic components [8, 108].

Solid ABC is a rare subtype which demonstrates the histologic features found in the solid portions of a classic ABC [113]. This lesion is essentially the same as the giant cell reparative granuloma, which classically presents in the jaw [114]. Solid ABC is most often seen in the hands or feet and rarely in the long bones, and there are isolated reports in the ribs [113–115]. MR imaging is nonspecific, demonstrating a solid-enhancing lesion, with or without a cystic component and typically without the fluid-fluid levels of a classic ABC [114].

Langerhans Cell Histiocytosis

Langerhans cell histiocytosis (LCH) is a spectrum of focal and systemic diseases characterized by proliferation of histiocytes. LCH confined to the bone was formerly called eosinophilic granuloma and most commonly presents as a solitary lesion [16, 102]. The imaging appearance of LCH varies based on disease activity. In the acute phase, lesions appear more aggressive with ill-defined borders, cortical destruction, and a soft tissue component [116] (Fig. 6.35). In the late or healing phase, lesions are better defined, with sclerotic margins.

MR imaging is particularly helpful in identifying the soft tissue component and can be used to monitor patients who are given therapy [117]. Lesions are hypointense on T1- and hyperintense on T2-weighted MR images, demonstrate diffuse enhancement, and are associated with adjacent bone marrow and soft tissue edema [102, 116]. Vertebral lesions may progress to uniform collapse ("vertebra plana") [118]. While skeletal survey or bone scan was traditionally used for extent-of-disease workup, whole-body MRI has been shown to identify more skeletal lesions as well as extraskeletal manifestations of LCH [119].

Malignant Primary Soft Tissue Neoplasms of the Chest Wall

Sarcoma

Soft tissue sarcomas of the pediatric chest wall are rare, including tumors such as rhabdomyosarcoma, fibrosarcoma, synovial sarcoma, hemangiopericytoma, malignant fibrous

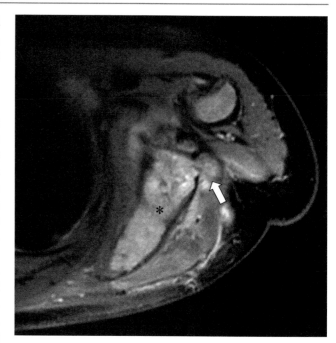

Fig. 6.35 Langerhans cell histiocytosis of the bone in a 12-month-old boy who presented with back and shoulder swelling. Axial non-enhanced T2-weighted fat-suppressed MR image demonstrates an aggressive-appearing, expansile lesion (∗) of the left scapula, with cortical destruction and soft tissue mass (*arrow*). There is edema of the surrounding musculature

histiocytoma, malignant peripheral nerve sheath tumor (MPNST), and others [108, 120]. These tumors are generally difficult to distinguish from one another by imaging, and the role of MR imaging is to assess tumor size, origin, and resectability [121]. Most sarcomas are large (>5 cm), hypointense on T1-weighted MR images, and hyperintense on T2-weighted MR images, with enhancement and peritumoral soft tissue edema [121]. Patient age and clinical presentation can assist with the differential diagnosis.

Rhabdomyosarcoma (RMS) is the most common childhood soft tissue sarcoma. It arises from primitive mesenchymal cells related to striated muscle, although it can occur in any body part excluding the bone [7, 120]. Most pediatric chest wall RMS are alveolar or embryonal type [120, 121]. On MR imaging, RMS is a nonspecific-appearing soft tissue mass, which enhances heterogeneously, and often demonstrates necrosis (Fig. 6.36).

Infantile Fibrosarcoma

Infantile fibrosarcoma (IF), also known as congenital fibrosarcoma, is a rare malignant tumor of spindled fibroblasts that falls within the spectrum of pediatric fibroblastic-myofibroblastic tumors, some of which have been discussed in the above section on benign neoplasms [122]. IF occurs in the extremities (especially the shoulder girdle), head-neck, and trunk, and is histologically similar to its adult counterpart but with more favorable prognosis. It presents in neonates and infants under the age of 1 year as a large mass that may undergo hemorrhage or necrosis [120, 123].

MR imaging of IF is nonspecific and demonstrates an infiltrative mass with heterogeneous contrast enhancement [121, 123] (Fig. 6.37). Blood products, foci of fibrous tissue, and calcification are sometimes present [123, 124]. The heterogeneous enhancement pattern helps distinguish this lesion from hemangioma of infancy, which has more homogeneous

enhancement or is highly vascularized with visible flow voids [7, 123]. Both lesions may result in skin discoloration [7, 121].

Malignant Peripheral Nerve Sheath Tumors

Malignant peripheral nerve sheath tumors (MPNST) are rare, particular within the thorax. MPNST is a high-grade spindle cell sarcoma of the nerve sheath, which may be sporadic but is associated with neurofibromatosis type 1 in 50% of cases [125]. MPNST often arises in a preexisting plexiform neurofibroma and is characterized by pain, rapid growth, and large size (>5 cm) [92, 97].

On MR imaging, it is variable in appearance depending on size and presence of hemorrhage or necrosis [97] (Fig. 6.38). MR imaging features that are more suggestive of MPNST over benign neurogenic tumors include a peripheral enhancement pattern, perilesional edema-like zone, intratumoral cysts, and lack of the target sign [125, 126]. Heterogeneity on T1-weighted MR images and substantially restricted diffusion favor a MPNST over neurofibroma [96, 126].

Malignant Primary Osseous Neoplasms of the Chest Wall

Ewing Sarcoma

The Ewing sarcoma (ES) family of tumors are the most common malignant chest wall malignancies in children and include classic Ewing sarcoma of bone, extraosseous Ewing sarcoma, and primitive neuroectodermal tumor (PNET) of the

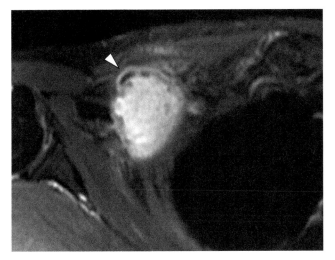

Fig. 6.36 Rhabdomyosarcoma in a 15-year-old girl who presented with a painful and rapidly growing chest wall mass. Axial enhanced T1-weighted MR image shows a large enhancing mass in the upper right chest wall and axilla, with ill-defined margins. There are small areas of necrosis (*arrowhead*) in the anterior margin of the tumor

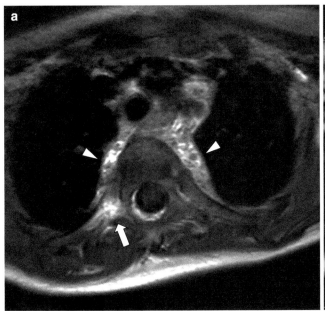 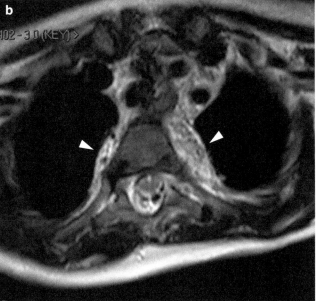

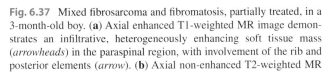

Fig. 6.37 Mixed fibrosarcoma and fibromatosis, partially treated, in a 3-month-old boy. (**a**) Axial enhanced T1-weighted MR image demonstrates an infiltrative, heterogeneously enhancing soft tissue mass (*arrowheads*) in the paraspinal region, with involvement of the rib and posterior elements (*arrow*). (**b**) Axial non-enhanced T2-weighted MR

image demonstrates punctate low-signal foci throughout the lesion (*arrowheads*) which may be due to fibrous tissue and/or calcification. There are no large flow voids to suggest a vascular anomaly. (Case courtesy of Benjamin H. Taragin, MD, Soroka Medical Center, Beersheba, Negev, Israel)

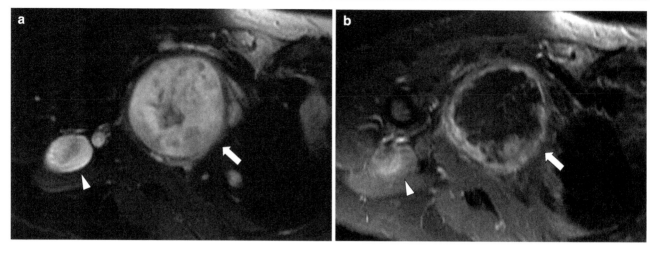

Fig. 6.38 Malignant peripheral nerve sheath tumor in an 18-year-old girl with neurofibromatosis type 1 who presented with an enlarging and palpable chest wall mass. (**a**) Axial non-enhanced T2-weighted fat-suppressed MR image demonstrates a dominant mass (*arrow*) in the upper right chest wall, which is T2 hyperintense but heterogeneous. Smaller neurofibromas (*arrowhead*) are seen in the nearby vicinity. (**b**) Axial enhanced T1-weighted fat-suppressed MR image shows peripheral enhancement of the dominant mass (*arrow*), which suggests malignancy. The nearby benign neurofibroma (*arrowhead*) demonstrates more homogeneous enhancement

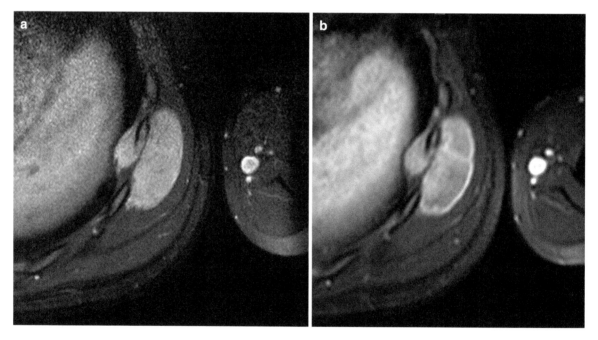

Fig. 6.39 Ewing sarcoma in an 8-year-old boy who presented with a chest wall mass. (**a**) Axial non-enhanced T2-weighted fat-suppressed MR image shows a hyperintense mass in the chest wall centered at the eighth rib, with cortical destruction but a large extraosseous compo-nent, typical of Ewing sarcoma. (**b**) Axial enhanced T1-weighted fat-suppressed MR image demonstrates diffuse enhancement of the mass with areas of faint hypoenhancement due to early necrosis

chest wall or Askin tumor [127]. ES tumors are aggressive small round blue cell tumors, thought to arise from embryonal neural crest cells, and are characterized by a balanced 11;22 chromosomal translocation [128]. Typical chest wall sites include the ribs, sternum, scapula, and clavicles [127]. Paravertebral lesions may have neural foraminal extension [8].

Soft tissue masses of ES are eccentric, large, and heterogeneous with necrosis and sometimes hemorrhage and only rarely calcify [108, 124, 127]. MR imaging demonstrates signal that is isointense or hyperintense to the muscle on T1-weighted MR images and hyperintense on T2-weighted MR images [108, 127] (Fig. 6.39). Post-contrast images demonstrate enhancement and areas of necrosis. The soft tissue component is typically larger than the intraosseous portion of the tumor [34].

Osteosarcoma

Osteosarcoma (OS) is a high-grade malignant bone-forming mesenchymal tumor seen in adolescents and young adults.

OS of the chest wall is rare, and sites of origin can include the ribs, sternum, scapula, and clavicles [8, 127, 128]. The rare extraosseous form can also present in the chest wall but is typically seen after radiation therapy in older adults [125]. OS of the chest wall is associated with greater recurrence and metastatic disease compared to OS of the extremities.

MR imaging is aimed at delineation of tumor extent [8]. OS is a large destructive soft tissue mass that is hypointense on T1-weighted MR images and hyperintense on T2-weighted MR images, although it may have heterogeneous signal due to hemorrhage or cystic change [127] (Fig. 6.40). Calcification in the lesion is hypointense on both T1- and T2-weighted MR imaging [124]. Contrast enhancement is heterogeneous and may demonstrate central necrosis, particularly after chemotherapy [125]. Correlation with radiograph and/or CT is important for appreciation of the osteoid matrix. The telangiectatic form of OS is rare in the chest wall but has a distinct appearance, being lytic on radiographs, and containing cystic spaces with fluid-fluid levels on MR imaging [8, 127].

Metastatic Disease of the Chest Wall

Metastatic disease constitutes a minority of chest wall lesions in children [124]. Metastases to the bones or soft tissues of the chest wall are usually seen in cases where widespread metastases are already present [127, 129]. The primary diagnostic consideration is neuroblastoma, which can directly extend to the chest wall from primary lesions of the posterior mediastinum but can also spread hematogeneously to form lytic lesions in the ribs and spine [124]. Additional tumors that can metastasize to the chest wall are rhabdomyosarcoma, lymphoma, and leukemia, among others. On MR imaging, osseous or soft tissue metastases generally demonstrate signal characteristics specific to the primary tumor from which they originate [127].

Vascular Anomalies of the Chest Wall

The classification scheme from the International Society for the Study of Vascular Anomalies (ISSVA) divides vascular lesions into two major categories: tumors and malformations [130]. Vascular tumors are subdivided into benign, locally aggressive or borderline, and malignant groups. Vascular malformations are subdivided into simple, combined, those of major named vessels, and those associated with other anomalies. A third broad category of provisionally unclassified vascular anomalies includes lesions with overlapping features of tumor and malformation. The following sections describe some of the important vascular lesions that may be encountered in MR imaging of the pediatric chest well.

Chest wall MR imaging examinations performed for suspected vascular lesions should include basic T1- and fat-suppressed T2-weighted or STIR MR imaging sequences for anatomic evaluation, heavily T2-weighted MR images to delineate lesion extent, and either contrast-enhanced MR angiography or dynamic time-resolved MR angiography using 3D fast gradient echo. The time-resolved technique is preferred because of its high temporal resolution [131].

Hemangioma

Hemangiomas are benign high-flow vascular neoplasms that can occur in two forms: infantile and congenital. Congenital hemangiomas are subdivided into rapidly involuting (RICH), noninvoluting (NICH), and partially involuting (PICH). Infantile hemangioma (IH) is the most common vascular anomaly in children and is more likely than a congenital hemangioma to present as a soft tissue lesion of the chest wall [132].

IH appears after birth as blue-red lesion, undergoes a proliferative phase of rapid growth in the first few months, and gradually involutes over the next few years with small residual fibrofatty tissue remaining [124, 132]. If IH is multiple with five or more skin lesions identified, affected pediatric patients must be screened for presence of liver hemangiomas [132]. IH stains positive for glucose transporter 1 (GLUT-1).

Diagnosis of IH can typically be made based on clinical grounds or on ultrasound with Doppler evaluation which

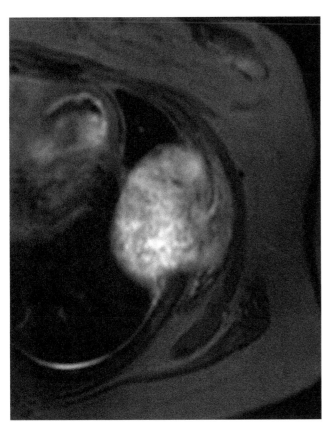

Fig. 6.40 Osteosarcoma in an 18-year-old girl who presented with left chest wall mass. Axial non-enhanced-T2-weighted fat-suppressed MR image shows a hyperintense mass arising from the left sixth rib. There are low-signal foci scattered throughout the lesion due to osteoid matrix

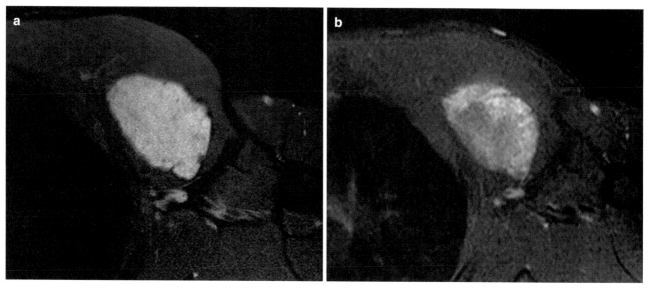

Fig. 6.41 Hemangioma in a 17-year-old boy who presented with left chest wall mass. (**a**) Axial non-enhanced T2-weighted fat-suppressed MR image demonstrates a T2 hyperintense, lobular mass within the left pectoralis musculature, with no surrounding edema. (**b**) Axial enhanced T1-weighted fat-suppressed MR image demonstrates enhancement of the mass; however, the pattern is somewhat heterogeneous rather than avidly homogeneous. This prompted biopsy of the lesion which confirmed a diagnosis of hemangioma

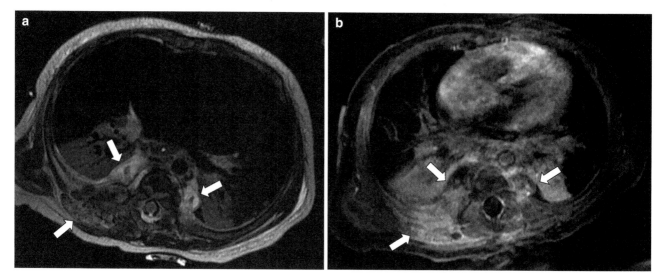

Fig. 6.42 Kaposiform hemangioendothelioma in a 5-month-old boy who presented with swelling and thrombocytopenia. (**a**) Axial non-enhanced T2-weighted MR image demonstrates a multi-compartmental infiltrative lesion (*arrows*) involving the right back and paraspinal region, extending to the posterior mediastinum, with destruction of the ribs and vertebrae. (**b**) Axial enhanced T1-weighted fat-suppressed MR image shows mostly intense, somewhat heterogeneous enhancement of the lesion (*arrows*)

demonstrates an echogenic lesion with diffuse vascularity [132]. At MR imaging during the proliferative phase, IH is hyperintense on T2-weighted MR imaging but less bright than fluid, may demonstrate internal flow voids, and has early avid enhancement [124, 132] (Fig. 6.41). During the involutional phase, enhancement decreases, and the lesion becomes heterogeneous with a more prominent fatty component [132].

Kaposiform Hemangioendothelioma

Kaposiform hemangioendothelioma (KHE) is a vascular neoplasm of borderline malignancy which presents in infants [132]. KHE can mimic IH clinically; however, unlike IH, it is an aggressive lesion, locally invasive, and strongly associated with Kasabach-Merritt phenomenon (70%) which causes thrombocytopenia, hemolytic anemia, and coagulopathy [132, 133]. KHE is immunonegative for GLUT-1.

On MR imaging, KHE is typically an infiltrative process with heterogeneous hyperintensity on T2-weighted MR images and shows intense enhancement [132, 133] (Fig. 6.42). KHE often demonstrates prominent vessels and/or flow voids, multi-compartment involvement, fat stranding, and sometimes bone destruction [124, 133].

Venous Malformation

Venous malformations (VM) are low-flow simple vascular malformations comprised of dysplastic blood-filled channels [131, 132]. Lesions may demonstrate bluish skin

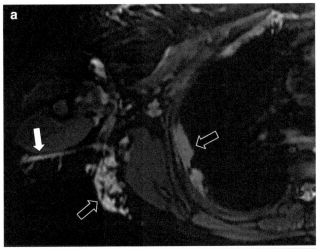

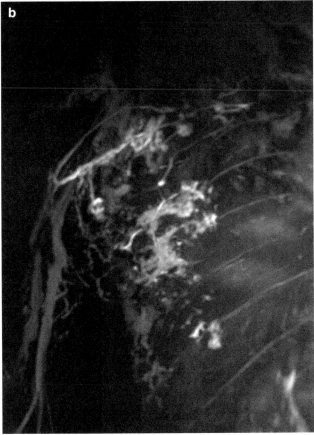

Fig. 6.43 Venous malformation in an 18-year-old girl who presented with chest wall mass. (**a**) Axial non-enhanced T2-weighted fat-suppressed MR image shows a lesion of the right chest wall with multiple lobular and tubular hyperintense components (*black arrows*) and an enlarged vein in the right arm (*white arrow*). (**b**) Coronal enhanced maximum intensity projection MR image from time-resolved MR angiography shows "puddling" of contrast throughout the lesion, consistent with a venous malformation

discoloration and enlarge with Valsalva or change in positioning [134]. VM can be found in subcutaneous tissue or in deeper structures such as the muscle, bone, and internal organs [128].

On MR imaging, VM appears as a lobulated or tubular lesion with fluid signal intensity on T1- and T2-weighted MR images, with thin septa, and sometimes with fluid-fluid levels from stagnant blood indicative of a low-flow lesion [132]. VM characteristically forms calcified phleboliths that are dark on all sequences, conspicuous on gradient sequences, and can be confirmed on radiographs [131]. On MR angiography, there is "puddling" of contrast over time resulting in near-complete enhancement of the lesion, with non-enhancement of venous channels that have undergone thrombosis [132] (Fig. 6.43).

Lymphatic Malformation

Lymphatic malformation (LM) is another low-flow simple vascular malformation consisting of dilated endothelial-lined channels or cysts [132]. LM are variable in overall size as well as in the size of the individual locules, which can be macrocystic (locules >1 cm), microcystic (locules <1 cm, solid-appearing), or combined [135]. LM can be confined to the subcutaneous tissue or extend transpatially into deeper structures. LM may grow in size in response to systemic viral infection, hemorrhage, or infection of the lesion itself.

On MR imaging, LM demonstrate multiple thin-walled fluid-filled cysts with minimal septal enhancement and no solid tissue [132, 135] (Fig. 6.44). Internal hemorrhage results in development of fluid-fluid levels, and T1 bright components may be present representing blood products and/or proteinaceous material [47]. Microcystic LM demonstrates mild diffuse solid-appearing enhancement due to high density of cyst walls [132].

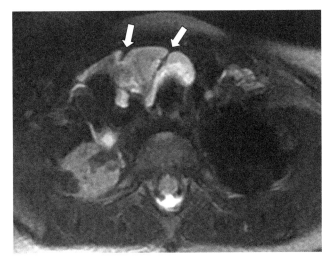

Fig. 6.44 Lymphatic malformation in an 11-month-old boy who presented with a mass of the chest and neck. Axial non-enhanced T2-weighted fat-suppressed MR image demonstrates a thin-walled hyperintense cystic lesion (*arrows*) in the anterior chest wall and base of the neck. Thin septations are present

Spectrum of Diaphragmatic Disorders

Congenital and Developmental Diaphragmatic Disorders

MR imaging is useful for prenatal and postnatal assessment of diaphragm morphology, particularly with regard to hernias. The following sections describe the spectrum of congenital and developmental disorders of the diaphragm.

Diaphragmatic Hernia

Congenital diaphragmatic hernias (CDH) are classified according to their location and include Bochdalek hernia (posterolateral), Morgagni hernia (parasternal), and hiatal hernia (central).

Bochdalek Hernia

Bochdalek-type hernias (BH) account for 90–95% of cases of congenital diaphragmatic hernias and have an incidence of 1 in 2000 to 1 in 5000 [2, 136]. The majority of BH (80–85%) are left-sided, and a minority are right-sided or bilateral. BH results from failure of the pleuroperitoneal fold and transverse septum to fuse with the intercostal muscles to form the posterolateral portion of the primordial diaphragm [137]. This leaves a "hole" in the diaphragm through which the abdominal viscera can herniate into the thoracic cavity and impede development of the lungs. The resultant pulmonary hypoplasia and subsequent development of pulmonary hypertension are key factors in the high morbidity associated with CDH. Pulmonary hypoplasia that is seen in these patients is likely in part due to genetic defects in pulmonary vascularization and alveolarization, rather than just the mechanical effects of the hernia [138].

MR imaging for CDH is performed primarily during fetal assessment but may also be used postnatally in patients with late presentation of CDH [21, 139]. Sonography is the mainstay of CDH imaging in the fetus; however, MR imaging is often recommended as adjunctive imaging to assess for fetal lung volumes, position of the liver, and other anomalies [136]. The additional information provided by fetal MR imaging is important for patient counseling and for guidance of potential therapies such as extracorporeal membrane oxygenation (ECMO) [21, 140].

Routine MR imaging protocols for assessments of the fetal chest and abdomen for CDH include axial, sagittal, and coronal T2-weighted rapid single-shot sequences, true fast imaging with steady-state precession (SSFP), and T1-weighted MR images. MR imaging should first be assessed to confirm the diagnosis of CDH and then to provide anatomic detail of the anomaly, including the location of the stomach (typically intrathoracic), small bowel loops and colon, spleen, and kidneys [140] (Fig. 6.45). The T1-weighted MR imaging sequence is important for identifying presence of liver tissue in the hernia, as the quantity of herniated liver correlates with patient outcome. The presence of a hernia "sac" portends a favorable prognosis and can be suggested by a sharp border between the hernia and the lung [140, 141].

Fetal MR imaging for CDH should include volumetric lung analysis based on the T2-weighted axial or coronal MR images, either by utilizing automated calculation on 3D workstation software or by freehand outline of lung tissue area on each slice multiplied by slice thickness [140, 142]. Typically the fetal lung volume is expressed as a ratio of "observed-to-expected total fetal lung volume" ("o/e TFLV") or "relative fetal lung volume," which can be obtained by measuring the fetal lung volumes against cited biometric formulas. Numerous studies have shown correlation between the o/e ratio, survival, and need for extracorporeal membrane oxygenation (ECMO) [140, 142–144].

MR imaging is also important for postoperative imaging of CDH [21]. CDH recurrence rates range from 3% to 22%, and CDH recurrence usually occurs within the first 6 months after surgery [145]. In cases of suspected recurrence, MR imaging can assess the integrity of the diaphragm patch or muscle flap repair and quantify the defect size and organ herniation [21, 146]. Expected findings after CDH repair include chest wall deformity, scoliosis, and decreased size and vascularity of the ipsilateral lung [147–149].

A minority (5–20%) of cases of CDH have a delayed presentation beyond the neonatal period [150]. MR imaging is often used to assess the diaphragm in these patients, as the diagnosis is challenging due to variability of both clinical presentation and radiographic appearance (Fig. 6.46).

Morgagni Hernia

Morgagni hernias (MH) account for 9–12% of cases of congenital diaphragmatic hernias [136]. The majority of MH are right-sided [2]. The foramen of Morgagni lies between the sternal and costal attachments of the diaphragm at the level of the eighth rib, and hernias at this location result from absence of fusion between the transverse septum and the lateral body wall, at the anteromedial portion of the diaphragm. Associated anomalies include pentalogy of Cantrell, congenital heart disease, and chromosomal abnormalities [2, 136].

Prenatal and postnatal MR imaging for Morgagni hernias is similar in use and methodology as described above for Bochdalek-type CDH. Most Morgagni hernias are detected in older children or adults and may be incidental [21]. The expected MR imaging findings include herniation of bowel and sometimes other viscera including the liver, spleen, and omentum.

Hiatal Hernia

Hiatal hernia occurs when a portion of the stomach ascends through the esophageal hiatus of the diaphragm into the

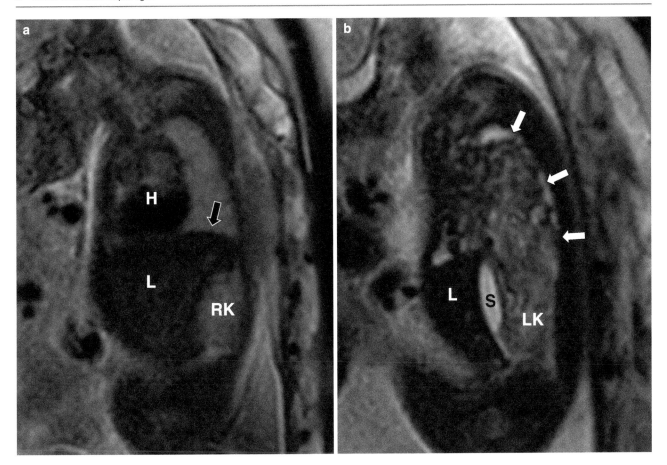

Fig. 6.45 Congenital left-sided diaphragmatic hernia in a 22-week gestation fetus referred for fetal lung volume assessment. (**a**) Sagittal non-enhanced T2-weighted MR image through the normal right hemithorax of the fetus demonstrates the intact diaphragm (*black arrow*) separating the liver (L) from the lung. RK right kidney, H heart. (**b**)

Sagittal non-enhanced T2-weighted MR image through the left hemithorax of the fetus demonstrates a large posterior diaphragmatic defect with bowel loops (*white arrows*) in the chest, consistent with a Bochdalek hernia. The liver (L), stomach (S), and kidney (LK) are in the abdomen

mediastinum. Three forms of hiatal hernia are recognized which may be acquired (most common) or congenital [21, 136]. In a sliding hernia, the widened hiatus allows the gastroesophageal (GE) junction and proximal stomach to move freely into the chest (Fig. 6.47). In a paraesophageal hernia, the GE junction maintains its normal position, and a portion of stomach ascends into the chest through the hiatus. In congenital short esophagus, the stomach is fixed in the chest above the diaphragm. While MR imaging can usually identify a hiatal hernia and its contents, the role of MR imaging is limited as the condition is usually diagnosed on plain radiograph or upper gastrointestinal series [21].

Diaphragmatic Eventration

Diaphragmatic eventration is a congenital weakening of the diaphragm due to deficiency of the muscle, leaving behind a layer of fibroelastic tissue [151]. The etiology is likely abnormal migration of myoblasts into the components of the fetal diaphragm. The body wall attachments of the diaphragm may also be deficient, and the affected portion of the diaphragm is elevated. While eventration can be

diffuse, it is most commonly focal and involves the anteromedial aspect of the right side [21]. Eventration is usually asymptomatic, but it can impair ventilation causing respiratory distress as well as chronic atelectasis and pneumonia [151].

On MR imaging, a focal eventration demonstrates a bulge of the diaphragmatic contour, and a diffuse eventration demonstrates elevation of an entire hemidiaphragm (Fig. 6.48). Eventration may result in hypokinesis, akinesis, or paradoxical motion of the diaphragm which can make it difficult to distinguish from paralysis [2, 151]. The finding may also be difficult to distinguish from diaphragmatic hernia. In such cases, MR imaging can help determine whether the diaphragm is intact but elevated, indicating eventration, or if abdominal viscera have herniated through an opening in the diaphragm as would be seen in CDH.

Diaphragm Duplication

Duplication of the diaphragm or accessory diaphragm occurs on the right side in frequent association with lobar agenesis-aplasia complex [152]. The duplicated diaphragm extends

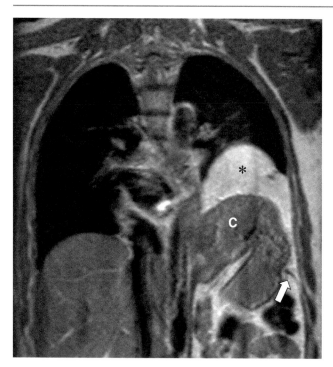

Fig. 6.46 Bochdalek hernia in a 17-year-old girl. Coronal non-enhanced T2-weighted MR image shows a large left posterior diaphragmatic hernia, containing colon (C) and fat (∗). There is discontinuity of the low-signal band of the diaphragm (arrow) consistent with the diaphragmatic defect

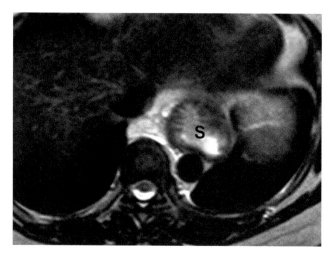

Fig. 6.47 Hiatal hernia in an 18-year-old girl. Axial non-enhanced T2-weighted MR image shows a widening of the diaphragmatic hiatus with stomach (S) projecting into the chest

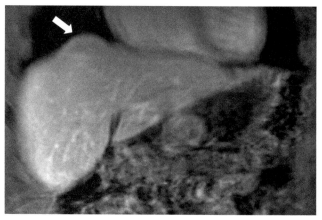

Fig. 6.48 Diaphragmatic eventration in a 17-year-old boy. Coronal enhanced T1-weighted fat-suppressed MR image shows a focal bulge (arrow) of the diaphragmatic contour consistent with a small eventration

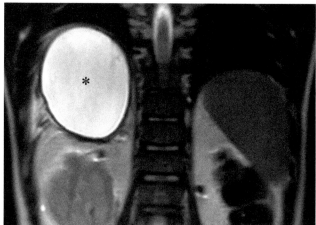

Fig. 6.49 Subphrenic abscess in a 9-year-old boy who presented with fever and chest pain after liver transplantation. Coronal non-enhanced T2-weighted MR image demonstrates a large thick-walled fluid collection (asterisk) in the right subphrenic space, causing elevation of the right hemidiaphragm

Infectious Diaphragmatic Disorders

Subphrenic Abscess

Infectious conditions of the chest or abdomen can result in abscess formations associated with the diaphragm. Subphrenic abscess is an important condition to recognize, as the imaging appearance can be confused with other causes of diaphragm elevation [153]. The right subphrenic space is a potential space between the right hepatic lobe and inferior surface of the diaphragm. Abscesses in this location typically arise from abdominopelvic infections, most commonly ruptured appendicitis, although they are less frequent in children than in adults [154]. MR imaging findings are similar to that of abscesses in other locations (Fig. 6.49). On axial MR imaging, the presence of aerated lung posterior

crescentically from the anterior aspect of the main diaphragm to the posterior chest wall. It consists of a thin fibromuscular band with a serosal lining and often has a central hiatus at its medial aspect [21, 152]. If the central hiatus is narrow and the separated lung is not aerated, the findings may appear as a mass on imaging. If the separated lung is aerated, the duplicated diaphragm appears as a band-like fissure.

to the abscess indicates that the collection is subphrenic in location [153].

Neoplastic Diaphragmatic Disorders

Neoplasms of the diaphragm are exceedingly rare in the pediatric population, and the majority are malignant [21]. MR imaging can play an important role in determining the site of origin of diaphragm lesions and distinguishing them from lesions of the liver, lung, spleen, and pericardium. Features of pediatric diaphragm masses are described in the following sections.

Benign Primary Neoplasms of the Diaphragm

Benign Cystic Lesions

Diaphragmatic mesothelial cysts are rare congenital benign cysts that are thought to arise from coelomic remnants [155]. On MR imaging, these lesions typically present as a thin-walled non-enhancing fluid-signal structure, located in the right posterolateral costophrenic angle attached to the diaphragm [156, 157] (Fig. 6.50). The origin may be difficult to determine given its proximity to the lung, pleura, and liver; however, diaphragmatic mesothelial cysts classically have a bi-lobulated configuration [156].

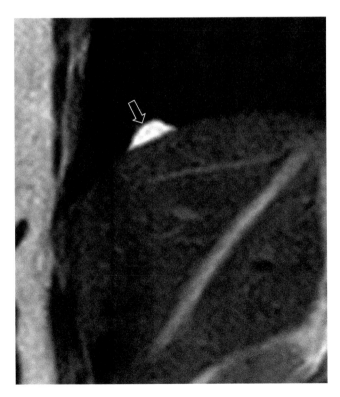

Fig. 6.50 Diaphragmatic mesothelial cyst in a 16-year-old girl. Coronal non-enhanced T2-weighted MR image demonstrates a small cyst (*arrow*) between the liver and pleura at the posterior aspect of the right hemidiaphragm, in a location typical for a mesothelial cyst

Bronchogenic cysts are congenital foregut duplication anomalies that are usually found in the mediastinum but rarely may occur in the diaphragm [157, 158]. On imaging, these lesions are similar to bronchogenic cysts of the mediastinum; however, resection is usually performed for diagnosis given their rarity. Diaphragmatic bronchogenic cysts are often found at the crus and appear as well-defined thin-walled and non-enhancing lesions [158–160]. Fluid signal intensity is seen on T2-weighted MR images, but the cyst may be intermediate or hyperintense on T1-weighted MR images due to proteinaceous or hemorrhagic material [160].

Benign Solid Lesions

Benign solid lesions of the diaphragm are rare and include hemangioma, lymphangioma, lipoma, myofibroma, and neurofibroma [21, 157]. The MR imaging characteristics of these lesions have been described in the prior section on chest wall imaging. Lipoma of the diaphragm occurs in two varieties. Sessile lipomas arise from mature fatty tissue, and hourglass-shaped lipomas arise from embryological undifferentiated tissue [157]. As with lipomas in other parts of the body, these lesions follow fat signal on all MR sequences. On imaging, a diaphragmatic lipoma can mimic a diaphragmatic hernia containing fat [157].

Malignant Primary Neoplasms of the Diaphragm

Malignant tumors that have been reported to affect the diaphragm include rhabdomyosarcoma, undifferentiated sarcoma, germ cell tumor, and extraosseous Ewing sarcoma [21, 161]. The most common of these is rhabdomyosarcoma. As discussed in the chest wall section of this chapter, rhabdomyosarcoma is a malignant neoplasm of embryonal mesenchymal cells related to skeletal muscle. Children with rhabdomyosarcoma of the diaphragm present more commonly with chest-associated symptoms (e.g., chest pain, shortness of breath) than abdomen-associated symptoms (e.g., abdominal pain, distention) [162]. The major challenge in MR imaging of these pediatric patients is correctly identifying the tumor origin site as being the diaphragm. The pattern of organ displacement and obtuse angle between the tumor and the diaphragm are clues leading toward the diaphragm as the site of origin.

Metastatic Disease of the Diaphragm

Metastases of the diaphragm include malignant thymoma of the anterior mediastinum and ovarian cancer, both of which are exceedingly rare in the pediatric population [157]. Direct extension of tumors into the diaphragm can occur with malignancies of the liver, kidneys, or retroperitoneum.

Diaphragmatic Movement Disorders

Abnormality of diaphragmatic motion can be caused by numerous conditions affecting the neuromuscular axis [1]. Examples include disorders affecting the cervical cord (e.g.,

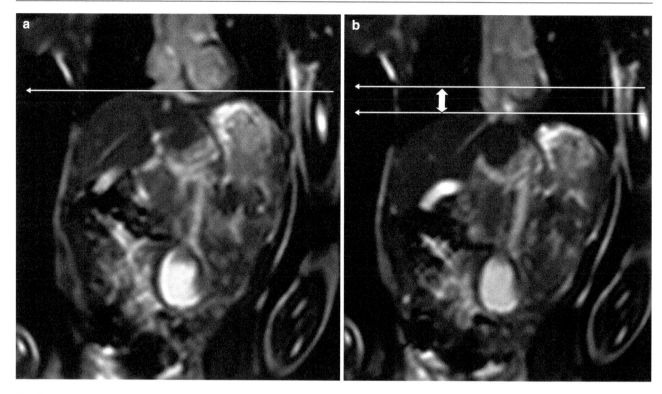

Fig. 6.51 Normal diaphragmatic motion on cinegraphic MR imaging in a 14-year-old boy. (**a**) Coronal non-enhanced balanced FFE MR image obtained in expiration shows the expected elevation of the diaphragm. (**b**) Coronal non-enhanced balanced FFE MR imaging obtained in inspiration shows the expected contraction of the diaphragm. By comparing this to the expiratory image, the diaphragmatic excursion can be measured (*double-headed arrow*)

trauma, tumors, amyotrophic lateral sclerosis, and others), phrenic nerve injuries (most commonly due to cardiac surgery or direct invasion by tumors), viral infections (e.g., West Nile virus), neuromuscular diseases such as myasthenia gravis, and myopathies such as muscular dystrophy.

Imaging of diaphragm motion was traditionally performed using fluoroscopy and more recently with ultrasonography. During real-time imaging, a paralyzed diaphragm exhibits absent or paradoxical motion, and a weak diaphragm exhibits lag in motion or hypokinesis. Dynamic MR imaging of the chest is not yet part of routine practice but is a promising tool for functional imaging assessment of the diaphragm. Some of the technical details of dynamic chest MR imaging have been described in the MR imaging protocol section at the beginning of this chapter. In general, fast dynamic GRE sequences performed in coronal and sagittal planes and viewed as cine loops are obtained to allow subjective or quantitative assessment of diaphragm motion. The technique is similar in principle to fluoroscopy; however, MR imaging is not "continuous," and temporal resolution is governed by the rate of image acquisition. Frequency of acquisition must be at least twice the respiratory rate in order to accurately represent diaphragmatic motion [10]. Quantitative assessment of motion can be obtained by measurement of diaphragmatic excursion on end-expiratory and end-inspiratory MR images (Fig. 6.51).

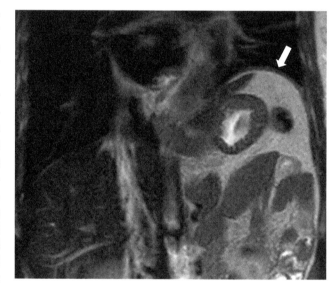

Fig. 6.52 Diaphragmatic paralysis in an 18-year-old boy with phrenic nerve impairment from a mediastinal tumor. Coronal T2-weighted MR image shows elevation of the left hemidiaphragm. The low-signal band of the diaphragmatic muscle (*arrow*) is noted to be intact

Diaphragmatic dysfunction typically causes an elevated appearance of the diaphragm on imaging [1] (Fig. 6.52). Diaphragmatic eventration is also associated with dysfunction but usually causes elevation of only a portion of a hemidiaphragm. Dysfunction can affect one hemidiaphragm or less commonly both hemidiaphragms. The condition may be asymptomatic or cause dyspnea on exertion, with restrictive pattern on pulmonary function test [1, 163].

Conclusion

The chest wall and diaphragm consist of multiple components and, therefore, are subject to a wide variety of pathologies in the pediatric population. MR imaging is a high-yield modality with the benefits of high contrast resolution and multiplanar capability. As discussed in this chapter, relatively basic MR imaging sequences can provide sufficient diagnostic information of chest wall and diaphragmatic disorders. MR imaging is particularly useful in delineating the anatomic extent and tissue characteristics of various benign and malignant lesions of the pediatric chest wall and diaphragm and for assessment of diaphragmatic motion. Familiarity with the typical clinical features and MR imaging characteristics of these conditions allows the practicing radiologist to make important contributions to the accurate diagnosis and optimal management of pediatric chest wall and diaphragmatic disorders.

References

1. Nason LK, Walker CM, McNeeley MF, Burivong W, Fligner CL, Godwin JD. Imaging of the diaphragm: anatomy and function. Radiographics. 2012;32(2):E51–70.
2. Restrepo R, Lee EY. The diaphragm. In: Coley BD, editor. Caffey's pediatric diagnostic imaging. 13th ed. Philadelphia: Elsevier; 2018. p. 587–92.
3. Antonov NK, Ruzal-Shapiro CB, Morel KD, Millar WS, Kashyap S, Lauren CT, et al. Feed and wrap MRI technique in infants. Clin Pediatr (Phila). 2017;56(12):1095–103.
4. Windram J, Grosse-Wortmann L, Shariat M, Greer ML, Crawford MW, Yoo SJ. Cardiovascular MRI without sedation or general anesthesia using a feed-and-sleep technique in neonates and infants. Pediatr Radiol. 2012;42(2):183–7.
5. Courtier J, Rao AG, Anupindi SA. Advanced imaging techniques in pediatric body MRI. Pediatr Radiol. 2017;47(5):522–33.
6. Kuhlman JE, Bouchardy L, Fishman EK, Zerhouni EA. CT and MR imaging evaluation of chest wall disorders. Radiographics. 1994;14(3):571–95.
7. Restrepo R, Lee EY. Updates on imaging of chest wall lesions in pediatric patients. Semin Roentgenol. 2012;47(1):79–89.
8. Lee TJ, Collins J. MR imaging evaluation of disorders of the chest wall. Magn Reson Imaging Clin N Am. 2008;16(2):355–79, x.
9. Mogalle K, Perez-Rovira A, Ciet P, Wens SC, van Doorn PA, Tiddens HA, et al. Quantification of diaphragm mechanics in Pompe disease using dynamic 3D MRI. PLoS One. 2016;11(7):e0158912.
10. Gierada DS, Curtin JJ, Erickson SJ, Prost RW, Strandt JA, Goodman LR. Diaphragmatic motion: fast gradient-recalled-echo MR imaging in healthy subjects. Radiology. 1995;194(3):879–84.
11. Iwasawa T, Kagei S, Gotoh T, Yoshiike Y, Matsushita K, Kurihara H, et al. Magnetic resonance analysis of abnormal dia-
12. Unal O, Arslan H, Uzun K, Ozbay B, Sakarya ME. Evaluation of diaphragmatic movement with MR fluoroscopy in chronic obstructive pulmonary disease. Clin Imaging. 2000;24(6):347–50.
13. Ryan S. Embryology and anatomy of the neonatal chest. In: Donoghue VB, editor. Radiological imaging of the neonatal chest. 2nd ed. Berlin Heidelberg: Springer; 2008. p. 1–10.
14. van der Merwe AE, Weston DA, Oostra RJ, Maat GJ. A review of the embryological development and associated developmental abnormalities of the sternum in the light of a rare palaeopathological case of sternal clefting. Homo. 2013;64(2):129–41.
15. Panicek DM, Benson CB, Gottlieb RH, Heitzman ER. The diaphragm: anatomic, pathologic, and radiologic considerations. Radiographics. 1988;8(3):385–425.
16. Restrepo R, Lee EY. The chest wall. In: Coley BD, editor. Caffey's pediatric diagnostic imaging. 13th ed. Philadelphia: Elsevier; 2018. p. 571–81.
17. Moore K, Dalley AF, Agure AMR. Clinically oriented anatomy. 8th ed. Philadelphia: Wolters Kluwer; 2018.
18. Kocjan J, Adamek M, Gzik-Zroska B, Czyzewski D, Rydel M. Network of breathing. Multifunctional role of the diaphragm: a review. Adv Respir Med. 2017;85(4):224–32.
19. Lennon EA, Simon G. The height of the diaphragm in the chest radiograph of normal adults. Br J Radiol. 1965;38(456):937–43.
20. Shin MS, Berland LL. Computed tomography of retrocrural spaces: normal, anatomic variants, and pathologic conditions. AJR Am J Roentgenol. 1985;145(1):81–6.
21. Chavhan GB, Babyn PS, Cohen RA, Langer JC. Multimodality imaging of the pediatric diaphragm: anatomy and pathologic conditions. Radiographics. 2010;30(7):1797–817.
22. Mak GZ, Speaker C, Anderson K, Stiles-Shields C, Lorenz J, Drossos T, et al. Median arcuate ligament syndrome in the pediatric population. J Pediatr Surg. 2013;48(11):2261–70.
23. Maish MS. The diaphragm. Surg Clin North Am. 2010;90(5): 955–68.
24. Schumpelick V, Steinau G, Schluper I, Prescher A. Surgical embryology and anatomy of the diaphragm with surgical applications. Surg Clin North Am. 2000;80(1):213–39, xi.
25. Donnelly LF, Frush DP. Abnormalities of the chest wall in pediatric patients. AJR Am J Roentgenol. 1999;173(6):1595–601.
26. Donnelly LF, Frush DP, Foss JN, O'Hara SM, Bisset GS 3rd. Anterior chest wall: frequency of anatomic variations in children. Radiology. 1999;212(3):837–40.
27. Kaneko H, Kitoh H, Mabuchi A, Mishima K, Matsushita M, Ishiguro N. Isolated bifid rib: clinical and radiological findings in children. Pediatr Int. 2012;54(6):820–3.
28. Yekeler E, Tunaci M, Tunaci A, Dursun M, Acunas G. Frequency of sternal variations and anomalies evaluated by MDCT. AJR Am J Roentgenol. 2006;186(4):956–60.
29. Fokin AA, Steuerwald NM, Ahrens WA, Allen KE. Anatomical, histologic, and genetic characteristics of congenital chest wall deformities. Semin Thorac Cardiovasc Surg. 2009;21(1):44–57.
30. Raikos A, Paraskevas GK, Tzika M, Faustmann P, Triaridis S, Kordali P, et al. Sternalis muscle: an underestimated anterior wall anatomical variant. J Cardiothorac Surg. 2011;6:73.
31. Bradley FM, Hoover HC Jr, Hulka CA, Whitman GJ, McCarthy KA, Hall DA, et al. The sternalis muscle: an unusual normal finding seen on mammography. AJR Am J Roentgenol. 1996;166(1):33–6.
32. Gale ME. Anterior diaphragm: variations in the CT appearance. Radiology. 1986;161(3):635–9.
33. Edwards DK 3rd, Berry CC, Hilton SW. Trisomy 21 in newborn infants: chest radiographic diagnosis. Radiology. 1988;167(2): 317–8.
34. Glass RB, Norton KI, Mitre SA, Kang E. Pediatric ribs: a spectrum of abnormalities. Radiographics. 2002;22(1):87–104.

35. Guttentag AR, Salwen JK. Keep your eyes on the ribs: the spectrum of normal variants and diseases that involve the ribs. Radiographics. 1999;19(5):1125–42.

36. Kurihara Y, Yakushiji YK, Matsumoto J, Ishikawa T, Hirata K. The ribs: anatomic and radiologic considerations. Radiographics. 1999;19(1):105–19; quiz 51–2.

37. Sheflin JR. Short rib(s). AJR Am J Roentgenol. 1995;165(6):1548–9.

38. Chang KZ, Likes K, Davis K, Demos J, Freischlag JA. The significance of cervical ribs in thoracic outlet syndrome. J Vasc Surg. 2013;57(3):771–5.

39. Henry BM, Vikse J, Sanna B, Taterra D, Gomulska M, Pekala PA, et al. Cervical rib prevalence and its association with thoracic outlet syndrome: a meta-analysis of 141 studies with surgical considerations. World Neurosurg. 2018;110:e965–e78.

40. Creswick HA, Stacey MW, Kelly RE Jr, Gustin T, Nuss D, Harvey H, et al. Family study of the inheritance of pectus excavatum. J Pediatr Surg. 2006;41(10):1699–703.

41. Fokin AA, Robicsek F. Poland's syndrome revisited. Ann Thorac Surg. 2002;74(6):2218–25.

42. Haller JA Jr, Kramer SS, Lietman SA. Use of CT scans in selection of patients for pectus excavatum surgery: a preliminary report. J Pediatr Surg. 1987;22(10):904–6.

43. Birkemeier KL, Podberesky DJ, Salisbury S, Serai S. Limited, fast magnetic resonance imaging as an alternative for preoperative evaluation of pectus excavatum: a feasibility study. J Thorac Imaging. 2012;27(6):393–7.

44. Lo Piccolo R, Bongini U, Basile M, Savelli S, Morelli C, Cerra C, et al. Chest fast MRI: an imaging alternative on pre-operative evaluation of pectus excavatum. J Pediatr Surg. 2012;47(3):485–9.

45. Marcovici PA, LoSasso BE, Kruk P, Dwek JR. MRI for the evaluation of pectus excavatum. Pediatr Radiol. 2011;41(6):757–8.

46. Lollert A, Funk J, Tietze N, Turial S, Laudemann K, Duber C, et al. Morphologic assessment of thoracic deformities for the preoperative evaluation of pectus excavatum by magnetic resonance imaging. Eur Radiol. 2015;25(3):785–91.

47. Laya BF, Zucker E, Liszewski MC, Restrepo R, Lee EY. Chest wall. In: Lee EY, editor. Pediatric thoracic imaging. Philadelphia: Wolters Kluwer; 2018. p. 289–326.

48. Jeung MY, Gangi A, Gasser B, Vasilescu C, Massard G, Wihlm JM, et al. Imaging of chest wall disorders. Radiographics. 1999;19(3):617–37.

49. Rosa RF, Travi GM, Valiatti F, Zen PR, Pinto LL, Kiss A, et al. Poland syndrome associated with an aberrant subclavian artery and vascular abnormalities of the retina in a child exposed to misoprostol during pregnancy. Birth Defects Res A Clin Mol Teratol. 2007;79(6):507–11.

50. Wright AR, Milner RH, Bainbridge LC, Wilsdon JB. MR and CT in the assessment of Poland syndrome. J Comput Assist Tomogr. 1992;16(3):442–7.

51. van Aalst JA, Phillips JD, Sadove AM. Pediatric chest wall and breast deformities. Plast Reconstr Surg. 2009;124(1 Suppl):38e–49e.

52. Lachman R. In: Lachman R, editor. Skeletal dysplasias. 5th ed. Philadelphia: Mosby; 2006/2007.

53. Cooper SC, Flaitz CM, Johnston DA, Lee B, Hecht JT. A natural history of cleidocranial dysplasia. Am J Med Genet. 2001;104(1):1–6.

54. Balioglu MB, Kargin D, Albayrak A, Atici Y. The treatment of cleidocranial dysostosis (Scheuthauer-Marie-Sainton Syndrome), a rare form of skeletal dysplasia, accompanied by spinal deformities: a review of the literature and two case reports. Case Rep Orthop. 2018;2018:4635761.

55. Hayeri MR, Ziai P, Shehata ML, Teytelboym OM, Huang BK. Soft-tissue infections and their imaging mimics: from cellulitis to necrotizing fasciitis. Radiographics. 2016;36(6):1888–910.

56. Kumar M, Meeks A, Kearl L. Necrotizing fasciitis of the chest wall: report of pediatric cases. Pediatr Emerg Care. 2015;31(9):656–60.

57. Fustes-Morales A, Gutierrez-Castrellon P, Duran-Mckinster C, Orozco-Covarrubias L, Tamayo-Sanchez L, Ruiz-Maldonado R. Necrotizing fasciitis: report of 39 pediatric cases. Arch Dermatol. 2002;138(7):893–9.

58. Fugitt JB, Puckett ML, Quigley MM, Kerr SM. Necrotizing fasciitis. Radiographics. 2004;24(5):1472–6.

59. Sakran W, Bisharat N. Primary chest wall abscess caused by *Escherichia coli* costochondritis. Am J Med Sci. 2011;342(3):241–6.

60. Otsuka T, Hosokai R, Watanabe T, Ishiwada N, Saitoh A. Subcutaneous chest wall abscess as a complication of BCG vaccination. Pediatr Int. 2017;59(11):1206–8.

61. Navarro OM, Laffan EE, Ngan BY. Pediatric soft-tissue tumors and pseudo-tumors: MR imaging features with pathologic correlation: part 1. Imaging approach, pseudotumors, vascular lesions, and adipocytic tumors. Radiographics. 2009;29(3):887–906.

62. Wong KS, Hung IJ, Wang CR, Lien R. Thoracic wall lesions in children. Pediatr Pulmonol. 2004;37(3):257–63.

63. Khanna G, Sato TS, Ferguson P. Imaging of chronic recurrent multifocal osteomyelitis. Radiographics. 2009;29(4):1159–77.

64. Gaude GS, Reyas A. Tuberculosis of the chest wall without pulmonary involvement. Lung India. 2008;25(3):135–7.

65. Teo HE, Peh WC. Skeletal tuberculosis in children. Pediatr Radiol. 2004;34(11):853–60.

66. Morris BS, Maheshwari M, Chalwa A. Chest wall tuberculosis: a review of CT appearances. Br J Radiol. 2004;77(917):449–57.

67. Boruah DK, Sanyal S, Sharma BK, Prakash A, Dhingani DD, Bora K. Role of cross sectional imaging in isolated chest wall tuberculosis. J Clin Diagn Res. 2017;11(1):TC01–TC6.

68. Chelli Bouaziz M, Jelassi H, Chaabane S, Ladeb MF, Ben Miled-Mrad K. Imaging of chest wall infections. Skeletal Radiol. 2009;38(12):1127–35.

69. Prasad A, Manchanda S, Sachdev N, Baruah BP, Manchanda V. Imaging features of pediatric musculoskeletal tuberculosis. Pediatr Radiol. 2012;42(10):1235–49.

70. Thompson AJ, Carty H. Pulmonary actinomycosis in children. Pediatr Radiol. 1979;8(1):7–9.

71. Wand A, Gilbert HM, Litvack B, Markisz JA. MRI of thoracic actinomycosis. J Comput Assist Tomogr. 1996;20(5):770–2.

72. Freeman AF, Ben-Ami T, Shulman ST. Streptococcus pneumoniae empyema necessitatis. Pediatr Infect Dis J. 2004;23(2):177–9.

73. Goussard P, Gie R, Janson J, Andronikou S. Empyema necessitans in a six-month-old girl. Paediatr Int Child Health. 2018;39:224–6.

74. Stein R, Manson D. Magnetic resonance imaging findings of empyema necessitatis in a child with a group A streptococcus infection. J Thorac Imaging. 2012;27(1):W13–4.

75. Hu HH, Yin L, Aggabao PC, Perkins TG, Chia JM, Gilsanz V. Comparison of brown and white adipose tissues in infants and children with chemical-shift-encoded water-fat MRI. J Magn Reson Imaging. 2013;38(4):885–96.

76. Deng J, Schoeneman SE, Zhang H, Kwon S, Rigsby CK, Shore RM, et al. MRI characterization of brown adipose tissue in obese and normal-weight children. Pediatr Radiol. 2015;45(11):1682–9.

77. Drubach LA, Palmer EL 3rd, Connolly LP, Baker A, Zurakowski D, Cypess AM. Pediatric brown adipose tissue: detection, epidemiology, and differences from adults. J Pediatr. 2011;159(6):939–44.

78. Gupta P, Babyn PS, Shammas A, Miller SF. Brown fat distribution in the chest wall of infants-normal appearance, distribution and evolution on CT scans of the chest. Pediatr Radiol. 2011;41(8):1020–7.

79. Atilla S, Eilenberg SS, Brown JJ. Hibernoma: MRI appearance of a rare tumor. Magn Reson Imaging. 1995;13(2):335–7.

80. Baskurt E, Padgett DM, Matsumoto JA. Multiple hibernomas in a 1-month-old female infant. AJNR Am J Neuroradiol. 2004;25(8):1443–5.

81. Lee JC, Gupta A, Saifuddin A, Flanagan A, Skinner JA, Briggs TW, et al. Hibernoma: MRI features in eight consecutive cases. Clin Radiol. 2006;61(12):1029–34.

82. Sheybani EF, Eutsler EP, Navarro OM. Fat-containing soft-tissue masses in children. Pediatr Radiol. 2016;46(13):1760–73.

83. Nam SJ, Kim S, Lim BJ, Yoon CS, Kim TH, Suh JS, et al. Imaging of primary chest wall tumors with radiologic-pathologic correlation. Radiographics. 2011;31(3):749–70.

84. Sargar KM, Sheybani EF, Shenoy A, Aranake-Chrisinger J, Khanna G. Pediatric fibroblastic and myofibroblastic tumors: a pictorial review. Radiographics. 2016;36(4):1195–214.

85. Xu H, Koo HJ, Lim S, Lee JW, Lee HN, Kim DK, et al. Desmoid-type fibromatosis of the thorax: CT, MRI, and FDG PET characteristics in a large series from a tertiary referral center. Medicine (Baltimore). 2015;94(38):e1547.

86. Lamboley JL, Le Moigne F, Proust C, Thivolet-Bejui F, Tronc F, Revel D, et al. Desmoid tumour of the chest wall. Diagn Interv Imaging. 2012;93(7–8):635–8.

87. McCarville MB, Spunt SL, Pappo AS. Rhabdomyosarcoma in pediatric patients: the good, the bad, and the unusual. AJR Am J Roentgenol. 2001;176(6):1563–9.

88. Kingston CA, Owens CM, Jeanes A, Malone M. Imaging of desmoid fibromatosis in pediatric patients. AJR Am J Roentgenol. 2002;178(1):191–9.

89. Murphey MD, Ruble CM, Tyszko SM, Zbojniewicz AM, Potter BK, Miettinen M. From the archives of the AFIP: musculoskeletal fibromatoses: radiologic-pathologic correlation. Radiographics. 2009;29(7):2143–73.

90. Naffaa L, Khalifeh I, Salman R, Itani M, Saab R, Al-Kutoubi A. Infantile myofibromatosis: review of imaging findings and emphasis on correlation between MRI and histopathological findings. Clin Imaging. 2019;54:40–7.

91. Koujok K, Ruiz RE, Hernandez RJ. Myofibromatosis: imaging characteristics. Pediatr Radiol. 2005;35(4):374–80.

92. Laffan EE, Ngan BY, Navarro OM. Pediatric soft-tissue tumors and pseudotumors: MR imaging features with pathologic correlation: part 2. Tumors of fibroblastic/myofibroblastic, so-called fibrohistiocytic, muscular, lymphomatous, neurogenic, hair matrix, and uncertain origin. Radiographics. 2009;29(4):e36.

93. Salerno S, Terranova MC, Rossello M, Piccione M, Ziino O, Re GL. Whole-body magnetic resonance imaging in the diagnosis and follow-up of multicentric infantile myofibromatosis: a case report. Mol Clin Oncol. 2017;6(4):579–82.

94. Soper JR, De Silva M. Infantile myofibromatosis: a radiological review. Pediatr Radiol. 1993;23(3):189–94.

95. Loyer EM, Shabb NS, Mahon TG, Eftekhari F. Fibrous hamartoma of infancy: MR-pathologic correlation. J Comput Assist Tomogr. 1992;16(2):311–3.

96. Soldatos T, Fisher S, Karri S, Ramzi A, Sharma R, Chhabra A. Advanced MR imaging of peripheral nerve sheath tumors including diffusion imaging. Semin Musculoskelet Radiol. 2015;19(2):179–90.

97. Pavlus JD, Carter BW, Tolley MD, Keung ES, Khorashadi L, Lichtenberger JP 3rd. Imaging of thoracic neurogenic tumors. AJR Am J Roentgenol. 2016;207(3):552–61.

98. Bhargava R, Parham DM, Lasater OE, Chari RS, Chen G, Fletcher BD. MR imaging differentiation of benign and malignant peripheral nerve sheath tumors: use of the target sign. Pediatr Radiol. 1997;27(2):124–9.

99. Lim R, Jaramillo D, Poussaint TY, Chang Y, Korf B. Superficial neurofibroma: a lesion with unique MRI characteristics in patients with neurofibromatosis type 1. AJR Am J Roentgenol. 2005;184(3):962–8.

100. Iyer RS, Chapman T, Chew FS. Pediatric bone imaging: diagnostic imaging of osteoid osteoma. AJR Am J Roentgenol. 2012;198(5):1039–52.

101. Rodallec MH, Feydy A, Larousserie F, Anract P, Campagna R, Babinet A, et al. Diagnostic imaging of solitary tumors of the spine: what to do and say. Radiographics. 2008;28(4):1019–41.

102. Hughes EK, James SL, Butt S, Davies AM, Saifuddin A. Benign primary tumours of the ribs. Clin Radiol. 2006;61(4):314–22.

103. Mizuno S, Anazawa U, Hotta H, Asano N, Susa M, Miyauchi J, et al. A rare case of an osteoid osteoma of the rib treated under computed tomography guidance: a case report and review of the literature. Case Rep Oncol. 2015;8(3):509–14.

104. Golant A, Lou JE, Erol B, Gaynor JW, Low DW, Dormans JP. Pediatric osteoblastoma of the sternum: a new surgical technique for reconstruction after removal: case report and review of the literature. J Pediatr Orthop. 2004;24(3):319–22.

105. Ye J, Liu L, Wu J, Wang S. Osteoblastoma of the rib with CT and MR imaging: a case report and literature review. World J Surg Oncol. 2012;10:49.

106. Galgano MA, Goulart CR, Iwenofu H, Chin LS, Lavelle W, Mendel E. Osteoblastomas of the spine: a comprehensive review. Neurosurg Focus. 2016;41(2):E4.

107. Bakhshi H, Kushare I, Murphy MO, Gaynor JW, Dormans JP. Chest wall osteochondroma in children: a case series of surgical management. J Pediatr Orthop. 2014;34(7):733–7.

108. Tateishi U, Gladish GW, Kusumoto M, Hasegawa T, Yokoyama R, Tsuchiya R, et al. Chest wall tumors: radiologic findings and pathologic correlation: part 1. Benign tumors. Radiographics. 2003;23(6):1477–90.

109. Meyer CA, White CS. Cartilaginous disorders of the chest. Radiographics. 1998;18(5):1109–23; quiz 241–2.

110. Chu L, Seed M, Howse E, Ryan G, Grosse-Wortmann L. Mesenchymal hamartoma: prenatal diagnosis by MRI. Pediatr Radiol. 2011;41(6):781–4.

111. Groom KR, Murphey MD, Howard LM, Lonergan GJ, Rosado-De-Christenson ML, Torop AH. Mesenchymal hamartoma of the chest wall: radiologic manifestations with emphasis on cross-sectional imaging and histopathologic comparison. Radiology. 2002;222(1):205–11.

112. Shah ZK, Peh WC, Koh WL, Shek TW. Magnetic resonance imaging appearances of fibrous dysplasia. Br J Radiol. 2005;78(936):1104–15.

113. Yamamoto T, Marui T, Akisue T, Mizuno K. Solid aneurysmal bone cyst in the humerus. Skeletal Radiol. 2000;29(8):470–3.

114. Matcuk GR Jr, Chopra S, Menendez LR. Solid aneurysmal bone cyst of the humerus mimics metastasis or brown tumor. Clin Imaging. 2018;52:117–22.

115. Gezer HO, Oguzkurt P, Temiz A, Demir S, Hicsonmez A. Solid variant of aneurysmal bone cyst of the rib presenting as a left intrathoracic mass without radiological bone destruction. Turk J Pediatr. 2014;56(3):303–6.

116. Jeh SK, Jee WH, Hong SJ, Kim JY, Sung MS, Ryu KN, et al. Extracranial skeletal Langerhans cell histiocytosis: MR imaging features according to the radiologic evolutional phases. Clin Imaging. 2012;36(5):466–71.

117. George JC, Buckwalter KA, Cohen MD, Edwards MK, Smith RR. Langerhans cell histiocytosis of bone: MR imaging. Pediatr Radiol. 1994;24(1):29–32.

118. Zaveri J, La Q, Yarmish G, Neuman J. More than just Langerhans cell histiocytosis: a radiologic review of histiocytic disorders. Radiographics. 2014;34(7):2008–24.

119. Goo HW, Yang DH, Ra YS, Song JS, Im HJ, Seo JJ, et al. Whole-body MRI of Langerhans cell histiocytosis: comparison with radiography and bone scintigraphy. Pediatr Radiol. 2006;36(10):1019–31.

120. van den Berg H, van Rijn RR, Merks JH. Management of tumors of the chest wall in childhood: a review. J Pediatr Hematol Oncol. 2008;30(3):214–21.

121. Stein-Wexler R. Pediatric soft tissue sarcomas. Semin Ultrasound CT MR. 2011;32(5):470–88.

122. Pandey A, Kureel SN, Bappavad RP. Chest wall infantile fibrosarcomas—a rare presentation. Indian J Surg Oncol. 2016;7(1):127–9.

123. Ainsworth KE, Chavhan GB, Gupta AA, Hopyan S, Taylor G. Congenital infantile fibrosarcoma: review of imaging features. Pediatr Radiol. 2014;44(9):1124–9.

124. Baez JC, Lee EY, Restrepo R, Eisenberg RL. Chest wall lesions in children. AJR Am J Roentgenol. 2013;200(5):W402–19.

125. Foran P, Colleran G, Madewell J, O'Sullivan PJ. Imaging of thoracic sarcomas of the chest wall, pleura, and lung. Semin Ultrasound CT MR. 2011;32(5):365–76.

126. Wasa J, Nishida Y, Tsukushi S, Shido Y, Sugiura H, Nakashima H, et al. MRI features in the differentiation of malignant peripheral nerve sheath tumors and neurofibromas. AJR Am J Roentgenol. 2010;194(6):1568–74.

127. Carter BW. MR imaging of chest and chest wall disease. Top Magn Reson Imaging. 2018;27(2):63–4.

128. Fefferman NR, Pinkney LP. Imaging evaluation of chest wall disorders in children. Radiol Clin North Am. 2005;43(2):355–70.

129. Franken EA Jr, Smith JA, Smith WL. Tumors of the chest wall in infants and children. Pediatr Radiol. 1977;6(1):13–8.

130. Wassef M, Blei F, Adams D, Alomari A, Baselga E, Berenstein A, et al. Vascular anomalies classification: recommendations from the International Society for the Study of Vascular Anomalies. Pediatrics. 2015;136(1):e203–14.

131. Flors L, Leiva-Salinas C, Maged IM, Norton PT, Matsumoto AH, Angle JF, et al. MR imaging of soft-tissue vascular malformations: diagnosis, classification, and therapy follow-up. Radiographics. 2011;31(5):1321–40; discussion 40–1.

132. Merrow AC, Gupta A, Patel MN, Adams DM. 2014 revised classification of vascular lesions from the International Society for the Study of Vascular Anomalies: radiologic-pathologic update. Radiographics. 2016;36(5):1494–516.

133. Ryu YJ, Choi YH, Cheon JE, Kim WS, Kim IO, Park JE, et al. Imaging findings of kaposiform hemangioendothelioma in children. Eur J Radiol. 2017;86:198–205.

134. Olivieri B, White CL, Restrepo R, McKeon B, Karakas SP, Lee EY. Low-flow vascular malformation pitfalls: from clinical examination to practical imaging evaluationDOUBLEHYPHEN-part 2, venous malformation mimickers. AJR Am J Roentgenol. 2016;206(5):952–62.

135. White CL, Olivieri B, Restrepo R, McKeon B, Karakas SP, Lee EY. Low-flow vascular malformation pitfalls: from clinical examination to practical imaging evaluationDOUBLEHYPHENpart 1, lymphatic malformation mimickers. AJR Am J Roentgenol. 2016;206(5):940–51.

136. Taylor GA, Atalabi OM, Estroff JA. Imaging of congenital diaphragmatic hernias. Pediatr Radiol. 2009;39(1):1–16.

137. Clugston RD, Klattig J, Englert C, Clagett-Dame M, Martinovic J, Benachi A, et al. Teratogen-induced, dietary and genetic models of congenital diaphragmatic hernia share a common mechanism of pathogenesis. Am J Pathol. 2006;169(5):1541–9.

138. Donahoe PK, Longoni M, High FA. Polygenic causes of congenital diaphragmatic hernia produce common lung pathologies. Am J Pathol. 2016;186(10):2532–43.

139. Mei-Zahav M, Solomon M, Trachsel D, Langer JC. Bochdalek diaphragmatic hernia: not only a neonatal disease. Arch Dis Child. 2003;88(6):532–5.

140. Kline-Fath BM. Current advances in prenatal imaging of congenital diaphragmatic [corrected] hernia. Pediatr Radiol. 2012;42(Suppl 1):S74–90.

141. Oliver ER, DeBari SE, Adams SE, Didier RA, Horii SC, Victoria T, et al. Congenital diaphragmatic hernia sacs: prenatal imaging and associated postnatal outcomes. Pediatr Radiol. 2019;49:593.

142. Busing KA, Kilian AK, Schaible T, Debus A, Weiss C, Neff KW. Reliability and validity of MR image lung volume measurement in fetuses with congenital diaphragmatic hernia and in vitro lung models. Radiology. 2008;246(2):553–61.

143. Jani J, Cannie M, Sonigo P, Robert Y, Moreno O, Benachi A, et al. Value of prenatal magnetic resonance imaging in the prediction of postnatal outcome in fetuses with diaphragmatic hernia. Ultrasound Obstet Gynecol. 2008;32(6):793–9.

144. Jani J, Keller RL, Benachi A, Nicolaides KH, Favre R, Gratacos E, et al. Prenatal prediction of survival in isolated left-sided diaphragmatic hernia. Ultrasound Obstet Gynecol. 2006;27(1):18–22.

145. Al-Iede MM, Karpelowsky J, Fitzgerald DA. Recurrent diaphragmatic hernia: modifiable and non-modifiable risk factors. Pediatr Pulmonol. 2016;51(4):394–401.

146. Kim W, Courtier J, Morin C, Shet N, Strauch E, Kim JS. Postnatal MRI for CDH: a pictorial review of late-presenting and recurrent diaphragmatic defects. Clin Imaging. 2017;43:158–64.

147. Kamata S, Usui N, Sawai T, Nose K, Kamiyama M, Fukuzawa M. Radiographic changes in the diaphragm after repair of congenital diaphragmatic hernia. J Pediatr Surg. 2008;43(12):2156–60.

148. Nasr A, Struijs MC, Ein SH, Langer JC, Chiu PP. Outcomes after muscle flap vs prosthetic patch repair for large congenital diaphragmatic hernias. J Pediatr Surg. 2010;45(1):151–4.

149. Saifuddin A, Arthur RJ. Congenital diaphragmatic herniaDOUBLEHYPHENa review of pre- and postoperative chest radiology. Clin Radiol. 1993;47(2):104–10.

150. Baglaj M, Dorobisz U. Late-presenting congenital diaphragmatic hernia in children: a literature review. Pediatr Radiol. 2005;35(5):478–88.

151. Wu S, Zang N, Zhu J, Pan Z, Wu C. Congenital diaphragmatic eventration in children: 12 years' experience with 177 cases in a single institution. J Pediatr Surg. 2015;50(7):1088–92.

152. Hidalgo A, Franquet T, Gimenez A. 16-MDCT and MR angiography of accessory diaphragm. AJR Am J Roentgenol. 2006;187(1):149–52.

153. Alexander ES, Proto AV, Clark RA. CT differentiation of subphrenic abscess and pleural effusion. AJR Am J Roentgenol. 1983;140(1):47–51.

154. Kahn AM, Weitzman JJ. Subphrenic and subhepatic abscess in the pediatric patient. J Pediatr Surg. 1969;4(2):256–62.

155. Esparza Estaun J, Gonzalez Alfageme A, Saenz Banuelos J. Radiological appearance of diaphragmatic mesothelial cysts. Pediatr Radiol. 2003;33(12):855–8.

156. Kahriman G, Ozcan N, Dogan S, Bayram A. Imaging findings and management of diaphragmatic mesothelial cysts in children. Pediatr Radiol. 2016;46(11):1546–51.

157. Kim MP, Hofstetter WL. Tumors of the diaphragm. Thorac Surg Clin. 2009;19(4):521–9.

158. Mubang R, Brady JJ, Mao M, Burfeind W, Puc M. Intradiaphragmatic bronchogenic cysts: case report and systematic review. J Cardiothorac Surg. 2016;11(1):79.

159. Fischbach R, Benz-Bohm G, Berthold F, Eidt S, Schmidt R. Infradiaphragmatic bronchogenic cyst with high CT numbers in a boy with primitive neuroectodermal tumor. Pediatr Radiol. 1994;24(7):504–5.

160. Rozenblit A, Iqbal A, Kaleya R, Rozenblit G. Case report: intradiaphragmatic bronchogenic cyst. Clin Radiol. 1998;53(12):918–20.

161. Raney RB, Anderson JR, Andrassy RJ, Crist WM, Donaldson SS, Maurer HM, et al. Soft-tissue sarcomas of the diaphragm: a report from the Intergroup Rhabdomyosarcoma Study Group from 1972 to 1997. J Pediatr Hematol Oncol. 2000;22(6):510–4.

162. Cada M, Gerstle JT, Traubici J, Ngan BY, Capra ML. Approach to diagnosis and treatment of pediatric primary tumors of the diaphragm. J Pediatr Surg. 2006;41(10):1722–6.

163. Kharma N. Dysfunction of the diaphragm: imaging as a diagnostic tool. Curr Opin Pulm Med. 2013;19(4):394–8.

Liver

Benjamin M. Kozak, Amirkasra Mojtahed,
and Michael S. Gee

Introduction

Magnetic resonance (MR) imaging is now commonly used in pediatric patients to evaluate focal and diffuse hepatic disorders. Various MR imaging techniques can greatly improve lesion detection and characterization compared to other imaging modalities without potentially harmful ionizing radiation exposure. In recent years, other technical advances have also helped minimize MR imaging acquisition time and motion-related image degradation.

This chapter reviews clinically important concepts related to up-to-date hepatic MR imaging techniques and MR imaging findings in a spectrum of congenital and acquired hepatic disorders. In addition, preoperative assessment and postoperative complications of liver transplantation in the pediatric population are also discussed.

Magnetic Resonance Imaging Techniques

Intravenous Contrast Agents

There are two main categories of intravenous contrast agents used in hepatic MR imaging: extracellular agents and hepatobiliary agents. Both categories are gadolinium-based.

B. M. Kozak (✉)
Department of Radiology, Massachusetts General Hospital, Harvard Medical School, Boston, MA, USA
e-mail: Bkozak@partners.org

A. Mojtahed
Division of Pediatric Imaging, Department of Radiology, Massachusetts General Hospital, Harvard Medical School, Boston, MA, USA

M. S. Gee
Division of Pediatric Imaging, Department of Radiology, Massachusetts General Hospital, Harvard Medical School, Boston, MA, USA

Extracellular Contrast Agents Extracellular agents distribute within the intravascular and extracellular spaces. There is no hepatocyte uptake and the agents are renally excreted [1]. These agents are excellent for both vascular and hepatic parenchymal evaluations, including in multiphase post-contrast imaging. Examples of FDA-approved extracellular agents include linear agents such as gadopentetate dimeglumine (Magnevist; Bayer, Whippany, NJ), gadoversetamide (Optimark; Guerbet, Villepinte, France), and gadodiamide (Omniscan; General Electric Healthcare, Waukesha, WI) as well as macrocyclic agents such as gadoterate meglumine (Dotarem; Guerbet, Villepinte, France), gadoteridol (Prohance; Bracco Diagnostics, Monroe Township, NJ), and gadobutrol (Gadavist; Bayer, Whippany, NJ).

Several recent studies have associated the use of gadolinium-based contrast agents with gadolinium tissue deposition within the central nervous system (CNS) in both adults and children, even in the setting of normal renal function [2]. The risk of CNS gadolinium deposition appears to be correlated with the number of contrast-enhanced MR examinations. Additionally, the risk appears increased with linear gadolinium-based contrast agents compared to macrocyclic agents, which is possibly related to the greater kinetic inertness of the latter [2]. Currently, the clinical significance of CNS gadolinium deposition remains unclear. However, concerns regarding potential effects of gadolinium deposition have led to reduced gadolinium use in MR imaging overall, with a shift toward use of macrocyclic agents when contrast is indicated.

Hepatobiliary Contrast Agents Hepatobiliary agents distribute within the extracellular space and can be used similarly to the extracellular agents [3, 4]. Additionally, they demonstrate uptake by hepatocytes and partial excretion into the biliary system. Consequently, hepatobiliary agents offer the added benefit of improved biliary system evaluation and can help further characterize hepatic lesions based upon hepatobiliary agent retention. For example, nearly all focal nodular hyperplasia lesions demonstrate hepatobiliary agent uptake, whereas most hepatic adenomas do not [5, 6]. Available agents include gadobenate dimeglumine

(MultiHance; Bracco Diagnostics, Monroe Township, NJ) and gadoxetate disodium (Eovist; Bayer, Whippany, NJ). Both agents are approved in the United States for use in the pediatric population, with gadoxetate approved for all ages and gadobenate approved for children 2 years of age and older [7–9]. Available studies have demonstrated a safety profile that is similar to extracellular agents [10]. The hepatobiliary phase is typically imaged between 60 and 90 minutes post-injection for gadobenate and 20 minutes for gadoxetate using T1-weighted fat-suppressed gradient echo (GRE) sequences.

MR Imaging Pulse Sequences and Protocols

Commonly used MR imaging protocols for evaluation of the liver are shown in Table 7.1. T2-weighted sequences form an important component of MR liver evaluations. Commonly acquired T2-weighted sequences in pediatric patients include fat-suppressed fast spin echo sequences acquired with respiratory triggering and single-shot fast spin echo sequences that can be acquired either free-breathing or with respiratory suspension. Diffusion-weighted and multiphase T1-weighted fat-suppressed post-contrast imaging are helpful for focal hepatic lesion characterization, while magnetic resonance cholangiopancreatography (MRCP) is a heavily T2-weighted

Table 7.1 Common MR imaging sequences used in pediatric hepatic imaging

Sequence	Plane	Motion correction	Acquisition time
2D radial or Cartesian T2-weighted fat-suppressed fast spin echo	Axial +/− coronal	Respiratory triggered +/− prospective motion correction	~3–5 minutes
Single-shot T2-weighted fast spin echo +/− fat suppression	Axial +/− coronal	Free breathing, breath-hold, or respiratory triggered	~30 seconds
3D heavily T2-weighted fast spin echo MRCP	Coronal	Respiratory triggered	~ 5 minutes
3D T1-weighted in-phase and opposed-phase gradient echo	Axial	Free breathing, breath-hold, or respiratory triggered	~20 seconds
PDFF/R2* relaxometry	Axial	Breath-hold	~20 seconds
Diffusion	Axial	Respiratory triggered or free breathing	~ 3–5 minutes
3D T1-weighted fat-suppressed multiphase post-contrast gradient echo	Axial	Free breathing, breath-hold, or respiratory triggered	~ 10–20 seconds per phase
MR elastography	Axial	Free breathing, breath-hold, or respiratory triggered	~ 1–2 minutes (~15 seconds per section)

sequence used to evaluate the biliary tree. A number of other sequences also have an important role in MR liver examinations that are less commonly used in other MR imaging protocols. These include T1-weighted in-phase and opposed-phase chemical shift GRE sequences for hepatic fat detection, multi-echo chemical shift GRE sequences for iron quantitation, proton density fat fraction imaging for fat quantitation, and MR elastography for fibrosis assessment.

Multiphase T1-Weighted Fat-Suppressed Post-Contrast Imaging The liver has a dual blood supply from the hepatic artery and portal vein. Focal hepatic lesions often demonstrate characteristic enhancement patterns at various time points following contrast administration based upon the blood supply to the lesion. Multiphasic post-contrast imaging permits the evaluation of these enhancement characteristics using volumetric GRE pulse sequences, including THRIVE (Philips, Best, Netherlands), LAVA (GE, Waukesha, WI), and VIBE (Siemens, Malvern, PA), which can be performed in a single breath-hold (10–20 seconds). In pediatric patients who cannot breath-hold, these sequences can be acquired free breathing using standard techniques such as signal averaging or respiratory triggering, with resultant loss of temporal resolution. Standard phases of image acquisition are timed relative to the start of injection and include pre-contrast, late hepatic arterial (25–35 seconds), portal venous (60–70 seconds when the liver parenchyma is uniformly enhanced), and equilibrium (120–180 seconds; contrast located in both vascular and extracellular compartments) phases (Fig. 7.1). A delayed hepatobiliary phase is also included if a hepatobiliary agent is used.

Liver Fat Quantitation Noninvasive quantification of hepatic steatosis can be helpful in a number of different clinical scenarios, including the detection and monitoring of nonalcoholic fatty liver disease and the assessment of hepatic fat content to monitor obesity and insulin resistance [11]. Chemical shift imaging is the most commonly used MR imaging technique for fat detection and is based on the difference in precessional frequencies of fat and water protons in a magnetic field [11]. A T1-weighted GRE sequence is performed at two echo times (corresponding to when fat and water protons are in the same phase or in an opposed phase), with signal loss on the opposed phase indicative of steatosis (Fig. 7.2).

Traditional chemical shift imaging provides a qualitative assessment of liver fat. A variant of the chemical shift technique, known as the Dixon method, separates the relative signal contributions of water and fat based on signal changes from the in- and opposed-phase sequences to generate water- and fat-only images [12, 13]. Dixon images can be interpreted visually to assess liver fat qualitatively, while quantitative assessment of hepatic fat can be performed using proton density fat fraction (PDFF): a more robust fat-only Dixon image that has been corrected for confounding factors such as T1 bias, T2* decay, and spectral complexity of fat. PDFF is FDA-approved for liver fat quantitation [14, 15] (Fig. 7.3). A unique

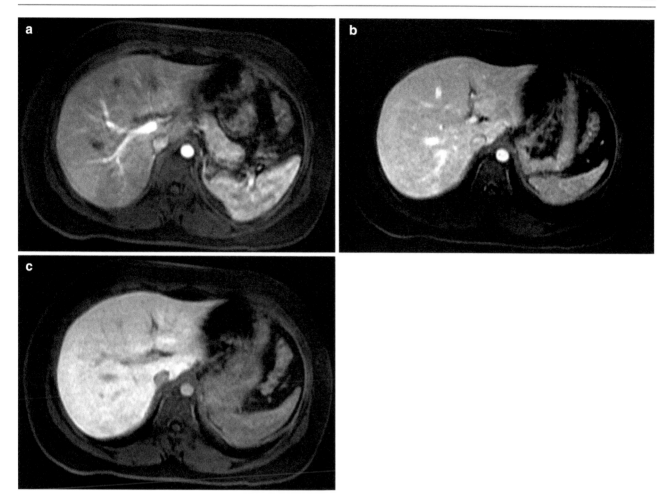

Fig. 7.1 Normal liver MR imaging in a 14-year-old girl. (**a**) Axial enhanced T1-weighted fat-suppressed GRE MR image acquired during the late arterial phase (35-second delay) shows contrast material within the arterial system and portal vein but not the hepatic veins. (**b**) Corresponding portal venous phase (70-second delay) MR image shows contrast material within the arterial system, portal vein, and hepatic veins. (**c**) Corresponding post-contrast MR image acquired during the equilibrium phase (180-second delay) MR image shows uniform parenchymal enhancement

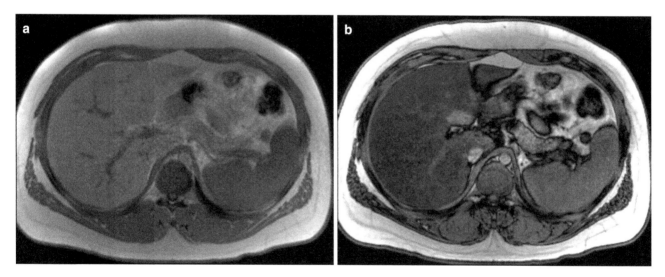

Fig. 7.2 Hepatic steatosis in a 17-year-old boy who presented after an abnormal abdominal ultrasound study. Axial T1-weighted GRE in-phase (**a**) and opposed-phase (**b**) MR images show loss of signal throughout the liver on the opposed-phase image consistent with diffuse hepatic steatosis

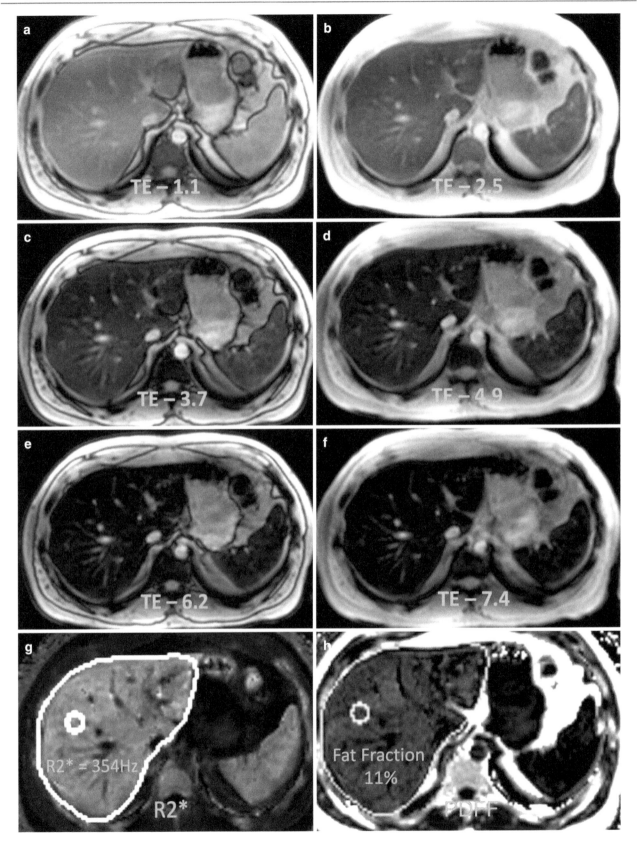

Fig. 7.3 Secondary hemosiderosis and hepatic steatosis in a 17-year-old boy with aplastic anemia and elevated serum ferritin following bone marrow transplant. (**a–f**) Axial non-enhanced T1-weighted GRE MR images obtained at multiple echo times (TE, measured in milliseconds) show progressively decreasing signal within the liver and spleen consistent with iron overload. Generated R2* (**g**) and PDFF maps (**h**) based on the sequence acquired in (**a–f**) confirm hepatic iron overload with a R2* value of 354 Hz within the segmented liver volume, which correlates with an estimated iron dry weight of 6 mg/g. Additionally, hepatic steatosis is present with an estimated fat fraction of 11% within the segmented liver volume. Of note, hepatic steatosis was not definitively evident when visually comparing the in-phase (**b**) and out-of-phase (**a**) images

artifact referred to as "fat-water swap" can occur with chemical shift-based water-fat separation methods. This artifact manifests as the incorrect assignment or "swapping" of fat and water signals in the generated fat-only and water-only images as a consequence of a computational phase error in areas of magnetic field inhomogeneity [16–18]. As this is a computational error, the original in- and opposed-phase images are unaffected and can be used for interpretation (Fig. 7.4).

Liver Iron Quantitation The liver is the primary storage organ for iron, and as total body iron increases in conditions such as hereditary hemochromatosis or hemosiderosis, a constant proportion of iron accumulates within the liver. Hepatic iron concentration is thus a good estimate of total body iron. Iron is paramagnetic and causes susceptibility-associated signal loss that is visible on $T2^*$-weighted imaging and increases with increased echo time (TE) [19] (Fig. 7.5). Relaxometry is a multi-echo MR imaging technique for quantifying liver iron concentration based on this principle. R2 relaxometry utilizes a free breathing spin echo sequence, while $R2^*$ relaxometry utilizes a breath-hold GRE sequence, with the rate of signal decay with increasing TE directly correlated with hepatic iron

concentration [20, 21]. Multi-echo GRE sequences are commercially available and can simultaneously quantify fat via PDFF and iron using $R2^*$ relaxometry [trade names include LiverLab (Siemens), IDEAL-IQ (GE), and mDixon Quant (Philips)] (see Fig. 7.3) [21, 22]. R2 relaxometry is the only FDA-approved MR-based iron quantitation method [20]. However, acquisition times (15–20 minutes) are longer than $R2^*$ relaxometry, and commercial off-site analysis is required with an average turnaround time of 2–3 days.

MR Elastography Chronic liver disease, regardless of etiology, can lead to hepatic fibrosis. If progressive, hepatic fibrosis can lead to cirrhosis. There is some evidence that early hepatic fibrosis is reversible, and therefore early detection may aid in the clinical management of these patients [23]. In recent years, MR elastography has emerged as an imaging technique for noninvasive measurement of hepatic fibrosis based on fibrosis-associated hepatic parenchymal stiffening causing increased velocity of propagated mechanical shear waves. A continuous acoustic vibration is generated outside of the scanner and transmitted through a passive driver resting on a patient over the liver, leading to propagation of shear waves through the

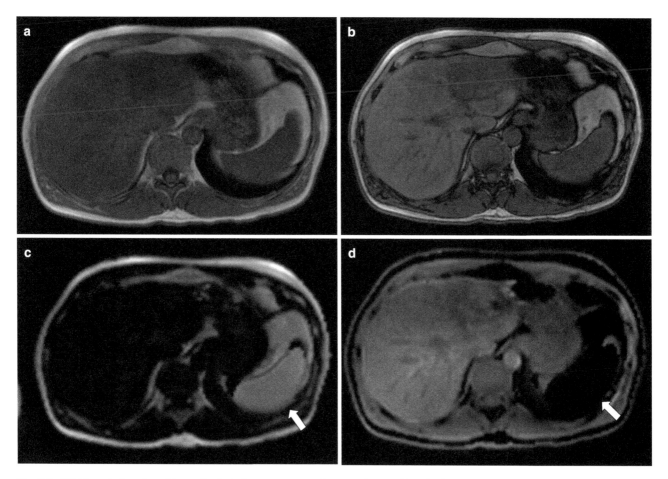

Fig. 7.4 Mild hepatic iron deposition and splenic fat-water swap artifact in a 16-year-old boy with chronic anemia related to chemotherapy. T1-weighted in-phase (**a**), out-of-phase (**b**), fat (**c**), and water (**d**) MR images were produced using the Dixon method. Mild signal loss is seen within the liver on the in-phase compared to the out-of-phase image consistent with mild hepatic iron deposition. Additionally, fat-water swap artifact is seen within the spleen (*arrows*) with abnormally high splenic signal on the fat image and low signal on the water image that resulted from a computation error. Note that the in-phase and out-of-phase images were not affected by this artifact

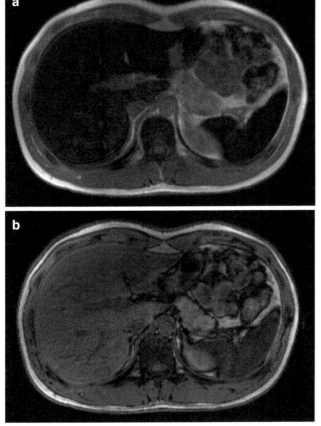

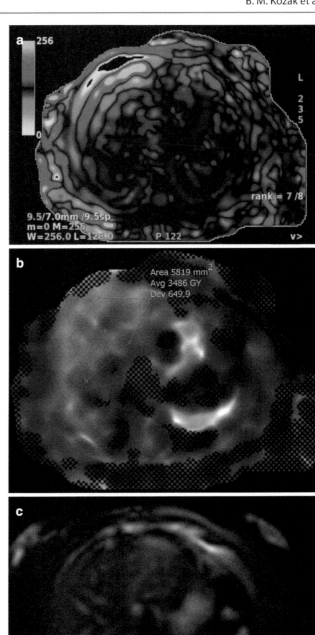

Fig. 7.5 Secondary hemosiderosis in a 15-year-old boy who presented with chronic pancytopenia related to chemotherapy for a hematologic malignancy. Axial non-enhanced T1-weighted GRE in-phase (**a**) and opposed-phase (**b**) MR images demonstrate diffuse loss of signal within the liver and spleen on the in-phase image compared to the opposed-phase image consistent with diffuse hemosiderosis from repeated blood transfusions

liver. The spatial location of the shear waves is encoded using a MR elastography sequence, most commonly a gradient-recalled echo sequence with motion-encoding gradients [24]. Magnitude and phase image sets are then generated and post-processed to yield a map of liver stiffness values (Fig. 7.6). Multiple studies have shown excellent correlation between MR elastographic stiffness values and the degree of fibrosis on biopsy in adults and children [24, 25].

Radial Non-Cartesian Techniques Degradation of images due to respiratory motion can be an important limitation in abdominal MR imaging, including evaluation of the liver. This is particularly true in young children who have more irregular and shallow respirations that can interfere with respiratory triggering. One strategy to minimize motion-related artifact is the use of radial K-space sampling, in which a series of radially oriented segments of K-space are acquired instead of the usual Cartesian linear order [26] (Fig. 7.7). This method oversamples the center of K-space, which encodes image contrast,

Fig. 7.6 Hepatic fibrosis in a 16-year-old girl with chronic viral hepatitis assessed by MR elastography. Wave (**a**) and elastogram (**b**) images were generated as part of an axial non-enhanced MR elastogram acquisition. The wave image shows propagation of shear waves through the liver with displacement of parenchymal tissue color coded with light blue representing the highest magnitudes of negative displacement and yellow representing highest magnitudes of positive displacement. The gray-scale elastogram represents hepatic stiffness in units of kilopascals (kPa). A region of interest drawn over the liver elastogram yields an average stiffness of 3.5 kPa. With MR elastography, clinically significant fibrosis (METAVIR stage ≥ F2) is considered when kPa is greater than 3 kPa. An axial non-enhanced T2-weighted fat-suppressed fast spin echo sequence acquired in the same study (**c**) demonstrates the anatomical correlate to the elastogram and wave images

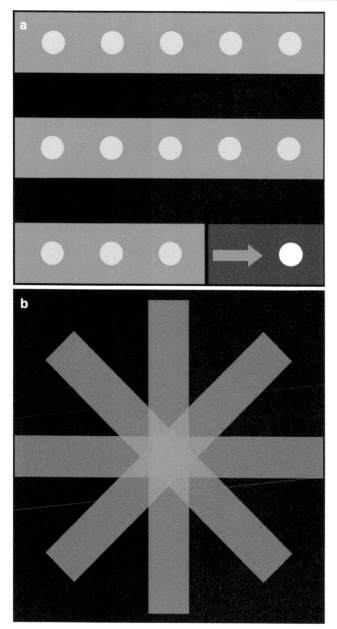

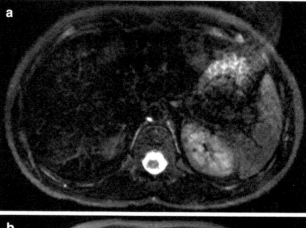

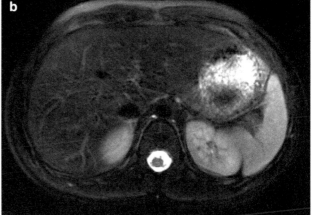

Fig. 7.8 Cartesian versus radial T2-weighted liver MR imaging in a 12-year-old boy. (**a**) T2-weighted fat-suppressed fast spin echo (FSE) image of the upper abdomen with respiratory triggering and standard Cartesian-based K-space sampling. (**b**) Axial T2-weighted fat-suppressed FSE image of the upper abdomen with respiratory triggering and radial-based K-space sampling. There is much less motion degradation with radial K-space sampling than Cartesian sampling

Fig. 7.7 Cartesian versus radial K-space sampling. (**a**) Conventional Cartesian K-space sampling results in line-by-line acquisition of K-space data. (**b**) Radial K-space sampling results in acquisition of radially oriented blades of K-space data that pass through central K-space

Anatomy

Embryology

resulting in a high signal-to-noise ratio and tissue contrast [19]. More importantly, in-plane respiratory motion is dispersed along the multiple radial axes rather than a single phase encoding direction, leading to less motion-related artifact (Fig. 7.8) [27]. Radial acquisitions are most commonly applied to T2-weighted sequences in liver imaging, although their applicability to multiphase enhanced T1-weighted acquisitions has also been demonstrated [28].

The liver, biliary system, and gallbladder form during the fourth week of gestation. They originate from the caudal aspect of the foregut near the duodenum as a ventral outpouching (hepatic diverticulum) (Fig. 7.9) [29]. The hepatic diverticulum grows rapidly and forms a cranial and caudal division. The larger cranial division forms the liver. The smaller caudal division forms the gallbladder and cystic duct. Hematopoietic cells, Kupffer cells, and the connective tissue of the liver develop from the mesoderm of the primitive diaphragm. The liver grows rapidly, and the biliary ductal system is complete by the 12th week of gestation [30].

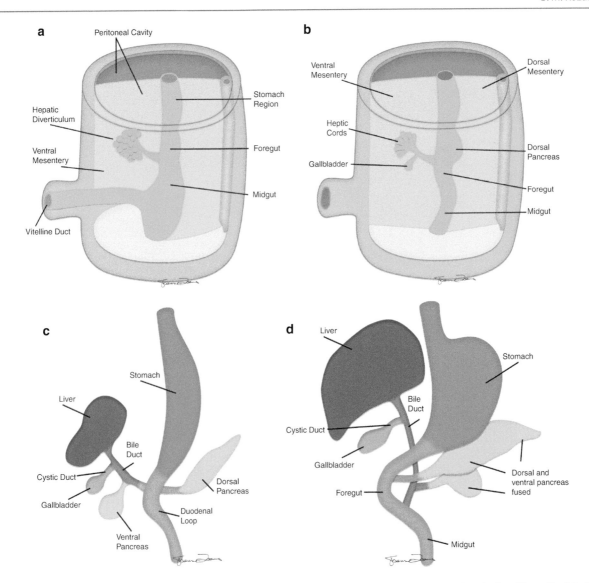

Fig. 7.9 Normal embryologic development of the liver. (**a**) The liver, biliary system, and gallbladder form during the fourth week of gestation from the hepatic diverticulum, which arises as a ventral outpouching from the caudal foregut. (**b–d**) The hepatic diverticulum grows to form a cranial and caudal division. The larger cranial division forms the liver. The smaller caudal division forms the gallbladder and cystic duct. The stalk of the hepatic diverticulum forms the common bile duct. The liver grows rapidly, and the biliary ductal system is complete by the 12th week of gestation when bile formation begins. (Image: Susanne L. Loomis, MS, FBCA; Department of Radiology, Massachusetts General Hospital, Boston, Massachusetts, USA)

Normal Development and Anatomy

The liver is located in the superior right aspect of the abdomen. It is nearly entirely covered by visceral peritoneum except at its posterosuperior portion, which directly contacts the diaphragm (bare area). The inferior aspect of the liver contains the porta hepatis through which the main portal vein, right and left branches of the hepatic artery, and right and left hepatic ducts enter or leave the liver. A unique feature of the liver is that it has a dual blood supply with approximately 25% supplied by the hepatic artery and 75% supplied by the portal vein.

Hepatic anatomy is commonly described in terms of segments. The Couinaud classification system is currently the most commonly used segmental classification scheme (Figs. 7.10 and 7.11) [29, 31]. The Couinaud system divides the liver into eight segments, each of which constitutes an independent functional unit with its own portal venous branch, hepatic arterial branch, and biliary and lymphatic drainage. The segments are delineated by vertical oblique planes drawn though the left, middle, and right hepatic veins as well as a horizontal plane through the portal vein at its bifurcation. The left hepatic and right hepatic lobes are separated by the middle hepatic vein as well as a plane drawn from the inferior vena cava to the gallbladder fossa (the Cantlie line).

The hepatic lobule serves as the basic functional unit of the liver, which is comprised of portal triads at the periphery (hepatic arteriole, portal venule, bile duct, lymphatics) and a central vein (Fig. 7.12) [32]. Sinusoids connect the portal triads to the central vein, which are surrounded by sheets of

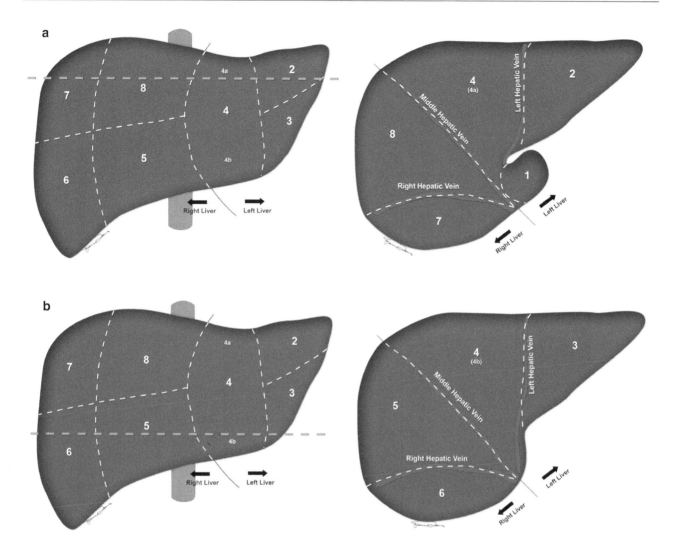

Fig. 7.10 Liver segmentation based on the Couinaud system. Segments are separated by vertical oblique lines drawn through the right, middle, and left hepatic veins as well as a horizontal line drawn through the portal vein. (**a**) Liver segments above the level of the portal vein. (**b**) Liver segments below the level of the portal vein. (Image: Susanne L. Loomis, MS, FBCA; Department of Radiology, Massachusetts General Hospital, Boston, Massachusetts, USA)

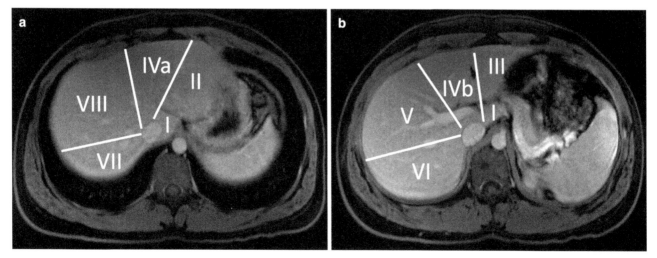

Fig. 7.11 MR imaging depiction of liver segmental anatomy in a 17-year-old boy. Axial enhanced T1-weighted fat-suppressed GRE images of the upper abdomen acquired in the portal venous phase above (**a**) and below (**b**) the level of the portal vein bifurcation demonstrate segmentation of the liver according to the Couinaud system. Oblique vertical planes represented as lines are drawn through the right, middle, and left hepatic veins

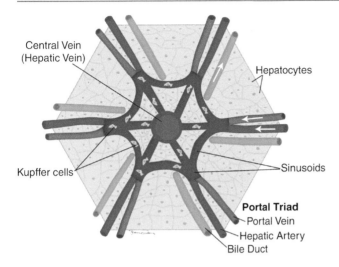

Fig. 7.12 Diagrammatic representation of the hepatic lobule. (Image: Susanne L. Loomis, MS, FBCA; Department of Radiology, Massachusetts General Hospital, Boston, Massachusetts, USA)

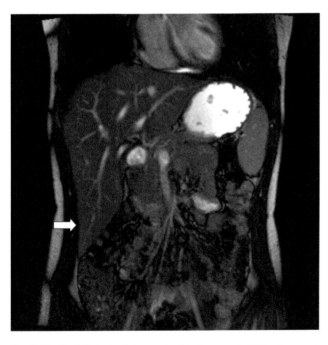

Fig. 7.13 Riedel lobe in a 16-year-old girl who presented following report of hepatic abnormality on a CT scan. A coronal balanced steady-state free precession MR image of the abdomen shows an inferior tongue-like elongation (*arrow*) of the right hepatic lobe consistent with a Riedel lobe

hepatocytes. Blood flows from the hepatic arterioles and portal venules into the sinusoids and then to the venules which drain to the hepatic veins.

There are four types of cells found within the liver: hepatocytes, endothelial cells lining sinusoids, Kupffer cells, and stellate cells. Hepatocytes perform biosynthesis (bile, proteins, glucose, biotransformation of toxins and drugs), Kupffer cells function as macrophages, and stellate cells store molecules such as fat and vitamin A [32, 33].

Anatomic Variants

A Riedel lobe is an anatomic variant in which there is downward tongue-like elongation of the right hepatic lobe (Fig. 7.13). Awareness of this variant is important to prevent misdiagnosis of a pathological mass. Prevalence of a Riedel lobe has been reported to be between 3% and 31% in different studies, and it is more commonly found in females [34].

Other anatomic variants are rare and include agenesis or hypoplasia of the left or right hepatic lobes, supradiaphragmatic liver, or the presence of additional hepatic lobes that may be connected to the liver or ectopic [30, 35].

Spectrum of Hepatic Disorders

Congenital Hepatic Disorders

Alagille Syndrome Alagille syndrome is a rare autosomal dominant disorder due to mutations in the Jag 1 and Notch signaling pathways [36]. It is a multi-system disorder that is diagnosed in the presence of at least three of five clinical features: chronic cholestasis, skeletal findings, cardiac disease, ocular abnormalities, and involvement of the face [37]. Within the liver, it is pathologically defined as a paucity of intrahepatic bile ducts. Most affected patients present with jaundice in early infancy. Bile duct paucity and hepatic fibrosis can progress over time ultimately leading to the need for liver transplantation in 20–50% of patients prior to adulthood [38].

MR imaging can be helpful in excluding the possibility of other etiologies of cholestasis when Alagille syndrome is suspected. Early findings can include a diminished appearance of the intrahepatic and extrahepatic biliary system. Differentiation between Alagille syndrome and biliary atresia may be difficult on MR imaging alone, with diagnosis relying upon a combination of biochemical, genetic, pathologic, and imaging tests [38]. Over time, findings consistent with fibrosis and portal hypertension can develop. Large regenerative nodules may be present, which are characteristically adjacent to the right portal vein (Fig. 7.14) [36].

Congenital Hepatic Fibrosis Congenital hepatic fibrosis belongs to a spectrum of fibrocystic liver diseases that include choledochal cysts, Caroli disease/syndrome, biliary hamartomas, and autosomal dominant polycystic disease. These abnormalities can also be associated with renal disease including autosomal recessive polycystic kidney disease [39]. The fibrocystic liver diseases are caused by aberrances in embryonic ductal plate development and can coexist with one another [40].

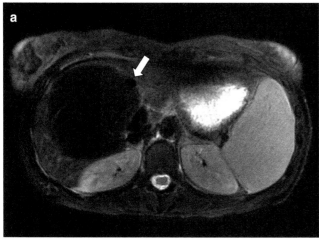

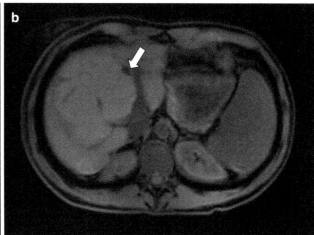

Fig. 7.14 Regenerative nodule in an 18-year-old female with Alagille syndrome. (**a**) Axial T2-weighted fat-suppressed fast spin echo (FSE) MR image with radial K-space acquisition demonstrates a large hypointense nodular mass (*arrow*) adjacent to the right portal vein. (**b**) Axial T1-weighted fat-suppressed GRE MR image shows the same hepatic mass (*arrow*) is isointense to slightly hyperintense compared to the surrounding hepatic parenchyma. These findings are consistent with a regenerative nodule in a characteristic location in a patient with Alagille syndrome

Histologically, the disease is characterized by progressive fibrosis between the ductal plate remnants and the adjacent biliary ducts as well as the presence of irregularly shaped bile ducts [40]. Clinical presentation is variable, although many affected patients present with clinical features of portal hypertension. Important complications include gastrointestinal bleeding from varices, hepatic failure, ascending cholangitis, hepatocellular carcinoma, and cholangiocarcinoma [36].

MR imaging can demonstrate morphologic features of the liver that can be suggestive of congenital hepatic fibrosis, including hypertrophy of the left lateral segment, normal size or hypertrophy of the left medial segment, and atrophy of the right hepatic lobe [41]. Enlargement or preservation in size of the left medial segment is less common in other causes of hepatic fibrosis. T2-weighted images may demonstrate periportal or more extensive patchy hyperintensity reflective of fibrosis. Other suggestive findings include sequelae of portal hypertension and the presence of other ductal plate abnormalities (Figs. 7.15 and 7.16).

Infectious Hepatic Disorders

Viral Hepatitis Viral hepatitis can be separated into acute and chronic (>6 months) stages. In the acute stage, disease severity can vary from subclinical infection to symptomatic disease. Less commonly, fulminant hepatitis can occur with diffuse immune-mediated destruction of infected hepatocytes. In pediatric patients who develop chronic hepatitis, cirrhosis can eventually develop.

In the neonatal period and early infancy, the most common etiologies of viral hepatitis are vertically transmitted infections including hepatitis B (HBV), cytomegalovirus (CMV), parvovirus, rubella, and herpes simplex virus (HSV). In childhood, the most common etiologies are hepatitis A (HAV), HBV, and hepatitis C (HCV) [42]. HBV, especially when acquired perinatally, and HCV infections are the most common etiologies that progress to chronic infection. Both chronic HBV and HCV infections independently increase the risk for hepatocellular carcinoma [43, 44].

MR imaging is not commonly used in the evaluation of acute hepatitis. Although imaging findings of acute hepatitis are non-specific but can include hepatomegaly, gallbladder wall thickening, heterogeneous signal on T2-weighted images, heterogeneous enhancement on arterial phase post-contrast images, and periportal edema [45]. In chronic viral hepatitis, imaging findings consistent with hepatic cirrhosis and portal hypertension can be present. Prior to the development of cirrhosis, the liver may appear unremarkable, or there can be heterogeneous enhancement, parenchymal heterogeneity, and surrounding lymphadenopathy.

Bacterial Infections The clinical presentation of pyogenic hepatic infections varies and can include subclinical hepatitis, symptomatic hepatitis, cholestatic jaundice, hepatic abscesses, and fulminant necrosis. Perinatally, *Escherichia coli* is the most common causative organism with other etiologies including streptococcus, *Listeria*, and syphilis [30]. Later in childhood, *Staphylococcus aureus*, *Streptococcus pyogenes*, and *E. coli* are the most common causes of hepatic abscesses [42] and are more common in the immunosuppressed. Other risk factors for hepatic infection include biliary obstruction, abdominal infectious or inflammatory processes secondary to pylephlebitis or contiguous spread, and particular animal exposures that increase the risk for

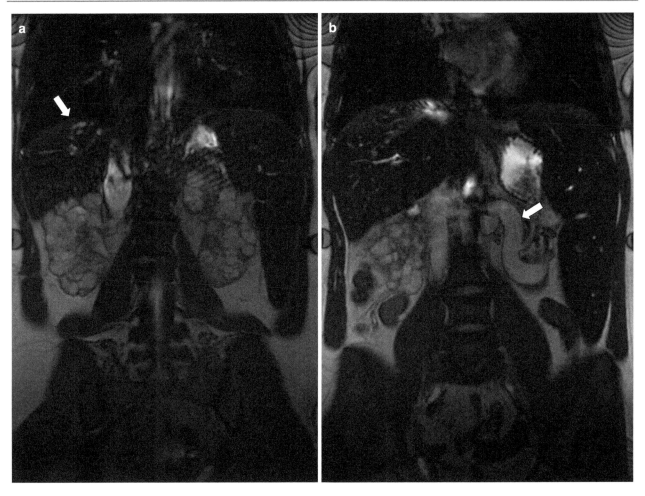

Fig. 7.15 Congenital hepatic fibrosis in an 18-year-old female who presented for surveillance imaging. (**a**) Coronal balanced steady-state free precession MR image shows a mildly nodular contour of the liver consistent with cirrhosis. Cystic dilation (*arrow*) of the bile ducts is seen at the hepatic dome, where there is geographic high signal intensity of the liver parenchyma consistent with confluent fibrosis. Innumerable cysts are also seen within both kidneys. (**b**) Coronal balanced steady-state free precession MR image more anteriorly demonstrates upper abdominal varices (*arrow*) and splenomegaly consistent with portal hypertension

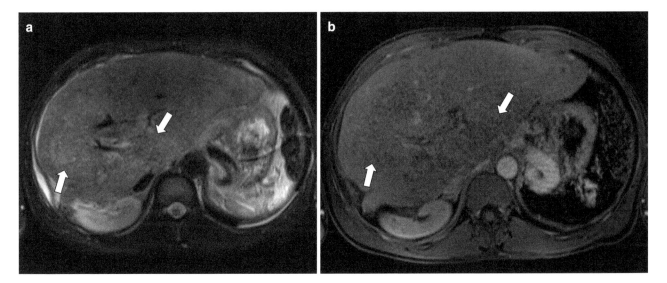

Fig. 7.16 An 18-year-old male with congenital hepatic fibrosis who presented for surveillance imaging. (**a**) Axial T2-weighted fat-suppressed fast spin echo (FSE) MR image demonstrates patchy T2 hyperintensity (*arrows*) throughout the liver. (**b**) Axial contrast-enhanced T1-weighted fat-suppressed GRE MR image acquired in the portal venous phase demonstrates decreased enhancement (*arrows*) in the same distribution as the patchy T2-weighted hyperintensity, consistent with confluent hepatic fibrosis

rickettsial organisms, leptospirosis, and bartonella. *S. aureus* is the most common cause of hepatic abscess in childhood, although most pyogenic liver abscesses are polymicrobial [46]. In endemic areas, tuberculosis is also an important cause of hepatic abscess [42].

The MR imaging findings for the majority of the above clinical scenarios are non-specific and can be normal or similar to those described for acute viral hepatitis. Hepatic abscesses can appear as a single non-loculated fluid collection, a multi-loculated cystic mass, multifocal lesions, diffuse microabscesses (such as with tuberculosis), or a phlegmonous process [47]. Small clustered abscesses can aggregate into a single large abscess (cluster sign). Hepatic abscesses demonstrate low internal signal on T1-weighted sequences, high internal signal intensity on T2-weighted sequences, and surrounding T2-weighted hyperintensity due to hepatic parenchymal edema. A double target appearance of the abscess wall is characteristic on T2-weighted images with an iso- to hypointense inner layer and a hyper-intense outer layer (Fig. 7.17). Following contrast administration, the inner layer demonstrates early and persistent enhancement, while the outer layer shows delayed enhancement. Restricted diffusion is often present [48]. Finally, air can be seen within the abscess.

Fungal Infections Hepatic fungal infections occur most frequently in the setting of disseminated infection in immunocompromised pediatric patients. The most common fungal etiologies are *Candida* species followed by *Aspergillus*, *Cryptococcus*, *Histoplasma*, and *Mucor* [47].

MR imaging is the imaging modality of choice when fungal infection of solid organs is suspected in pediatric patients given its high sensitivity and lack of ionizing radiation [42]. Imaging may demonstrate hepatomegaly with possible splenomegaly but no focal lesions. However, diffuse microabscesses are commonly observed and demonstrate marked T2-weighted hyperintensity (Fig. 7.18). Arterial phase rim enhancement can be present depending on the degree of neutropenia [49]. Diffusion-weighted restriction can also be seen [48].

Amebic Infections Amebic infections occur worldwide but are endemic in Africa, Southeast Asia, and Central and South America [47]. *Entamoeba histolytica* is the most commonly implicated amebic protozoan. Infection occurs after ingestion of contaminated food or water. The protozoan can disseminate via the portal vein to the liver, where abscesses can form. Most amebic hepatic abscesses occur in children less than 3 years old [30]. Amebic hepatic abscesses are usually unilocular and solitary. They occur most commonly in the right hepatic lobe near the liver capsule. Extension through the diaphragm into the thorax is highly suggestive of an amebic hepatic abscess [50].

On MR imaging, an amebic hepatic abscess is usually centrally T1-weighted hypointense and T2-weighted hyperintense. Peri-abscess edema is frequently seen, and rim enhancement is often present [51] (Fig. 7.19).

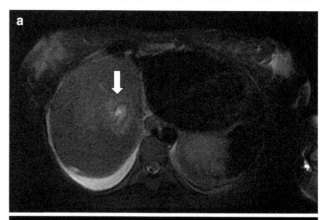
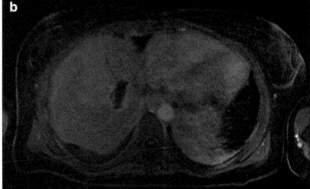
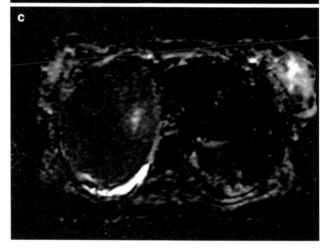

Fig. 7.17 Hepatic abscess in a 17-year-old girl with nausea, fever, and back pain. (**a**) Axial T2-weighted fat-suppressed MR image shows a hyperintense lesion (*arrow*), an outer hyperintense layer (target sign), as well as surrounding parenchymal edema. (**b**) Axial contrast-enhanced T1-weighted fat-suppressed MR image demonstrates thick rim enhancement. (**c**) Axial diffusion-weighted MR image shows restricted diffusion within the lesion. These findings were suspicious for a hepatic abscess. Cultures from the lesion eventually grew *Klebsiella*

Echinococcus Echinococcal (also referred to as hydatid) infections are caused by the tapeworm *Echinococcus granulosus* and less commonly by *Echinococcus multilocularis* [42]. The liver is the most commonly involved organ [47].

MR imaging can demonstrate a unilocular cyst or a cyst with adjacent smaller daughter cysts. On T1- and T2-weighted images, the pericyst (fibrous capsule formed

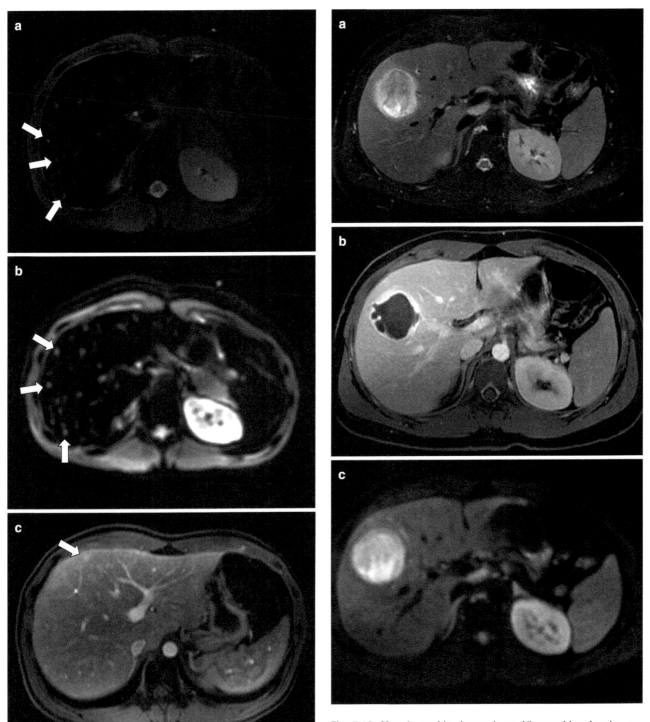

Fig. 7.18 Hepatic fungal microabscesses in a 14-year-old boy with acute myeloid leukemia undergoing treatment with fever and neutropenia. (a) Axial T2-weighted fat-suppressed MR image shows numerous small hyperintense lesions (*arrows*) within the liver. Diffusely low signal intensity of the liver and spleen is consistent with iron overload from repeated blood transfusions. (b) Axial diffusion-weighted MR image demonstrates high signal intensity within the majority of the lesions (*arrows*) consistent with restricted diffusion. (c) Axial contrast-enhanced T1-weighted, fat-suppressed MR image acquired during the portal venous demonstrates rim enhancement of one of these small lesions (*arrow*). Beta-D-glucan levels were elevated, and fungal blood cultures eventually grew *Trichophyton* species

Fig. 7.19 Hepatic amebic abscess in an 18-year-old male who presented with fevers and abdominal pain. (a) Axial T2-weighted fat-suppressed MR image shows a large heterogeneous lesion in the right hepatic lobe with surrounding edema. (b) Axial contrast-enhanced T1-weighted fat-suppressed MR image acquired in the equilibrium phase demonstrates thick peripheral enhancement of the lesion. (c) Axial diffusion-weighted MR image shows high signal intensity within the lesion consistent with restricted diffusion. These findings were considered suspicious for a hepatic abscess, with cultures growing *Entamoeba histolytica*

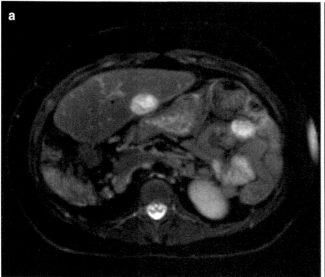
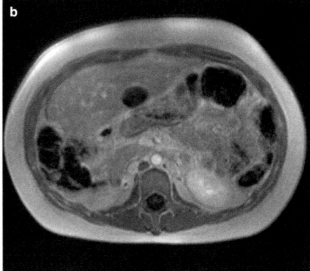

Fig. 7.20 Echinococcal hepatic infection in a 12-year-old girl status post liver transplant who presented with fever and abdominal pain. (**a**) Axial T2-weighted fat-suppressed MR image show a hyperintense lesion in the liver with an internal hypointense floating membrane. There is no substantial surrounding hepatic parenchymal edema. (**b**) Axial enhanced T1-weighted non-fat-suppressed MR image shows mild peripheral enhancement but no internal enhancement within this lesion. Pathology following excision confirmed an echinococcal infection

by host response) is hypointense due to its fibrous composition [52]. The cyst matrix typically has low to intermediate signal intensity on T1-weighted images and high to intermediate signal intensity on T2-weighted images [52]. Debris can be seen within the matrix from ruptured daughter cysts. Daughter cysts usually have lower signal intensity on T1-weighted images and higher signal intensity on T2-weighted images compared to the cyst matrix. There is no enhancement of the cyst contents or septa following contrast administration, although some delayed enhancement of the pericyst may be present.

If the hydatid cyst ruptures into the pericyst, floating internal membranes can be identified, which is referred to as the water lily sign (Fig. 7.20). Chronic hydatid cysts demonstrate progressive calcification of their walls and internal contents with complete calcification indicative of a non-viable cyst [42].

Diffuse Hepatic Parenchymal Disorders

Metabolic Disorders

Glycogen Storage Disease Glycogen storage diseases (GSDs) are a collection of autosomal recessive diseases characterized by enzymatic defects involved in glycogen metabolism. In the GSDs that involve the liver, the enzymatic defects lead to the hepatic buildup of glycogen or its metabolites, hepatomegaly, and hypoglycemia. The most common GSD with hepatic involvement is type I GSD (von Gierke disease). It is caused by a deficiency in glucose 6-phosphatase. Other GSDs with hepatic involvement are type 0 (glycogen synthetase defect), type III (Cori disease, glycogen debranching enzyme defect),

and type IV (Andersen disease, glycogen branching enzyme defect) [53].

Type I GSD manifests around 3 months of age with hypoglycemia and hepatomegaly [54]. Hepatic steatosis often develops, and hepatic adenomas are also common, with up to 75% of patients with type I GSD developing adenomas by the second decade of life (Fig. 7.21) [55]. The imaging features of adenomas are discussed later in this chapter. Routine surveillance imaging is recommended to assess for development of adenomas, usually ultrasound every 1–2 years until 16 years of age [56]. If adenomas are present, contrast-enhanced MR imaging or CT is recommended every 3–6 months to assess risk of adenoma hemorrhage or malignant transformation [53]. Progression to fibrosis and cirrhosis is not commonly observed in type I GSD but common with the other GSDs described above [53].

Gaucher Disease Gaucher disease is an autosomal recessive lysosomal storage disease that results from a deficiency in the lysosomal enzyme glucocerebrosidase. This deficiency causes the accumulation of glucosylceramide within the lysosomes of reticuloendothelial cells. Three clinical subtypes exist, with over 90% of cases classified as type I [57, 58]. This subtype has no neurologic symptoms and occurs most commonly in people of Ashkenazi-Jewish descent. The age of presentation ranges from childhood to adulthood, and clinical manifestations include hepatosplenomegaly, anemia, thrombocytopenia, and bone disease (bone crises, avascular necrosis, and fractures) [58].

MR imaging of the liver in affected pediatric patients shows hepatomegaly, which is often less marked than the degree of splenomegaly (Fig. 7.22) [59]. Lipid-laden macro-

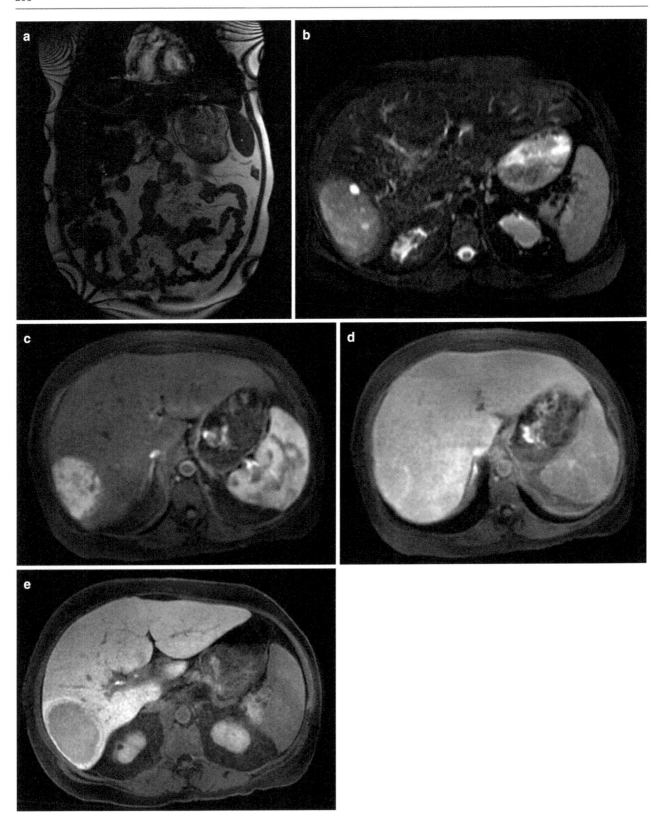

Fig. 7.21 Hepatic adenoma in an 18-year-old female with known von Gierke disease who presented with abdominal pain. (**a**) Coronal balanced steady-state free precession MR image demonstrates hepatomegaly. (**b**) Axial T2-weighted fat-suppressed MR image shows a mildly hyperintense mass in the right hepatic lobe with cystic change. (**c**) Axial enhanced T1-weighted fat-suppressed MR image obtained in the arterial phase shows heterogeneous hyperenhancement of the mass. (**d**) Axial enhanced T1-weighted fat-suppressed MR image obtained in the equilibrium phase shows isointensity of the mass relative to the hepatic parenchyma. (**e**) Axial enhanced T1-weighted fat-suppressed MR image obtained in the hepatobiliary phase shows hypointensity of the mass. These MR imaging findings are suggestive of a hepatic adenoma

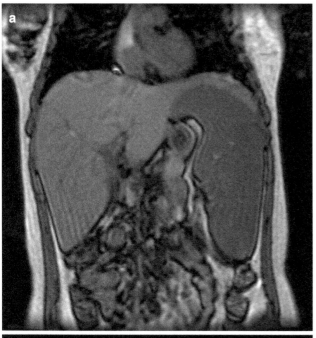

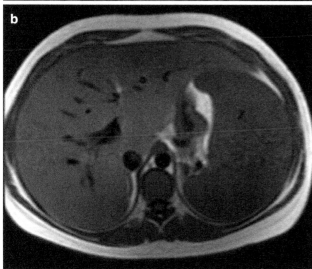

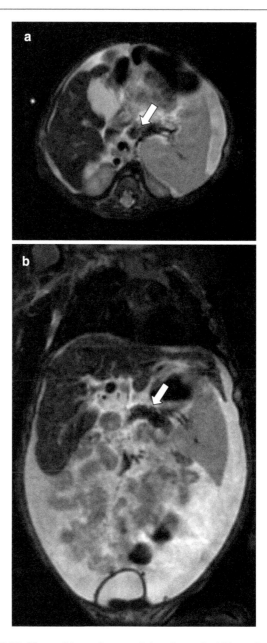

Fig. 7.22 Hepatosplenomegaly in an 18-year-old female with known Gaucher disease who presented with abdominal pain. Coronal (**a**) and axial (**b**) T1-weighted GRE MR images demonstrate hepatosplenomegaly

Fig. 7.23 Neonatal hemochromatosis in a 2-month-old boy who presented with liver function test abnormalities. Axial (**a**) and coronal (**b**) T2-weighted fat-suppressed MR images show cirrhotic morphology of the liver and ascites, with diffusely decreased intensity of the liver and pancreas (*arrow*) and sparing of the spleen suggestive of iron overload from hereditary hemochromatosis

phages (Gaucher cells) may form nodules that appear hypointense on T1-weighted images and hyperintense on T2-weighted images. Areas of fibrosis can also be seen.

Iron Deposition in the Liver

Hereditary Hemosiderosis Hereditary hemochromatosis is an autosomal recessive disease that results in parenchymal iron deposition. It is caused by a mutation in the HFE (high iron Fe) gene resulting in increased gastrointestinal iron

absorption. Eventually, this excess iron is deposited intracellularly within various organs, particularly the liver, pancreas, heart, pituitary gland, synovium of joints, and skin. Within the cell, iron can catalyze the production of free radicals leading to cellular damage. Symptoms typically begin in adulthood; however, a neonatal form of hemosiderosis does exist that can present with hepatic failure along with pancreatic and cardiac abnormalities (Fig. 7.23) [59].

Within the liver, iron accumulation may lead to hepatomegaly and eventual cirrhosis. Hepatocellular carcinoma and cholangiocarcinoma are late complications [60]. MR imaging is the modality of choice to quantify parenchymal iron deposition [59] and assess the need for therapeutic phlebotomy (see *Liver Iron Quantitation*).

Secondary Hemosiderosis Secondary hemosiderosis refers to iron overload usually from frequent blood transfusions, iron-loading anemia, or frequent iron transfusions. In comparison to hereditary hemochromatosis where excess iron predominantly deposits within parenchymal cells, the iron in transfusions is primarily taken up by reticuloendothelial cells in the liver, bone marrow, and spleen. Hepatic dysfunction from secondary hemosiderosis is less common [61].

MR imaging findings in secondary hemosiderosis are similar to those with hereditary hemochromatosis with the exception of the typical organs involved. In secondary hemosiderosis, the liver, bone marrow, and spleen usually demonstrate iron overload (Fig. 7.24). Hereditary hemochromatosis, by contrast, tends to spare the spleen but involves the pancreas. MR-based liver iron quantitation is beginning to replace liver biopsy as a noninvasive diagnostic tool in determining which hemosiderosis patients are candidates for iron chelation therapy.

Hepatic Steatosis

Nonalcoholic fatty liver disease (NAFLD) is the most common form of hepatic steatosis in pediatric patients. It is also the most common cause of chronic hepatic disease in this patient population. NAFLD can manifest as hepatic steatosis, nonalcoholic steatohepatitis (NASH), fibrosis, and cirrhosis [62]. Other possible etiologies of hepatic

steatosis include viral hepatitis, medication side effects (corticosteroids, valproic acid, amiodarone, methotrexate, various chemotherapy agents), total parental nutrition, extreme malnutrition, familial hyperlipoproteinemia, and glycogen storage diseases [63].

Hepatic steatosis is easily identified by MR imaging using T1-weighted in-phase and opposed-phase GRE sequences (Fig. 7.25). These sequences demonstrate loss of signal on the opposed-phase images in regions of hepatic steatosis. MR spectroscopy has also been demonstrated to be highly accurate for quantifying hepatic fat [11] but is limited by spatial coverage. MR-based proton density fat fraction (PDFF) is FDA-approved and provides whole liver fat quantitation (see *Liver Fat Quantitation*).

Hepatic steatosis can be diffuse or heterogeneous with focal areas of fatty deposition or fatty sparing. Typical locations for focal fatty deposition or fatty sparing include adjacent to the falciform ligament, gallbladder fossa, porta hepatis, or in subcapsular regions. In comparison to mass lesions, areas of focal fatty deposition or focal sparing do not exhibit mass effect, have a geographic distribution, and have ill-defined or angulated margins.

Hepatic Cirrhosis

Cirrhosis represents end-stage liver disease that can result from any chronic or repetitive hepatic injury. Etiologies include various infectious, metabolic, biliary, and vascular processes (Table 7.2) [64]. Hepatic cirrhosis is characterized by progressive hepatic fibrosis and the presence of regenerative nodules. Complications include sequelae of portal hypertension, coagulopathies, hepatorenal syndrome, and hepatocellular carcinoma.

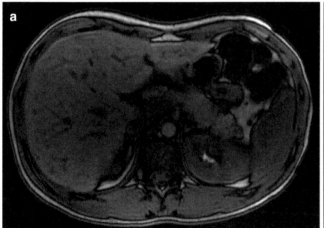
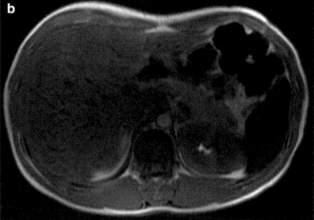

Fig. 7.24 Secondary hemosiderosis in a 16-year-old boy with acute myeloid leukemia requiring repeated transfusions for chronic anemia who presented with abdominal pain. Axial T1-weighted GRE MR images obtained out-of-phase (**a**) and in-phase (**b**) demonstrate decreased signal in the liver and spleen on the in-phase image. There is no change in MR signal within the pancreas. These findings are consistent with iron overload from secondary hemosiderosis

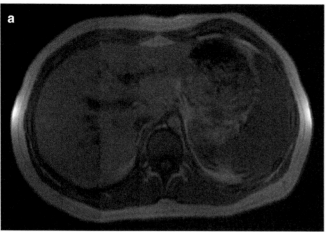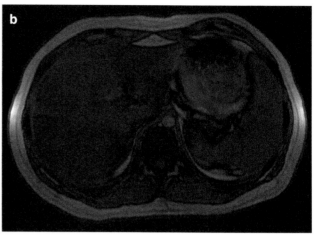

Fig. 7.25 Hepatic steatosis in a 17-year-old boy with obesity who presented with abnormal liver function tests. Axial T1-weighted GRE MR images obtained in-phase (**a**) and out-of-phase (**b**) demonstrate diffuse loss of signal intensity in the liver parenchyma on opposed-phase images consistent with steatosis

Table 7.2 Etiologies of hepatic cirrhosis in pediatric patients

Nonalcoholic fatty liver disease
Biliary atresia
Primary biliary cirrhosis
Primary sclerosing cholangitis
Budd-Chiari syndrome
Alagille syndrome
Congenital hepatic fibrosis
Hereditary hemochromatosis or secondary hemosiderosis
Chronic viral hepatitis
Glycogen storage disease
Wilson disease
Tyrosinemia
Galactosemia
Fructosemia
Cystic fibrosis
Autosomal recessive polycystic kidney disease
Drugs and toxins
Total parental nutrition
Cardiomyopathies and constrictive pericarditis

The morphologic changes characteristic of cirrhosis are well demonstrated on MR imaging. These changes include a nodular liver contour, hypertrophy of the caudate lobe and left lateral segment, atrophy of the right hepatic lobe with posterior notching, and widening of the gallbladder fossa and other hepatic fissures. Sequelae of portal hypertension can be present.

Hepatic fibrosis manifests as areas of hyperintensity on T2-weighted images and hypointensity on T1-weighted images. Post-contrast images demonstrate reduced enhancement in the arterial phase followed by increased enhancement in the portal venous and equilibrium phases.

Nodules are usually present in the cirrhotic liver. The majority of these nodules are benign regenerative nodules reflecting reparative efforts of the hepatic parenchyma. They have variable signal on T1-weighted images and are usually isointense or hypointense on T2-weighted images. Regenerative nodules are isointense or hypointense to hepatic parenchyma on post-contrast images, without arterial hyperenhancement (Fig. 7.26) [65].

Dysplastic nodules contain abnormal but noncancerous cells on histology. Low-grade dysplastic nodules can be indistinguishable from regenerative nodules on MR imaging. High-grade dysplastic nodules can be difficult to distinguish from well-differentiated hepatocellular carcinoma. They are often hyperintense on T2-weighted images and may demonstrate arterial phase enhancement without washout on the portal venous on post-contrast imaging. Dysplastic nodules are also more likely to demonstrate microscopic fat or siderosis. Siderotic nodules refer to the presence of iron in regenerative and dysplastic nodules, which are associated with low signal intensity on T1-weighted GRE and T2-weighted fast spin echo (FSE) imaging.

Neoplastic Hepatic Disorders

Benign Hepatic Neoplasms

Hepatic Hemangioma Hepatic hemangiomas (previously called infantile hemangioendotheliomas) are vascular tumors that are the most common benign liver masses in children. They are divided into congenital and infantile subtypes. Congenital hemangiomas develop perinatally and do not proliferate after birth. Congenital hemangiomas are further divided into rapidly involuting congenital hemangiomas (RICH) and non-involuting congenital hemangiomas (NICH). The former involute entirely, usu-

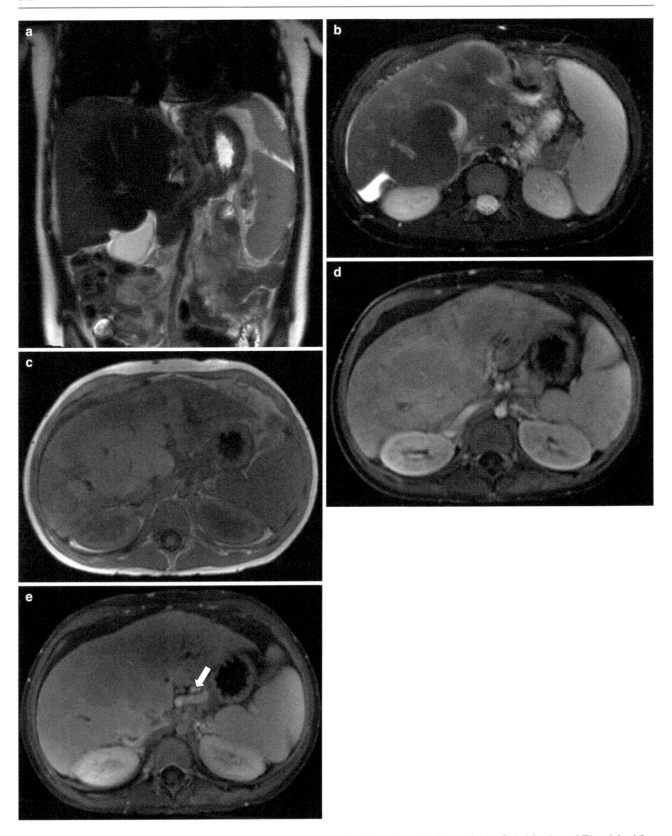

Fig. 7.26 Hepatic cirrhosis in a 10-year-old boy with secondary sclerosing cholangitis. (**a**) Coronal T2-weighted MR image demonstrates nodular contour of the liver and splenomegaly consistent with hepatic cirrhosis with multiple hypointense nodules. There is gallbladder wall thickening and pericholecystic fluid, which are likely reactive changes related to cirrhosis. (**b**) Axial T2-weighted fat-suppressed MR image redemonstrates hypointense nodules within the liver with small-volume ascites adjacent to the liver. (**c**) Axial T1-weighted GRE MR image demonstrates mildly increased signal intensity to the liver nodules. (**d**) Axial enhanced T1-weighted fat-suppressed MR image acquired during the arterial phase shows no enhancement of the liver nodules. (**e**) Axial enhanced T1-weighted fat-suppressed MR image acquired during the portal venous phase again shows no enhancement or washout of the liver nodules. Together, the imaging features of the liver nodules are consistent with regenerative nodules. Upper abdominal varices (*arrow*) are evident. Irregular dilation of bile ducts in the left hepatic lobe is consistent with sclerosing cholangitis

ally by 14 months of age [66]. The latter does not involute and may grow proportionally to the patient. Infantile hemangiomas develop shortly after birth and can grow rapidly in the first few months of life. An involuting phase then ensues, typically beginning around 12 months of life. The majority of hemangiomas are clinically occult. Infantile hemangiomas are often associated with cutaneous hemangiomas [67].

Congenital hemangiomas are usually solitary lesions. On MR imaging, they demonstrate T1-weighted hypointensity and T2-weighted hyperintensity, although hemorrhage and calcification can alter signal intensity on both sequences. Post-contrast images demonstrate early peripheral nodular enhancement and classically exhibit progressive centripetal enhancement on delayed images [68, 69]. Infantile hemangiomas are usually multifocal or diffuse. Hepatomegaly may be present. Signal intensity and enhancement patterns are similar to those for congenital hemangiomas, although lesions can show more homogeneous enhancement (Figs. 7.27 and 7.28). Flow voids can be present within or adjacent to these lesions reflecting enlarged contributory hepatic arteries and veins. Enlargement of the upper abdominal aorta, celiac trunk, hepatic arteries, and inferior vena cava may be evident [68, 69].

Mesenchymal Hamartoma Mesenchymal hamartomas are the second most common benign liver mass in children [70].

These tumors reflect uncoordinated mesenchymal proliferation that also contain unencapsulated cysts, bile ducts, and hepatocytes [71]. The majority of mesenchymal hamartomas are identified in pediatric patients younger than 2 years of age with 95% discovered by 5 years of age [68].

On MR imaging, mesenchymal hamartomas can range from predominantly cystic masses to predominantly solid masses. The solid portions of the tumor tend to have decreased signal intensity on both T1-weighted and T2-weighted images because of fibrosis [68]. Solid components and septa demonstrate mild enhancement (Fig. 7.29). Calcification and hemorrhage are uncommon.

Focal Nodular Hyperplasia Focal nodular hyperplasia (FNH) is uncommonly seen in pediatric patients [71]. The average age of diagnosis is between 2 and 5 years [72]. FNH is comprised of hyperplastic hepatocytes, biliary ductules that do not connect to the biliary tree, Kupffer cells, and a central stellate fibrous scar that contains malformed vessels [71]. Necrosis and hemorrhage are uncommon.

On MR imaging, FNH is commonly homogeneous in appearance with iso- to slight hypointensity on T1-weighted images and iso- to slight hyperintensity on T2-weighted images. The central scar, if present, is hypointense on T1-weighted images and hyperintense on T2-weighted images. Post-contrast images demonstrate uniform hyperenhancement

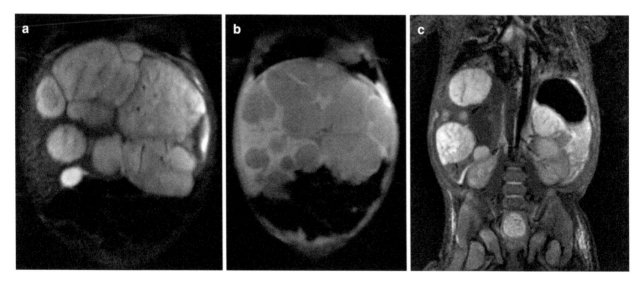

Fig. 7.27 Hepatic infantile hemangiomas in a 2-month-old boy who presented with multiple cutaneous hemangiomas and increasing hepatomegaly. (**a**) Coronal T2-weighted fat-suppressed MR image shows multiple large hyperintense masses within an enlarged liver containing flow voids. (**b**) Coronal T1-weighted fat-suppressed MR image shows the masses to be hypointense to surrounding liver. (**c**) Coronal fast spin echo (FSE) inversion recovery MR image redemonstrates multiple flow voids within the hepatic masses. Additionally, there is abrupt decrease in caliber of the aorta following the takeoff of the celiac trunk

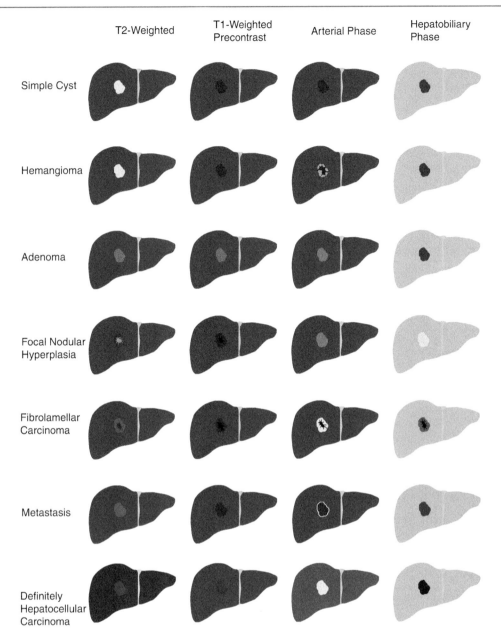

Fig. 7.28 Common MR imaging characteristics for different benign and malignant hepatic lesions. T2-weighted, pre-contrast T1-weighted, post-contrast arterial phase, and hepatobiliary phase signal characteristics are shown for a simple cyst, hemangioma, adenoma, focal nodular hyperplasia, fibrolamellar hepatocellular carcinoma, metastasis, and hepatocellular carcinoma. Note that while these lesions commonly have these MR imaging patterns, their signal characteristics can be variable

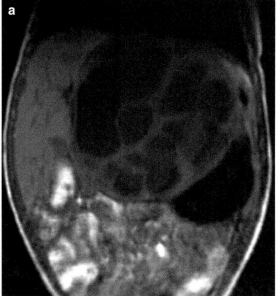

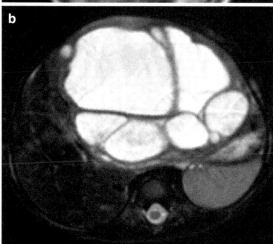

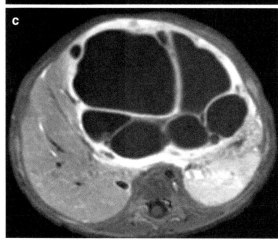

on the arterial phase as well as isointensity on the portal venous and equilibrium phases. On the equilibrium phase, there is enhancement of the central scar [68]. If a hepatobiliary contrast agent is used, hepatobiliary phase images show retention of contrast within the lesion, often in a spoked wheel configuration because of the central scar (Fig. 7.30 and see Fig. 7.28) [71]. Pediatric patients with a prior history of malignancy treated with chemotherapy are known to have a higher likelihood of developing FNH or FNH-like lesions in the years following treatment, possibly as a response to therapy-induced hepatic vascular injury. It is important to distinguish delayed FNH development from metastatic disease in this population [73].

Hepatocellular Adenoma Hepatocellular adenomas are uncommon benign tumors in the pediatric population composed of hepatocytes arranged in sheets or cords that can have increased concentrations of fat and glycogen. Large peritumoral arteries supply the sinusoids within the mass, which are believed to increase the risk for hemorrhage [68]. Several different subtypes of adenomas have been described based on genetic and histopathologic features. These subtypes can have different biological behavior as well as imaging characteristics [74].

Inflammatory adenomas are the most common subtype and mainly seen in females with obesity/metabolic syndrome or oral contraceptive (OCP) use. They have the highest risk for bleeding. The most common MR imaging features are T2-weighted hyperintensity (which can be marked and more prominent peripherally) and arterial phase hyperenhancement that persists on the portal venous phase. Delayed washout is not typical. Inflammatory adenomas can have variable degrees of intralesional fat and variable contrast uptake on the hepatobiliary phase [74, 75] (Fig. 7.31 and see Fig. 7.28).

Hepatocyte nuclear factor 1-α (alpha) inactivated (HNF-1α) adenomas are the second most common subtype and are almost exclusively seen in females with oral contraceptive use. They have the lowest risk of malignant transformation to hepatocellular carcinoma. MR imaging features include T2-weighted isointensity, arterial phase hyperenhancement that does not persist on the portal venous phase, and without delayed washout. The presence of intralesional lipid

Fig. 7.29 Mesenchymal hamartoma in an 11-month-old boy who presented with abdominal distension. (**a**) Coronal T1-weighted fat-suppressed MR image shows a large multi-cystic mass in the left hepatic lobe. (**b**) Axial T2-weighted fat-suppressed MR image redemonstrates the predominantly cystic mass with multiple septa. (**c**) Axial contrast-enhanced T1-weighted fat-suppressed MR image shows enhancement of the solid components of the cystic mass. These findings are consistent with a mesenchymal hamartoma

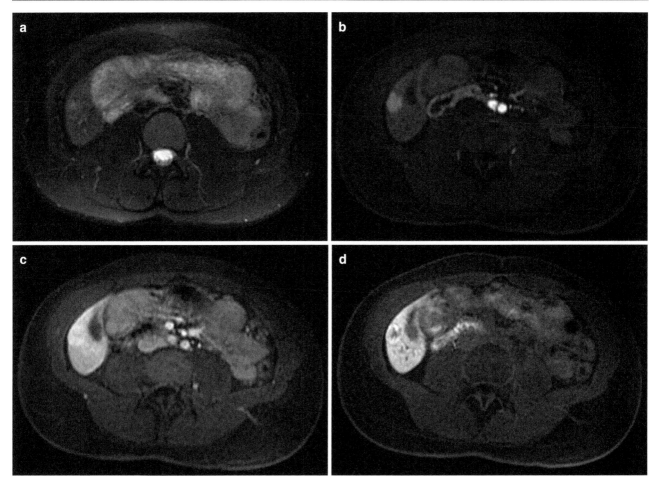

Fig. 7.30 Focal nodular hyperplasia in a 15-year-old boy who presented after incidental detection of a hepatic mass on a spine MR imaging. (**a**) Axial T2-weighted fat-suppressed MR image shows a hyperintense focus in the right hepatic lobe. (**b**) Axial enhanced T1-weighted fat-suppressed MR image acquired in the late arterial phase shows the lesion to be hyperenhancing. (**c**) Axial enhanced T1-weighted fat-suppressed MR image acquired in the portal venous shows the lesion to be isointense. (**d**) Axial enhanced T1-weighted fat-suppressed MR image acquired in the hepatobiliary phase shows retention of contrast within the lesion, with central hypointensity that may reflect a scar

exhibiting signal loss on opposed-phase chemical shift imaging is the most specific MR imaging feature [74, 75]. This subtype is almost always hypointense on the hepatobiliary phase.

The β (beta)-catenin-mutated adenomas are the least common subtype. They occur more frequently in males with glycogen storage diseases or anabolic steroid use. They have the highest risk for malignant transformation. There are no characteristic imaging features that help distinguish this subtype from the others, but they are more likely to demonstrate suspicious imaging features such as delayed contrast washout or pseudocapsule (Table 7.3) [74, 75].

Angiomyolipoma The liver is the second most common site for angiomyolipomas (AMLs) following the kidney. There is an association with tuberous sclerosis, although not as strong as with renal AMLs [76]. Histologically, AMLs reflect an unencapsulated lesion comprised of varying amounts of fat, smooth muscle, and vascular tissue.

On MR imaging, AMLs are typically T1-weighted hyperintense due to intra-tumoral fat. The diagnosis of AML on MR imaging is based on signal loss within the lesion on T1-weighted or T2-weighted images with fat suppression, although lipid-poor AMLs without detectable fat are common. Signal loss on opposed-phase T1-weighted imaging is not sufficient to diagnose AMLs, as hepatocellular carcinomas can also demonstrate intracellular lipid. AMLs are typically hyperintense on T2-weighted images, although lipid-poor AMLs often show low T2-weighted signal intensity (Fig. 7.32). Post-contrast imaging most commonly demonstrates arterial phase hyperenhancement with portal venous and equilibrium phase washout [77]. There is usually no retention of hepatobiliary contrast agents during the hepatocyte phase.

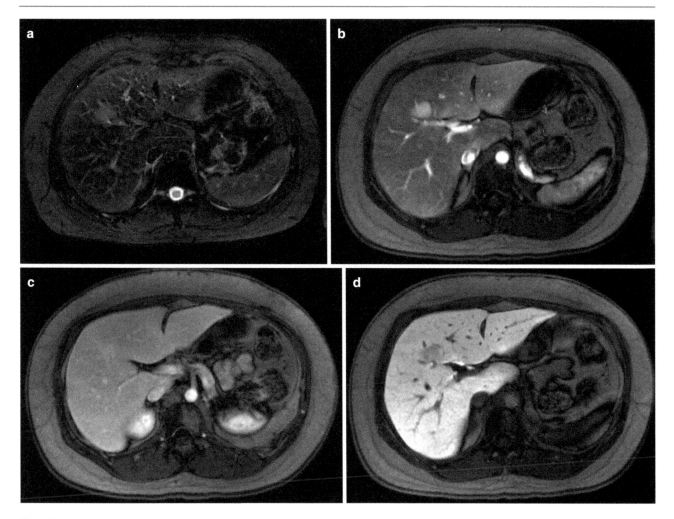

Fig. 7.31 Hepatic adenoma in an 18-year-old female on oral contraceptives. (**a**) Axial T2-weighted fat-suppressed MR image shows a hyperintense focus in the liver. (**b**) Axial enhanced T1-weighted fat-suppressed MR image acquired in the late arterial phase shows the lesion to be hyperenhancing. (**c**) Axial enhanced T1-weighted fat-suppressed MR image acquired in the portal venous shows the lesion to be isointense to mildly hyperintense. (**d**) Axial enhanced T1-weighted fat-suppressed MR image acquired in the hepatobiliary phase shows lack of contrast retention within the lesion

Table 7.3 Subtypes of hepatic adenomas

Subtype	Risk factors	Clinical features	T2WI	T1WI	T1WI in−/ out-of-phase	DWI	Post-contrast
Inflammatory	• OCPs • Obesity • Metabolic syndrome	• Highest-risk for bleeding • Elevated C-reactive protein • Leukocytosis • Fever • Chronic anemia	Hyperintense, possibly more prominent in the periphery	Hypointense	Uncommon signal loss on out-of-phase due to intralesional fat	Restriction	• Arterial phase hyperenhancement that persists on the portal venous and delayed phases • Variable retention of contrast on hepatobiliary phase
Hepatocyte nuclear factor 1α (HNF-1α) inactivated	OCPs	Most indolent	Iso- or mildly hyperintense	Hyperintense	Loss of signal on out-of-phase due to intralesional fat	No restriction	• Arterial phase hyperenhancement that does not persist on the portal venous and delayed phases • Hypointense on hepatobilliary phase
β-Catenin mutated	• Glycogen storage disease • Anabolic steroid use	Highest risk for transformation to HCC	Variable but most often hyperintense	Variable but most often hypointense	Variable	Variable	• Arterial phase hyperenhancement with variable persistence on the portal venous and delayed phases • Variable retention of contrast on hepatobiliary phase

DWI diffusion-weighted imaging, *OCPs* oral contraceptives, *HCC* hepatocellular carcinoma

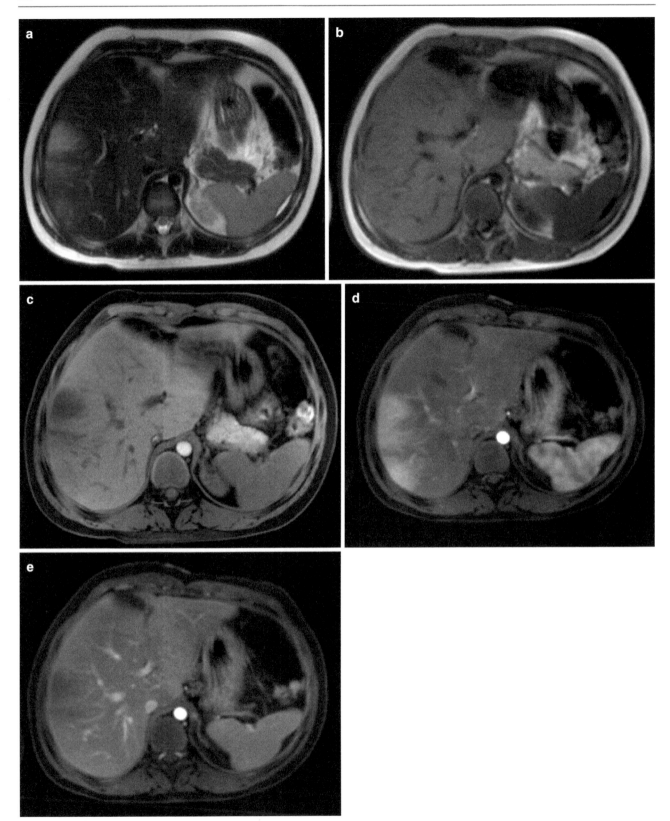

Fig. 7.32 Hepatic angiomyolipoma in a 13-year-old boy with tuberous sclerosis who presented for surveillance imaging. (**a**) Axial T2-weighted MR image shows a hyperintense lesion in the right hepatic lobe. Axial T1-weighted non-fat-suppressed (**b**) and fat-suppressed (**c**) MR images show loss of signal within the lesion on the fat-suppressed image consistent with intralesional fat. (**d**) Axial enhanced T1-weighted fat-suppressed MR image acquired in the arterial phase shows hyperenhancement of the lesion. (**e**) Axial enhanced T1-weighted fat-suppressed MR image acquired in the portal venous phase shows contrast washout

Nodular Regenerative Hyperplasia Nodular regenerative hyperplasia (NRH) is characterized by the presence of regenerative nodules surrounded by atrophied and non-fibrotic liver. It can occur in patients of any age and has been reported in children [78, 79]. The etiology is unknown but may reflect compensatory hyperplasia adjacent to areas of atrophy that result from decreased blood flow. Associated conditions include hematologic disorders, autoimmune disorders, collagen vascular disease, and Budd-Chiari syndrome [68]. NRH may be asymptomatic or can cause portal hypertension.

MR imaging features of NRH are variable. Nodules are most commonly mildly hyperintense on T1-weighted imaging with variable signal on T2-weighted images. A T2-weighted hyperintense rim can be present. T1-weighted chemical shift sequences may demonstrate the presence of lipid within the nodule. Contrast enhancement tends to follow the normal hepatic parenchyma (Fig. 7.33) [68].

Malignant Hepatic Neoplasms

Hepatoblastoma Hepatoblastoma is the most common primary malignant liver tumor in the pediatric population. Approximately 68% of cases are diagnosed prior to 2 years of age, and 90% are diagnosed prior to 5 years of age [70, 80]. There is a male-to-female ratio of 2:1. Hepatoblastomas are associated with Beckwith-Wiedemann syndrome, familial adenomatous polyposis, trisomy 18, Gardner syndrome, fetal alcohol syndrome, and type IA glycogen storage diseases [81]. There is also an association with prematurity and low birth weight [71]. There are two main histological types, epithelial and mixed epithelial, which have different imaging features. Serum alpha fetoprotein (AFP) levels are usually elevated.

On imaging, hepatoblastomas are usually well-defined masses that can be singular or multifocal. However, they can also appear as diffusely infiltrative lesions. Focal lesions are more commonly located in the right hepatic lobe [81]. Epithelial hepatoblastomas are most commonly homogeneously T1-weighted hypointense and T2-weighted hyperintense. Mixed tumors have more heterogeneous signal due to calcification, hemorrhage, fibrotic septa, and necrosis. Both types demonstrate heterogeneous contrast enhancement including washout compared with normal parenchyma on venous or equilibrium phase imaging (Fig. 7.34) [71, 82].

Vascular invasion from hepatoblastoma can be present, more commonly affecting the portal vein than the hepatic veins. Distant metastases are present in less than 10% of cases, most commonly involving the lungs [71]. The

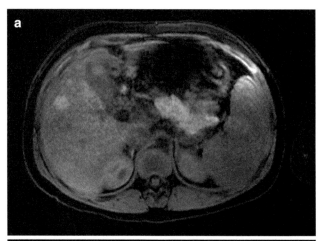

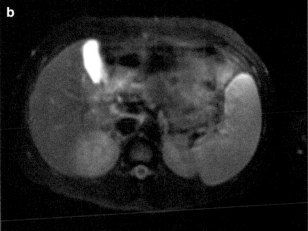

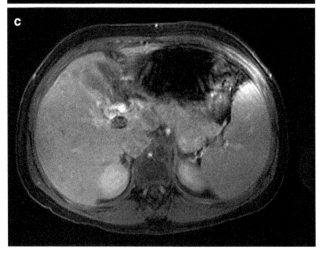

Fig. 7.33 Nodular regenerative hyperplasia in an 11-year-old boy with Budd-Chiari syndrome who presented for surveillance imaging. (**a**) Axial T1-weighted fat-suppressed MR image shows a hyperintense mass in the right hepatic lobe. (**b**) Axial non-enhanced T2-weighted fat-suppressed MR image shows isointensity of the lesion to surrounding liver. (**c**) Axial enhanced T1-weighted fat-suppressed MR image shows similar enhancement of the lesion compared to the background hepatic parenchyma

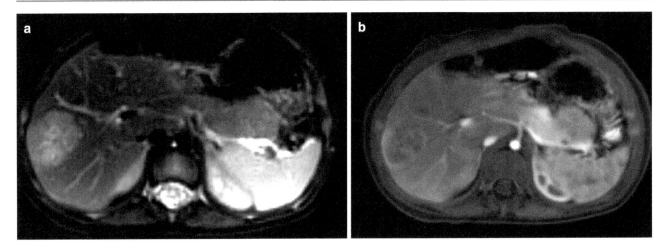

Fig. 7.34 Hepatoblastoma in an 11-month-old girl with Beckwith-Wiedemann syndrome who presented for surveillance imaging. (a) Axial T2-weighted fat-suppressed MR image demonstrates a heteroge-neously T2-weighted hyperintense mass in the right hepatic lobe. (b) Axial enhanced T1-weighted fat-suppressed MR image shows hetero-geneous enhancement of the mass

PRETEXT classification system is commonly used in the staging of hepatoblastoma based on imaging. PRETEXT staging has been shown to predict overall survival in patients with hepatoblastoma and can be helpful in treatment planning [83]. In PRETEXT, the liver is divided into four sections: left lateral (segments II/III), left medial (IVa/IVb), right anterior (V/VIII), and right posterior (VI/VII). A PRETEXT group (I–IV) is assigned based on the number of sections involved by the tumor. Additional annotation factors can also be assigned to help further risk stratify based on the presence of other findings such as vascular involvement, distant metastases, and caudate lobe involvement [83].

Hepatocellular Carcinoma Hepatocellular carcinoma (HCC) is the most common primary hepatic malignancy in adolescence and the second most common primary hepatic malignancy in pediatric patients [82]. HCC most commonly occurs in patients aged 10–14 years [81]. Unlike in adults, HCC in pediatric patients does not usually occur in the setting of underlying liver disease/cirrhosis [84]. Similar to hepatoblastomas, AFP levels are commonly elevated.

On MR imaging, typical features of HCC include avid arterial phase enhancement, hypointensity to the liver parenchyma on the portal venous and equilibrium phases (washout), an enhancing fibrous pseudocapsule on portal venous and equilibrium phases, and hypointensity on the hepatobiliary phase [85] (Fig. 7.35 and see Fig. 7.28). HCC is usually slightly T2-weighted hyperintense and T1-weighted hypoin-

tense. Heterogeneity may be present due to the presence of hemorrhage, fat, calcification, and necrosis. HCC has a propensity for vascular invasion, occurring in approximately 75% of cases [71]. Metastases are most common to the lung, brain, and bones.

Fibrolamellar Carcinoma Fibrolamellar carcinoma (FLC) is a variant of HCC that occurs in young adults and adolescents with 85% of affected patients diagnosed prior to 35 years of age [71]. FLC can occur in children as young as 10 years [86]. Affected patients typically do not have underlying liver disease. Outcomes are similar between HCC and FLC in patients without underlying liver disease [86, 87].

MR imaging typically demonstrates a large well-defined hepatic mass that is T1-weighted hypo- to isointense and T2-weighted hyperintense. There is avid heterogeneous enhancement on the arterial phase with washout on the portal venous and equilibrium phases [81]. FLC appears hypointense on the hepatobiliary phase, which distinguishes it from FNH. A fibrous central scar can be present, which is hypointense on T1-/T2-weighted imaging and does not enhance (Fig. 7.36 and see Fig. 7.28) [82].

Metastasis A number of different pediatric neoplasms can metastasize to the liver, the most common of which include neuroblastoma, Wilms tumor, and lymphoma. Hepatic metastases can present as single or multiple masses. Less often, hepatic metastasis can be diffusely infiltrative with

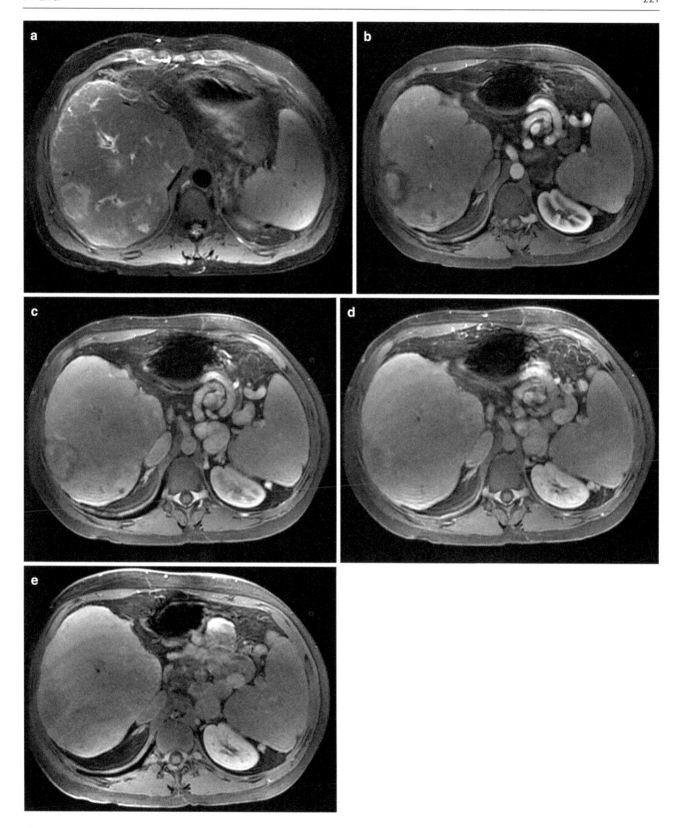

Fig. 7.35 Hepatocellular carcinoma in an 18-year-old male with biliary atresia complicated by cirrhosis. (**a**) Axial T2-weighted fat-suppressed MR image shows a heterogeneous mass in the right hepatic lobe. The liver contour is nodular, consistent with cirrhosis. (**b**) Axial enhanced T1-weighted fat-suppressed MR image obtained in the arterial phase shows hyperenhancement of the lesion. Upper abdominal varices are present. (**c**) Axial enhanced T1-weighted fat-suppressed MR image obtained in the portal venous phase shows isointensity of the lesion. (**d**) Axial enhanced T1-weighted fat-suppressed MR image obtained in the equilibrium phase shows washout and a delayed enhancing pseudocapsule. (**e**) Axial enhanced T1-weighted fat-suppressed MR image obtained in the hepatobiliary phase shows a lack of contrast retention in the lesion

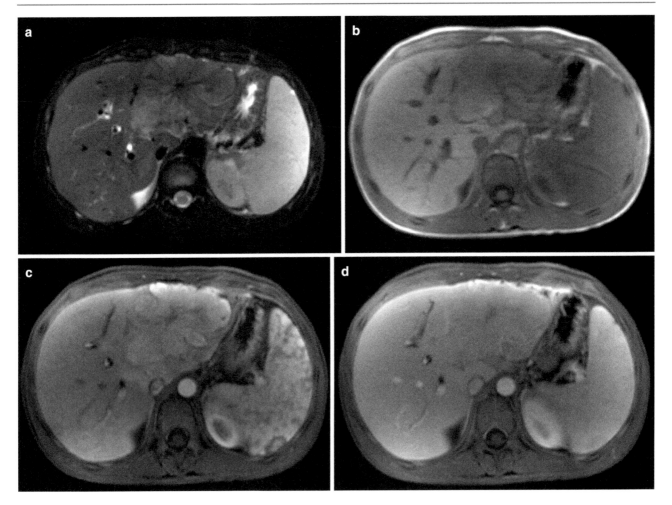

Fig. 7.36 Fibrolamellar carcinoma in a 14-year-old boy who presented with abdominal pain. (**a**) Axial T2-weighted fat-suppressed MR image shows a hyperintense mass in the left hepatic lobe with a radiating central hypointense fibrotic scar. (**b**) Axial T1-weighted fat-suppressed MR image shows a slightly hypointense mass in the left hepatic lobe with a radiating central hypointense fibrotic scar. (**c**) Axial enhanced T1-weighted fat-suppressed MR image obtained in the arterial phase shows a hyperenhancing mass in the left hepatic lobe. The central scar is non-enhancing. (**d**) Axial enhanced T1-weighted fat-suppressed MR image obtained in the portal venous phase shows an iso-enhancing mass in the left hepatic lobe. The central scar remains non-enhancing

hepatomegaly and architectural distortion, most commonly with neuroblastoma [71].

MR imaging features of hepatic metastasis are variable depending on the primary malignancy (Figs. 7.37 and 7.38, and see Fig. 7.28), but metastases tend to be T1-weighted hypointense and T2-weighted hyperintense. They may demonstrate restricted diffusion. Hypervascular hepatic metastases can be hyperenhancing on arterial phase images with isointensity or hypointensity on portal venous and equilibrium phase images. Meanwhile, hypovascular metastases may be most conspicuous on portal venous phase images where they are hypointense to surrounding hepatic parenchyma. Hypovascular metastases can also demonstrate a thin rim of hyperenhancement on post-contrast images. Metastases are typically hypointense compared with normal liver on the hepatobiliary phase [8].

Hepatic lymphoma is usually secondary as primary hepatic lymphoma is rare. Both Hodgkin and non-Hodgkin lymphomas involve the liver in more than half of patients [71]. Hepatic lymphomas can be solitary, multifocal, or diffusely infiltrative. MR imaging features are variable, with lesions more likely to demonstrate low signal intensity on T2-weighted images compared with other malignancies. Restricted diffusion can be present. Enhancement characteristics of hepatic lymphoma are variable, but some solid lesion enhancement should be present [88] (Fig. 7.39). The presence of lymphadenopathy and splenic lesions can help raise suspicion for this etiology.

Undifferentiated Embryonal Sarcoma Undifferentiated embryonal sarcoma (UES) is the third most common pri-

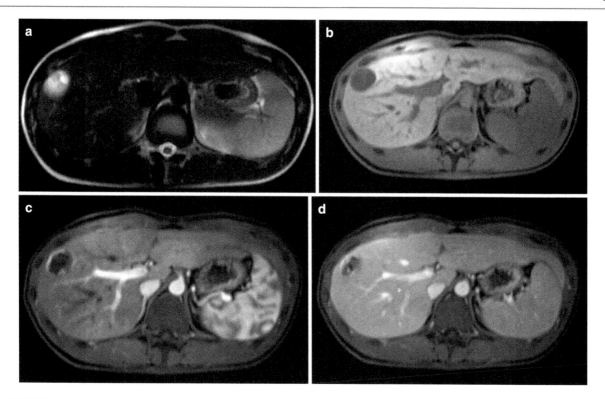

Fig. 7.37 Hepatic metastasis in an 18-year-old male with testicular rhabdomyosarcoma. (a) Axial T2-weighted fat-suppressed MR image shows a hyperintense lesion in the right hepatic lobe. (b) Axial T1-weighted fat-suppressed MR image shows the lesion is hypointense. (c) Axial enhanced T1-weighted fat-suppressed MR image acquired during the late arterial phase demonstrates lesional rim enhancement. (d) Axial enhanced T1-weighted fat-suppressed MR image demonstrates persistent rim enhancement on the portal venous phase with central hypointensity. A biopsy confirmed a hepatic metastasis

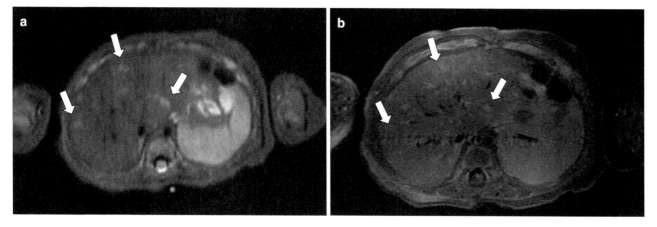

Fig. 7.38 Hepatic metastases in a 4-month-old boy with neuroblastoma. (a) Axial STIR MR image shows multiple hyperintense lesions (*arrows*) in the liver. (b) Axial enhanced T1-weighted fat-suppressed MR image shows mild lesion hyperenhancement (*arrows*)

mary malignant tumor in children [71]. It most commonly affects children between 6 and 10 years of age [81]. AFP levels are usually normal.

It is an aggressive tumor that is usually large and solitary at diagnosis. On MR imaging, UES is usually hypointense on T1-weighted images and hyperintense on T2-weighted images. Hemorrhage, necrosis, cystic change, and fluid-fluid levels can be present, resulting in heterogeneity [81]. Calcification is uncommon. A pseudocapsule can be present, which is T1−/T2-weighted

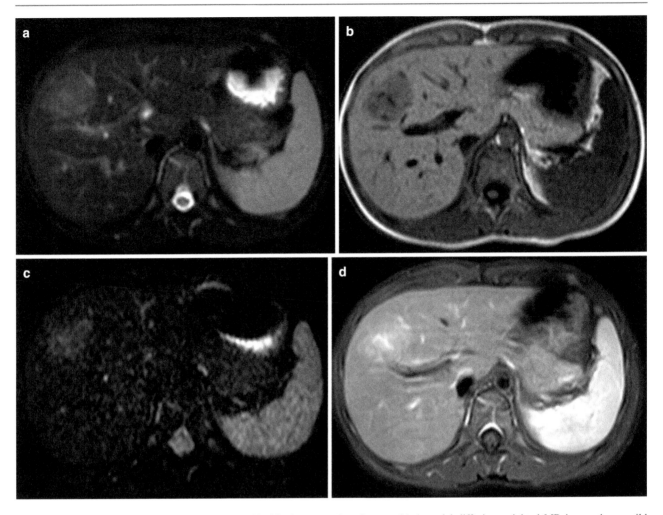

Fig. 7.39 Primary hepatic lymphoma in a 6-year-old girl who pre-sented with abdominal pain. (a) Axial T2-weighted fat-suppressed MR image shows a heterogeneous mildly hyperintense mass in the right hepatic lobe. (b) Axial T1-weighted MR image shows the mass to be hypointense. (c) An axial diffusion-weighted MR image shows mild restricted diffusion within the mass. (d) An axial enhanced T1-weighted fat-suppressed MR image shows mild hyperenhancement. Biopsy con-firmed the diagnosis of primary hepatic lymphoma

hypointense. There is usually heterogeneous enhancement [89, 90] (Fig. 7.40).

Rhabdomyosarcoma Embryonal rhabdomyosarcomas are rare, highly aggressive tumors within the liver that arise from the biliary tree. They occur most commonly in patients under the age of 5 years [81]. The most common clinical presenta-tion is cholestasis, and AFP levels are usually normal. Metastatic disease can be present at diagnosis in up to 30% of cases [81], most commonly to the liver, pericardium, and bones. These tumors most commonly arise as polypoid-like projections into the lumen of the common bile duct. However, they can also originate from the intrahepatic biliary ducts, cys-tic duct, or gallbladder.

MR imaging can demonstrate a T1-weighted hypointense and T2-weighted hyperintense intraductal mass that has het-erogeneous enhancement (Fig. 7.41). Intralesional cysts can be present. MRCP can help further delineate the intraductal mass or may demonstrate a mass adjacent to the bile ducts with biliary duct mural irregularity [81].

Vascular Hepatic Disorders

Budd-Chiari Syndrome Budd-Chiari syndrome (BCS) is caused by post-sinusoidal hepatic venous outflow obstruc-tion, which can occur at the level of the small hepatic veins to the most superior aspect of the inferior vena cava. The result is severe hepatic congestion, ascites, hepatic dysfunction, the development of intrahepatic and extrahepatic collaterals, and portal hypertension. Primary causes include caval webs, thrombosis due to hypercoagulable states, vessel wall fibro-sis, and liver transplantation. Secondary BCS can be caused by external compression or venous tumor invasion [91–93].

In acute BCS (less than 4 weeks), there is hepatomegaly. T2-weighted sequences show heterogeneously increased sig-nal in the hepatic periphery. On T1-weighted fat-suppressed post-contrast images, there is heterogeneous enhancement. A characteristic finding of acute BCS is relative hypoen-hancement of the hepatic periphery with relative hyperen-hancement of the caudate lobe on the late arterial phase [94]. The arterial phase hyperenhancement of the caudate lobe is

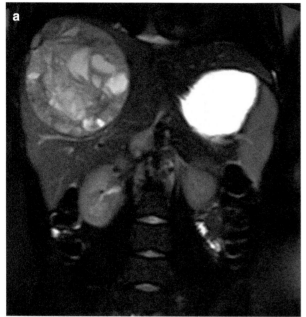

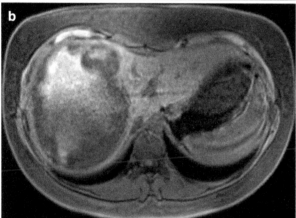

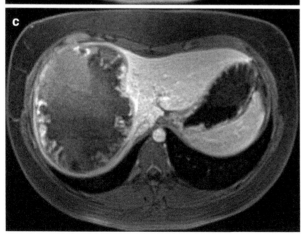

Fig. 7.40 Undifferentiated embryonal sarcoma of in a 15-year-old girl who presented with a palpable abdominal mass and pain. (**a**) Coronal T2-weighted fat-suppressed MR image shows a heterogeneous large mass in the right hepatic lobe with cystic change and hemorrhage. (**b**) Axial T1-weighted fat-suppressed MR image shows central hyperintensity within the mass consistent with hemorrhage. There is a peripheral pseudocapsule. (**c**) An axial enhanced T1-weighted fat-suppressed MR image shows heterogeneous and predominantly peripheral enhancement of the mass

a result of its independent venous drainage to the inferior vena cava (Fig. 7.42). The occluded hepatic veins or inferior vena cava is not visualized or shows lack of opacification on post-contrast images. In chronic BCS, there can be hepatic fibrosis and hypertrophy of the caudate lobe. Enhancement patterns are more variable, and the differences seen in the acute phase are usually less prominent [94]. Large intrahepatic and extrahepatic collaterals, splenomegaly, regenerative nodules, and ascites may be evident.

Hepatic Veno-occlusive Disease Hepatic veno-occlusive disease is a severe toxin-induced obstructive hepatic vascular disorder that predominantly affects the sinusoids. It most commonly occurs following myeloablative procedures for hematopoietic stem cell transplants, usually within 40 days of the procedure [95]. MR imaging features are non-specific but can include hepatomegaly, heterogeneous parenchymal signal intensity, and heterogeneous enhancement. Periportal edema may be present as periportal T2-weighted hyperintensity [96, 97]. Gallbladder wall thickening, ascites, and pleural effusions may also be present. Collateral vessels may be identified as rounded foci of enhancement in the portal venous and delayed phases.

Portal Hypertension Portal hypertension is defined by an increase in portal venous pressures by 10 mm Hg or more. Obstructive etiologies are generally classified into pre-sinusoidal, sinusoidal, and post-sinusoidal categories. Portal hypertension can also result from increased inflow pressures (Table 7.4) [95, 98]. Complications can include ascites, gastrointestinal bleeding, and spontaneous bacterial peritonitis.

MR imaging findings of portal hypertension include splenomegaly and ascites (see Fig. 7.25). The portal vein may become abnormally enlarged or narrowed. A variety of different portosystemic collateral draining veins may become apparent, including paraumbilical, gastric, peri-splenic, retroperitoneal, and esophageal varices [99]. Cavernous transformation of the portal vein results from the development of portoportal collaterals in the setting of thrombosis or stenosis of the portal vein (Fig. 7.43). On MR imaging, it manifests as numerous tortuous venous channels at the liver hilum and along a variable extent of the intrahepatic portal venous course [99]. Portal gastropathy, enteropathy, and colopathy may appear as abnormal thickening of the stomach, small bowel, or colon. The ascending colon is most commonly involved. There can also be gallbladder wall thickening. MR imaging may demonstrate the underlying etiology of portal hypertension, such as venous thrombosis or cirrhosis.

Liver Transplantation

Liver transplantation in pediatric patients accounts for approximately 8% of all liver transplantations in the United States

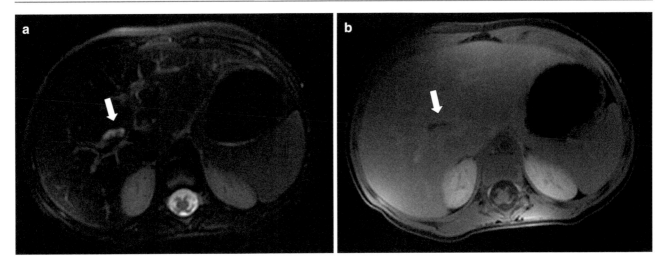

Fig. 7.41 Biliary rhabdomyosarcoma in a 3-year-old girl who presented with jaundice. (**a**) Axial T2-weighted, fat-suppressed MR image shows focal dilation of the right common intrahepatic bile duct with a partial filling defect (*arrow*). (**b**) Axial enhanced T1-weighted fat-suppressed MR image acquired in the equilibrium phase shows the filling defect (*arrow*) which has intrinsic enhancement

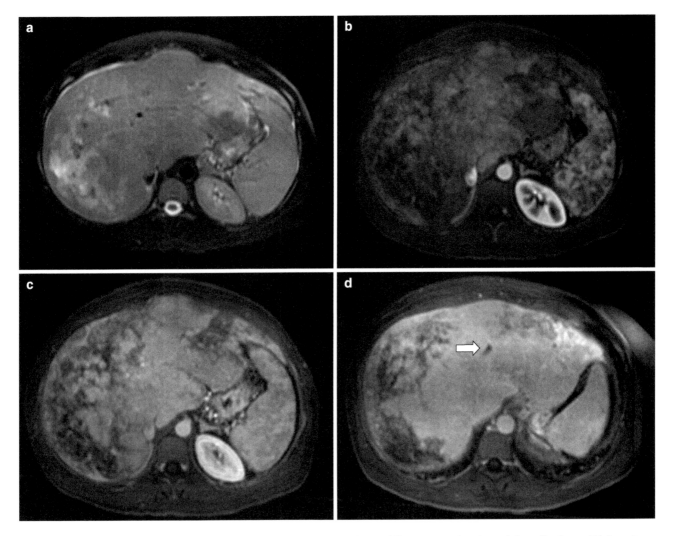

Fig. 7.42 Budd-Chiari syndrome in an 18-year-old female with polycythemia vera who presented with abdominal pain. (**a**) T2-weighted fat-suppressed MR image shows patchy peripheral hyperintensity and caudate lobe enlargement. Axial enhanced T1-weighted fat-suppressed MR images obtained in the arterial (**b**), portal venous (**c**), and equilibrium (**d**) phases show relative hyperenhancement of the caudate lobe and central liver compared to the periphery. On the equilibrium phase, there is non-enhancement of the hepatic veins (*arrow*) suggestive of thrombus. (**e**) An axial enhanced T1-weighted fat-suppressed MR image obtained at 4 minutes show subtle relative hypoenhancement of the caudate lobe relative to the liver periphery

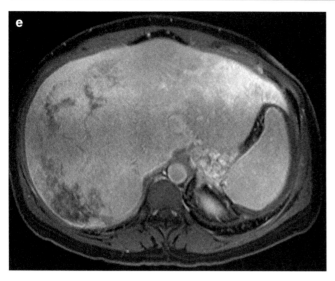

Fig. 7.42 (continued)

Table 7.4 Causes of portal hypertension in children

Pre-sinusoidal	Extrahepatic portal vein thrombosis or occlusion (e.g., tumor infiltration)
	Splenic vein occlusion
	Portal vein stenosis or thrombosis post-transplantation
	Schistosomiasis
	Cystic fibrosis-related liver disease
Sinusoidal	Biliary atresia
	Cirrhosis
	Hepatitis
	Sclerosing cholangitis
	Cystic fibrosis-related liver disease
	Nonalcoholic fatty liver disease
	Congenital hepatic fibrosis
	Caroli disease
Post-sinusoidal	Budd-Chiari syndrome
	Congestive heart failure
	Veno-occlusive disease
Increased portal venous blood flow	Hepatic arterial to portal vein fistulae
	Pulmonary sequestration with portal venous drainage
	Total anomalous pulmonary venous return to the portal system
Idiopathic	

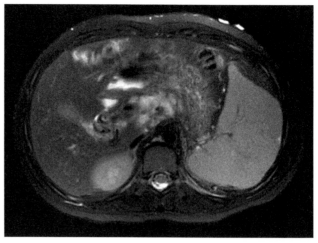

Fig. 7.43 Cavernous transformation of the portal vein in an 8-year-old girl with idiopathic portal hypertension who presented following hematemesis. Axial T2-weighted fat-suppressed MR image shows multiple collateral vessels within the porta hepatis. The portal vein and splenic vein were not visualized suggestive of portal vein and splenic vein thrombosis. There is also splenomegaly

extent of liver disease and its sequelae, and identifying any possible contraindications to transplant surgery [102].

Important anatomic details for surgical planning include the patency, caliber, and any variance to the typical configuration of the hepatic vasculature and inferior vena cava. Delineation of visceral and biliary system anatomy is also useful. Absolute contraindications to liver transplant include (1) unresectable extrahepatic malignancy, (2) rapid progression of hepatocellular carcinoma, and (3) severe portopulmonary hypertension not responsive to therapy. Malignant invasion of venous structures is a relative contraindication [100].

Ultrasound is the first-line imaging modality in preoperative transplant assessment. MR imaging can serve as a useful problem-solving tool for evaluating the hepatic vasculature and the extent of hepatic disease. MR imaging can be particularly useful in assessing the biliary system with MRCP and the use of hepatobiliary contrast agents [101]. In liver transplant donors, MR imaging can be useful for assessing hepatic iron and fat content as well as delineating biliary anatomy.

[100]. Common indications include cholestatic disease (such as biliary atresia), metabolic and genetic disorders, fulminant liver failure, and malignancies [101]. A full discussion of the technical considerations related to the liver transplant surgery in pediatric patients is beyond the scope of this text. However, liver transplants may involve an entire cadaveric liver, split adult cadaveric grafting, or living-donor transplant.

Preoperative Assessment Preoperative imaging assessment in the transplant recipient is aimed at evaluating anatomic features that are important for surgical planning, evaluating the

Postoperative Complications Approximately 40% of pediatric transplant recipients develop postoperative complications [103]. Early diagnosis of these complications is important for graft and patient survival [101]. Complications may be related to the graft vasculature, biliary system, peri-graft fluid collections, infection, rejection, and post-transplantation lymphoproliferative disease.

Hepatic artery complications include thrombosis, stenosis, aneurysms or pseudoaneurysms, and arteriovenous fistulas. Hepatic artery thrombosis is the most common vascular complication, occurring in up to 26% of cases [104]. Biliary ischemia can also develop, leading to biliary leaks and stric-

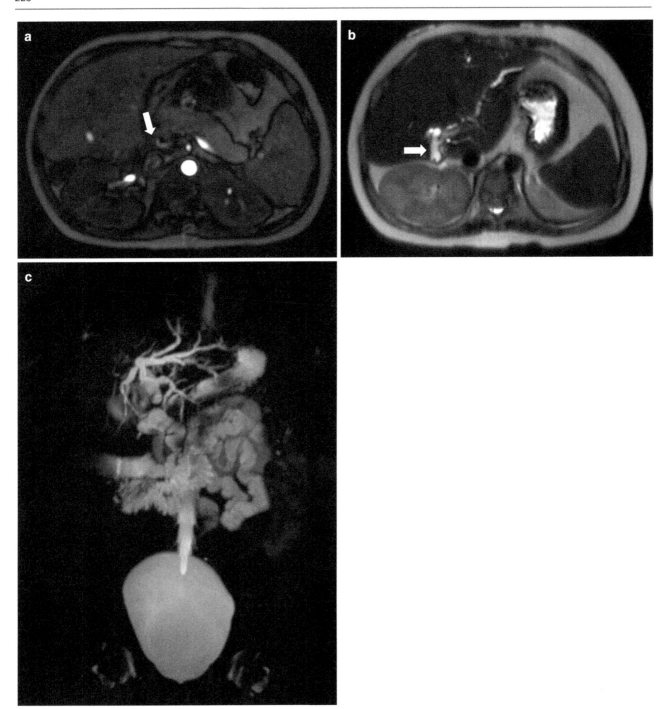

Fig. 7.44 Hepatic artery stenosis and biliary stenosis in a 4-year-old girl status post liver transplant. (**a**) Axial time-of-flight (TOF) MR angiogram shows the extrahepatic artery which is not well seen distal to the segment marked by the *arrow*, suggestive of a long segment of hepatic artery stenosis. (**b**) Axial T2-weighted MR image shows dila- tion of several bile ducts. There is an intraluminal filling defect within the common bile duct at the hepaticojejunal anastomosis (*arrow*). An ERCP showed fibrotic stenosis at this site. (**c**) MRCP image shows intrahepatic biliary ductal dilation

tures. Hepatic artery stenosis most commonly occurs at the anastomosis and is usually diagnosed within the first 100 days of the procedure [101]. Ultrasound is the main imaging modality used to evaluate for hepatic artery compli- cations. In inconclusive cases, further evaluation with mag- netic resonance angiography (MRA) can be useful in further delineating hepatic artery patency, caliber, and associated complications (Fig. 7.44).

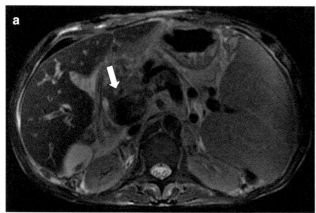

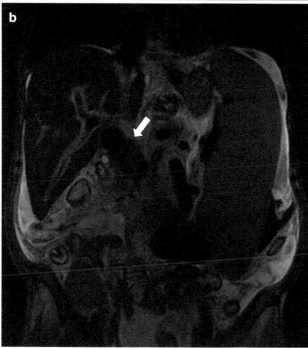

Fig. 7.45 Portal vein thrombosis in a 17-year-old girl status post liver transplant who presented with worsening ascites. Axial (**a**) and coronal (**b**) T2-weighted fat-suppressed MR images show a mildly hyperintense filling defect (*arrows*) in a dilated portal vein. There is associated splenomegaly, ascites, and upper abdominal varices consistent with portal hypertension

Portal vein complications include thrombosis and stenosis. Portal vein thrombus most commonly occurs in the first month following transplant [101] (Fig. 7.45). Portal vein stenosis usually occurs at the anastomosis or in extension grafts. Clinical manifestations can include portal hypertension and hepatic failure. Chronic thrombosis or stenosis may lead to the development of collateral vessels (cavernous transformation) [102]. These findings can be well demonstrated on MR/MRA if ultrasound findings are indeterminate [102].

Complications related to the hepatic veins and inferior vena cava occur less frequently [105] and may also manifest as thrombosis or stenosis. Stenosis and thrombosis are most common at surgical anastomoses. Piggyback anastomoses are more susceptible to hemorrhage and Budd-Chiari syndrome due to inadequate drainage [101]. Focal narrowing, luminal thrombus, and post-stenotic dilation are well demonstrated on MR/MRA [106, 107].

Biliary complications are the second most common cause of graft dysfunction [104]. Early biliary complications are usually related to technical surgical issues, while later biliary complications are usually related to hepatic ischemia [102]. Specific complications can include biliary strictures at anastomotic or non-anastomotic sites. Bile leaks, biliary stones, and cast syndrome can also develop. Cast syndrome occurs when hardened material containing bilirubin fills the biliary tree causing obstruction [108, 109]. Chronic rejection can also cause loss of bile ducts and mild chronic dilation [102]. MRCP can be helpful in assessing the biliary tree for strictures and obstruction (see Fig. 7.44). Cast syndrome appears as T2-weighted hypointense material within the biliary ducts on MRCP images, which is also hyperintense on T1-weighted images.

Rejection is the most common cause of graft failure, most often occurring within the first year [101]. However, imaging findings of rejection are non-specific, and the main utility of imaging is to exclude other causes of graft injury.

Peri-graft fluid collections and ascites are common in the first few weeks post-transplant. Most are transient and may reflect seromas, hematomas, or bilomas. Differentiating between these collections is not always possible on imaging. More concerning fluid collections can include abscesses, biliary leaks, hematomas with active hemorrhage, and collections related to bowel perforation. MR imaging with hepatobiliary agents and MRCP are particularly useful for evaluating biliary leaks (Fig. 7.46).

Finally, post-transplantation lymphoproliferative disease (PTLD) more commonly occurs in children post-transplant than adults [110]. PTLD is a collection of lymphoid proliferation abnormalities ranging from polyclonal B cell proliferation to monoclonal B cell lymphoma. The majority of pediatric cases are associated with Epstein-Barr virus [102]. The average time to development is approximately 8 months [111]. A periportal mass and mesenteric lymphadenopathy are common [101]. MR imaging features are similar to those for lymphoma [112] (Fig. 7.47).

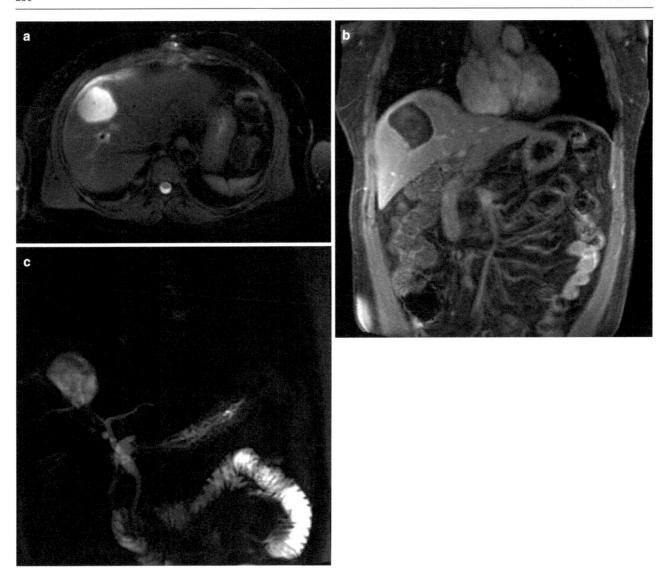

Fig. 7.46 Biloma in a 17-year-old boy status post liver transplant with an abnormal ultrasound study. (**a**) Axial T2-weighted fat-suppressed MR image shows a fluid collection in the right hepatic lobe. (**b**) Coronal enhanced T1-weighted fat-suppressed MR image shows mild rim enhancement to the collection. (**c**) Coronal non-enhanced MRCP image shows connection of the fluid collection to the right intrahepatic bile duct suggestive of a biloma. An ERCP confirmed the presence of a biloma

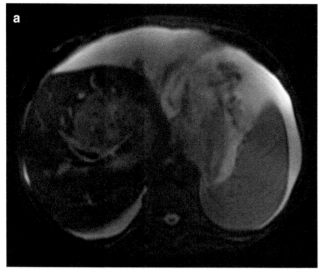

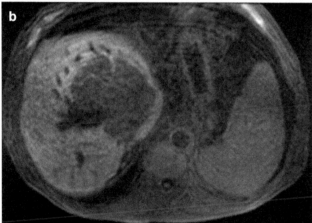

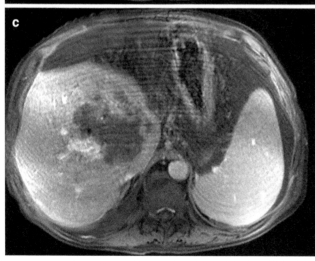

Fig. 7.47 Post-transplant lymphoproliferative disease in a 16-year-old boy status post liver transplant. (**a**) Axial T2-weighted fat-suppressed MR image shows a mildly hyperintense mass within the liver. There is ascites. (**b**) Axial T1-weighted fat-suppressed MR image shows the mass is hypointense. (**c**) Axial enhanced T1-weighted fat-suppressed MR image shows mild heterogeneous enhancement of the mass. Biopsy confirmed this mass to be post-transplant lymphoproliferative disease

Conclusions

MR imaging can play an important role in the diagnosis and surveillance of a variety of congenital and acquired hepatic pathological conditions in the pediatric population. Particularly useful tools include multiphase post-contrast imaging, MR elastography, and fat and iron detection and quantitation. Clear knowledge of up-to-date MR imaging techniques and characteristic MR imaging findings is essential for accurate imaging diagnosis and optimal pediatric patient management.

References

1. Gandhi SN, Brown MA, Wong JG, Aguirre DA, Sirlin CB. MR contrast agents for liver imaging: what, when, how. Radiographics. 2006;26(6):1621–36.
2. Gale EM, Caravan P, Rao AG, McDonald RJ, Winfeld M, Fleck RJ, et al. Gadolinium-based contrast agents in pediatric magnetic resonance imaging. Pediatr Radiol. 2017;47(5):507–21.
3. Kuwatsuru R, Kadoya M, Ohtomo K, Tanimoto A, Hirohashi S, Murakami T, et al. Comparison of gadobenate dimeglumine with gadopentetate dimeglumine for magnetic resonance imaging of liver tumors. Investig Radiol. 2001;36(11):632–41.
4. Huppertz A, Haraida S, Kraus A, Zech CJ, Scheidler J, Breuer J, et al. Enhancement of focal liver lesions at gadoxetic acid–enhanced MR imaging: correlation with histopathologic findings and spiral CT--initial observations. Radiology. 2005;234(2):468–78.
5. Grazioli L, Morana G, Kirchin MA, Schneider G. Accurate differentiation of focal nodular hyperplasia from hepatic adenoma at gadobenate dimeglumine–enhanced MR imaging: prospective study. Radiology. 2005;236(1):166–77.
6. Grazioli L, Bondioni MP, Haradome H, Motosugi U, Tinti R, Frittoli B, et al. Hepatocellular adenoma and focal nodular hyperplasia: value of gadoxetic acid–enhanced MR imaging in differential diagnosis. Radiology. 2012;262(2):520–9.
7. Chavhan GB, Mann E, Kamath BM, Babyn PS. Gadobenate-dimeglumine-enhanced magnetic resonance imaging for hepatic lesions in children. Pediatr Radiol. 2014;44(10):1266–74.
8. Meyers AB, Towbin AJ, Serai S, Geller JI, Podbersky DJ. Characterization of pediatric liver lesions with gadoxetate disodium. Pediatr Radiol. 2011;41(9):1183–97.
9. Rozenfeld MN, Podbersky DJ. Gadolinium-based contrast agents in children. Pediatr Radiol. 2018;48(9):1188–96.
10. Schneider G, Schürholz H, Kirchin MA, Bücker A, Fries P. Safety and adverse effects during 24 hours after contrast-enhanced MRI with gadobenate dimeglumine (MultiHance) in children. Pediatr Radiol. 2013;43(2):202–11.
11. Ma X, Holalkere N-S, R AK, Mino-Kenudson M, Hahn PF, Sahani DV. Imaging-based quantification of hepatic fat: methods and clinical applications. Radiographics. 2009;29(5):1253–77.
12. Dixon WT. Simple proton spectroscopic imaging. Radiology. 1984;153(1):189–94.
13. Glover GH. Multipoint Dixon technique for water and fat proton and susceptibility imaging. J Magn Reson Imaging. 1991;1(5):521–30.
14. Idilman IS, Aniktar H, Idilman R, Kabacam G, Savas B, Elhan A, et al. Hepatic steatosis: quantification by proton density fat fraction with MR imaging versus liver biopsy. Radiology. 2013;267(3):767–75.

15. Reeder SB, Cruite I, Hamilton G, Sirlin CB. Quantitative assessment of liver fat with magnetic resonance imaging and spectroscopy. J Magn Reson Imaging. 2011;34(4):729–49.

16. Bley TA, Wieben O, François CJ, Brittain JH, Reeder SB. Fat and water magnetic resonance imaging. J Magn Reson Imaging. 2010;31(1):4–18.

17. Hernando D, Levin YS, Sirlin CB, Reeder SB. Quantification of liver iron with MRI: state of the art and remaining challenges. J Magn Reson Imaging. 2014;40(5):1003–21.

18. Sharma SD, Artz NS, Hernando D, Horng DE, Reeder SB. Improving chemical shift encoded water-fat separation using object-based information of the magnetic field inhomogeneity. Magn Reson Med. 2015;73(2):597–604.

19. Mitchell DG, Cohen M. MRI principles. 2nd ed. Philadelphia: Elsevier; 2004.

20. Labranche R, Gilbert G, Cerny M, Vu K-N, Soulières D, Olivié D, et al. Liver iron quantification with MR imaging: a primer for radiologists. Radiographics. 2018;38(2):392–412.

21. Wood JC, Enriquez C, Ghugre N, Tyzka JM, Carson S, Nelson MD, et al. MRI R2 and R2* mapping accurately estimates hepatic iron concentration in transfusion-dependent thalassemia and sickle cell disease patients. Blood. 2005;106(4):1460–5.

22. Serai SD, Fleck RJ, Quinn CT, Zhang B, Podberesky DJ. Retrospective comparison of gradient recalled echo R2* and spin-echo R2 magnetic resonance analysis methods for estimating liver iron content in children and adolescents. Pediatr Radiol. 2015;45(11):1629–34.

23. Srinivasa Babu A, Wells ML, Teytelboym OM, Mackey JE, Miller FH, Yeh BM, et al. Elastography in chronic liver disease: modalities, techniques, limitations, and future directions. Radiographics. 2016;36(7):1987–2006.

24. Venkatesh SK, Yin M, Ehman RL. Magnetic resonance elastography of liver: technique, analysis, and clinical applications. J Magn Reson Imaging. 2013;37(3):544–55.

25. Singh S, Venkatesh SK, Wang Z, Miller FH, Motosugi U, Low RN, et al. Diagnostic performance of magnetic resonance elastography in staging liver fibrosis: a systematic review and meta-analysis of individual participant data. Clin Gastroenterol Hepatol. 2015;13(3):440–51.

26. Pipe JG. Motion correction with PROPELLER MRI: application to head motion and free-breathing cardiac imaging. Magn Reson Med. 1999;42(5):963–9.

27. Jaimes C, Kirsch JE, Gee MS. Fast, free-breathing and motion-minimized techniques for pediatric body magnetic resonance imaging. Pediatr Radiol. 2018;48(9):1197–208.

28. Chandarana H, Block KT, Winfeld MJ, Lala SV, Mazori D, Giuffrida E, et al. Free-breathing contrast-enhanced T1-weighted gradient-echo imaging with radial k-space sampling for paediatric abdominopelvic MRI. Eur Radiol. 2014;24(2):320–6.

29. McPherson AM, Anthony EY. Embryology, anatomy, and normal findings. In: Coley BD, Dillman JR, Frush DP, Hernanz-Schulman M, Hutchison LH, Khanna G, et al., editors. Caffey's pediatric diagnostic imaging. 13th ed. Philadelphia: Elsevier; 2019. p. 751–60.

30. Parker B, Blickman JG. Accessory organs of digestion. In: Blickman JG, Parker BR, Barnes PD, editors. Pediatric radiology. 3rd ed. Philadelphia: Mosby Elsevier; 2009. p. 103–20.

31. Majno P, Mentha G, Toso C, Morel P, Peitgen HO, Fasel JHD. Anatomy of the liver: an outline with three levels of complexity—a further step towards tailored territorial liver resections. J Hepatol. 2014;60(3):654–62.

32. Chavhan GB, Shelmerdine S, Jhaveri K, Babyn PS. Liver MR imaging in children: current concepts and technique. Radiographics. 2016;36(5):1517–32.

33. Piñeiro-Carrero VM, Piñeiro EO. Liver. Pediatrics. 2004;113(4 Suppl):1097–106.

34. Yano K, Ohtsubo M, Mizota T, Kato H, Hayashida Y, Morita S, et al. Riedel's lobe of the liver evaluated by multiple imaging modalities. Intern Med. 2000;39(2):136–8.

35. Chen Y-Y, Huang T-W, Chang H, Hsu H-H, Lee S-C. Intrathoracic caudate lobe of the liver: a case report and literature review. World J Gastroenterol. 2014;20(17):5147–52.

36. Chavhan GB. Congenital hepatobiliary anomalies. In: Coley BD, Dillman JR, Frush DP, Hernanz-Schulman M, Hutchison LH, Khanna G, et al., editors. Caffey's pediatric diagnostic imaging. 13th ed. Philadelphia: Elsevier; 2019. p. 810–5.

37. Subramaniam P, Knisely A, Portmann B, Qureshi S, Aclimandos W, Karani J, et al. Diagnosis of Alagille syndrome—25 years of experience at King's College Hospital. J Pediatr Gastroenterol Nutr. 2011;52(1):84–9.

38. Han S, Jeon TY, Hwang SM, Yoo S-Y, Choe YH, Lee S-K, et al. Imaging findings of Alagille syndrome in young infants: differentiation from biliary atresia. Br J Radiol. 2017;90(1077):20170406.

39. Venkatanarasimha N, Thomas R, Armstrong EM, Shirley JF, Fox BM, Jackson SA. Imaging features of ductal plate malformations in adults. Clin Radiol. 2011;66(11):1086–93.

40. Brancatelli G, Federle MP, Vilgrain V, Vullierme M-P, Marin D, Lagalla R. Fibropolycystic liver disease: CT and MR imaging findings. Radiographics. 2005;25(3):659–70.

41. Zeitoun D, Brancatelli G, Colombat M, Federle MP, Valla D, Wu T, et al. Congenital hepatic fibrosis: CT findings in 18 adults. Radiology. 2004;231(1):109–16.

42. Hilmes MA. Infectious causes of liver disease. In: Coley BD, Dillman JR, Frush DP, Hernanz-Schulman M, Hutchison LH, Khanna G, et al., editors. Caffey's pediatric diagnostic imaging. 13th ed. Philadelphia: Elsevier; 2019. p. 830–7.

43. Ganem D, Prince AM. Hepatitis B virus infection--natural history and clinical consequences. N Engl J Med. 2004;350(11):1118–29.

44. Hu K-Q, Tong MJ. The long-term outcomes of patients with compensated hepatitis C virus-related cirrhosis and history of parenteral exposure in the United States. Hepatology. 1999;29(4):1311–6.

45. Faria SC, Mazhar SM, Peterson MR, Shiehmorteza M, Sirlin CB. Hepatitis. In: Sahani DV, Samir AE, editors. Abdominal imaging. Maryland Heights MO: Saunders Elsevier; 2011. p. 641–53.

46. Huang CJ, Pitt HA, Lipsett PA, Osterman FA, Lillemoe KD, Cameron JL, et al. Pyogenic hepatic abscess. Changing trends over 42 years. Ann Surg. 1996;223(5):600–7.

47. Bächler P, Baladron MJ, Menias C, Beddings I, Loch R, Zalaquett E, et al. Multimodality imaging of liver infections: differential diagnosis and potential pitfalls. Radiographics. 2016;36(4):1001–23.

48. Chan JH, Tsui EY, Luk SH, Fung AS, Yuen MK, Szeto ML, et al. Diffusion-weighted MR imaging of the liver: distinguishing hepatic abscess from cystic or necrotic tumor. Abdom Imaging. 2001;26(2):161–5.

49. Semelka RC, Kelekis NL, Sallah S, Worawattanakul S, Ascher SM. Hepatosplenic fungal disease: diagnostic accuracy and spectrum of appearances on MR imaging. Am J Roentgenol. 1997;169(5):1311–6.

50. Radin D, Ralls P, Colletti P, Halls J. CT of amebic liver abscess. Am J Roentgenol. 1988;150(6):1297–301.

51. Elizondo G, Weissleder R, Stark DD, Todd LE, Compton C, Wittenberg J, et al. Amebic liver abscess: diagnosis and treatment evaluation with MR imaging. Radiology. 1987;165(3):795–800.

52. Mortelé KJ, Segatto E, Ros PR. The infected liver: radiologic-pathologic correlation. Radiographics. 2004;24(4):937–55.

53. Mazhar SM, Stein LL, Faria SC, Peterson MR, Sirlin CB. Hepatic storage disorders. In: Sahani DV, Samir AE, editors. Abdominal imaging. Maryland Heights MO: Saunders Elsevier; 2011. p. 630–40.

54. Rake J, Visser G, Labrune P, Leonard J, Ullrich K, Smit P. Glycogen storage disease type I: diagnosis, management, clinical

course and outcome. Results of the European Study on Glycogen Storage Disease Type I (ESGSD I). Eur J Pediatr. 2002;161(Suppl 1):S20–34.

55. Howell RR, Stevenson RE, Ben-Menachem Y, Phyliky RL, Berry DH. Hepatic adenomata with type 1 glycogen storage disease. JAMA. 1976;236(13):1481–4.

56. Limmer J, Fleig WE, Leupold D, Bittner R, Ditschuneit H, Berger H-G. Hepatocellular carcinoma in type I glycogen storage disease. Hepatology. 1988;8(3):531–7.

57. Grabowski GA, Andria G, Baldellou A, Campbell PE, Charrow J, Cohen IJ, et al. Pediatric non-neuronopathic Gaucher disease: presentation, diagnosis and assessment. Consensus statements. Eur J Pediatr. 2004;163(2):58–66.

58. Simpson WL, Hermann G, Balwani M. Imaging of Gaucher disease. World J Radiol. 2014;6(9):657–68.

59. Cox M, Epelman M, Podberesky DJ. Parenchymal liver disease. In: Coley BD, Dillman JR, Frush DP, Hernanz-Schulman M, Hutchison LH, Khanna G, et al., editors. Caffey's pediatric diagnostic imaging. 13th ed. Philadelphia: Elsevier; 2019. p. 822–9.

60. Morcos M, Dubois S, Bralet M-P, Belghiti J, Degott C, Terris B. Primary liver carcinoma in genetic hemochromatosis reveals a broad histologic spectrum. Am J Clin Pathol. 2001;116(5):738–43.

61. Patton HM, Mazhar SM, Peterson MR, Hanna R, Ganesan K, Sirlin CB. Hepatic iron overload. In: Sahani DV, Samir AE, editors. Abdominal imaging. Maryland Heights MO: Saunders Elsevier; 2011. p. 621–9.

62. Schwimmer JB, Behling C, Newbury R, Deutsch R, Nievergelt C, Schork NJ, et al. Histopathology of pediatric nonalcoholic fatty liver disease. Hepatology. 2005;42(3):641–9.

63. Mazhar SM, Patton HM, Scuderi RT, Yokoo T, Faria SC, Sirlin CB. Fatty liver disease. In: Sahani DV, Samir AE, editors. Abdominal imaging. Maryland Heights MO: Saunders Elsevier; 2011. p. 595–606.

64. Pinto RB, Schneider ACR, da Silveira TR. Cirrhosis in children and adolescents: an overview. World J Hepatol. 2015;7(3):392–405.

65. Hussain SM, Zondervan PE, IJzermans JNM, Schalm SW, de Man RA, Krestin GP. Benign versus malignant hepatic nodules: MR imaging findings with pathologic correlation. Radiographics. 2002;22(5):1023–36.

66. Restrepo R, Palani R, Cervantes LF, Duarte AM, Amjad I, Altman NR. Hemangiomas revisited: the useful, the unusual and the new. Pediatr Radiol. 2011;41(7):895–904.

67. Kulungowski AM, Alomari AI, Chawla A, Christison-Lagay ER, Fishman SJ. Lessons from a liver hemangioma registry: subtype classification. J Pediatr Surg. 2012;47(1):165–70.

68. Chung EM, Cube R, Lewis RB, Conran RM. From the archives of the AFIP: Pediatric liver masses: radiologic-pathologic correlation. Part 1. Benign tumors. Radiographics. 2010;30(3):801–26.

69. Kassarjian A, Zurakowski D, Dubois J, Paltiel HJ, Fishman SJ, Burrows PE. Infantile hepatic hemangiomas: clinical and imaging findings and their correlation with therapy. Am J Roentgenol. 2004;182(3):785–95.

70. Stocker JT. Hepatic tumors in children. Clin Liver Dis. 2001;5(1):259–81.

71. Dubois J, Ditchfield M. Neoplasia. In: Coley BD, Dillman JR, Frush DP, Hernanz-Schulman M, Hutchison LH, Khanna G, et al., editors. Caffey's pediatric diagnostic imaging. 13th ed. Philadelphia: Elsevier; 2019. p. 838–50.

72. Meyers RL. Tumors of the liver in children. Surg Oncol. 2007;16(3):195–203.

73. Smith EA, Salisbury S, Martin R, Towbin AJ. Incidence and etiology of new liver lesions in pediatric patients previously treated for malignancy. Am J Roentgenol. 2012;199(1):186–91.

74. Dharmana H, Saravana-Bawan S, Girgis S, Low G. Hepatocellular adenoma: imaging review of the various molecular subtypes. Clin Radiol. 2017;72(4):276–85.

75. Grazioli L, Olivetti L, Mazza G, Bondioni MP. MR imaging of hepatocellular adenomas and differential diagnosis dilemma. Int J Hepatol. 2013;2013:374170.

76. Cha I, Cartwright D, Guis M, Miller TR, Ferrell LD. Angiomyolipoma of the liver in fine-needle aspiration biopsies: its distinction from hepatocellular carcinoma. Cancer. 1999;87(1):25–30.

77. Lee SJ, Kim SY, Kim KW, Kim JH, Kim HJ, Lee MG, et al. Hepatic angiomyolipoma versus hepatocellular carcinoma in the noncirrhotic liver on gadoxetic acid–enhanced MRI: a diagnostic challenge. Am J Roentgenol. 2016;207(3):562–70.

78. Casillas C, Martí-Bonmatí L, Galant J. Pseudotumoral presentation of nodular regenerative hyperplasia of the liver: imaging in five patients including MR imaging. Eur Radiol. 1997;7(5):654–8.

79. Dachman A, Ros P, Goodman Z, Olmsted W, Ishak K. Nodular regenerative hyperplasia of the liver: clinical and radiologic observations. Am J Roentgenol. 1987;148(4):717–22.

80. Ishak KG, Goodman ZD, Stocker J. Tumors of the liver and intrahepatic bile ducts. Washington, D.C: Armed Forces Institute of Pathology; 2001.

81. Chung EM, Lattin GE, Cube R, Lewis RB, Marichal-Hernández C, Shawhan R, et al. From the archives of the AFIP: Pediatric liver masses: radiologic-pathologic correlation. Part 2. Malignant tumors. Radiographics. 2011;31(2):483–507.

82. Shelmerdine SC, Roebuck DJ, Towbin AJ, McHugh K. MRI of paediatric liver tumours: how we review and report. Cancer Imaging. 2016;16(1):21.

83. Towbin AJ, Meyers RL, Woodley H, Miyazaki O, Weldon CB, Morland B, et al. 2017 PRETEXT: radiologic staging system for primary hepatic malignancies of childhood revised for the Paediatric Hepatic International Tumour Trial (PHITT). Pediatr Radiol. 2018;48(4):536–54.

84. Siegel MJ, Chung EM, Conran RM. Pediatric liver: focal masses. Magn Reson Imaging Clin N Am. 2008;16(3):437–52.

85. Cruite I, Schroeder M, Merkle EM, Sirlin CB. Gadoxetate disodium–enhanced MRI of the liver: part 2. Protocol optimization and lesion appearance in the cirrhotic liver. Am J Roentgenol. 2010;195(1):29–41.

86. Torbenson M. Review of the clinicopathologic features of fibrolamellar carcinoma. Adv Anat Pathol. 2007;14(3):217–23.

87. Liu S, Chan KW, Wang B, Qiao L. Fibrolamellar hepatocellular carcinoma. Am J Gastroenterol. 2009;104(10):2617–24.

88. Hegde SV, Dillman JR, Lopez MJ, Strouse PJ. Imaging of multifocal liver lesions in children and adolescents. Cancer Imaging. 2013;12:516–29.

89. Buetow PC, Buck JL, Pantongrag-Brown L, Marshall WH, Ros PR, Levine MS, et al. Undifferentiated (embryonal) sarcoma of the liver: pathologic basis of imaging findings in 28 cases. Radiology. 1997;203(3):779–83.

90. Yoon W, Kim JK, Kang HK. Hepatic undifferentiated embryonal sarcoma: MR findings. J Comput Assist Tomogr. 1997;21(1):100–2.

91. Plessier A, Valla DC. Budd-Chiari syndrome. Semin Liver Dis. 2008;28(3):259–69.

92. Cura M, Haskal Z, Lopera J. Diagnostic and interventional radiology for Budd-Chiari syndrome. Radiographics. 2009;29(3):669–81.

93. Darwish Murad S, Plessier A, Hernandez-Guerra M, Fabris F, Eapen CE, Bahr MJ, et al. EN-Vie (European network for vascular disorders of the liver). Etiology, management, and outcome of the Budd-Chiari syndrome. Ann Intern Med. 2009;151(3):167–75.

94. Brancatelli G, Vilgrain V, Federle MP, Hakime A, Lagalla R, Iannaccone R, et al. Budd-Chiari syndrome: spectrum of imaging findings. Am J Roentgenol. 2007;188(2):W168–76. Review.

95. Rivard DC, Bacon PN. Vascular abnormalities of the liver. In: Coley BD, Dillman JR, Frush DP, Hernanz-Schulman M, Hutchison LH, Khanna G, et al., editors. Caffey's pediatric diagnostic imaging. 13th ed. Philadelphia: Elsevier; 2019. p. 851–61.

96. Mortelé KJ, Van Vlierberghe H, Wiesner W, Ros PR. Hepatic veno-occlusive disease: MRI findings. Abdom Imaging. 2002;27(5):523–6.

97. van den Bosch MA, van Hoe L. MR imaging findings in two patients with hepatic veno-occlusive disease following bone marrow transplantation. Eur Radiol. 2000;10(8):1290–3.

98. Vogel CB. Pediatric portal hypertension. Nurse Pract. 2017;42(5):35–42.

99. Gallego C, Velasco M, Marcuello P, Tejedor D, De Campo L, Friera A. Congenital and acquired anomalies of the portal venous system. Radiographics. 2002;22(1):141–59.

100. Squires RH, Ng V, Romero R, Ekong U, Hardikar W, Emre S, Mazariegos GV, American Association for the Study of Liver Diseases, American Society of Transplantation, North American Society for Pediatric Gastroenterology, Hepatology, and Nutrition. Evaluation of the pediatric patient for liver transplantation: 2014 practice guideline by the American Association for the Study of Liver Diseases, American Society of Transplantation and the North American Society for Pediatric Gastroenterology, Hepatology, and Nutrition. Hepatology. 2014;60(1):362–98.

101. Horvat N, Marcelino ASZ, Horvat JV, Yamanari TR, Batista Araújo-Filho JDA, Panizza P, et al. Pediatric liver transplant: techniques and complications. Radiographics. 2017;37(6):1612–31.

102. Rivard DC, Khanna G. Liver transplantation in children. In: Coley BD, Dillman JR, Frush DP, Hernanz-Schulman M, Hutchison LH, Khanna G, et al., editors. Caffey's pediatric diagnostic imaging. 13th ed. Philadelphia: Elsevier; 2019. p. 862–72.

103. Goldstein MJ, Salame E, Kapur S, Kinkhabwala M, LaPointe-Rudow D, Harren P, et al. Analysis of failure in living donor liver transplantation: differential outcomes in children and adults. World J Surg. 2003;27(3):356–64.

104. Seda-Neto J, Antunes da Fonseca E, Pugliese R, Candido HL, Benavides MR, Carballo Afonso R, et al. Twenty years of experience in pediatric living donor liver transplantation. Transplantation. 2016;100(5):1066–72.

105. Berrocal T, Parrón M, Álvarez-Luque A, Prieto C, Santamaría ML. Pediatric liver transplantation: a pictorial essay of early and late complications. Radiographics. 2006;26(4):1187–209.

106. Caiado AHM, Blasbalg R, Marcelino ASZ, da Cunha Pinho M, Chammas MC, da Costa Leite C, et al. Complications of liver transplantation: multimodality imaging approach. Radiographics. 2007;27(5):1401–17.

107. Singh AK, Nachiappan AC, Verma HA, Uppot RN, Blake MA, Saini S, et al. Postoperative imaging in liver transplantation: what radiologists should know. Radiographics. 2010;30(2):339–51.

108. Starzl TE, Putnam CW, Hansbrough JF, Porter KA, Reid HA. Biliary complications after liver transplantation: with special reference to the biliary cast syndrome and techniques of secondary duct repair. Surgery. 1977;81(2):212–21.

109. Shah JN, Haigh WG, Lee SP, Lucey MR, Brensinger CM, Kochman ML, et al. Biliary casts after orthotopic liver transplantation: clinical factors, treatment, biochemical analysis. Am J Gastroenterol. 2003;98(8):1861–7.

110. Jain A, Nalesnik M, Reyes J, Pokharna R, Mazariegos G, Green M, et al. Posttransplant lymphoproliferative disorders in liver transplantation: a 20-year experience. Ann Surg. 2002;236(4):429–36.

111. George TI, Jeng M, Berquist W, Cherry AM, Link MP, Arber DA. Epstein-Barr virus-associated peripheral T-cell lymphoma and hemophagocytic syndrome arising after liver transplantation: case report and review of the literature. Pediatr Blood Cancer. 2005;44(3):270–6.

112. Camacho JC, Moreno CC, Harri PA, Aguirre DA, Torres WE, Mittal PK. Posttransplantation lymphoproliferative disease: proposed imaging classification. Radiographics. 2014;34(7):2025–38.

Bile Duct and Gallbladder

Nathan C. Hull, Gary R. Schooler, and Edward Y. Lee

Introduction

Disorders of the gallbladder and bile ducts are not uncommon in children. Ultrasound is typically the first-line imaging modality employed in the workup of right upper quadrant pain or suspected hepatobiliary diseases. However, magnetic resonance (MR) imaging offers multiple advantages for evaluation of bile duct and gallbladder disorders in pediatric patients, including its lack of ionizing radiation as well as its ability to provide excellent visualization of these structures and allow comprehensive evaluation of the biliary system and possible concurrent liver disease. MR imaging sequences such as magnetic resonance cholangiopancreatography (MRCP) and the use of hepatobiliary contrast agents provide a noninvasive way of evaluating the intrahepatic and extrahepatic bile ducts.

Several important factors including proper patient preparation, the need for sedation, and appropriate coil selection should be carefully considered when performing MR imaging in the pediatric population to ensure an optimal examination. Up-to-date working knowledge of techniques and tools available to perform MR imaging of the biliary system and familiarity with common disease processes that are encountered in the pediatric population is essential. Therefore, in this chapter, MR imaging techniques for evaluating bile duct and gallbladder anatomy are discussed followed by the review of bile duct and gallbladder anatomy including embryology, normal development, and anatomic variants. In addition, various congenital and acquired disorders affecting infants and children are discussed including clinical features and characteristic MR imaging findings.

Magnetic Resonance Imaging Techniques

Patient Preparation

Patient preparation is essential to facilitate optimal imaging of pediatric patients. Each MR examination should be tailored to the age, size, and expected level of understanding and cooperation of the child. In order to minimize bowel peristalsis artifact and ensure the gallbladder is distended, patients should have nothing by mouth for 4 hours prior to the examination. Child life specialists may meet with the patient and parents prior to imaging to explain what to expect and answer questions. Providing breath-hold instructions and practicing with consistency helps to improve image quality [1]. Adequate peripheral venous access should be obtained if power injection of contrast is needed for the examination.

Sedation Careful consideration should be given for a patient's need for sedation or anesthesia during MR imaging. Infants (<3 months of age) can often be imaged without sedation using the "feed and wrap" method where the child is fed, tightly swaddled, and laid on the scanner table with hearing protection in place [2]. Typically children less than 6 years old require some degree of sedation to minimize the amount of voluntary motion during the examination. In children between the ages of 6 and 8, MR imaging-compatible goggles can be utilized that allow patients to watch movies during the examination and can help reduce the need for sedation.

N. C. Hull (✉)
Department of Radiology, Mayo Clinic, Rochester, MN, USA
e-mail: hull.nathan@mayo.edu

G. R. Schooler
Department of Radiology, Duke University Medical Center, Durham, NC, USA

E. Y. Lee
Division of Thoracic Imaging, Department of Radiology, Boston Children's Hospital, Harvard Medical School, Boston, MA, USA

© Springer Nature Switzerland AG 2020
E. Y. Lee et al. (eds.), *Pediatric Body MRI*, https://doi.org/10.1007/978-3-030-31989-2_8

Children older than 6 years of age should be evaluated on a case-by-case basis to determine if sedation is necessary.

Hardware

For MR biliary imaging, both 1.5 Tesla (T) and 3T field strength magnets can be used, although smaller patients may benefit from the higher signal in 3T machines [3]. The smallest possible radiofrequency coil that covers the anatomy of interest should be utilized. Usually used are 16–32 channel phased-array body coils. For the majority of children, smaller coils such as cardiac phased array coils work well, although older pediatric patients usually require a larger body or torso array coil [3].

MR Imaging Pulse Sequences and Protocols

Standard Sequences

MR imaging sequences should be tailored to the individual pediatric patient and the specific clinical query including the field of view, slice thickness, and matrix parameters. MR imaging of the gallbladder and bile ducts usually occurs with concurrent evaluation of the liver and upper abdomen. Standard sequences which should be included to evaluate the gallbladder and bile ducts are discussed below and in Table 8.1.

T2-Weighted Sequences

T2-weighted imaging (T2WI) of the hepatobiliary system is usually obtained using fast-spin echo (FSE) or turbo-spin echo (TSE), three-dimensional isotropic or single-shot fast-spin echo (SSFE) sequences [1]. Conventional T2WI with fat suppression is usually acquired in the axial plane using two-dimensional (2D) FSE utilizing respiratory-triggered or navigator-gated sequences and provides high contrast evaluation of abdominal anatomy with higher signal-to-noise ratio (SNR). This sequence allows good visualization of the liver, gallbladder, and bile ducts and can be especially helpful when evaluating intrahepatic lesions. Echo times (TEs) for 1.5T are usually 80–90 milliseconds (msec) and around 70–80 msec for 3T. Due to the required acquisition time and breath-hold needed for this sequence, it can be prone to respiratory motion artifact if not optimized.

SSFE T2WI can be acquired in just seconds with reasonably good spatial resolution [4]. Because of its rapid acquisition, it is less prone to motion artifact and has a higher signal-to-noise ratio than FSE, due to less "noise" from motion [5]. However, SSFE contrast resolution is poorer and focal hepatic lesions are less conspicuous compared with FSE imaging. SSFE sequences in the abdomen are optimally performed using either breath-hold or respiratory triggering technique; however, diagnostic quality images can often still be obtained as a non-triggered acquisition in free-breathing patients. SSFE are usually acquired in the coronal and axial planes [6].

Table 8.1 Commonly used MR imaging sequences in evaluating the bile duct and gallbladder

Sequence	Visualization	Plane(s)	Advantages	Disadvantages
T2-weighted, fat-suppressed FSE/TSE	Intrahepatic lesions	Axial, +/− coronal	High SNR and image quality	Longer acquisition time Motion artifact
Single-shot fast-spin echo	Fluid containing structures: bile ducts, gallbladder	Coronal, +/− axial	Good spatial resolution Less prone to motion artifact Rapid acquisition	Poorer contrast resolution
SSFP	Fluid-filled structures are hyperintense	Axial and/or coronal	Rapid acquisition Good SNR and spatial resolution	Blood vessels and ducts are both hyperintense
MRCP	Bile and pancreatic ducts	Coronal	Noninvasive visualization of pancreaticobiliary tree	Image blurring from long echo train lengths Flow artifacts may mimic stones
Contrast-enhanced, fat-suppressed volumetric T1-weighted GRE with hepatobiliary contrast	Periductal inflammation Mass enhancement Dynamic cholangiogram	Axial and/or coronal	Dynamic visualization of biliary ducts Characterize enhancement of hepatobiliary abnormalities	Motion artifact

FSE Fast-spin echo, *TSE* Turbo-spin echo, *SNR* Signal-to-noise ratio, *SSFP* Steady-state free precession, *MRCP* Magnetic resonance cholangio-pancreatography, *GRE* Gradient recalled echo

Balanced steady-state free precession (SSFP) images also offer the advantages of rapid acquisition and motion resistance with good SNR and spatial resolution. This sequence offers a combination of T1- and T2-weighting and shows biliary ducts well, although a disadvantage is that blood vessels also appear as hyperintense structures, making distinction between hepatic vessels and intrahepatic bile ducts challenging [6].

Additional Sequences

T1-Weighted Images / Spoiled Gradient Pre-contrast three-dimensional T1-weighted gradient recalled (GRE) echo fat-suppressed images can be helpful for anatomical visualization and comparison with post-contrast images to assess for focal hepatic lesion enhancement or peribiliary enhancement suggestive of cholangitis. These sequences offer rapid volumetric acquisition in a single breath-hold with high-resolution but have lower SNR than traditional T1-weighted imaging (T1WI).

MR Cholangiopancreatography MR cholangiopancreatography (MRCP) is an effective noninvasive manner of visualizing gallbladder and pancreaticobiliary ductal disease in pediatric patients with diagnostic accuracy around 90–100% [7–12]. MRCP consists of FSE heavily weighted T2WI with long TEs (up to 1000 msec) to allow visualization of the gallbladder and pancreaticobiliary ducts. The coronal and axial imaging planes are typically employed with respiratory triggering. These are usually acquired as thin-slice 2D images from which a single maximum-intensity-projection (MIP) reconstruction is generated. Alternatively, 3D isotropic MRCP imaging can be performed, with images acquired in the coronal plane and then reformatted into axial, coronal, and oblique planes as needed. The coronal oblique plane along the axis of the liver hilum and common bile duct is especially useful as a global assessment of the intrahepatic and extrahepatic biliary tree. The axial plane is helpful in evaluation of punctate calculi or ductal filling defects [6]. FSE imaging is prone to respiratory motion artifacts, and, for patients with rapid or shallow breathing, a thick (3–5 cm) slab SSFE image with long TE can be acquired in less than 1 second and provides similar information.

Negative (T1- and T2-weighted hypointense) oral contrast may be used in nonsedated children to help reduce the high signal intensity of gastric or intestinal fluid. It has been shown to improve image quality without significant adverse reactions [6]. The addition of intravenous secretin to an MRCP examination is usually primarily employed to improve visualization of the pancreatic duct [6, 13, 14].

Post-Contrast Images and Contrast Selection T1-weighted fat-suppressed contrast-enhanced images can be valuable in characterizing biliary stones, in evaluating inflammation, and in the staging of malignancies. Often used are 3D GRE sequences (THRIVE; Philips, VIBE; Siemens, LAVA; GE Healthcare) that have short acquisition times (10–20 seconds) and can be acquired as a breath-hold acquisition [1]. These can be performed using signal averaging in children who cannot suspend respiration. Radial filling of k-space with free-breathing 3D GRE sequences, such as StarVIBE (Siemens) may be utilized to help diminish respiratory motion artifact [15].

Both extracellular and hepatobiliary gadolinium-based agents are available and commonly used in hepatobiliary imaging. The clinical indication should guide the decision of which contrast agent should be used. While extracellular contrast agents are the most commonly used agents and are excreted via the kidneys, hepatobiliary contrast agents (gadobenate dimeglumine (Multihance, Bracco Diagnostics) or gadoxetate (Eovist or Primovist; Bayer Healthcare)) are partially excreted through the biliary system and produce contrast-enhanced functional and anatomic cholangiography images. Cholangiography images can be obtained approximately 15–40 minutes after injection of gadoxetate and up to 60 minutes after gadobenate injection [1, 16]. These contrast agents can also be helpful in determining if cystic structures or fluid collections communicate with the biliary tract. Of note, hepatobiliary contrast agents have poor hepatic uptake and excretion in the setting of poorly functioning hepatocytes (bilirubin level > 3 mg/dl) and may not be effective imaging agents in patients with hepatic dysfunction [17].

Anatomy

Embryology

Early in the mid 4th week of intrauterine development, a hepatic diverticulum in the ventral wall of the primitive midgut forms [18]. Later in the 4th week, two buds are present (Fig. 8.1). The cranial bud gives rise to the liver and extrahepatic biliary tree, while the caudal bud divides into a superior

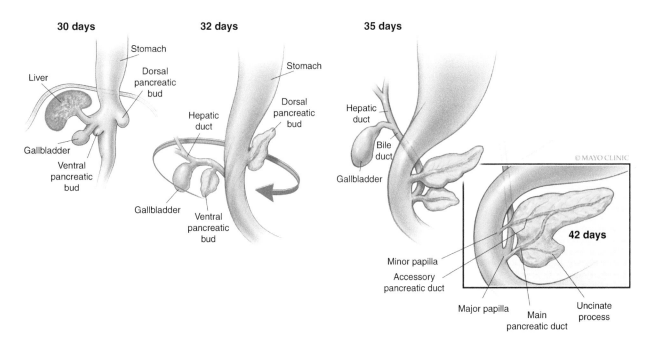

Fig. 8.1 Diagram showing the development of the pancreaticobiliary ducts. Between 30 and 35 days of gestation, a hepatic diverticulum forms from the primitive midgut and divides into two buds. The cranial bud gives rise to the liver and extrahepatic biliary tree. The gallbladder, cystic duct, and pancreas arise from the caudal bud. © Mayo Clinic. (Used with permission of Mayo Foundation for Medical Education and Research. All rights reserved)

and inferior bud [19]. The gallbladder and cystic duct arise from the superior bud, and the dorsal and ventral pancreas from the inferior bud. By 35–42 days, all elements of the biliary tree are recognizable [19]. The common duct undergoes an elongation process as its lumen is plugged by epithelial cells, and then a subsequent recanalization. The common duct and central pancreatic bud then rotate 180° around the duodenum clockwise by the 6th week, which then allows for entrance of the common duct into the left posterior surface of the duodenum [19].

Normal Development and Anatomy

Approximately 60% of the population has what is considered to be classic biliary anatomy; meaning the right and left ducts drain their respective lobes [20, 21]. Small segmental ducts drain segments II–IV to form the left hepatic duct. The right duct is formed from the fusion of the right posterior duct, which usually has a horizontal course and drains segments VI and VII, and the more vertically oriented right anterior duct draining segments V and VIII [20]. The caudate lobe may drain to the right hepatic duct or originate from the left duct. The cystic duct typically drains into the lateral portion of the common hepatic duct inferior to its origin [22].

Anatomic Variants

While the majority of patients have classic biliary anatomy, it is important to recognize variations and report them accurately. Branching patterns of the bile ducts can be classified and have been described by Choi [21] (Fig. 8.2). Type 1 represents the most common or classic branching pattern as discussed above. Variants include trifurcation (Type 2), the right posterior duct draining to the left duct (Type 3A) or to the common duct (Type 3B) or cystic duct (Type 3C), the right duct draining to the cystic duct (Type 4), or accessory ducts which drain into the common duct (Type 5A), or right duct (Type 5B), or finally separate segmental ducts which drain the left lobe to the confluence or common duct (Type 6). Type 2 and Type 3A each occur in approximately 10% of individuals, while the remaining variations occur in 6% or less [21].

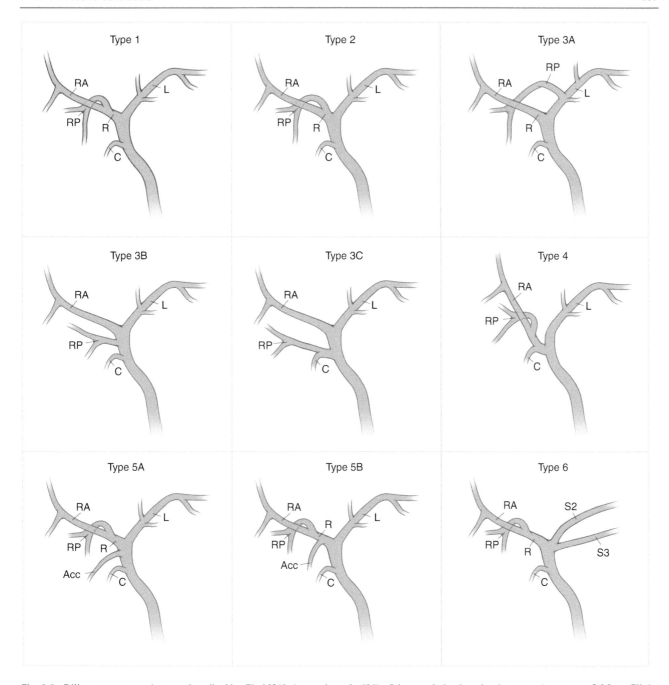

Fig. 8.2 Biliary anatomy variants as described by Choi [21]. Approximately 60% of the population has classic or type 1 anatomy. © Mayo Clinic. (Used with permission of Mayo Foundation for Medical Education and Research. All rights reserved)

Spectrum of Bile Duct and Gallbladder Disorders

Congenital Bile Duct and Gallbladder Disorders

Biliary Atresia Biliary atresia (BA) is a congenital obliterative cholangiopathy seen in neonates that involves the intrahepatic and extrahepatic ducts leading to cholestasis and jaundice and eventually to cirrhosis and death if not treated. This disorder is usually suspected clinically due to jaundice and high serum bilirubin levels. However, other conditions including neonatal hepatitis may manifest with similar symptoms. Kasai portoenterostomy, which involves excision of the central fibrotic bile duct with anastomosis of a Roux-en-Y jejunal limb to the porta hepatis, is usually the initial surgical intervention in BA patients. However, the majority of patients with Kasai portoenterostomy eventually require liver transplantation.

Imaging is helpful for evaluation for BA and its alternative diagnoses although definitive diagnosis is usually confirmed with biopsy and/or intraoperative cholangiogram. Commonly, hepatobiliary scintigraphy with Technetium-99m iminodiacetic acid (HIDA) is performed to visualize uptake of radiotracer into the liver and if tracer is excreted into the bowel. MR cholangiography can be used to evaluate children suspected to have BA with a high degree of sensitivity and accuracy with nonvisualization of either the common bile duct or common hepatic duct [23, 24]. MR imaging is also the current imaging modality of choice in the longitudinal follow-up of pediatric patients after Kasai portoenterostomy. Typical MR imaging findings of Kasai portoenterostomy failure include bile duct dilatation, bile lakes due to bile pseudocysts caused by damaged bile ducts, regenerative nodules as hepatic cirrhosis progresses, and enlarged portal vein, splenomegaly, varices, and ascites due to portal hypertension (Fig. 8.3).

Biliary Hamartoma Biliary hamartomas are benign ductal plate malformations of the small bile ducts and are composed of disorganized cystic and dilated bile ducts surrounded by fibrocollagenous stroma. The ducts within these lesions range in caliber from narrow to ectatic and more marked dilation may lead to a cyst that can be large enough to see macroscopically [25]. Bile duct hamartomas are also referred to as von Meyenburg complex, as these lesions were first described by von Meyenburg in 1918 [26]. Biliary hamartomas are most commonly multiple, small lesions measuring 1–10 mm and are found in a subcapsular location. These are asymptomatic masses seen incidentally in the liver on imaging in most cases, although jaundice and portal hypertension can occur from mass effect [27], and there are some reports of an association between multiple hamartomas and cholangiocarcinomas [28, 29].

On MR imaging, biliary hamartomas are hypointense on T1WI, isointense to slightly hyperintense on T2WI, and hypointense on post-contrast MR images (Fig. 8.4). MRCP may be helpful in showing both the lesion number and extent [26]. Because the imaging appearance is often nonspecific, a definitive diagnosis may require histologic analysis to exclude other lesions which may have a similar appearance such as hepatic metastases or microabscesses. Usually no treatment is required but follow-up imaging should be considered due to rare possibility of malignancy.

Choledochal Cystic Disease Choledochal cysts are congenital segmental fusiform or saccular cystic dilations that can affect intrahepatic or extrahepatic ducts. The etiology is thought to be related to ductal plate malformations, although other theories include obstruction of the distal biliary duct, prenatal rupture of the duct with subsequent healing, or reflux of pancreatic juices due to anomalous insertion of the pancreatic duct into the common bile duct [30–32]. The classic triad of symptoms of choledochal cystic disease are recurrent right upper quadrant abdominal pain, jaundice, and a palpable mass. Ascending cholangitis is the most common complication [33], with calculi and cyst rupture also possible [34]. Long-term complications include hepatic cirrhosis and cholangiocarcinoma. The lifetime risk of developing a secondary cholangiocarcinoma is 10–15% and surgery with hepatojejunostomy is the recommended treatment to minimize this risk [35–37].

There are five types as classified by the Todani classification (Table 8.2). Type 1 is the most common subtype seen in 80–90% of cases [38] and consists of a variable degree of

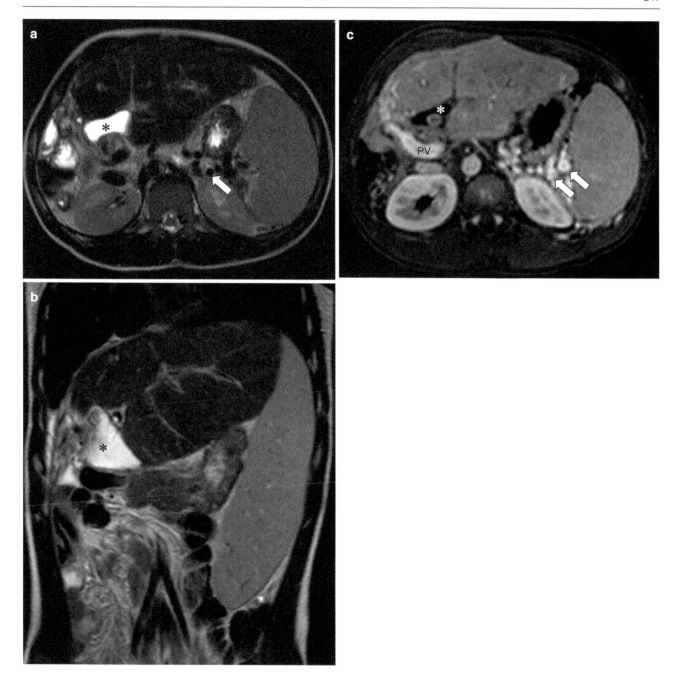

Fig. 8.3 Portal hypertension in a 2-year-old boy with a history of biliary atresia status post Kasai procedure. (**a, b**) Axial and coronal T2-weighted MR images show the mildly dilated portoenterostomy (*). There are signs of portal hypertension with enlarged spleen and varices (*arrow*). (**c**) Axial contrast-enhanced T1-weighted fat-suppressed MR image shows the portoenterostomy (*), a dilated portal vein (PV), and multiple small varices (*arrows*) near the spleen

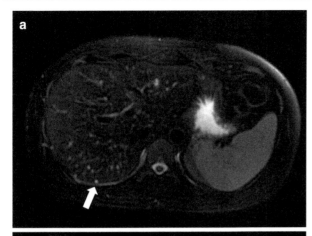

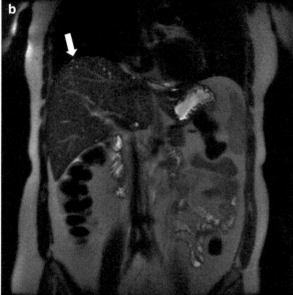

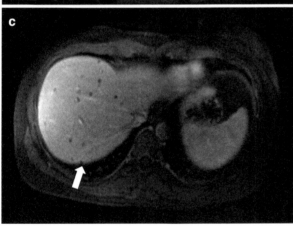

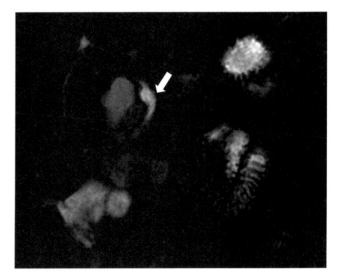

Table 8.2 Todani classification of choledochal cysts. Note Type I accounts for 80–90% of choledochal cysts

Type	Malformation
I	Dilation of the common bile duct (CBD)
II	Diverticula of the CBD
III	Cyst-like dilation of the distal CBD, choledochocele
IV	Intra- and extrahepatic cystic ductal dilations typically
V (Caroli disease)	Intrahepatic cystic ductal dilations

Fig. 8.5 Choledochal cyst in a 12-year-old girl who presented with right upper quadrant pain and elevated liver enzymes. Coronal MR cholangiopancreatography (MRCP) image shows a focal dilation (*arrow*) of the common bile duct below the cystic duct (Todani type 1B)

Fig. 8.4 Incidental biliary hamartomas in a 19-year-old woman who underwent MR imaging for evaluation of metastatic disease from rectal cancer. (**a, b**) Axial non-enhanced T2-weighted fat-suppressed and coronal single-shot T2-weighted MR images show multiple round hyperintense cyst-like small nodules (*arrows*) in the liver; many are subcapsular in location. (**c**) Axial enhanced T1-weighted fat-suppressed MR image shows no enhancement of the lesions (*arrow*) despite normal hepatic parenchymal enhancement

dilation of the common duct. Type I can be further subdivided into types IA (cystic dilation of the common bile duct), IB (segmental dilation below the cystic duct) (Fig. 8.5), and IC (fusiform dilation of the common bile duct). Type II is seen as diverticula of the common bile duct and is seen in only 2% of cases [39]. Todani type III cyst accounts for 1–5% of cases and is often referred to as a "choledochocele" as it forms a cyst-like mass at the intraduodenal portion of the duct (Fig. 8.6) [39]. Type IVA has multiple intra- and extrahepatic cystic dilations and occurs in approximately 10% of patients with choledochal cysts [39, 40], while type IVB only has extrahepatic biliary cysts without intrahepatic involvement and is rare. Type V, also known as Caroli disease, is characterized with intrahepatic biliary cysts and is discussed further below.

MRCP is an excellent noninvasive way to assess the hepatobiliary tree and characterize choledochal cystic disease. The choledochal cysts are hypointense on T1WI and hyperintense on T2WI and have no significant wall enhancement on post-contrast MR images. Suspicious imaging findings for infection or malignancy include mural nodularity, wall

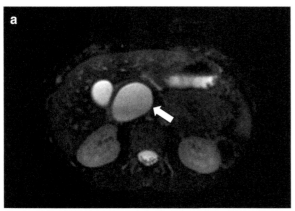

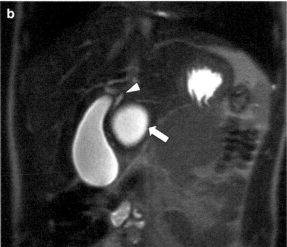

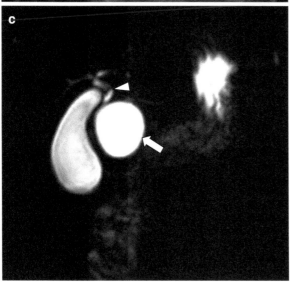

Table 8.3 Fibrocystic liver disease from malformation of embryonic ductal plates and size of ducts

Disorder	Duct size
Caroli disease	Large intrahepatic
Choledochal cyst	Large extrahepatic
Polycystic liver disease	Medium
Congenital hepatic fibrosis	Small
Biliary hamartoma	Small

Adapted from Knowlton et al. [30], with permission

thickening, or increased wall enhancement. Non-enhancing T2-weighted hypointense filling-defects within the bile ducts are highly suggestive of choledocholithiasis.

Ascending cholangitis in pediatric patients with choledochal cysts can be treated as needed with antibiotics. Other medical therapies to decrease the risk of cholestasis and stone formation can also be employed. If substantial liver damage and cirrhosis occur, liver transplantation may be required.

Caroli Disease Caroli disease, also known as Todani type V choledochal cyst, is an autosomal recessive disease characterized by non-obstructive segmental dilation of the large intrahepatic bile ducts. Caroli disease can be further subdivided into two types: Caroli disease proper and Caroli syndrome. Both Caroli disease proper and Caroli syndrome have ectatic cyst-like biliary ducts in continuity with the biliary system. In Caroli syndrome, however, congenital hepatic fibrosis is also present. Caroli disease proper is thought to result from arrested remodeling of the ductal plates of the large intrahepatic ducts (Table 8.3). Caroli syndrome is also thought to be from arrested remodeling of the bile ducts both during embryogenesis and later as more peripheral ducts are formed [33].

Complications of Caroli disease are usually due to stagnant bile leading to cholangitis, calculi formation, hepatic abscess, and rarely cholangiocarcinoma [41]. While the disease is present at birth, affected patients may not come to medical attention until symptoms of these complications occur. Pediatric patients with Caroli syndrome may also have complications that are associated with the concurrent congenital hepatic fibrosis such as portal hypertension and hemorrhage from esophageal varices. In addition to congenital hepatic fibrosis, pediatric patients with Caroli syndrome also have autosomal recessive polycystic kidney disease.

On MR imaging, Carol disease has multiple T1-weighted hypointense/T2-weighted hyperintense cyst-like structures in the liver representing the ectatic intrahepatic bile ducts. The adjacent portal vein radicles protrude into the lumen of the dilated ducts and create the so called "central dot" sign (Fig. 8.7). These portal vein radicles show enhancement on post-contrast images. MRCP can show the communication between the biliary tree and the cystic dilations and help confirm the diagnosis.

Fig. 8.6 Choledochocele in a 12-year-old boy who presented with jaundice and history of cholangitis. (**a, b**) Axial non-enhanced T2-weighted fat-suppressed and coronal T2-weighted single-shot MR images show normal caliber of the proximal common bile duct (*arrowhead*) with cystic dilation (*arrows*) of the distal duct near the junction with the pancreatic duct (Todani type III choledochocele). Note, no upstream dilation of the intrahepatic bile ducts or pancreatic duct is seen. (**c**) Coronal MR cholangiopancreatography (MRCP) maximum intensity projection (MIP) image shows the cystic dilation (*arrow*) of the distal common bile duct and normal proximal common bile duct (*arrowhead*)

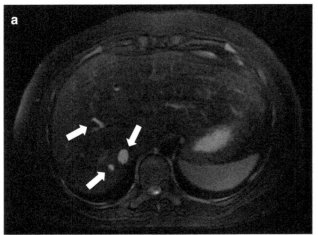

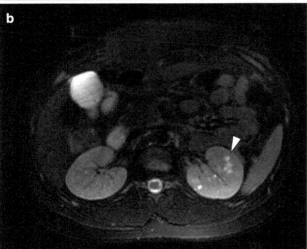

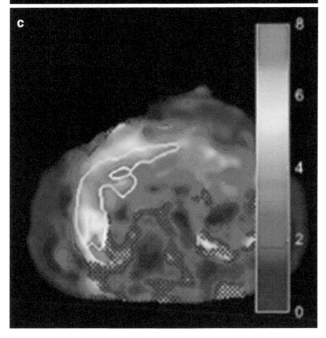

Duplicated Gallbladder Gallbladder duplication, or bilobed gallbladder, is a rare congenital malformation which occurs in approximately 1 per 4000 individuals [42]. It is believed to be due to extra budding of the biliary tree when the developing caudal bud of the hepatic diverticulum divides [43, 44]. Variations of gallbladder duplication can be discussed according to the Boyden classifications (Fig. 8.8) including the vesica fellea divisa (bifid or bilobed gallbladder), or vesica fellea duplex (double gallbladder with either a shared cystic duct or duplicated gallbladder each with their own cystic duct entering separately into the common duct) [42, 43, 45]. Due to possible associated variants of the cystic duct and hepatic artery, this abnormality is important to identify and report accurately, especially if surgery is planned to avoid biliary injuries [45]. Bilobed or duplicated gallbladders can either be asymptomatic or associated with right upper quadrant pain and may predispose to cholelithiasis and cholecystitis [20].

Bifid or duplicated gallbladder is well-defined on MR imaging with T2WI (Fig. 8.9) as well as MRCP and has the typical MR imaging features of the normal gallbladder. Surgical removal of both gallbladders is recommended to avoid cholelithiasis or cholecystitis in the remaining organ [46, 47].

Acquired Bile Duct and Gallbladder Disorders

Acute Cholecystitis Acute cholecystitis is less common in children than in adults. It may occur secondary to obstruction of the outflow of the gallbladder lumen at the gallbladder neck or cystic duct, leading to a sequence of luminal dilation, edema, ischemia, necrosis, and finally perforation. Although cholelithiasis may lead to acute cholecystitis, only a small percentage of children develop cholecystitis from cholelithiasis [48]. Most cases of acute cholecystitis in children, up to 50–70%, is seen with acalculous cholecystitis [48]. Acalculous cholecystitis may occur from biliary stasis, dehydration, or gallbladder ischemia and is often seen in patients with serious illnesses in the intensive care unit like severe trauma or burns, sepsis, or postoperative state [49].

Fig. 8.7 Caroli syndrome in a 15-year-old boy who presented with elevated liver enzyme. (**a, b**) Axial T2-weighted fat-suppressed MR images show segmental dilation (*arrows*) of intrahepatic biliary ducts with the "central dot" sign, and multiple small cysts in the kidneys (*arrowhead*). (**c**) Axial color map from an MR elastogram shows an elevated liver stiffness of 4.2 kiloPascals, corresponding to grade 3–4 hepatic fibrosis

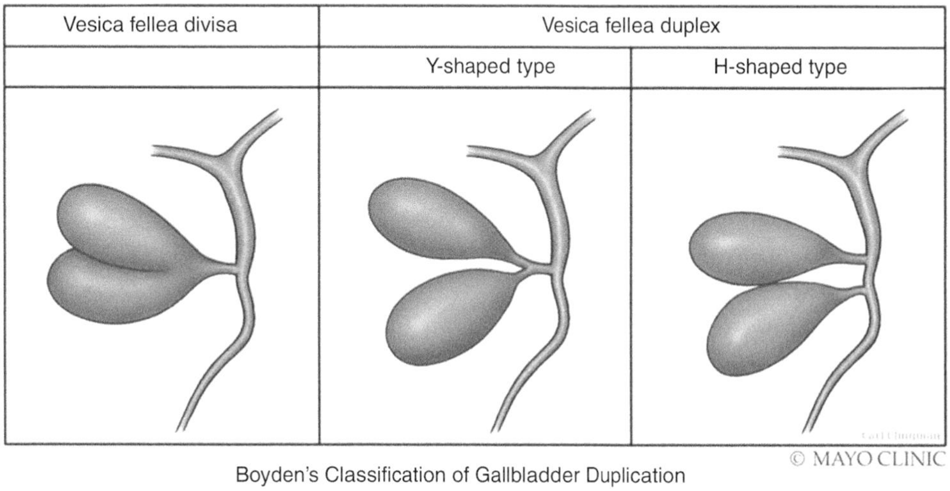

Fig. 8.8 Variations of gallbladder duplication according to the Boyden classifications, including the vesica fellea divisa (bifid or bilobed gallbladder), or vesica fellea duplex (double gallbladder with either a shared cystic duct or duplicated gallbladder each with their own cystic duct entering separately into the common duct). © Mayo Clinic. (Used with permission of Mayo Foundation for Medical Education and Research. All rights reserved)

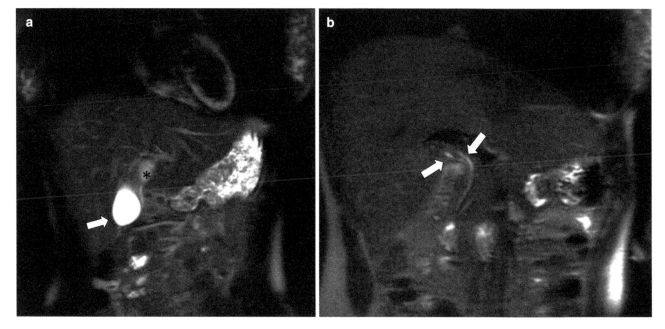

Boyden's Classification of Gallbladder Duplication

© MAYO CLINIC

Fig. 8.9 Duplicated gallbladder in a 16-year-old boy with right upper quadrant pain and clinical concern for cholecystitis. (**a**) Coronal single-shot T2-weighted MR image shows the normal gallbladder (white *arrow*) and an additional cystic structure (∗) along the undersurface of the mid liver representing a duplicated gallbladder. (**b**) Coronal single-shot T2-weighted MR image shows two small ducts converging (*arrows*) that can be traced back to a gallbladder

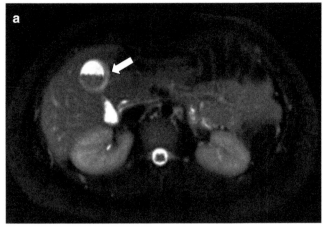
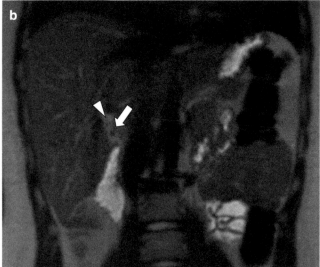

Fig. 8.10 Cholelithiasis and early cholecystitis in a 17-year-old boy who presented with right upper quadrant pain. (**a**) Axial T2-weighted fat-suppressed MR image shows multiple, small dependent gallbladder stones and gallbladder wall thickening measuring 5 mm (*arrow*). (**b**) Coronal single-shot T2-weighted MR image shows cholelithiasis with a stone in the gallbladder neck (*arrow*) and mild surrounding pericholecystic fluid (*arrowhead*)

While ultrasound is typically the first line for imaging if cholecystitis is suspected, MR imaging can be valuable in both making the diagnosis and evaluating for potential causes or sequelae. Thickening of the gallbladder wall with increased signal on T2-weighted fat-suppressed MR images suggests acute inflammation (Fig. 8.10) [50–52]. Other MR imaging findings include reticular or patchy T2-weighted signal intensity and contrast enhancement of pericholecystic adipose tissue, enhancement of the gallbladder wall, and the presence of pericholecystic fluid. MRCP images may also show filling defects in the gallbladder lumen or in the common bile duct if the cause of inflammation is related to biliary stones. Laparoscopic or open cholecystectomy is usually the treatment of choice.

Choledocholithiasis Choledocholithiasis occurs when biliary stones migrate and become lodged within the hepatic or common bile duct. Most affected pediatric patients are symptomatic with epigastric or right upper quadrant pain, nausea, and vomiting. Symptoms usually occur due to intermittent or total obstruction of the common bile duct. As the stones pass into the distal common bile duct, this can cause inflammation of the adjacent pancreas and/or occlusion of the pancreatic duct leading to secondary pancreatitis, also called gallstone pancreatitis. Obstruction of the common bile duct may also lead to cholangitis.

MR imaging is a highly useful and noninvasive tool in the diagnosis of choledocholithiasis [9, 53]. Bile is markedly hyperintense on T2WI, while ductal stones are hypointense, making them conspicuous filling defects seen both on

standard T2WI and MRCP (Fig. 8.11). MRCP has been shown to be accurate when compared with direct cholangiopancreatography in detecting stones and may help guide in planning of endoscopic retrograde cholangiopancreatography (ERCP) [7, 8, 54].

Impacted stones may be removed via ERCP or intraoperatively if cholecystectomy is planned in the setting of concomitant cholecystitis.

Cholangitis Cholangitis is inflammation or infection of the bile ducts. Etiologies include infectious, idiopathic, iatrogenic from chemotherapy, or autoimmune related. One form of cholangitis, primary sclerosing cholangitis (PSC), is an idiopathic condition thought to be autoimmune related and is highly associated with inflammatory bowel disease, particularly ulcerative colitis [55, 56]. PSC causes obliterative inflammation of the bile ducts. Boys are more often affected than girls and usually present in the second decade of life [30]. Affected pediatric patients may present with abdominal pain, jaundice, and hepatomegaly.

MR imaging and MRCP can show findings of cholangitis of irregularity of the bile ducts, strictures or ductal wall enhancement. MRCP is highly accurate for detecting findings of PSC which include irregularity of the bile duct with areas of mild dilation and intermittent strictures giving a "beaded" appearance [1, 57] (Fig. 8.12). Other patterns that may be seen include the cobblestone pattern (course mural irregularities), pruned-tree appearance (dilation of only central ducts), or pseudodiverticula [30]. Cholangitis may some-

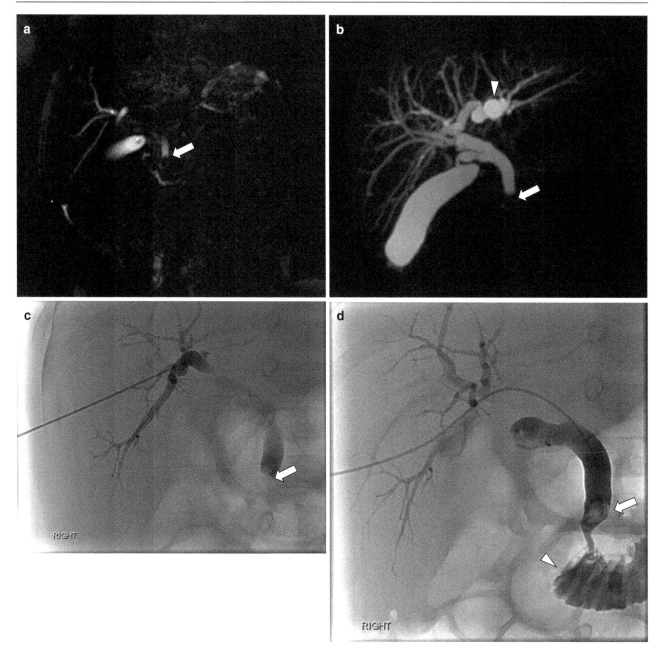

Fig. 8.11 Choledocholithiasis in a 3-month-old girl who presented with elevated bilirubin. (**a**) Coronal MR cholangiopancreatography (MRCP) image shows an ovoid filling defect (*arrow*) in the distal common bile duct occluding the ampulla. (**b**) 3D MRCP maximum intensity projection (MIP) image shows secondary dilation of the central intrahepatic ducts (*arrowhead*) and abrupt attenuation of the distal common bile duct with a filling defect (*arrow*). (**c**) Frontal projection from percutaneous cholangiogram that was performed to relieve the obstruction after initial endoscopic retrograde cholangiopancreatography (ERCP) was unsuccessful shows a large filling defect (*arrow*) in the common bile duct without flow of contrast into the duodenum. (**d**) After some manipulation, the stone was dislodged with contrast now flowing into the duodenum (*arrowhead*). Note the stone remains in the distal common bile duct as a filling duct (*arrow*)

times be segmental, although the entire biliary tract is usually involved and intrahepatic ductal involvement is present in all cases, while extrahepatic ducts are involved in only 60% of cases [30, 58].

Therapy for cholangitis is directed towards the underlying cause. Treatment of PSC focuses on managing complications and monitoring damage to the liver. Other treatments may help with symptoms such as ursodeoxycholic acid (to help bile flow), antibiotics, and antihistamines. Portal hypertension, secondary cholangitis, biliary cirrhosis, and cholangiocarcinoma are complications which can be seen with PSC. Ultimately, liver transplantation may be necessary with a median reported time to transplant of 12.7 years from diagnosis [55, 59].

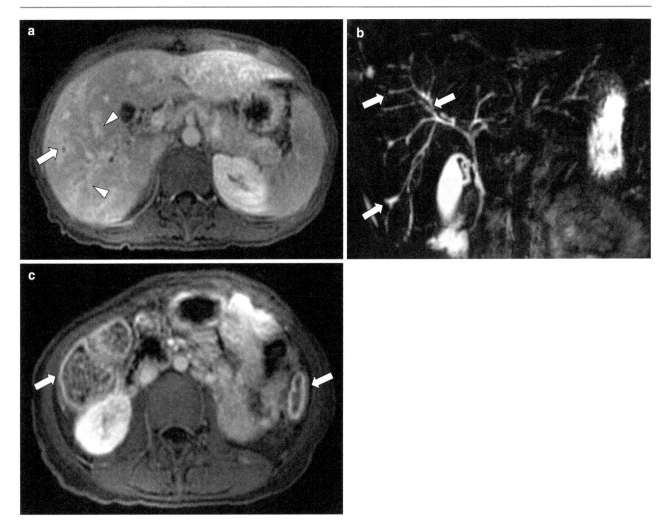

Fig. 8.12 Primary sclerosing cholangitis in a 14-year-old girl who presented with acute on chronic abdominal pain suspected to have inflammatory bowel disease. (**a**) Axial contrast-enhanced gradient volumetric T1-weighted fat-suppressed MR image shows peri-ductal enhancement (*arrowheads*) compatible with inflammation. The visualized intrahepatic bile ducts show mural thickening and enhancement (*arrow*). (**b**) Coronal MR cholangiopancreatography (MRCP) maximum intensity projection (MIP) image shows irregularity of the intrahepatic bile ducts with intermittent narrowing and dilation (*arrows*) with a "beaded" appearance compatible with primary sclerosing cholangitis. (**c**) Axial contrast-enhanced gradient volumetric T1-weighted fat-suppressed MR image inferior to the level of the liver shows hyperenhancement of the hepatic flexure and descending colon (*arrows*) compatible with concurrent inflammatory bowel disease

Neoplastic Bile Duct and Gallbladder Disorder

Cholangiocarcinoma Cholangiocarcinoma is a somewhat rare malignant neoplasm arising from the biliary tract. It accounts for fewer than 1% of all carcinomas [30]. It is usually seen in children as a complication of other hepatobiliary disorders such as choledochal cysts, Caroli disease, and sclerosing cholangitis (Fig. 8.12), although it usually occurs late in these diseases. It is thought to occur as a sequela of chronic inflammation. Cholangiocarcinoma can manifest in three different morphologic types: mass-forming, periductal infiltrating, and intraductal [60].

On MR imaging, the mass-forming type can appear as an intrahepatic hyperintense mass on T2WI and hypointense on T1WI, with peripheral and centripetal enhancement. Enhancement is often seen on delayed post-contrast MR images (>10 minutes) (Fig. 8.13), which should be acquired if there is suspicion of possible cholangiocarcinoma. Associated findings may include capsular retraction, satellite nodules, hepatolithiasis, and vascular encasement without gross tumor

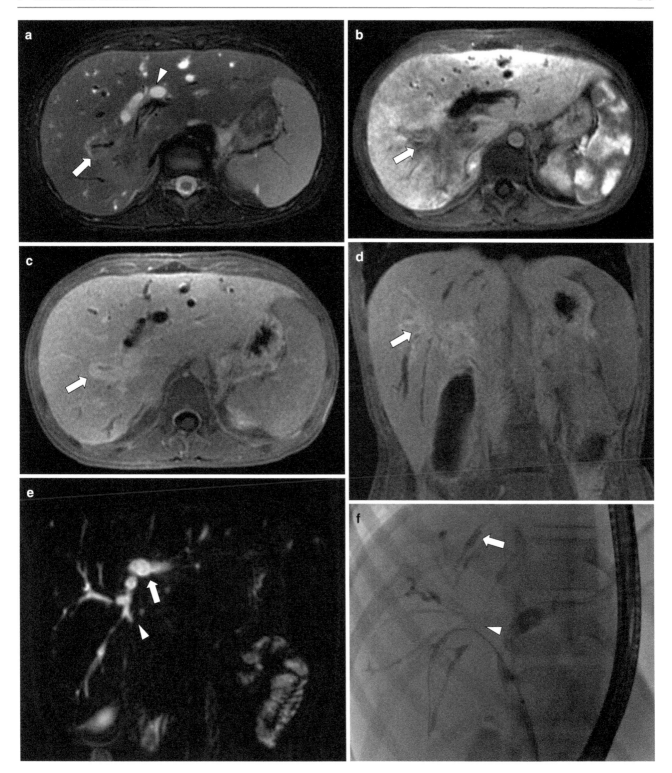

Fig. 8.13 Primary sclerosing cholangitis and biopsy proven hilar cholangiocarcinoma in a 16-year-old girl who presented with weight loss and abdominal pain. (**a**) Axial T2-weighted fat-suppressed MR image shows ill-defined increased T2-weighted signal intensity (*arrow*) in the right hepatic lobe and biliary ductal dilation (*arrowhead*). (**b**) Axial arterial phase post-contrast T1-weighted fat-suppressed MR image with hepatobiliary contrast agent shows an ill-defined mass (*arrow*) with enhancement less than the adjacent hepatic parenchyma. (**c, d**) Axial and coronal 15-minute delayed T1-weighted fat-suppressed MR images with hepatobiliary contrast shows delayed hyperenhancement of an ill-defined mass (*arrows*) in the right hepatic lobe. (**e, f**) Coronal MR cholangiopancreatography (MRCP) and frontal ERCP images show dilation of the central intrahepatic ducts (*arrows*) and attenuation of the ducts as they approach the hilum (*arrowheads*)

thrombus [60]. The periductal infiltrating form of the tumor may have a small mass-like lesion or diffuse bile duct thickening. Diffuse periductal thickening and enhancement may also be present, with irregular narrowed ducts and/or ductal dilation [60]. The intraductal form has diffuse duct ectasia with an intraductal mass which enhances or a more focal stricture-like lesion with proximal ductal dilation [60].

Treatment of cholangiocarcinoma usually entails surgical resection and systemic chemotherapy.

Traumatic Bile Duct and Gallbladder Disorder

Bile Leak Bile leaks may occur in the setting of abdominal trauma or as a complication of surgical intervention. Because of the insulating effect of the liver, isolated bile leaks are rare with abdominal trauma but often occur with injuries from abrupt deceleration such as motor vehicle collision or from traumatic hepatic elevation and stretching of the common bile duct [61–63]. The injury commonly occurs at a sight of anatomic fixation like the intrapancreatic portion of the common bile duct. Substantial liver lacerations can also injure intrahepatic ducts leading to bile leakage (Fig. 8.14).

Iatrogenic leaks have been associated with multiple procedures including open or laparoscopic cholecystectomy, liver transplantation, partial hepatic resection, or liver biopsy [64, 65]. Slippage of the cystic duct clip or ligature and misidentification of biliary anatomy, sometimes in the setting of an accessory or anomalous duct, are the most common causes of leak following laparoscopic cholecystectomy [66, 67]. Risk factors for iatrogenic bile leak include intrahepatic position of the gallbladder, anomalous anatomy, or chronic inflammatory changes of cholecystitis with friable or adherent gallbladder [63]. Biliary leaks may also be seen with manipulation or migration of external drainage tubes or at the sites of choledochocholedochostomy following liver transplantation or hepaticojejunostomy [63, 68]. Bile leaks are often manifested within 7 days of surgery with nonspecific clinical symptoms such as abdominal pain, anorexia, and malaise [63]. The resultant bilomas are at risk of becoming superinfected and affected patients may present with infectious symptoms.

MR imaging can be useful tool in evaluating suspected bile leaks in the pediatric population. The combination of MRCP images with traditional MR images with the use of hepatobiliary contrast agents provide a dynamic anatomic evaluation of the biliary system (including biliary-enteric anastomoses) and have been demonstrated to increase diagnostic accuracy in leak site localization when compared to

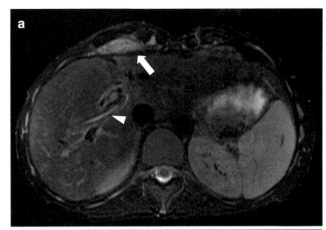

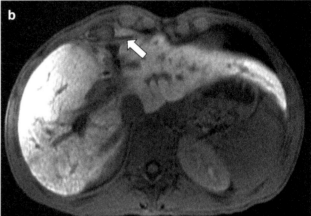

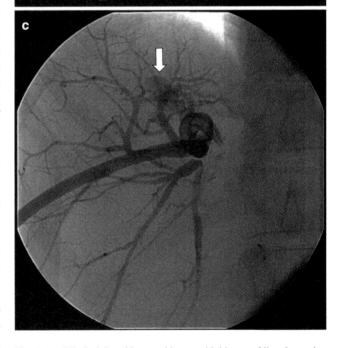

Fig. 8.14 Bile leak in a 20-year-old man with history of liver laceration from motocross accident. (**a**) Axial T2-weighted fat-suppressed MR image shows a hyperintense fluid collection (*arrow*) anterior to the liver. Partially visualized drainage catheter (*arrowhead*) is also present. (**b**) Axial 20-minute delayed T1-weighted fat-suppressed MR image with hepatobiliary contrast shows contrast pooling in the fluid collection (*arrow*) anterior to the liver proving a connection to the biliary tree. (**c**) Frontal projection fluoroscopic image from cholangiogram via the patient's drain shows an irregular ovoid focus of contrast (*arrow*) that connects to the biliary tree

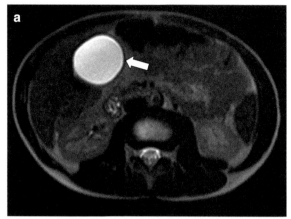

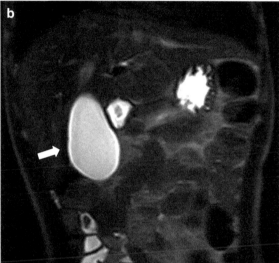

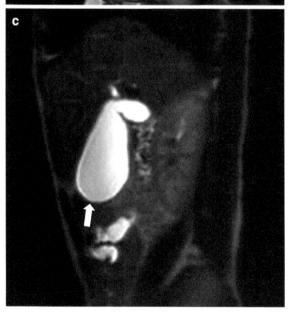

Fig. 8.15 Gallbladder hydrops in a 10-year-old boy with a history of inflammatory bowel disease and elevated transaminase levels. (**a**) Axial T2-weighted MR image without fat suppression shows an enlarged, dilated, and fluid-filled gallbladder (*arrow*). Note: no associated inflammatory changes are present. (**b, c**) Coronal and sagittal single-shot T2-weighted MR images show an enlarged and dilated gallbladder (*arrows*) extending inferior to the margin of the liver to nearly the level of the inferior pole of the right kidney

traditional MRCP [69]. It can also help in differentiating biliary versus non-biliary fluid collections with a high sensitivity and specificity [63, 70]. These are obvious advantages to ERCP or scintigraphy.

Small, asymptomatic bilomas tend to resolve spontaneously, while larger collections often require percutaneous drainage [63]. Surgical intervention or revision may be needed to correct large leaks or if prior ERCP attempts are unsuccessful.

Miscellaneous Bile Duct and Gallbladder Disorder

Gallbladder Hydrops Hydrops of the gallbladder is characterized as abnormal dilation of the gallbladder thought to be secondary to transient or chronic cholestasis and obstruction of the cystic duct. This leads to sterile accumulation of mucin and dilation of the gallbladder which can extend inferiorly below the liver edge into the pelvis. It may be associated with a preceding infection, most notably Kawasaki disease, or parenteral nutrition [30]. Gallbladder hydrops typically presents between the ages of 17 months and 7 years of age and is more common in males [71]. Affected patients may present with a palpable right sided mass, abdominal pain, jaundice, or vomiting [71].

On MR imaging, the gallbladder appears dilated and lengthened and may lose its normal contours (Fig. 8.15) in the setting of gallbladder hydrops. The gallbladder should be without wall thickening or other inflammatory findings. The remainder of the biliary tree should appear normal. In infants, a normal gallbladder length is 1.5–3 cm (<1 year of age), and 3–7 cm in older children [30, 72].

Typically, gallbladder hydrops resolves with conservative therapy; however, perforation of the gallbladder has been reported in patients with Kawasaki disease [30, 72].

Conclusion

Disorders involving the gallbladder and bile duct are not uncommon in infants and children. Although ultrasound is typically the first-line imaging modality, MR imaging, which is a powerful tool to evaluate the gallbladder and biliary ducts in pediatric patients, can be also utilized. MR imaging, particularly MRCP and use of hepatobiliary contrast agents, can provide excellent noninvasive anatomic visualization and evaluation as well as can help in the diagnosis and management of congenital and acquired biliary disease processes in the pediatric population.

References

1. Chavhan GB, Shelmerdine S, Jhaveri K, Babyn PS. Liver MR imaging in children: current concepts and technique. Radiographics. 2016;36(5):1517–32.

2. Antonov NK, Ruzal-Shapiro CB, Morel KD, Millar WS, Kashyap S, Lauren CT, et al. Feed and wrap MRI technique in infants. Clin Pediatr. 2017;56(12):1095–103.

3. Mitchell CL, Vasanawala SS. An approach to pediatric liver MRI. AJR Am J Roentgenol. 2011;196(5):W519–26.

4. Glockner JF. Hepatobiliary MRI: current concepts and controversies. J Magn Reson Imaging. 2007;25(4):681–95.

5. Vitellas KM, Keogan MT, Spritzer CE, Nelson RC. MR cholangiopancreatography of bile and pancreatic duct abnormalities with emphasis on the single-shot fast spin-echo technique. Radiographics. 2000;20(4):939–57; quiz 1107-8, 12.

6. Chavhan GB, Babyn PS, Manson D, Vidarsson L. Pediatric MR cholangiopancreatography: principles, technique, and clinical applications. Radiographics. 2008;28(7):1951–62.

7. Delaney L, Applegate KE, Karmazyn B, Akisik MF, Jennings SG. MR cholangiopancreatography in children: feasibility, safety, and initial experience. Pediatr Radiol. 2008;38(1):64–75.

8. Tipnis NA, Dua KS, Werlin SL. A retrospective assessment of magnetic resonance cholangiopancreatography in children. J Pediatr Gastroenterol Nutr. 2008;46(1):59–64.

9. Tipnis NA, Werlin SL. The use of magnetic resonance cholangiopancreatography in children. Curr Gastroenterol Rep. 2007;9(3):225–9.

10. Fitoz S, Erden A, Boruban S. Magnetic resonance cholangiopancreatography of biliary system abnormalities in children. Clin Imaging. 2007;31(2):93–101.

11. Shimizu T, Suzuki R, Yamashiro Y, Segawa O, Yamataka A, Kuwatsuru R. Magnetic resonance cholangiopancreatography in assessing the cause of acute pancreatitis in children. Pancreas. 2001;22(2):196–9.

12. Suzuki M, Shimizu T, Kudo T, Suzuki R, Ohtsuka Y, Yamashiro Y, et al. Usefulness of nonbreath-hold 1-shot magnetic resonance cholangiopancreatography for the evaluation of choledochal cyst in children. J Pediatr Gastroenterol Nutr. 2006;42(5):539–44.

13. Trout AT, Podberesky DJ, Serai SD, Ren Y, Altaye M, Towbin AJ. Does secretin add value in pediatric magnetic resonance cholangiopancreatography? Pediatr Radiol. 2013;43(4):479–86.

14. Trout AT, Wallihan DB, Serai S, Abu-El-Haija M. Secretin-enhanced magnetic resonance cholangiopancreatography for assessing pancreatic secretory function in children. J Pediatr. 2017;188:186–91.

15. Courtier J, Rao AG, Anupindi SA. Advanced imaging techniques in pediatric body MRI. Pediatr Radiol. 2017;47(5):522–33.

16. Yeh BM, Liu PS, Soto JA, Corvera CA, Hussain HK. MR imaging and CT of the biliary tract. Radiographics. 2009;29(6):1669–88.

17. Fidler J, Hough D. Hepatocyte-specific magnetic resonance imaging contrast agents. Hepatology (Baltimore, Md). 2011;53(2):678–82.

18. Bremer JL. Description of a 4 mm human embryo. Am J Anat. 1906;5:459–80.

19. Ando H. Embryology of the biliary tract. Dig Surg. 2010;27(2):87–9.

20. Catalano OA, Sahani DV, Kalva SP, Cushing MS, Hahn PF, Brown JJ, et al. MR imaging of the gallbladder: a pictorial essay. Radiographics. 2008;28(1):135–55; quiz 324.

21. Choi JW, Kim TK, Kim KW, Kim AY, Kim PN, Ha HK, et al. Anatomic variation in intrahepatic bile ducts: an analysis of intraoperative cholangiograms in 300 consecutive donors for living donor liver transplantation. Korean J Radiol. 2003;4(2):85–90.

22. Mortele KJ, Ros PR. Anatomic variants of the biliary tree: MR cholangiographic findings and clinical applications. AJR Am J Roentgenol. 2001;177(2):389–94.

23. Han SJ, Kim MJ, Han A, Chung KS, Yoon CS, Kim D, et al. Magnetic resonance cholangiography for the diagnosis of biliary atresia. J Pediatr Surg. 2002;37(4):599–604.

24. Jaw TS, Kuo YT, Liu GC, Chen SH, Wang CK. MR cholangiography in the evaluation of neonatal cholestasis. Radiology. 1999;212(1):249–56.

25. Lev-Toaff AS, Bach AM, Wechsler RJ, Hilpert PL, Gatalica Z, Rubin R. The radiologic and pathologic spectrum of biliary hamartomas. AJR Am J Roentgenol. 1995;165(2):309–13.

26. Zheng RQ, Zhang B, Kudo M, Onda H, Inoue T. Imaging findings of biliary hamartomas. World J Gastroenterol. 2005;11(40):6354–9.

27. Wohlgemuth WA, Bottger J, Bohndorf K. MRI, CT, US and ERCP in the evaluation of bile duct hamartomas (von Meyenburg complex): a case report. Eur Radiol. 1998;8(9):1623–6.

28. Bornfors M. The development of cholangiocarcinoma from multiple bile-duct adenomas. Report of a case and review of the literature. Acta Pathol Microbiol Immunol Scand A. 1984;92(4):285–9.

29. Horton KM, Bluemke DA, Hruban RH, Soyer P, Fishman EK. CT and MR imaging of benign hepatic and biliary tumors. Radiographics. 1999;19(2):431–51.

30. Knowlton JQ, Lowe LH. Chapter 88: congenital hepatobiliar anomalies; Reading BD, Lowe LH. Chapter 89: acquired biliary tract disease. In: Coley BD, Bates DG, Faerber EN, Hernanz-Schulman M, Kan H, Lee EY, Panigrahy A, Rigsby C, editors. Caffey's pediatric diagnostic imaging. 12th ed. Philadelphia: Elsevier. p. 906–20.

31. Kim OH, Chung HJ, Choi BG. Imaging of the choledochal cyst. Radiographics. 1995;15(1):69–88.

32. Wiedmeyer DA, Stewart ET, Dodds WJ, Geenen JE, Vennes JA, Taylor AJ. Choledochal cyst: findings on cholangiopancreatography with emphasis on ectasia of the common channel. AJR Am J Roentgenol. 1989;153(5):969–72.

33. Brancatelli G, Federle MP, Vilgrain V, Vullierme MP, Marin D, Lagalla R. Fibropolycystic liver disease: CT and MR imaging findings. Radiographics. 2005;25(3):659–70.

34. de Vries JS, de Vries S, Aronson DC, Bosman DK, Rauws EA, Bosma A, et al. Choledochal cysts: age of presentation, symptoms, and late complications related to Todani's classification. J Pediatr Surg. 2002;37(11):1568–73.

35. Lazaridis KN, Gores GJ. Cholangiocarcinoma. Gastroenterology. 2005;128(6):1655–67.

36. Zheng LX, Jia HB, Wu DQ, Shang H, Zhong XY, Wang QS, et al. Experience of congenital choledochal cyst in adults:treatment, surgical procedures and clinical outcome in the Second Affiliated Hospital of Harbin Medical University. J Korean Med Sci. 2004;19(6):842–7.

37. Watanabe Y, Toki A, Todani T. Bile duct cancer developed after cyst excision for choledochal cyst. J Hepato-Biliary-Pancreat Surg. 1999;6(3):207–12.

38. Gubernick JA, Rosenberg HK, Ilaslan H, Kessler A. US approach to jaundice in infants and children. Radiographics. 2000;20(1):173–95.

39. Carneiro RC, Fordham LA, Semelka RC. MR imaging of the pediatric liver. Magn Reson Imaging Clin N Am. 2002;10(1):137–64.

40. Todani T, Watanabe Y, Narusue M, Tabuchi K, Okajima K. Congenital bile duct cysts: classification, operative procedures, and review of thirty-seven cases including cancer arising from choledochal cyst. Am J Surg. 1977;134(2):263–9.

41. Jung G, Benz-Bohm G, Kugel H, Keller KM, Querfeld U. MR cholangiography in children with autosomal recessive polycystic kidney disease. Pediatr Radiol. 1999;29(6):463–6.

42. Boyden EA. The accessory gallbladder: an embryological and comparative study of aberrant biliary vesicles occurring in man and the domestic mammals. Am J Anat. 1926;38:177–231.

43. Lamah M, Karanjia ND, Dickson GH. Anatomical variations of the extrahepatic biliary tree: review of the world literature. Clin Anat. 2001;14(3):167–72.

44. Kothari PR, Kumar T, Jiwane A, Paul S, Kutumbale R, Kulkarni B. Unusual features of gall bladder duplication cyst with review of the literature. Pediatr Surg Int. 2005;21(7):552–4.

45. Desolneux G, Mucci S, Lebigot J, Arnaud JP, Hamy A. Duplication of the gallbladder. A case report. Gastroenterol Res Pract. 2009;2009:483473.

46. Horattas MC. Gallbladder duplication and laparoscopic management. J Laparoendosc Adv Surg Tech A. 1998;8(4):231–5.

47. Gigot J, Van Beers B, Goncette L, Etienne J, Collard A, Jadoul P, et al. Laparoscopic treatment of gallbladder duplication. A plea for removal of both gallbladders. Surg Endosc. 1997;11(5):479–82.

48. Tsakayannis DE, Kozakewich HP, Lillehei CW. Acalculous cholecystitis in children. J Pediatr Surg. 1996;31(1):127–30; discussion 30-1.

49. Barie PS, Fischer E. Acute acalculous cholecystitis. J Am Coll Surg. 1995;180(2):232–44.

50. Watanabe Y, Nagayama M, Okumura A, Amoh Y, Katsube T, Suga T, et al. MR imaging of acute biliary disorders. Radiographics. 2007;27(2):477–95.

51. Watanabe Y, Dohke M, Ishimori T, Amoh Y, Oda K, Okumura A, et al. High-resolution MR cholangiopancreatography. Crit Rev Diagn Imaging. 1998;39(2–3):115–258.

52. Kim KW, Park MS, Yu JS, Chung JP, Ryu YH, Lee SI, et al. Acute cholecystitis at T2-weighted and manganese-enhanced T1-weighted MR cholangiography: preliminary study. Radiology. 2003;227(2):580–4.

53. Guarise A, Baltieri S, Mainardi P, Faccioli N. Diagnostic accuracy of MRCP in choledocholithiasis. Radiol Med. 2005;109(3):239–51.

54. Arcement CM, Meza MP, Arumanla S, Towbin RB. MRCP in the evaluation of pancreaticobiliary disease in children. Pediatr Radiol. 2001;31(2):92–7.

55. Feldstein AE, Perrault J, El-Youssif M, Lindor KD, Freese DK, Angulo P. Primary sclerosing cholangitis in children: a long-term follow-up study. Hepatology. 2003;38(1):210–7.

56. Sisto A, Feldman P, Garel L, Seidman E, Brochu P, Morin CL, et al. Primary sclerosing cholangitis in children: study of five cases and review of the literature. Pediatrics. 1987;80(6):918–23.

57. Ferrara C, Valeri G, Salvolini L, Giovagnoni A. Magnetic resonance cholangiopancreatography in primary sclerosing cholangitis in children. Pediatr Radiol. 2002;32(6):413–7.

58. Debray D, Pariente D, Urvoas E, Hadchouel M, Bernard O. Sclerosing cholangitis in children. J Pediatr. 1994;124(1):49–56.

59. Ibrahim SH, Lindor KD. Current management of primary sclerosing cholangitis in pediatric patients. Paediatr Drugs. 2011;13(2):87–95.

60. Chung YE, Kim MJ, Park YN, Choi JY, Pyo JY, Kim YC, et al. Varying appearances of cholangiocarcinoma: radiologic-pathologic correlation. Radiographics. 2009;29(3):683–700.

61. Gupta A, Stuhlfaut JW, Fleming KW, Lucey BC, Soto JA. Blunt trauma of the pancreas and biliary tract: a multimodality imaging approach to diagnosis. Radiographics. 2004;24(5):1381–95.

62. Wittenberg A, Minotti AJ. CT diagnosis of traumatic gallbladder injury. AJR Am J Roentgenol. 2005;185(6):1573–4.

63. Melamud K, LeBedis CA, Anderson SW, Soto JA. Biliary imaging: multimodality approach to imaging of biliary injuries and their complications. Radiographics. 2014;34(3):613–23.

64. Zimmitti G, Roses RE, Andreou A, Shindoh J, Curley SA, Aloia TA, et al. Greater complexity of liver surgery is not associated with an increased incidence of liver-related complications except for bile leak: an experience with 2,628 consecutive resections. J Gastrointest Surg. 2013;17(1):57–64; discussion p.-5.

65. Kapoor V, Baron RL, Peterson MS. Bile leaks after surgery. AJR Am J Roentgenol. 2004;182(2):451–8.

66. Hoeffel C, Azizi L, Lewin M, Laurent V, Aube C, Arrive L, et al. Normal and pathologic features of the postoperative biliary tract at 3D MR cholangiopancreatography and MR imaging. Radiographics. 2006;26(6):1603–20.

67. Valek V, Kala Z, Kysela P. Biliary tree and cholecyst: post surgery imaging. Eur J Radiol. 2005;53(3):433–40.

68. Ernst O, Sergent G, Mizrahi D, Delemazure O, L'Hermine C. Biliary leaks: treatment by means of percutaneous transhepatic biliary drainage. Radiology. 1999;211(2):345–8.

69. Kantarci M, Pirimoglu B, Karabulut N, Bayraktutan U, Ogul H, Ozturk G, et al. Non-invasive detection of biliary leaks using Gd-EOB-DTPA-enhanced MR cholangiography: comparison with T2-weighted MR cholangiography. Eur Radiol. 2013;23(10):2713–22.

70. Aduna M, Larena JA, Martin D, Martinez-Guerenu B, Aguirre I, Astigarraga E. Bile duct leaks after laparoscopic cholecystectomy: value of contrast-enhanced MRCP. Abdom Imaging. 2005;30(4):480–7.

71. Egritas O, Nacar N, Hanioglu S, Soyer T, Tezic T. Early but prolonged gallbladder hydrops in a 7-month-old girl with Kawasaki syndrome: report of a case. Surg Today. 2007;37(2):162–4.

72. Suddleson EA, Reid B, Woolley MM, Takahashi M. Hydrops of the gallbladder associated with Kawasaki syndrome. J Pediatr Surg. 1987;22(10):956–9.

Pancreas

Monica Johnson, Sudha A. Anupindi, and Michael S. Gee

Introduction

The discovery of the pancreas is attributed to the ancient Greek physician Herophilus (335–380 BC). Unlike other larger abdominal organs, such as the liver, the pancreas was largely ignored in early medicine, relegated as a "cushion of the stomach and pad supporting the vessels" [1]. In 1642, the German surgeon Johann Georg Wirsung discovered the main pancreatic duct, and subsequent experiments established that the pancreas was a complex and essential organ whose dysfunction could lead to illness and death [1]. Today, the pancreas is known to serve vital roles in the both the digestive and endocrine systems. Pancreatic disease has a lower incidence in children compared to adults, but pathologies such as pancreatitis have been increasing in the pediatric population and are associated with significant morbidity and mortality [2].

Diagnostic imaging plays an important role in evaluating pancreatic disorders in children and adolescents. Ultrasound and magnetic resonance (MR) imaging are preferred modalities over computed tomography (CT), in large part because both methods avoid ionizing radiation. MR imaging, in particular, offers additional advantages including multiplanar imaging capability and superior soft tissue contrast. Technologic advancements have made diagnostic-quality MR imaging examinations faster and more feasible for pediatric patients.

The adept radiologist should be familiar with the normal development of the pancreas and the various manifestations

of disease that are seen in and often unique to children. Some pathologies (e.g., acute pancreatitis) are similar in imaging appearance to their adult counterparts, but often have different etiologies. Meanwhile, some congenital anomalies and certain neoplasms are almost exclusively seen in children.

The overarching goal of this chapter is to discuss the up-to-date and fundamental basics of pediatric pancreatic MR imaging protocols, the normal and abnormal development of the pancreas, and MR imaging features of pancreatic disorders in the pediatric population.

Magentic Resonance Imaging Techniques

In recent years, MR imaging has become increasingly useful for evaluating pancreatitis and pancreatic tumors in the pediatric population. The superior soft tissue contrast and its ability to image the pancreas in multiple contrast-enhanced phases make MR imaging ideally suited to evaluating both diffuse and focal pancreatic pathology. MR cholangiopancreatography (MRCP) is a specialized MR imaging technique that provides excellent noninvasive evaluation of the pancreaticobiliary tree and often serves as an imaging alternative to endoscopic retrograde cholangiopancreatography (ERCP), which is invasive and often requires general anesthesia when performed in the pediatric population. Secretin is a hormone that is produced by the duodenum and stimulates pancreatic exocrine secretion. Synthetic secretin-enhanced MRCP is a technique that improves sensitivity for visualizing pancreatic duct abnormalities due to secretin-induced ductal dilation [3]. Pancreatic exocrine function can also be assessed by secretin MRCP by visualizing or quantifying secretin-induced duodenal fluid [3].

Patient Preparation

As with all pediatric studies, MR imaging of the pancreas should be tailored to the clinical question and the patient's

M. Johnson (✉)
Department of Radiology, Massachusetts General Hospital, Harvard Medical School, Boston, MA, USA
e-mail: mjohnson86@partners.org

S. A. Anupindi
Department of Radiology, The Children's Hospital of Philadelphia, Perelman School of Medicine, University of Pennsylvania, Philadelphia, PA, USA

M. S. Gee
Division of Pediatric Imaging, Department of Radiology, Massachusetts General Hospital, Harvard Medical School, Boston, MA, USA

age, size, and ability to cooperate. MR imaging of the pancreas is challenging in young children because of potential image quality degradation from respiratory motion and patient movements. During the examination, child life specialists, engagement and education of patients and families, and distraction techniques like music and video goggles can help relax pediatric patients and decrease motion artifacts [4]. These environmental factors and faster MR imaging sequences often reduce the need for anesthesia, thus making examinations faster and safer for pediatric patients. Deep sedation or general anesthesia may be required, particularly for young children between 6 months and 6 years of age [4].

No specific patient preparation is required for pancreatic MR imaging, although fasting 3–5 hours before an MRCP is beneficial to empty the stomach, decrease bowel motility, and fully distend the gallbladder and biliary tree [2]. Secretin, if used, is administered using a weight-based protocol at a dose of 0.2 mg/kg as a slow infusion over 1 minute [3]. Negative oral contrast agents that decrease the signal inten-

sity of stomach and duodenal contents on T2-weighted images can also improve visualization of the pancreatic duct and ampulla on MRCP [2]. Pediatric patients who require sedation or anesthesia for MR imaging needs to adhere to institutional specific guidelines for NPO (nothing per oral) status to minimize the risk of aspiration.

MR Imaging Pulse Sequences and Protocols

The pancreas is intrinsically hyperintense on T1-weighted images due the high amounts of protein and paramagnetic ions (e.g., manganese) within pancreatic cells [5]. Therefore, the pancreas is well-evaluated on T1-weighted fat-suppressed images, even in the absence of intravenous contrast. Most pancreatic parenchymal abnormalities result in low signal intensity on T1-weighted fat-suppressed images. The normal pancreas enhances avidly on arterial and venous phases and appears similar to the liver on delayed imaging (Fig. 9.1).

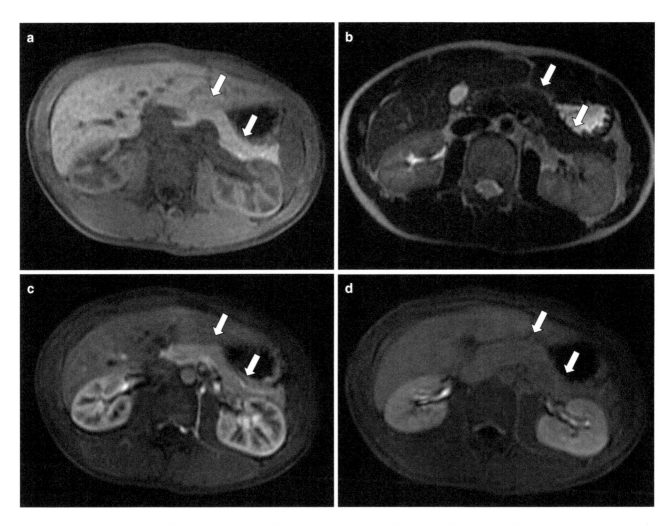

Fig. 9.1 Normal pancreas in a 13-year-old boy. Axial T1-weighted MR image (**a**) shows a uniformly hyperintense pancreas *(arrows)*. T2 signal intensity is uniform and similar to the liver on the axial single-shot image (**b**, *arrows*). Post-contrast, the pancreas demonstrates early arterial enhancement (**c**, *arrows*) and appears similar in intensity to the liver on delayed imaging (**d**, *arrows*)

Unlike adult exams, pediatric MR imaging must be tailored to the size of the patient and may require a reduced field of view and smaller slice thickness. MR imaging of the pancreas is usually performed using a multi-channel phased-array cardiac or body coil, depending on the size of the child. The smallest coil that fits the anatomic region should be used, as this permits a smaller field of view and better resolution [6].

The standard pediatric pancreatic protocol includes T1-weighted in- and opposed-phase breath-hold and T2-weighted fat-suppressed fast-spin echo respiratory-triggered sequences to evaluate the pancreas and adjacent abdominal organs. Volumetric T1-weighted fat-suppressed gradient echo sequences can be acquired in a single breath-hold acquisition (10–20 seconds) and are helpful for evaluating the pancreatic parenchyma for both focal and diffuse abnormalities [2]. This same sequence (also known as VIBE/LAVA/eTHRIVE) can be used for multi-phase post-contrast evaluation of the pancreas, which increases sensitivity for detecting subtle pancreatic lesions, pancreatic vascularity in cases of suspected necrosis in the setting of pancreatitis, and peripancreatic inflammatory changes [7]. Signal averaging is often used for T1-weighted sequences in infants and young children who are unable to suspend respiration. Additional sequences in a pancreatic MR imaging protocol include balanced steady-state free precession (bSSFP) sequences that provide excellent visualization of peripancreatic inflammatory changes, as well as diffusion-weighted imaging (DWI) with B-values up to 800–1000 s/mm^2 that are useful for focal lesion detection as well as abscesses associated with pancreatitis [7, 8].

The optimal timing for pancreatic evaluation is late arterial (35–55 seconds post-injection), as the pancreaticoduodenal arteries are end branches of the celiac and superior mesenteric arteries. Additional post-contrast imaging time points include portal venous (60–70 seconds) and delayed venous (2–3 minutes) phases [2, 6].

MRCP consists of a heavily T2-weighted pulse sequence with a long echo time (TE range 500–1000 ms), which increases the conspicuity of bile in the pancreaticobiliary tree while suppressing background signal from soft tissues and vascular structures. Typically, MRCP is a 3D volumetric fast-spin echo sequence, acquired with respiratory triggering in the coronal oblique plane, designed to view the pancreatic duct in its entirety. In secretin MRCP, coronal oblique single-shot T2-weighted images that include the entire pancreatic duct are acquired every 30–60 seconds after secretin administration for a period of 5–10 minutes, with peak pancreatic duct dilatation typically occurring at 3–5 minutes [9]. In children who are breathing fast or irregularly, MRCP image quality can be degraded and thick-slab single-shot T2-weighted imaging can be performed instead to freeze motion [7].

Non-Cartesian radial pulse sequences can also be used to reduce respiratory motion artifacts on T2-weighted and T1-weighted fat-suppressed post-contrast imaging [7, 10]. In these sequences, in-plane K-space is acquired in a spoke-wheel fashion, which leads to oversampling of the center and undersampling of the periphery of K-space. Oversampling the center of k-space, which encodes for image contrast, results in high signal-to-noise and contrast-to-noise ratios. Because the phase-encoding direction shifts with the rotating lines of radial k-space acquisition, respiratory motion is dispersed over multiple axes, leading to less reduction in visual image quality compared with standard Cartesian sequences [7]. These sequences are particularly helpful for young children who are unable to suspend respiration.

Anatomy

Embryology

The pancreas emerges at approximately 3–4 weeks gestation [11]. Pancreatic development begins with formation of ventral and dorsal pancreatic buds or anlagen (Fig. 9.2a), which originate from the endodermal lining of the duodenum. The dorsal pancreatic bud or anlage forms below the greater curvature of the stomach, eventually becoming the neck, body, and tail of the pancreas. At the same time, the ventral bud becomes the head and uncinate process. The dorsal bud initially drains into the dorsal duct of Santorini and then into the minor papilla of the duodenum, above the insertion site of the common bile duct (CBD). The ventral bud is drained by the ventral duct of Wirsung into the major papilla of the duodenum, at the same level as the CBD [12].

At about 7 weeks gestation, the stomach and duodenum rotate, pulling the ventral bud posteriorly and inferiorly, while the dorsal bud moves anteriorly and superiorly, resulting in the final position of the pancreas (Fig. 9.2b). The ventral and dorsal ducts fuse in the pancreatic head [11].

Normal Development and Anatomy

The pancreas is a retroperitoneal organ, located posterior to the lesser sac (Fig. 9.3). The pancreas is divided into the head, uncinate process, neck, body, and tail. The head is the thickest part of the pancreas, surrounded by the duodenum, and to the right of the superior mesenteric artery (SMA) and superior mesenteric vein (SMV). The uncinate process emerges from the back of the pancreatic head, posterior to the SMA and SMV. The neck, between the head and body, is the thinnest part of the pancreas and lies in front of the SMA and SMV, anterior to the portosplenic confluence. The body is the largest portion. The tail abuts the splenic hilum.

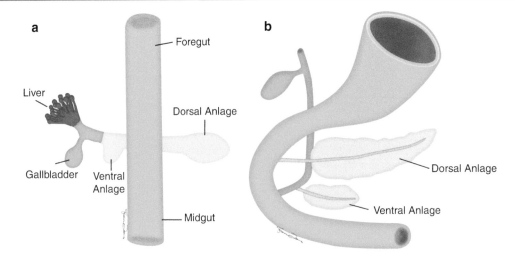

Fig. 9.2 Early development of the pancreas. At approximately 3–4 weeks gestation (**a**), the ventral and dorsal anlagen or buds develop from the endodermal lining of the duodenum, which arises at the junction between the foregut and midgut. At about 7 weeks gestation (**b**), the stomach and duodenum rotate, pulling the ventral anlage posteriorly and inferiorly, and the dorsal bud anteriorly and superiorly. (Images: Susanne L. Loomis, MS, FBCA; Department of Radiology, Massachusetts General Hospital, Boston, Massachusetts, USA)

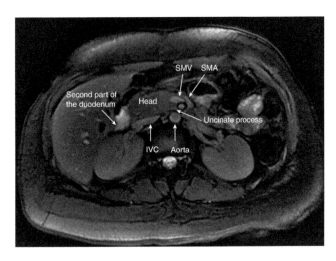

Fig. 9.3 Normal MR imaging pancreatic anatomy in a 16-year-old girl. Normal appearance of the pancreatic head, uncinate process, and surrounding structures (*labeled*). The pancreatic body and tail are not visualized on this image. SMV, superior mesenteric vein; SMA, superior mesenteric artery; IVC, inferior vena cava

The pancreas has both endocrine and exocrine functions. The endocrine glands are composed of discrete units called islets of Langerhans, which secrete hormones, including insulin, glucagon, somatostatin. The exocrine glands, a network of acinar cells, secrete pancreatic fluid into the duodenum via the pancreatic duct; bicarbonate neutralizes gastric acid and enzymes aid with digestion [11, 12].

Anatomic Variants

Anatomic anomalies of the pancreas arise due to failed fusion of the ventral and dorsal buds or abnormal rotation.

Often, these are incidental discoveries in asymptomatic pediatric patients. However, it is important to recognize these structural anomalies as some lead to pathology, such as recurrent pancreatitis or duodenal obstruction, and may require surgical correction. MRCP demonstrates the course and drainage pattern of the pancreatic duct and is helpful in diagnosing developmental anomalies. In recent years, MRCP has replaced ERCP as the primary diagnostic tool for evaluating pancreatic ductal anatomy in pediatric patients.

Pancreas Divisum Pancreas divisum is the most common congenital pancreatic abnormality, seen in about 10% of the population [13]. It is caused by non-fusion of the ventral and dorsal pancreatic ducts, which retain their primitive drainage patterns (Fig. 9.4). This is identified on MRCP by the "crossing" sign, when the common bile duct crosses the dorsal pancreatic duct as it courses to join the ventral duct [12].

In complete pancreas divisum, the main (dorsal) pancreatic duct drains into the minor papilla without communicating with the ventral duct (Fig. 9.5). Complete pancreas divisum may be a cause of recurrent pancreatitis in pediatric patients. In incomplete divisum, some communication remains between the dorsal and ventral ducts [12]. Incomplete pancreas divisum is considered a normal anatomic variant and not associated with pathology [13].

Annular Pancreas Annular pancreas is rare and occurs when the ventral bud does not fully rotate and a part of the pancreas wraps around the second portion of duodenum [11] (Fig. 9.6). There are two types of annular pancreas: extramural and intramural. In the extramural type, the ventral duct encircles the duodenum and joins the main duct. This presents with duodenal obstruction in infancy and is one etiology of the classic "double-bubble" sign in neonates. In the intramural type, pan-

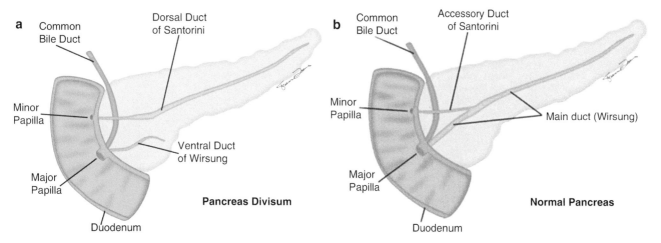

Fig. 9.4 Pancreas divisum anatomy. In pancreas divisum (a), the ventral and dorsal ducts do not fuse, retaining their early drainage patterns. The normal drainage pattern is shown as comparison (b). (Images: Susanne L. Loomis, MS, FBCA; Department of Radiology, Massachusetts General Hospital, Boston, Massachusetts, USA)

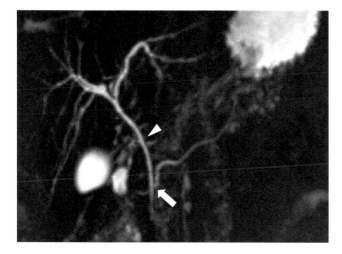

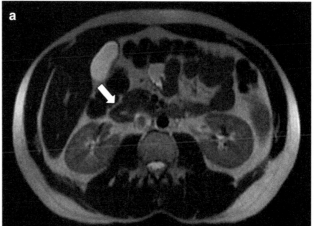

Fig. 9.5 Pancreas divisum in an 18-year-old female with ulcerative colitis and primary sclerosing cholangitis. 3D thick maximum intensity projection MR image demonstrates the crossing sign of pancreas divisum. The main pancreatic duct (*arrow*) crosses over the common bile duct (*arrowhead*) into drains into the minor papilla via the dorsal duct of Santorini. Note the additional beading of the intrahepatic bile ducts, characteristic of primary sclerosing cholangitis

creatic tissue is within the walls of the duodenum, and small ducts drain directly into the duodenum. These children may present with peptic ulcer disease, without duodenal obstruction [12]. One-half to two-thirds of all patients with annular pancreas are asymptomatic [14].

Pancreatic Agenesis and Hypoplasia (Congenital Short Pancreas) Complete agenesis of the pancreas is rare and lethal. Partial agenesis is still very rare but compatible with life and usually involves the dorsal rather than ventral pancreas. In dorsal agenesis or hypoplasia, the pancreatic head appears enlarged and widened, with a partially or completely absent pancreatic body and tail [12] (Fig. 9.7). Patients with dorsal pancreatic agenesis are at risk of developing abdomi-

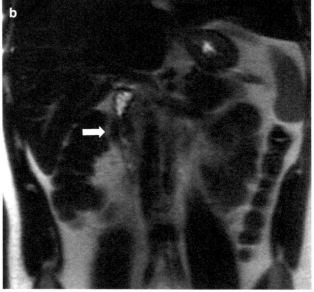

Fig. 9.6 Annular pancreas in an asymptomatic 16-year-old boy. Axial (a) and coronal (b) single-shot T2-weighted MR images show the pancreas (*arrows*) wrapped around the second portion of the duodenum. A small amount of fluid is seen in the distended duodenum proximal to the annulus

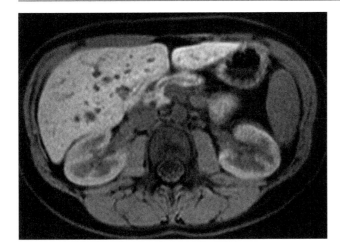

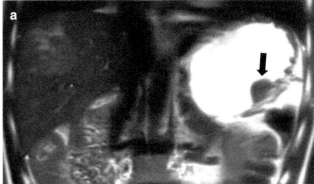

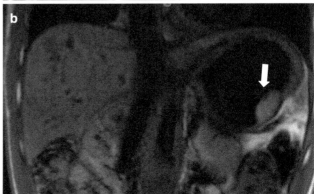

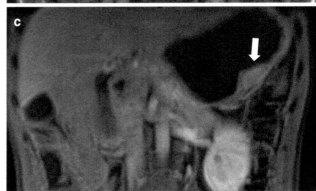

Fig. 9.7 Dorsal agenesis of the pancreas in an asymptomatic 17-year-old girl. Axial T1-weighted fat-suppressed MR image demonstrates the dorsal pancreas is truncated, with an absent pancreatic tail. The main pancreatic duct is mildly prominent

nal pain, hypoglycemia, and pancreatitis related to problems with pancreatic drainage [15].

Ectopic Pancreas Residual primitive cells from the ventral and dorsal buds can migrate to nearby structures and mature, leading to ectopic pancreatic tissue in locations such as the gastric antrum or duodenum (Fig. 9.8). Ectopic pancreatic tissue is subject to the same inflammatory and neoplastic processes affecting the orthotropic pancreas. Rarely, cystic dystrophy can occur, which represents cystic dilatation of the ectopic ducts and occurs most often in the second portion of the duodenum [12, 13].

Intrapancreatic Splenic Tissue Accessory spleens, or splenules, are congenital foci of normal splenic tissue separate from the main spleen. These are distinguished from splenosis, which is autotransplantation of splenic tissue, usually after splenectomy or trauma. The tail of the pancreas is the second most common site of an accessory spleen (the splenic hilum is the most common location). This is usually an incidental finding on CT or MR imaging and is important not to mistake for a mass. The accessory spleen typically has the same signal characteristics as the spleen on all MR pulse sequences (Fig. 9.9) [12].

Pancreatic Cyst A true congenital pancreatic cyst is very rare. As opposed to cystic dilatation of the pancreatic duct or pseudocysts, true pancreatic cysts are lined by epithelium and do not communicate with the pancreatic ducts. These may be idiopathic or associated with systemic diseases like von Hippel-Lindau disease, Beckwith-Wiedemann syndrome, or polycystic kidney disease [12].

Fig. 9.8 Ectopic pancreas in a 17-year-old girl with abdominal pain and vomiting. Coronal single-shot T2-weighted (**a**) and T1-weighted fat-suppressed pre- (**b**) and post-contrast (**c**) MR images demonstrate a T2-weighted hypointense, T1-weighted hyperintense, mildly enhancing lesion (*arrows*) in the stomach. The lesion consistent with ectopic pancreas on biopsy. Incidental note is made of a hepatic mass found to be a focal nodular hyperplasia

Spectrum of Pancreatic Disorders

Congenital Pancreatic Disorders

von Hippel-Lindau Disease von Hippel-Lindau (VHL) disease is a rare autosomal dominant disorder caused by a mutation in the VHL tumor suppressor gene on chromosome 3. Patients with VHL are at high risk for various malignan-

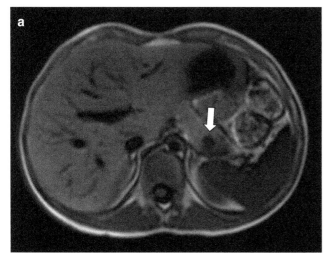

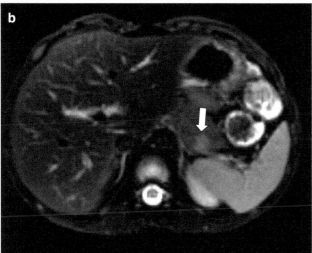

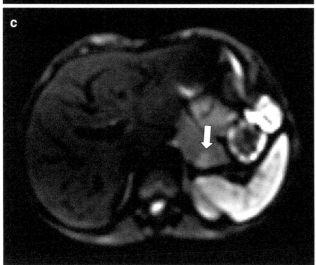

cies, including neuroendocrine tumors and serous cystadenomas in the pancreas. The disease is also associated with bilateral or multifocal renal cell carcinomas, adrenal pheochromocytomas, skull base endolymphatic sac tumors, and hemangioblastomas involving the brainstem, cerebellum, and spinal cord. Numerous cysts can be seen in the kidneys, pancreas, and liver [12].

Cystic Fibrosis Cystic fibrosis (CF) is an autosomal recessive disease caused by a gene defect encoding the CF transmembrane conductance regulator (CFTR), which is a chloride and bicarbonate channel. Abnormal chloride metabolism causes glands to produce abnormally thick, viscous material. This is mostly seen in the exocrine glands of the tracheobronchial tree, pancreas, sweat glands, and seminal vesicles of boys. The pancreas is one of the organs earliest affected by CF [12, 16].

In patients with CF, thickened secretions result in plugging of the proximal pancreatic ducts, leading to exocrine insufficiency, which is seen in approximately 85–90% of CF patients. Endocrine dysfunction is seen in about 30–50% of patients [16]. Fatty infiltration is the most common manifestation of CF in the pancreas, usually seen in adolescence or early adulthood. This can progress to complete pancreatic lipomatosis (Fig. 9.10). Pancreatic cystosis can also be seen, which is diffuse replacement of the pancreas with cysts of varying sizes (Fig. 9.11). On MR imaging, the cysts demonstrate typical low T1-weighted and high T2-weighted signal [16]. Various abnormalities of the ducts can occur, including strictures, dilatation, and obstruction [17].

Fig. 9.9 Intrapancreatic splenule in a 16-year-old girl. Axial T1-weighted (**a**), T2-weighted fat-suppressed (**b**), and diffusion-weighted (**c**) MR images demonstrate a small lesion (*arrows*) in the tail of the pancreas, which has the same signal characteristics as the spleen on all sequences

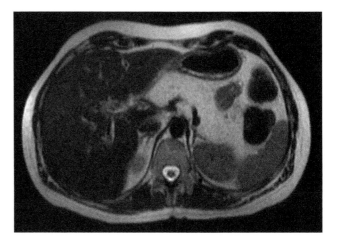

Fig. 9.10 Pancreatic lipomatosis in a 17-year-old girl with cystic fibrosis. Axial single-shot T2-weighted MR image shows fatty replacement of the pancreas, which is indistinct with the adjacent retroperitoneal fat

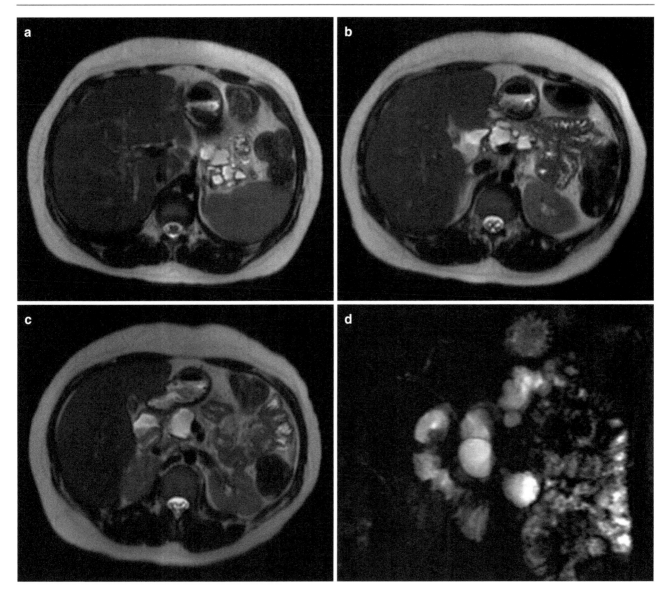

Fig. 9.11 Pancreatic cystosis in a 17-year-old girl with cystic fibrosis. Axial single-shot T2-weighted (**a–c**) and coronal MRCP (**d**) MR images show numerous cysts of various size replacing normal pancreas, in keeping with pancreatic cystosis

Shwachman-Diamond Syndrome Shwachman-Diamond syndrome is a rare, autosomal recessive disease, caused by a mutation in the Shwachman-Bodian-Diamond gene, the function of which is unknown. It is a multisystem disease, which involves the bones, bone marrow, and pancreas, often manifesting as pancreatic exocrine insufficiency, neutropenia, and bone dysplasia [18]. It is the second most common cause of childhood pancreatic atrophy, following CF [12]. The characteristic imaging feature is fatty replacement of the pancreas, which is well-visualized on MR imaging using paired T1-weighted or T2-weighted sequences with and without fat suppression. Unlike other causes of fatty pancreatic atrophy, the pancreas in Shwachman-Diamond syndrome is normal in size [18].

Congenital Hyperinsulinism Congenital hyperinsulinism (CHI), otherwise known as *persistent hyperinsulinemic hypoglycemia of infancy*, is an uncommon (1:50,0000 live births) but important cause of severe neonatal hypoglycemia. CHI was previously known as nesidioblastosis, meaning the persistence of nesidioblasts, which are fetal pancreatic cells [12]. CHI is attributable to a range of mutations that regulate insulin secretion, resulting in proliferation of B islet cells and pancreatic ducts. CHI is typically sporadic but can be associated with genetic conditions, including Beckwith-Wiedemann and Sotos syndromes [19].

Affected patients typically present with recurrent hypoglycemia refractory to feeds. CHI can be either diffuse or

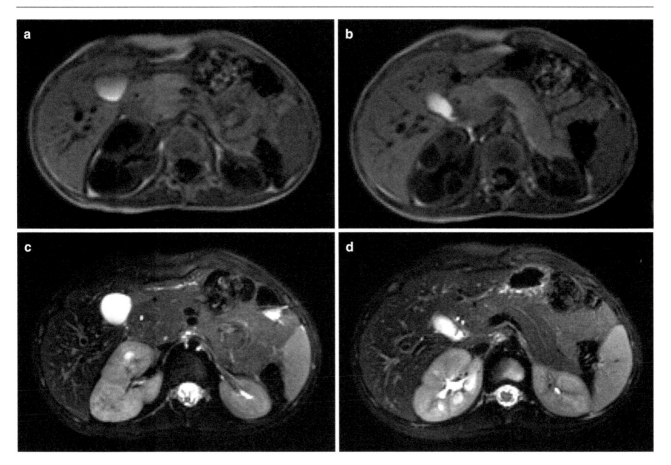

Fig. 9.12 Congenital hyperinsulinism in a 2-year-old girl with Beckwith-Wiedemann syndrome and hypoglycemia. Axial T1-weighted (**a**, **b**) and T2-weighted fat-suppressed (**c**, **d**) MR images demonstrate focal enlargement of the pancreatic head, without a discrete mass, in keeping with congenital hyperinsulinism

focal, with MRI being helpful to identify the extent of parenchymal enlargement, usually without an identifiable discrete mass [12] (Fig. 9.12), although MR imaging may not be definitive. As much, it is important to know that the diagnosis of CHI is usually made by F-DOPA PET imaging. It is important to distinguish the two forms of CHI because the focal form typically is treated by subtotal pancreatectomy, while diffuse CHI is typically managed medically [20].

Inflammatory Pancreatic Disorders

Acute Pancreatitis Pancreatitis, which is defined as inflammation of the pancreas, is the most common pancreatic disorder in children and adults. Three categories of pancreatitis have been defined: acute pancreatitis, acute recurrent pancreatitis, and chronic pancreatitis, based on the number of pancreatitis episodes and the presence or absence of irreversible features of pancreatitis [21]. Acute pancreatitis is diagnosed clinically when two of the following are present: abdominal pain compatible with acute pancreatitis,

serum amylase or lipase more than three times the upper limit of normal, and imaging findings consistent with acute pancreatitis [22]. The incidence of acute pancreatitis has increased in the pediatric population, which may be related to increased frequency of testing and childhood obesity. Pancreatitis occurs in all age groups, including infants, although studies have shown that it is more common in children more than 5 years old [2].

Pancreatitis in children is associated with significant morbidity and mortality. About one-quarter of children develop severe complications and the mortality rate is estimated to be 4% [2, 22]. Therefore, it is important for radiologists to have a broad awareness of pancreatitis in children in order to help guide appropriate treatment.

Imaging has a pivotal role in diagnosing pancreatitis. For children, ultrasound is the primary imaging modality of choice, although CT is also widely used. MR imaging with MRCP is becoming increasingly helpful and may soon replace CT, as it is able to provide exquisite anatomic delineation of the pancreatic parenchyma and pancreaticobiliary duct system. Acute pancreatitis in children looks similar to

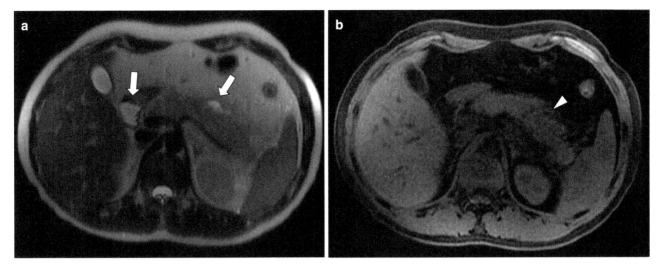

Fig. 9.13 Acute pancreatitis in an 18-year-old male who presented with acute abdominal pain. Axial single-shot T2-weighted MR image (**a**) demonstrates a swollen pancreas with small peripancreatic fluid collections (*arrows*). Fat-suppressed T1-weighted MR image (**b**) demonstrates areas of low signal intensity within the pancreatic body (*arrowhead*) consistent with edema in the context of acute pancreatitis

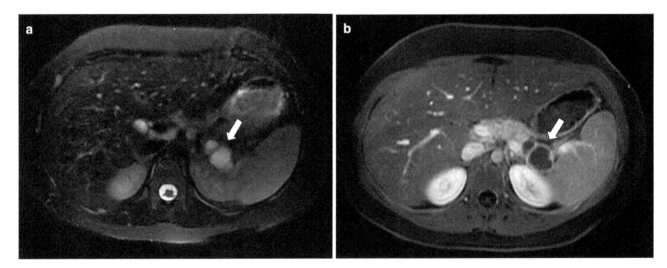

Fig. 9.14 Pancreatic pseudocyst in a 13-year-old boy with a history of acute pancreatitis. A lobulated cystic lesion (*arrow*) is seen in the pancreatic tail on an axial T2-weighted fat-suppressed MR image (**a**). This demonstrates a rim of enhancement (*arrow*) on a T1-weighted fat-suppressed post-contrast MR image (**b**). The patient's history of acute pancreatitis favors a diagnosis of a pseudocyst, which was confirmed when the lesion resolved on subsequent imaging

that in adults. The most common imaging feature of acute pancreatitis is an edematous enlarged pancreas, which in early or mild cases may be identified only as a subtle contour abnormality or increased signal intensity on T2-weighted imaging [23, 24]. The pancreas demonstrates loss of its intrinsic T1-weighted signal intensity, instead becoming heterogeneous and hypointense. Peripancreatic edema and fluid collections are often seen [2, 23] (Fig. 9.13).

Complications of Acute Pancreatitis Pseudocysts are the most common complication of acute pancreatitis, and the most common lesions seen within the pancreas. They are T2-weighted hyperintense and may have high T1-weighted

signal intensity due to internal debris or hemorrhage. There may be peripheral enhancement surrounding the cyst but no internal enhancement (Fig. 9.14), which would suggest a mass [2].

Necrotizing pancreatitis is uncommon in children but is important to be aware of because it is associated with increased morbidity and mortality [25]. Classic MR imaging features include focal areas of non-enhancement on post-contrast sequences that typically show high signal intensity on T1-weighted imaging. Gas can also be a feature of more severe necrotizing pancreatitis and can be difficult to identify on MR imaging, appearing as punctate low signal foci on T1- and T2-weighted images. Gradient recalled echo imaging

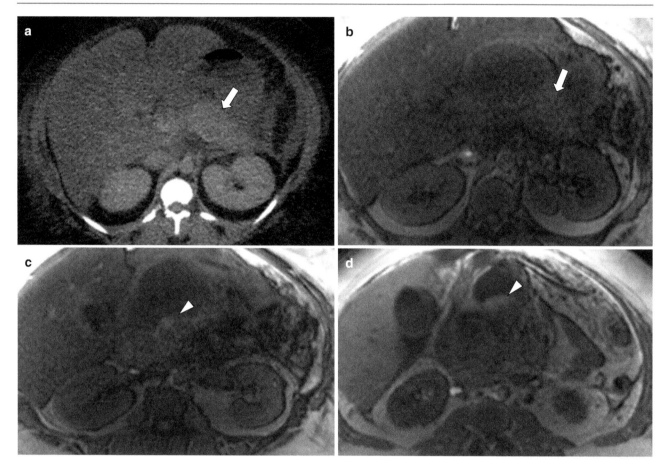

Fig. 9.15 Hemorrhagic pancreatitis in a 15-year-old girl with obesity and gallstones. Axial CT (**a**) and T1-weighted MR image (**b**) demonstrate an edematous pancreas (*arrows*). Additional T1-weighted axial MR images (**c, d**) demonstrate a high signal intensity hemorrhagic peripancreatic collection (*arrowheads*)

(such as T1-weighted fat-suppressed pre-contrast imaging) can be helpful to identify susceptibility artifact from air associated with pancreatic necrosis [2, 24, 25]. Hemorrhagic changes may also be seen in necrotizing pancreatitis, which may affect the pancreas itself or surrounding fatty tissue (Fig. 9.15).

Pancreaticopleural fistulas are extremely rare, occurring in less than 1% of patients with pancreatitis. This complication should be considered if the patient has large, recurrent pleural effusions despite resolution of his or her acute symptoms. T2-weighted and contrast-enhanced sequences may show a fistulous connection between the pancreatic duct and pleural space. The diagnosis can be confirmed by high amylase levels in the pleural fluid aspirate [2].

Vascular complications, including splenic vein thrombosis or splenic artery pseudoaneurysms, arise due to the close proximity of these vascular structures to inflamed pancreatic tissue. These are best detected on sequential contrast-enhanced T1-weighted fat-suppressed sequences [2, 23].

Causes of Pancreatitis About 10–20% of pediatric patients have recurrent episodes of pancreatitis. Many of these causes are treatable and thus it is important to identify on imaging if possible. Biliary disease is one of the most common causes of acute pancreatitis in children, accounting for approximately 10–30% of cases (although compared to more than 80% of adult pancreatitis). Obesity is both a risk factor for developing gallstones and an independent risk factor for developing gallstone pancreatitis. Pancreaticobiliary anomalies, including pancreas divisum, have been associated with recurrent pancreatitis. Approximately 50% of patients with acute recurrent pancreatitis have genetic pancreatitis predisposition mutations, with mutations in cystic fibrosis transmembrane conductance regulator (CFTR) and pancreatic secretory trypsin inhibitor (SPINK1) being among the most common [26]. Other less common but important causes of acute pancreatitis in children include trauma, autoimmune disorders, medications (e.g., valproic acid, prednisone, L-asparaginase, and 6-mercaptopurine), and certain systemic diseases like CF, chronic renal failure, and diabetes [2, 27].

Chronic Pancreatitis Chronic pancreatitis is relatively uncommon in children compared to adults. Children with chronic pancreatitis usually have genetic risk factors or con-

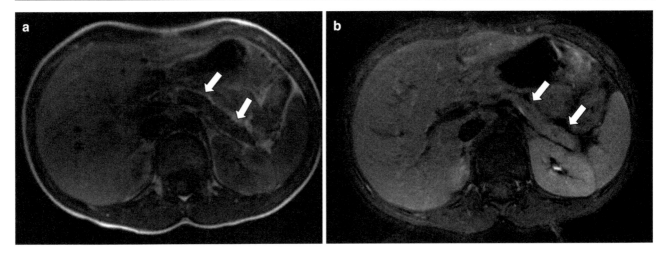

Fig. 9.16 Chronic pancreatitis in a 7-year-old boy with recurrent abdominal pain. Axial T1-weighted MR image (**a**) demonstrates pancreatic atrophy (*arrows*), with hypo-enhancement and pancreatic duct prominence on the T1-weighted fat-suppressed post-contrast MR images (**b**), indicative of chronic pancreatitis

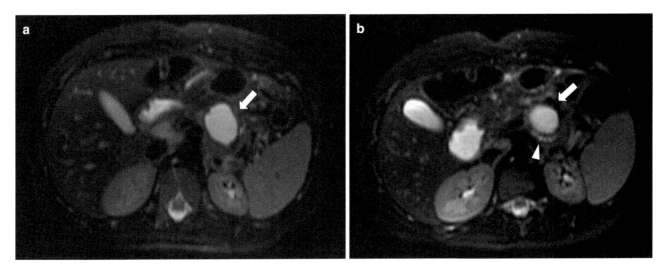

Fig. 9.17 Chronic pancreatitis and pseudocyst in an 11-year-old boy. Axial T2-weighted fat-suppressed MR images demonstrate a pseudocyst (**a**, **b**; *arrows*) anterior to an atrophic pancreas. The main pancreatic duct can be seen posterior to the pseudocyst and is dilated and beaded in appearance (**b**; *arrowhead*). Overall these findings are consistent with chronic pancreatitis

genital anomalies leading to chronic obstruction (e.g., pancreas divisum). Chronic pancreas can be debilitating in children and associated with significant morbidity, including chronic pain, frequent emergency room visits, hospitalizations, as well as lost time from school [28].

On MR imaging, the afflicted pancreas demonstrates low T1-weighted signal intensity and atrophy (Fig. 9.16), with MRCP ideally suited to show pancreatic duct tortuosity and dilatation (Fig. 9.17) as well as increased visibility of pancreatic duct side branches [23, 24]. Parenchymal calcifications associated with chronic pancreatitis are difficult to identify on MR imaging but appear as punctate foci of low signal intensity on T1-weighted and T2-weighted images causing susceptibility artifact on GRE imaging (similar to air). Acute on chronic pancreatitis has features of acute pancreatitis (edema, peripancreatic fluid) superimposed on chronic changes (abnormal duct morphology) (Fig. 9.18).

Autoimmune Pancreatitis Autoimmune pancreatitis is a rare entity in adults, and even more uncommon in children, although the disease is increasing being recognized in both demographic groups. Unlike the adult form, autoimmune pancreatitis in children is less frequently associated with an

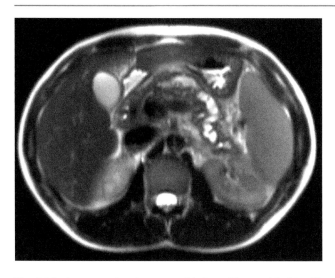

Fig. 9.18 Acute on chronic pancreatitis in a 15-year-old girl with abdominal pain. The main pancreatic duct is markedly dilated with a gradual transition at the pancreatic neck, as seen on this single-shot T2-weighted MR image. There is peripancreatic edema (note blurred parenchymal margins). Findings are consistent with acute on chronic pancreatitis

Table 9.1 Pediatric pancreatic neoplasms

Epithelial tumors	Pancreatoblastoma
	Solid pseudopapillary tumor
	Endocrine (islet cell) tumor
	Acinar cell carcinoma
	Ductal adenocarcinoma (exceedingly rare)
Non-epithelial tumors (rare)	Lymphoma (secondary > primary)
	Mesenchymal tumors

elevated IgG4, seen in 22% of children with the disease [29]. On MR imaging, the pancreas typically demonstrates low signal intensity on T1-weighted images and be globally or focally enlarged. Focal or segmental autoimmune pancreatitis may mimic a pancreatic mass. Other imaging features to look out for in the setting of autoimmune pancreatitis include irregularity of the main pancreatic duct and narrowing of the common bile duct, which are seen in the majority of cases [23, 29]. Most children respond well to steroids, with accompanying normalization of the pancreas on imaging.

Neoplastic Pancreatic Disorders

Pancreatic tumors are relatively rare in children compared with adults. In general, they have distinct histologic patterns and fortunately better prognoses compared to their adult counterparts. Pancreatic neoplasms can be divided into those of epithelial origin and those of non-epithelial origin (Table 9.1).

Pancreatic neoplasms in general occur less frequently in children compared with adults. This section focuses on pancreatic neoplasms that are most likely to occur in pediatric patients, acknowledging that several of these tumors are very rare and MRI is often not the primary imaging modality for diagnosis.

Epithelial Pancreatic Neoplasms

Pancreatoblastoma Pancreatoblastoma, formerly infantile pancreatic carcinoma, is the most common pancreatic tumor in children, representing approximately 25% of pancreatic tumors. However, this tumor is still extremely rare, with an incidence of less than 1 per 1,000,000 children [30]. Pancreatoblastoma may be slightly more common in males and usually occurs in the first decade of life (mean age is 5 years old). The tumor is often quite large (2–20 cm) at diagnosis, and clinical presentation is variable based on mass effect, ranging from abdominal pain and nausea and vomiting to jaundice. Alpha-fetoprotein (AFP) is usually elevated. While there is some association with Beckwith-Wiedemann syndrome, most cases are sporadic [30].

On MR imaging, pancreatoblastomas are usually large mixed solid-cystic masses with well-defined margins. They usually arise from the pancreatic head and tend to protrude into the lesser sac (Fig. 9.19). Pancreatoblastomas demonstrate low to intermediate T1-weighted signal intensity and heterogeneously increased T2-weighted signal intensity due to hemorrhage and necrosis [31]. Calcifications are often present and better seen on CT. About one-third of patients have metastases at presentation, usually to the liver [30].

Solid Pseudopapillary Tumor In contrast to pancreatoblastomas, which are usually seen in male children less than 10 years old, solid pseudopapillary tumors (SPT; also known as solid pseudopapillary epithelial neoplasms) are more common in young women in their second or third decade of life. Affected patients may present with abdominal pain but are often asymptomatic [30].

SPN is a mixed solid and cystic, slow-growing tumor, often large at diagnosis (>5 cm). The most common location is the pancreatic head. Key imaging features include a fibrous capsule and internal hemorrhage. The fibrous capsule typically demonstrates low signal intensity on

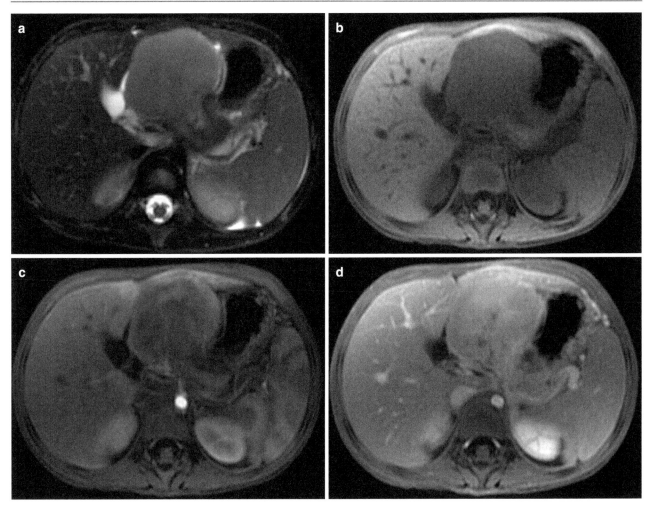

Fig. 9.19 Pancreatoblastoma in a 4-year-old boy. Axial T2-weighted (**a**) and T1-weighted (**b**) fat-suppressed MR images demonstrate a large, well-circumscribed low signal mass originating from the pancreatic head/neck, protruding into the lesser sac. The mass demonstrates enhancement on arterial and venous phase T1-weighted fat-suppressed post-contrast MR images (**c, d**) and was shown to be a pancreatoblastoma on histology

T1-weighted and T2-weighted imaging (Fig. 9.20). The solid components can demonstrate hemorrhage, particularly at larger sizes [30, 31]. Although usually benign, the tumor has malignant potential and therefore is treated with surgical resection. Vascular invasion and capsule disruption are aggressive features. Metastases are uncommon and are most common in the liver [30].

Neuroendocrine (Islet Cell) Tumors Islet cell tumors are neuroendocrine tumors seen in older children. In general, tumors that are large at presentation are typically non-functioning as they do not cause symptoms until they compress adjacent structures. Conversely, hormonally active neuroendocrine cell tumors are often small at diagnosis. Clinical features of islet cell tumors are summarized in Table 9.2.

The most common islet cell tumor is the insulinoma, accounting for approximately 50% of cases. These tumors often present at a very small size due to their clinical symptoms related to hypoglycemia. Insulinomas are often seen in the body or tail of the pancreas [30]. Gastrinomas are the second most common islet cell tumor, representing 30% of cases. These tend to occur in the "gastrinoma triangle," between the

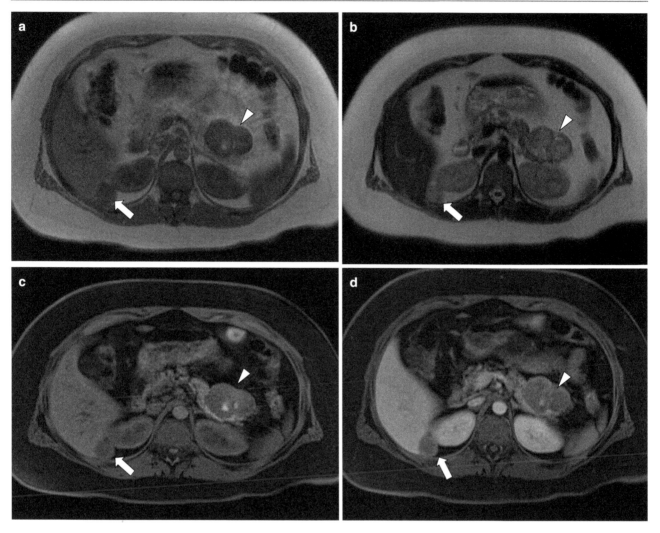

Fig. 9.20 Pancreatic solid pseudopapillary tumor and liver metastasis in an 18-year-old female. Axial T1-weighted (**a**) and T2-weighted (**b**) MR images demonstrate a large, well-circumscribed, heterogeneous, mass originating from the pancreatic body/tail (*arrowheads*; **a–d**). Intrinsic T1-weighted hyperintensity likely represents hemorrhage. T1-weighted fat-suppressed pre- (**c**) and post-contrast (**d**) images show heterogeneous enhancement of the mass. There is also a hypoenhancing hepatic lesion (*arrows*; **a–d**) consistent with a hepatic metastasis

Table 9.2 Clinical features of pancreatic endocrine tumors

Tumor type	Clinical features
Insulinoma	Hyperinsulinemic hypoglycemia
Gastrinoma	Zollinger-Ellison syndrome: duodenal ulcers, gastroesophageal reflux, diarrhea
ACTHoma	Cushing syndrome
VIPoma	Profuse watery diarrhea, hypokalemia, achlorhydria
Somatostatinoma	Diabetes, steatorrhea, gallbladder disease
Glucagonoma	Diabetes, stomatitis, necrolytic migratory erythema

junction of the cystic duct and CBD, duodenum, and neck and body of the pancreas [30]. While the majority of islet cell tumors arising in children occur sporadically, there is an association with genetic conditions such as multiple endocrine neoplasia type 1 and von Hippel-Lindau syndrome [23]. More recently, an association has been established with tuberous sclerosis complex in which nonfunctional pancreatic islet cells are incidentally discovered during renal imaging surveillance. The current data suggest that the islet cell tumors arising in this context are indolent [32].

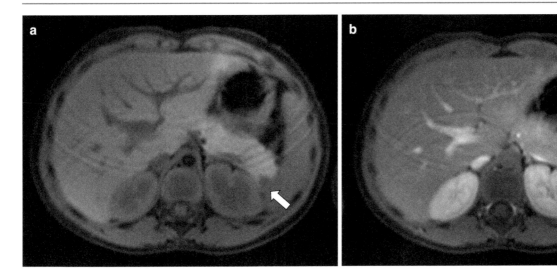

Fig. 9.21 Pancreatic insulinoma in an 8-year-old girl who presented with hypoglycemia. Axial T1-weighted fat-suppressed MR image (**a**) shows a hypointense lesion (*arrows*) in the tail of the pancreas, with avid arterial enhancement post-contrast (**b**), in keeping with a neuroendocrine tumor. Pathology was compatible with an insulinoma

On MR imaging, islet cell tumors are typically solid, hypervascular masses that avidly enhance on arterial-phase sequences (Fig. 9.21). They can be inconspicuous to background parenchyma on delayed sequences, which emphasizes the importance of arterial phase imaging. They often demonstrate heterogeneous signal intensity on T2-weighted images, including central areas of necrosis when the tumors become large in size [30, 31].

Non-epithelial Pancreatic Neoplasms

Lymphoma Pancreatic involvement of lymphoma is the most common non-epithelial tumor of the pancreas. Although very rare, most cases of pancreatic lymphoma are non-Hodgkin lymphoma. Burkitt lymphoma, an aggressive B-cell non-Hodgkin lymphoma that is associated with translocation of the MYC oncogene, can present as a rapidly growing pancreatic mass associated with pancreatitis [33]. Primary (isolated to the pancreas) and secondary (present in both the pancreas and lymphatic organs) pancreatic lymphoma have similar imaging features. Presenting symptoms are nonspecific and may include a palpable abdominal mass, weight loss, and obstructive jaundice [30].

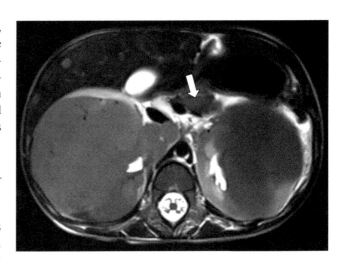

Fig. 9.22 Burkitt lymphoma in a 2-year-old boy. Axial T2-weighted MR image demonstrates low and intermediate signal intensity masses in the pancreas (*arrow*), kidneys, and liver

Lymphoma of the pancreas has two morphologic patterns: focal and diffuse. The focal form most often involves the pancreatic head, with low T1-weighted signal intensity and intermediate T2-weighted signal intensity (Fig. 9.22). Post-contrast sequences may demonstrate either absent or mild enhancement [30, 31].

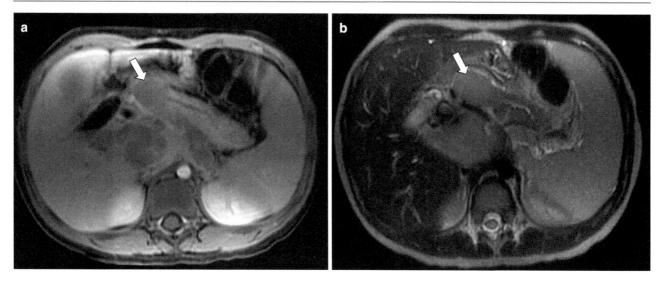

Fig. 9.23 Neuroblastoma invading the pancreas in a 4-year-old boy. Axial T1-weighted post-contrast fat-suppressed (**a**) and Axial T2-weighted fat-suppressed (**b**) MR images demonstrate T1-weighted mildly hypointense, T2-weighted isointense masses (*arrows*) invading the pancreatic head and neck

The diffuse form leads to glandular enlargement and could mimic acute pancreatitis. There is typically global low signal intensity on T1-weighted images and high signal intensity on T2-weighted images. The pancreas typically demonstrates diffuse enhancement with small foci or decreased or no enhancement. Compression of the biliary tree may be seen [31]. Diffusion restriction on DWI sequences is also characteristic and related to the high nuclear to cytoplasmic ratio of the tumor cells.

Metastases Non-pancreatic tumors within the pancreas typically occur due to local invasion from contiguous organs, most commonly neuroblastoma from the adrenal gland [30] (Fig. 9.23). Metastases to the pancreas is very rare.

Mimics and Pitfalls of Pancreatic Neoplasms

It is important to understand that non-neoplastic pathologies (e.g., splenules, pseudocysts, focal pancreatitis), discussed earlier in the chapter, may present as mass-like lesions. For example, fatty infiltration of the pancreas can be focal

or diffuse and could mimic a neoplasm. In such a case, T1-weighted in- and out-of-phase MR imaging confirms the diagnosis (Fig. 9.24). True pancreatic lesions do not contain fat except for pancreatic lipomas, which are uncommon but benign. Duodenal diverticula are rare in children, but are another potential pitfall. It is important to recognize that air causes inhomogeneities in the magnetic field and blooming artifacts on in-phase images due to their longer TE. Often the clinical presentation (e.g., fever, abdominal pain) would favor pancreas over a mass lesion, although follow-up imaging may be required.

Inflammatory myofibroblastic tumors (IMTs), previously known as inflammatory pseudotumors, are unusual pseudosarcomatous lesions that can mimic a malignant mass. Composed of inflammatory myofibroblastic spindle cells, these are most often seen in children and young adults. The lungs and orbits are most often involved, but cases have been reported in nearly every organ [34]. While IMT does not demonstrate aggressive features (Fig. 9.25), imaging cannot currently confidently distinguish IMT from a malignancy, especially in the pancreas where very few cases have been reported. As such, treatment is currently surgical resection.

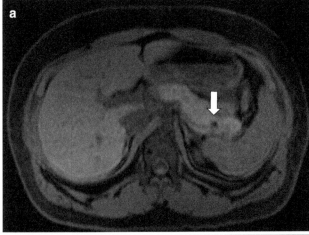

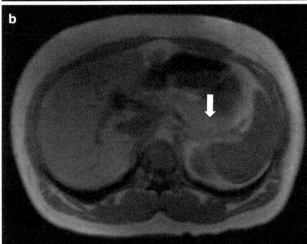

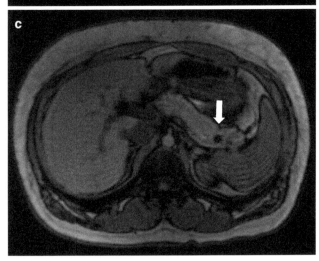

Fig. 9.24 Incidental pancreatic lipoma in an 18-year-old female. Axial T1 fat-suppressed MR image (**a**) demonstrates a small low signal intensity lesion (*arrow*) in the tail of the pancreas. T1-weighted chemical shift in-phase (**b**) and opposed phase (**c**) MR images demonstrate signal loss on the opposed phase image (**c**, *arrow*), at the interface between the lipoma and the surrounding normal pancreas

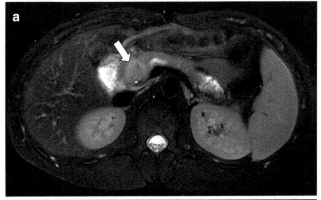

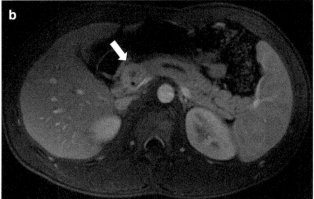

Fig. 9.25 Myofibroblastic pancreatic tumor in a 17-year-old boy. Axial T2-weighted fat-suppressed (**a**) and T1-weighted fat-suppressed post-contrast (**b**) MR images show a well-circumscribed enhancing mass (*arrows*) in the head of the pancreas. There is no infiltration of surrounding structures. Pathology demonstrated a myofibroblastic tumor, previously known as an inflammatory pseudotumor

Table 9.3 Pancreatic injury grading

Injury type	Clinical features
Grade 1	Contusion or laceration with intact duct
Grade 2	Deep laceration or transection with duct injury
Grade 3	Severe laceration or crush injury to head of pancreas
Grade 4	Pancreaticoduodenal injuries

Traumatic Pancreatic Injury

Pancreatic injury occurs in 5–10% of children with blunt abdominal trauma and is almost never isolated. The pancreas is vulnerable to injury given its fixed position in the retroperitoneum. Two-thirds of injuries occur in the pancreatic body, which is the largest pancreatic segment. Trauma to the pancreas has a grading system, listed in Table 9.3. Unexplained pancreatic injury, especially in an infant, should raise concern for child abuse [23, 24].

Pancreatic injury is associated with direct blunt force trauma to the abdomen, often handlebar injuries or second-

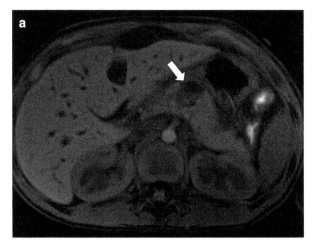

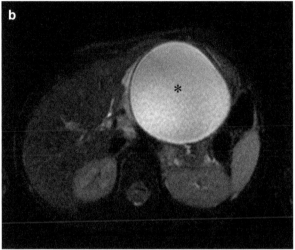

Fig. 9.26 Handle bar injury in an 8-year-old boy. Axial T1-weighted fat-suppressed MR image (**a**) demonstrates a hematoma in the pancreatic body (*arrow*), on a background of contusion, disrupting the path of the main pancreatic duct. Four months later, axial T2-weighted MR image (**b**) shows this area had matured into a pseudocyst (asterisk)

ary to child abuse in children. Lacerations and hematoma can be seen (Fig. 9.26). Direct signs of injury (e.g., lacerations) are often subtle and difficult to detect, so it is important to look for secondary signs of injury. These include peripancreatic fluid in the anterior pararenal space or lesser sac and findings of pancreatitis (Fig. 9.27).

Treatment of pancreatic injury is somewhat controversial in children, with the standard of care currently being medical management. Although CT is often the initial imaging modality diagnosing traumatic injury of the pancreas in the setting of blunt abdominal trauma, MRI often plays an important role in assessing for development of peripancreatic fluid collections suggesting pancreatic duct injury, as well as MRCP direct assessment of pancreatic duct integrity [35].

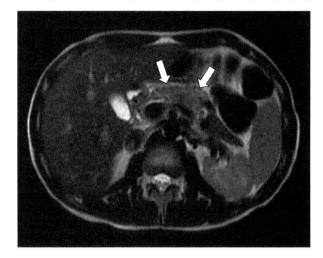

Fig. 9.27 Focal pancreatitis in an 18-year-old male with abdominal trauma. Axial single-shot T2-weighted MR image demonstrates swelling and focal high signal in the body of the pancreas (*arrows*), consistent with focal pancreatitis secondary to trauma. Note the diminished size of the uninvolved pancreatic tail for comparison

Conclusion

Clear knowledge of normal development and various disorders of the pediatric pancreas is important to allow for generating appropriate differential diagnoses and facilitating optimal care for pediatric patients. In summary, pancreatic disorders are relatively uncommon and often incidental in the pediatric population but are important to recognize as they may cause acute or recurrent symptoms. These are best diagnosed with MR imaging including MRCP. Pancreatitis in children is becoming more common and is important to keep on the differential diagnosis of a pediatric patient with abdominal pain. Pancreatitis can be subtle on imaging and is important to diagnose before complications arise. Pancreatic tumors are very rare in the pediatric population but can often be differentiated on the basis of MR imaging features, patient age/gender, and clinical presentation.

References

1. Howard JM, Hess W. History of the 9ancreas: mysteries of a hidden organ. 2nd ed. New York: Springer; 2002.
2. Restrepo R, Hagerott HE, Kulkarni S, Yasrebi M, Lee EY. Acute pancreatitis in pediatric patients: demographics, etiology, and diagnostic imaging. Am J Roentgenol. 2016;206(3):632–44.
3. Trout AT, Podberesky DJ, Serai SD, Ren Y, Altaye M, Towbin AJ. Does secretin add value in pediatric magnetic resonance cholangiopancreatography? Pediatr Radiol. 2013;43(4):479–86.

4. Jaimes C, Gee MS. Strategies to minimize sedation in pediatric body magnetic resonance imaging. Pediatr Radiol. 2016;46(6):926–7.

5. Semelka RC, Ascher SM. MR imaging of the pancreas. Radiology. 1993;188(3):593–602.

6. Nievelstein RA, Robben SGF, Blickman JG. Hepatobiliary and pancreatic imaging in children—techniques and an overview of neo-neoplastic disease entities. Pediatr Radiol. 2011;41(1):55–75.

7. Jaimes C, Kirsch JE, Gee MS. Fast, free-breathing and motion-minimized techniques for pediatric body magnetic resonance imaging. Pediatr Radiol. 2018;48(9):1197–208.

8. Chavhan GB, AlSabban Z, Babyn PS. Diffusion-weighted imaging in pediatric body mr imaging: principles, techniques, and emerging applications. Radiographics. 2014;34(3):E73–88.

9. Manfredi R, Pozzi Mucelli R. Secretin-enhanced MR imaging of the pancreas. Radiology. 2016;279(1):29–43.

10. Chavhan GB, Babyn PS, Vasanawala SS. Abdominal MR imaging in children: motion compensation, sequence optimization, and protocol organization. Radiographics. 2013;33(3):703–19.

11. Sadler TW. Langman's medical embryology. 11th ed. Philadelphia: Lippincott Williams and Wilkins; 2010.

12. Borghei P, Sokhandon F, Shirkhoda A, Morgan DE. Anomalies, anatomic variants, and sources of diagnostic pitfalls in pancreatic imaging. Radiology. 2013;266(1):28–36.

13. Bülow R, Simon P, Thiel R, Thamm P, Messner P, Lerch MM, et al. Anatomic variants of the pancreatic duct and their clinical relevance: an MR-guided study in the general population. Eur Radiol. 2014;24(12):3142–9.

14. Sandrasegaran K, Patel A, Fogel E, Zyromski NJ, Pitt HA. Annular pancreas in adults. AJR Am J Roentgenol. 2009;193(2):455–60.

15. Schnedl WJ, Piswanger-Soeklner C, Wallner SJ, Reittner P, Krause R, Lipp RW, et al. Agenesis of the dorsal pancreas and associated diseases. Dig Dis Sci. 2009;54(3):481–7.

16. Berrocal T, Pajares MP, Zubillaga AF. Pancreatic cystosis in children and young adults with cystic fibrosis: sonographic, CT, and MRI findings. AJR Am J Roentgenol. 2005;184(4):1305–9.

17. Fields TM, Michel SJ, Butler CL, Kriss VM, Albers SL. Abdominal manifestations of cystic fibrosis in older children and adults. AJR Am J Roentgenol. 2006;187(5):1199–203.

18. Toivianinen-Salo S, Raade M, Durie PR, Ip W, Marttinen E, Savilahti MO. Magnetic resonance imaging findings of the pancreas with Shwachman-Diamond syndrome and mutations in the SBDS gene. J Pediatr. 2008;152(3):434–6.

19. Arnoux JB, de Lonlay P, Ribeiro MJ, Hussain K, Blankenstein O, Mohnike K, et al. Congenital hyperinsulinism. Early Hum Dev. 2010;86(5):287–94.

20. Adzick NS, De Leon DD, States LJ, Lord K, Bhatti TR, Becker SA, Stanley CA. Surgical treatment of congenital hyperinsulinism: results from 500 pancreatectomies in neonates and children. J Pediatr Surg. 2019;54(1):27–32.

21. Shukla-Udawatta M, Madani S, Kamat D. An update on pediatric pancreatitis. Pediatr Ann. 2017;46(5):e207–11.

22. Morinville VD, Husain SZ, Bai H, Barth B, Alhosh R, Durie PR, et al. Definitions of pediatric pancreatitis and survey on present clinical practices. J Pediatr Gastroenterol Nutr. 2012;55(3):261–5.

23. Anupini SA, Chauvin NA, Khwaja A, Biko DM. Magnetic resonance imaging of pancreaticobiliary diseases in children: from technique to practice. Pediatr Radiol. 2016;46(6):778–90.

24. Thai TC, Riherd DM, Rust KR. MRI manifestations of pancreatic disease, especially pancreatitis, in the pediatric population. AJR Am J Roentgenol. 2013;201(6):W877–92. Review.

25. Raizner A, Phatak UP, Baker K, Patel MG, Husain SZ, Pashankar DS. Acute necrotizing pancreatitis in children. J Pediatr. 2013;162(4):788–92.

26. Kumar S, Ooi CY, Werlin S, Abu-El-Haija M, Barth B, Bellin MD, et al. Risk factors associated with pediatric acute recurrent and chronic pancreatitis: lessons from INSPPIRE. JAMA Pediatr. 2016;170(6):562–9.

27. Bai HX, Lowe ME, Hussain SZ. What have we learned about acute pancreatitis in children? J Pediat Gastroenterol Nutr. 2011;52(3):262–70.

28. Schwarzenberg SJ, Bellin M, Husain SZ, Monika A, Barth B, Davis H, et al. Pediatric chronic pancreatitis is associated with genetic risk factors and substantial disease burden. J Pediatr. 2015;166(4):890–6.

29. Scheers I, Palermo JJ, Freedman S, Wilschanski M, Shah U, Abu-El-Haij M, et al. Autoimmune pancreatitis in children: characteristic features, diagnosis, and management. Am J Gastroenterol. 2017;112(10):1604–11.

30. Chung EM, Travis MD, Conran RM. Pancreatic tumors in children: radiologic-pathologic correlation. Radiographics. 2006;26:1211–38.

31. Shet NS, Cole BL, Iyer RS. Imaging of pediatric pancreatic neoplasms with radiologic histopathologic correlation. AJR Am J Roentgenol. 2014;202:1337–48.

32. Koc G, Sugimoto S, Kuperman R, Kammen BF, Karakas SP. Pancreatic tumors in children and young adults with tuberous sclerosis complex. Pediatr Radiol. 2016;47(1):39–45.

33. Amodio J, Brodsky JE. Pediatric Burkitt lymphoma presenting as acute pancreatitis: MRI characteristics. Pediatr Radiol. 2010;40(5):770–2.

34. Kim SJ, Kim WS, Cheon JE, Shin SM, Youn BJ, Kim IO, Yeon KM. Inflammatory myofibroblastic tumors of the abdomen as mimickers of malignancy: imaging features in nine children. AJR Am J Roentgenol. 2009;193:1419–24.

35. Sivit CJ. Imaging children with abdominal trauma. AJR Am J Roentgenol. 2009;192(5):1179–89.

Spleen

10

Gary R. Schooler, Alison R. Hart, Nathan C. Hull, and Edward Y. Lee

Introduction

The spleen is the largest accumulation of lymphoid tissue in the human body. It is composed of red pulp responsible for managing worn-out, damaged, or otherwise deranged red blood cells and white pulp that activates the immune response when antigens and antibodies are presented in the blood [1]. A wide variety of disorders may be encountered in the pediatric spleen, including congenital, neoplastic, infectious, and traumatic abnormalities. The spleen also manifests abnormalities related to systemic disorders.

Magnetic resonance (MR) imaging can yield important diagnostic information regarding an array of pediatric splenic disorders. This chapter provides up-to-date MR imaging techniques; reviews splenic anatomy including embryology, normal development, and anatomic variants; and highlights clinically important disorders affecting the spleen in the pediatric population.

Magnetic Resonance Imaging Techniques

Patient Preparation

Sedation The majority of children under 6–7 years of age, as well as any child who is unable to comply with MR imaging technologist instructions, require some form of sedation or anesthesia to successfully complete an abdominal MR imaging examination. Voluntary motion is a major source of artifacts in patients, especially those less than 6–7 years of age. Sedation or anesthesia may also be necessary to mitigate involuntary motion, predominantly respiratory, when imaging the abdomen in patients who are unwilling or unable to comply with breath hold instructions. In some pediatric patients, the use of respiratory triggering and fast free-breathing sequences may permit successful completion of abdominal MR imaging without the use of sedation or anesthesia [2–4]. Children less than 6 months of age may successfully be imaged with a feed and swaddle technique, thus obviating the need for sedation [5].

Intravenous Contrast Material Complete evaluation of the majority of splenic disorders is aided by the use of an intravenously administered gadolinium-based contrast agent (GBCA). Dynamic or multiphase contrast-enhanced images using a GBCA have been shown to significantly improve the conspicuity of splenic lesions by providing differential contrast enhancement compared to normal splenic tissue [6]. Dynamic enhancement characteristics can help distinguish among splenic lesion types. The decision to incorporate a GBCA into the imaging protocol for splenic evaluation should be made on an individual patent basis, weighing potential risks and benefits of GBCAs in children [7].

MR Imaging Pulse Sequences and Protocols

MR imaging of the pediatric abdomen can be adequately performed on either 1.5 Tesla (T) or 3T MR imaging systems. However, 3T imaging can provide higher signal-to-noise ratio (SNR), which may be of benefit in pediatric patients, especially infants and smaller children. Using a smaller voxel size results in better spatial resolution with the same acquisition time at 3T as compared with 1.5T imaging. Combining the inherent benefits of 3T imaging with parallel imaging and compressed sensing is expected to decrease imaging time and help improve tolerance of examinations in younger children [4, 8, 9].

G. R. Schooler (✉)
Department of Radiology, Duke University Medical Center, Durham, NC, USA
e-mail: gary.schooler@duke.edu

A. R. Hart
Diagnostic Imaging, Rhode Island Hospital, Brown University, Providence, RI, USA

N. C. Hull
Department of Radiology, Mayo Clinic, Rochester, MN, USA

E. Y. Lee
Division of Thoracic Imaging, Department of Radiology, Boston Children's Hospital, Harvard Medical School, Boston, MA, USA

© Springer Nature Switzerland AG 2020
E. Y. Lee et al. (eds.), *Pediatric Body MRI*, https://doi.org/10.1007/978-3-030-31989-2_10

Construction of a protocol for evaluation of the spleen should incorporate T1- and T2-weighted images. Fast spin-echo (FSE) T2-weighted images are helpful for characterizing most splenic lesions. In children with substantial image degradation by respiratory motion artifact, sequences that utilize radial k-space filling can help mitigate the effects of motion by dispersing motion artifact across multiple radial planes. T1-weighted images are often acquired using a gradient recalled echo (GRE) sequence that is faster than FSE and can be obtained in a single breath hold, although they can suffer from a relatively lower SNR [4]. Volumetric acquisition of T1-weighted GRE sequences, especially those acquired using radial sampling of k-space, permit motion robust assessment of the spleen in multiple phases of contrast enhancement. Sequences such as diffusion-weighted imaging (DWI) and T1-weighted in-opposed phase Dixon imaging may provide additional information about lesion composition. Ultimately, priority should be given to those sequences best suited to answer the specific clinical question, attempting to avoid a nondiagnostic assessment should the child not be able to complete the full examination.

Anatomy

Embryology

The spleen originates from the intraembryonic splanchnic mesoderm where it develops from either a single or multiple outpouchings of embryonic mesenchymal tissue that subsequently fuse together inside the dorsal mesogastrium. The rotation of the stomach and development of the dorsal mesogastrium between the six and seventh weeks of development results in migration of the spleen from the median plane to the left upper quadrant. The spleen is fixed by two large ligaments, the gastrosplenic and phrenicosplenic, in the left upper quadrant of the abdominal cavity and is intraperitoneal in location [1, 10] (Fig. 10.1).

Normal Development and Anatomy

Hematopoietic stem cells migrate into the spleen during the first trimester of development, and the spleen functions exclusively as a hematopoietic organ until the 14th week of gestation. Lymphoid colonization occurs later, between the 15th and 18th weeks of development, around the time the spleen assumes its characteristic shape. Lymphatic follicles are formed by B-lymphocytes beginning around the 23rd week of gestation. During most of fetal life, the spleen functions as a hematopoietic organ, gradually decreasing during the eighth month of fetal development [10].

Postnatally, the combination of red and white pulp elements results in the characteristic appearance of the spleen on imaging (Fig. 10.2). Normal development and maturation of the spleen result in an evolving appearance on MR imaging in

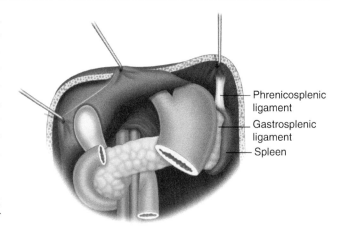

Fig. 10.1 Normal relationship and anatomic positioning of the spleen in the left upper quadrant, fixed in an intraperitoneal location by two large ligaments, the gastrosplenic and phrenicosplenic ligaments

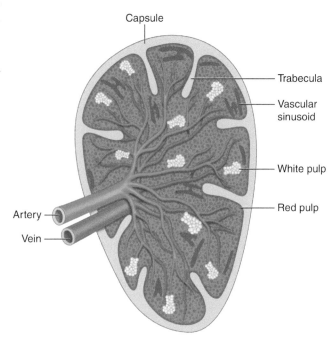

Fig. 10.2 Schematic rendering of normal splenic anatomy with red and white pulp components

neonates. In adults, normal splenic signal on MR imaging is higher than that of the liver on T2-weighted images and lower than that of the liver on T1-weighted images [11]. The neonatal spleen, particularly during the first week of life, is equal to or less than the liver in signal intensity on T2-weighted images (Fig. 10.3) and approximately equal to that of the liver on T1-weighted images. Not until approximately 8 months of life on T2-weighted images and approximately 1 month of life on T1-weighted images does the signal assume the normal adult signal pattern. This change in signal characteristics is believed to be due to maturation and evolution of the red pulp/white pulp ratio and should not be interpreted as pathologic [12].

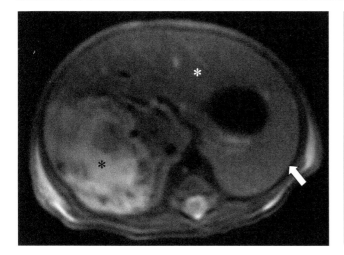

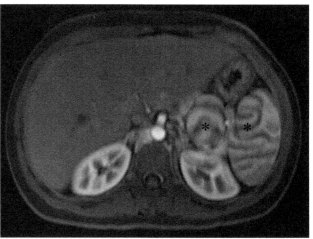

Fig. 10.3 Normal neonatal spleen appearance in an 11-day-old boy imaged with MR imaging to evaluate the congenital hepatic hemangioma (*black asterisk*). Axial T2-weighted MR image shows isointensity of the spleen (*white arrow*) compared to the adjacent liver (*white asterisk*), typical for neonates

Fig. 10.4 Polysplenia in a 17-year-old girl who presented with abdominal pain. Axial T1-weighted fat-suppressed contrast-enhanced MR image demonstrates multiple rounded homogeneous masses (*asterisks*) in the left upper quadrant with a serpentine or arciform enhancement pattern compatible with polysplenia

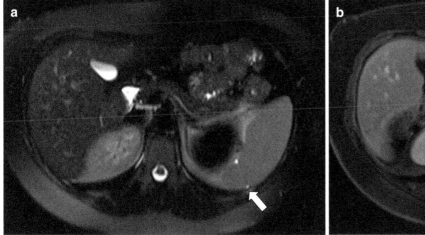

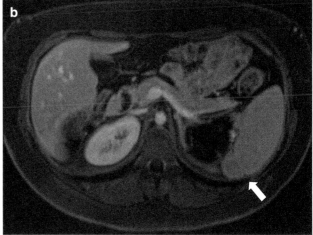

Fig. 10.5 Splenic cleft in a 15-year-old girl who presented with abdominal pain. (**a**) Axial T2-weighted fat-suppressed and (**b**) axial T1-weighted fat-suppressed contrast-enhanced MR images demonstrate an incidental splenic cleft (*white arrows*) at the posterior mid spleen

Blood flow to the spleen is provided by the splenic artery, a branch of the celiac artery. The splenic artery divides into multiple segmental arterial branches near the splenic hilum. Venous drainage of the spleen is provided by the splenic vein which courses along the posterior and inferior margin of the pancreas to join the superior mesenteric vein and form the main portal vein. The spleen exhibits a unique appearance on images obtained early (25–45 seconds) after IV contrast administration. Images typically reveal alternating hyper- and hypoenhancing bands of tissue, resulting in a serpentine or arciform pattern of enhancement (Fig. 10.4). The enhancement pattern becomes more homogeneous approximately 60–90 seconds after contrast material administration [13].

The spleen exhibits the greatest diffusion restriction – high signal on diffusion-weighted images (DWI) and low signal on the apparent diffusion coefficient (ADC) map – of the upper abdominal organs [14].

Anatomic Variants

Splenic Clefts

Clefts in the spleen are normally present in the lobulated fetal spleen but disappear before birth [15]. However, they may persist beyond fetal life and, when present, are usually seen along the medial border of the spleen [15]. The clefts are generally sharply defined and may be as deep as 2–3 cm (Fig. 10.5). These splenic clefts may be mistaken for a mass, traumatic injury, or sequelae of infarct if they are not recognized.

Accessory Spleen

An accessory spleen, also known as a splenule or supernumerary spleen, is a congenital focus of splenic tissue separate from the main splenic organ, arising from a failure of the splenic primordia to completely fuse [15]. Accessory spleens may be single or multiple. They are most commonly found near the splenic hilum but may be identified along the splenic vessels, within the gastrosplenic or splenorenal ligaments, within the pancreatic tail, within the gastric or bowel wall, and within the pelvis or scrotum [10]. Most splenules are asymptomatic and incidentally discovered. However, the tissue may become clinically important when unrecognized and not removed at the time of splenectomy for a hematologic or autoimmune disorder, potentially leading to recurrence of the disease [16]. When the splenic tissue is ectopically positioned beyond the splenic hilum, it may mimic a neoplastic entity especially when encountered in the pancreas [15]. Accessory splenic tissue shares the same signal and enhancement characteristics as the normal spleen on MR imaging, a key to its recognition (Fig. 10.6).

Spectrum of Splenic Disorders

Congenital Splenic Disorders

Asplenia and Polysplenia Congenital absence of the spleen, or asplenia, is one of the two major categories in the spectrum of abnormalities known as heterotaxia. Asplenia is more commonly seen in males and is associated with congenital heart disease in nearly 100% of patients, resulting in a very high mortality rate in the first year of life [15]. The liver is frequently midline, and there may be a truncated pancreas and an interrupted inferior vena cava with azygous continuation [15]. Without a spleen, patients are susceptible to life-threatening sepsis caused by encapsulated bacteria [10]. On MR imaging, the absence of the spleen as well as the above-described associated anomalies is evident (Fig. 10.7).

Polysplenia, or more than one spleen, is a complex congenital anomaly characterized by partial visceral heterotaxia and levoisomerism. As with asplenia, affected pediatric patients may have concomitant congenital heart disease, a midline liver, and a truncated pancreas [15]. Malrotation is also a reported association [17]. On imaging, there is a wide range of splenic appearances, ranging from numerous small spleens to a dominant multi-lobular spleen with very small accessory spleens. The spleens always reside on the same side as the stomach, usually along its greater curvature [1]. Signal characteristics and

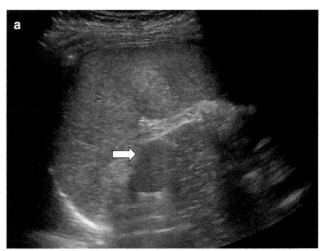
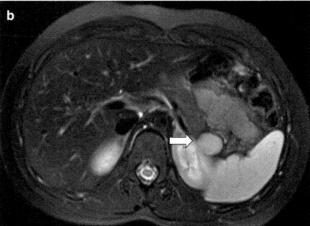
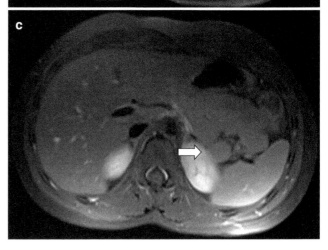

Fig. 10.6 Splenule in a 9-year-old boy who presented with nausea. (**a**) Transverse grayscale ultrasound image demonstrates a lobulated lesion (*white arrow*) at the splenic hilum isoechoic to the spleen which may represent a splenule or mass. (**b**) Axial T2-weighted fat-suppressed MR image and (**c**) axial T1-weighted fat-suppressed contrast-enhanced MR image demonstrate a homogenous round mass at the splenic hilum with identical signal characteristics to the spleen on all sequences compatible with a splenule (*white arrows*)

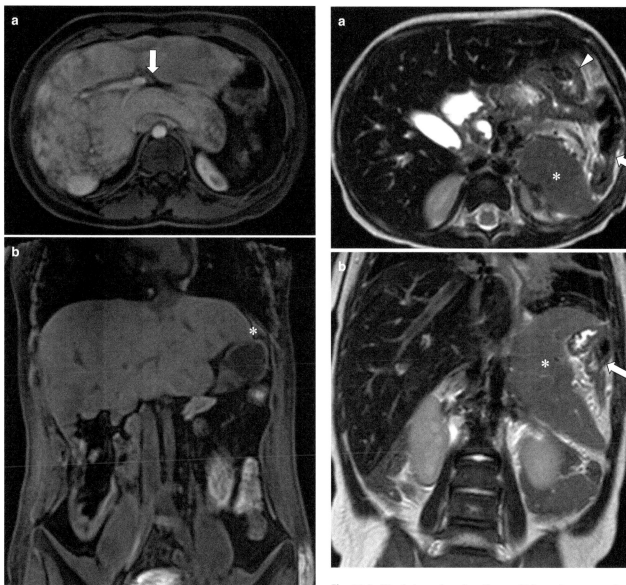

Fig. 10.7 Asplenia in an 18-year-old female with hypoplastic left heart and known heterotaxy/asplenia. (a) Axial T1-weighted fat-suppressed and (b) coronal T1-weighted fat-suppressed MR images demonstrate congenital absence of the splenic vein (*white arrow*) and an empty splenic fossa (*asterisk*), compatible with asplenia

Fig. 10.8 Wandering spleen in a 7-year-old boy who presented with non-specific abdominal pain. (a) Axial and (b) coronal T2-weighted MR images demonstrate an abnormally positioned spleen (*asterisks*) in the left upper quadrant that is posterior and medial to the stomach (*white arrowhead*) and splenic flexure of the colon (*white arrows*), consistent with a wandering spleen

enhancement patterns of the splenic tissue are uniform among the spleens (see Fig. 10.4).

Wandering Spleen Wandering spleen is a rare condition of abnormal splenic ligament laxity, permitting abnormal splenic mobility. This condition is found in both pediatric and adult patients. In the pediatric patient population, it is observed in males and females with equal incidence and thought to be due to congenital ligamentous laxity [18]. While this condition is often asymptomatic and frequently found incidentally, the ligamentous laxity predisposes to splenic torsion and infarction, in which case the affected pediatric patient presents with acute abdominal symptoms.

On MR imaging, the wandering spleen may be found in the pelvis, abdomen, or left upper quadrant with an abnormal rotation (Fig. 10.8). When torsion of the spleen around the vascular pedicle is present, MR imaging may reveal swirling of the vascular pedicle, thrombosis of the splenic vein, ascites, and perisplenic edema on T2-weighted and T1-weighted fat-suppressed contrast-enhanced images [18, 19].

Hereditary Spherocytosis Hereditary spherocytosis is a congenital splenic disorder caused by mutations in the genes encoding various red blood cell membrane proteins. Such genetic mutations result in sphere-shaped red blood cells that display a decreased surface area to volume ratio and are unusually fragile [20]. The abnormal red blood cells are trapped and destroyed in the spleen, the main cause of hemolysis in these pediatric patients. Affected individuals generally present with anemia, jaundice, and splenomegaly [21]. Splenomegaly is the most common finding on imaging and is seen in 50% of infants and 75% to 95% of older children and adults [22]. On MR imaging, splenomegaly can range from mild to substantial (Fig. 10.9). The affected pediatric patient may also have cholelithiasis as a result of increased red blood cell turnover. Affected infants and children are generally treated symptomatically, though total or partial splenectomy may be indicated in patients with severe disease [20, 21].

Epidermoid Cyst Splenic cysts can be either congenital or acquired. Epidermoid cysts are uncommon congenital, epithelial-cell-lined cysts [23, 24]. Differentiation of epidermoid cysts from other cysts that can be found in the spleen is not possible on the basis of imaging alone. Epidermoid cysts rarely show calcification in the wall and may have internal septations or wall trabeculation. These cysts may have simple internal fluid or fluid containing cholesterol crystals, inflammatory debris, or hemorrhage [17]. The internal contents affect the signal characteristics on MR imaging. Splenic cysts with simple internal fluid appear homogeneously hyperintense on T2-weighted images and hypointense on T1-weighted images (Fig. 10.10). Epidermoid cysts with fluid containing cholesterol have higher signal on T1-weighted images, and those with internal hemorrhage have T1-weighted and T2-weighted signal intensities that reflect the chemical state of the hemoglobin within [17, 25] (Table 10.1).

Post-traumatic Pseudocyst Post-traumatic pseudocysts are a rare complication of prior splenic trauma and are thought to develop in the setting of prior hematoma. In distinction to the splenic epidermoid (congenital) cyst described previously, splenic pseudocysts have a fibrous wall rather than an endothelial lining. Post-traumatic pseudocysts are generally well-defined lesions with imperceptible walls on MR imaging, though they can have calcifications within the wall. The fluid within the cyst usually has MR imaging signal characteristics on T1- and T2-weighted images compatible with that of simple fluid. However, some cysts may have

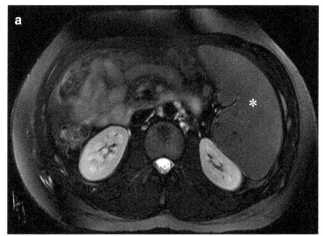

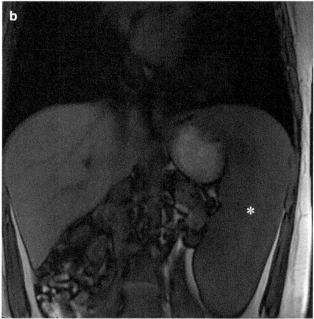

Fig. 10.9 Hereditary spherocytosis in a 16-year-old boy who presented with splenomegaly and elevated hepatic enzymes 2 weeks after cholecystectomy. (**a**) Axial T2-weighted fat-suppressed and (**b**) coronal T1-weighted fat-suppressed contrast-enhanced MR images demonstrate marked enlargement of the spleen (*asterisks*)

debris or septations within the cyst from hemorrhage or infection that result in variable MR signal characteristics [26, 27] (see Table 10.1). Post-traumatic pseudocysts may be difficult to distinguish from epidermoid cysts on the basis of imaging alone.

Infectious Splenic Disorders

Viral Infections Epstein-Barr virus (EBV), a ubiquitous herpes virus, is the most common cause of infectious mononucleosis [28]. Pediatric patients infected with the virus may be asymptomatic or present with the classic symptoms of fever, pharyngitis, and cervical lymphadenopathy.

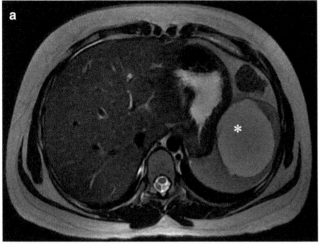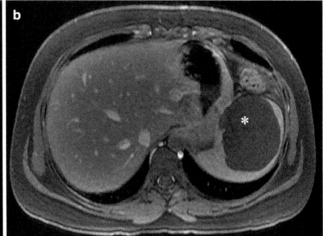

Fig. 10.10 Epidermoid cyst in a 14-year-old girl who initially presented with vomiting and was incidentally found to have a cystic lesion in the spleen on ultrasound. (**a**) Axial T2-weighted and (**b**) axial T1-weighted fat-suppressed contrast-enhanced MR images demonstrate a unilocular T2-weighted hyperintense lesion (*asterisks*) in the spleen without contrast enhancement. Histologic analysis following surgical resection was compatible with an epidermoid cyst

Table 10.1 Most common splenic lesions encountered in pediatric patients

Lesion	MR imaging characteristics[a]	Distinguishing features
Bacterial infection	Hypointense on T1-weighted images Hyperintense on T2-weighted images Peripheral/perilesional enhancement	Usually larger than microabscesses associated with fungal infections
Fungal infection	Acute: Hyperintense on T2-weighted images; No peripheral enhancement With treatment: Intermediate to high signal on T1- and T2-weighted images; perilesional ring of hypointense signal	Typically manifests as microabscesses a few millimeters in diameter
Hemangioma	Hypo- to isointense on T1-weighted images Hyperintense on T2-weighted images Small lesions tend to show immediate homogenous post-contrast enhancement Larger lesions tend to show peripheral enhancement with or without progressive centripetal enhancement	Centripetal enhancement, when present, can help distinguish from other lesions
Lymphoma	Hypo- to isointense on T1-weighted images Hyperintense on T2-weighted images Hypoenhancing on contrast-enhanced images	Splenomegaly; focal lesions may be small or large, multiple or singular
Cysts	Generally hypointense on T1-weighted images and markedly hyperintense on T2-weighted images; no central enhancement	Thin or imperceptible wall with fluid signal intensity centrally; cyst contents may be complicated by septations, internal hemorrhage, or infection

[a]Signal characteristics of the lesions are in reference to normal splenic tissue signal

Many pediatric patients with infectious mononucleosis have splenomegaly that, on MR imaging, may be mild or severe [28] (Fig. 10.11). Pediatric patients with infectious mononucleosis and splenomegaly are at risk of splenic rupture that may be spontaneous or induced by trauma, with most of the observed splenic ruptures occurring during the initial 3 weeks of infection [28, 29].

Bacterial Infections Bacterial infections involving the spleen are rare in healthy children. They are more common in pediatric patients with compromised immune function or other risk factors such as those with hemoglobinopathies (e.g., sickle cell disease), bacterial endocarditis, trauma, and splenic infarction [30]. Presenting symptoms are vague but include

abdominal pain and fever. Typically, any abscesses complicating bacterial infections are discovered on MR imaging. Pyogenic abscesses may be single or multiple and are usually larger than the micro-abscesses observed in fungal infections. When large, abscesses may exhibit internal septations and/or complex fluid. Splenic abscesses generally have low signal intensity on T1-weighted MR images and high signal on T2-weighted MR images, with peripheral and perilesional enhancement visible on post-contrast images [23, 31] (see Table 10.1).

Cat scratch disease is caused by the Gram-negative organism *Bartonella henselae*. The infection is usually caused by a scratch from a kitchen or cat, most commonly on the upper extremity. A minority of patients may develop a systemic

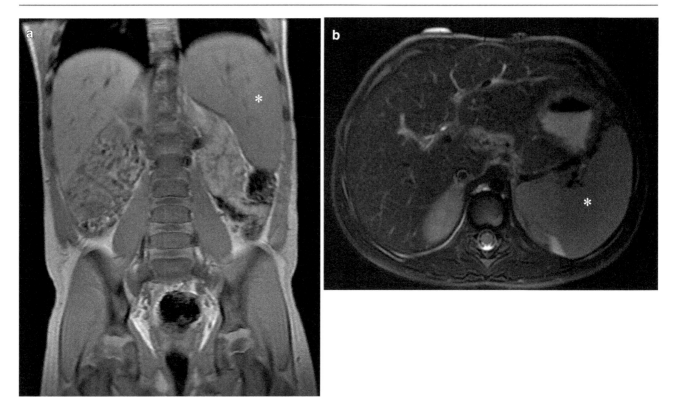

Fig. 10.11 Splenomegaly in a 4-year-old girl with Epstein-Barr virus mononucleosis found to have splenomegaly with the spleen measuring up to 12.5 cm. (**a**) Coronal T1-weighted and (**b**) axial T2-weighted fat-suppressed MR images demonstrate splenomegaly (*asterisks*)

infection that can involve the liver and spleen. When present, splenic infection generally manifests as multiple abscesses, sharing MR imaging characteristics with other pyogenic abscesses. Lesions may exhibit calcification during resolution [30].

Fungal Infections Fungal infections within the spleen typically manifest as micro-abscesses that are a few millimeters in diameter. Similar to pyogenic abscesses, fungal abscesses are generally seen in those pediatric patients that are immune compromised, typically due to chemotherapy, bone marrow transplantation, or organ transplantation (Fig. 10.12). The most common fungal organisms causing splenic infection are *Candida*, *Aspergillus*, and *Cryptococcus* [32]. Acute fungal micro-abscesses appear hyperintense on T2-weighted fat-suppressed images and usually do not show peripheral enhancement on post-contrast images because of the immunosuppressed state of the patient [31, 33] (Fig. 10.13). With treatment, splenic fungal abscesses are intermediate to high signal intensity on T1- and T2-weighted sequences with a perilesional ring of hypointense signal representing sequelae of therapy and immune response [33].

Splenic infection, with the ubiquitous and endemic fungal pathogen *Histoplasma capsulatum*, may be seen in immunocompetent or immunocompromised patients. MR imaging during the acute and subacute phases of the infection typically reveals numerous lesions within the spleen that are hypointense on both T1- and T2-weighted images [13] (see Table 10.1).

Splenic involvement in *Mycobacterium tuberculosis* (TB) infection is uncommon, though when identified is likely due to hematogenous dissemination of the primary infection. TB infection in the spleen may appear micronodular or macronodular on imaging. The miliary form of the disease may only produce splenomegaly or generate findings similar to fungal micro-abscesses. The macronodular form of the disease is rare and may show diffuse splenic involvement with multiple lesions or a single large lesion that, on MR imaging, displays variable signal intensities and enhancement patterns after IV contrast administration, with the variability thought to represent different phases of disease progression [34, 35].

Splenic calcifications may be a manifestation of subacute or remote splenic fungal and TB infections. On MR imaging, these splenic calcifications are hypointense on both T1- and T2-weighted images and may show blooming artifacts, especially on GRE sequences with long echo times [13].

Parasitic Infections Parasitic infection of the spleen is rare but classically caused by systemic dissemination or intraperitoneal spread of a ruptured hepatic (hydatid) cyst caused by *E. granularis* [17]. The cysts appear similar to those

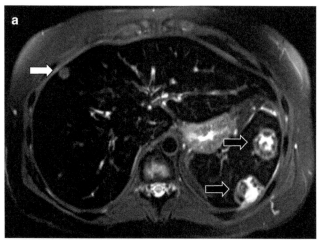

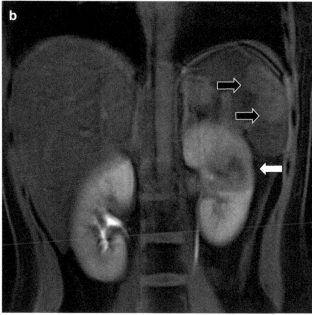

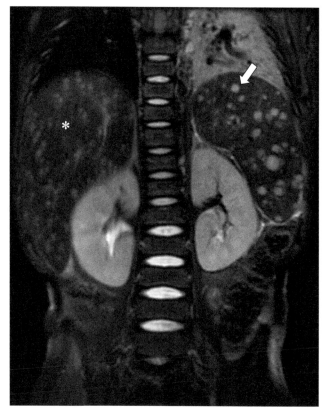

Fig. 10.13 Candida micro-abscesses in a 6-year-old boy with B cell acute lymphoblastic leukemia and blood culture compatible with disseminated candida infection. Coronal T2-weighted fat-suppressed MR image demonstrates numerous hyperintense lesions compatible with acute fungal micro-abscess (*white arrow*). The liver is also involved (*asterisk*)

Fig. 10.12 Splenic abscesses in a 17-year-old girl with acute lymphoblastic leukemia who found to have biopsy-proven mucor infection in the spleen, kidney, and liver. (**a**) Axial T2-weighted fat-suppressed MR image demonstrates centrally T2-weighted hyperintense lesions within the spleen with irregular walls (*black arrows*). An associated T2-weighted hyperintense lesion is noted at the periphery of the liver (*white arrow*). (**b**) Coronal T1-weighted fat-suppressed contrast-enhanced MR image demonstrates enhancement of the splenic abscesses (*black arrows*) with a lesion of similar characteristics within the left kidney (*white arrow*)

observed in the liver and are usually solitary but may have daughter cysts or peripheral calcification depending on the stage of the infection [36]. Simple cysts appear hypointense on T1-weighted images and markedly hyperintense on T2-weighted images. The cyst wall and internal septations may enhance [36]. Hydatid cysts may not be distinguishable from other splenic cysts on the basis of imaging alone, though the likely presences of concomitant disease elsewhere in the body may help confirm the diagnosis.

Neoplastic Splenic Disorders

Hemangioma Hemangiomas are the most common benign primary neoplasm of the spleen, usually identified incidentally in pediatric patients without symptoms, and thought to arise from sinusoidal epithelium [37]. Splenic hemangiomas may be solitary or multiple and can vary in size, though most tend to be less than 2 cm in diameter. Hemangiomas rarely can diffusely infiltrate the spleen, replacing the normal splenic parenchyma in diffuse angiomatosis. Splenic hemangiomas tend to increase in size with time and can become large, rarely resulting in Kasabach-Merritt syndrome [38].

Splenic hemangioma appearance on MR imaging may be solid or cystic, depending on the gross morphology. Smaller splenic hemangiomas tend to be solid, while larger splenic hemangiomas tend to be cystic due to underlying thrombosis, infarction, and cystic degeneration due to necrosis [37]. Splenic hemangiomas are usually hypo- to isointense to the normal spleen on T1-weighted images and hyperintense to the normal spleen on T2-weighted images. On contrast-enhanced images, smaller lesions tend to show immediate homogenous enhancement, whereas larger lesions may show progressive centripetal enhancement or peripheral enhancement with non-enhancement of the center of the lesion due to hemorrhage, necrosis, etc. (Fig. 10.14). When a central scar is present, it may or may not show enhancement [39] (see Table 10.1).

Hamartoma Hamartomas are rare benign neoplasms of the spleen composed of an anomalous mixture of normal red pulp elements without organized lymphatic follicles [37, 40]. Splenic hamartomas are often an incidental finding, and most affected pediatric patients manifest no symptoms. Uncommonly, larger lesions may present with a palpable mass, splenomegaly, rupture, thrombocytopenia, or anemia [37]. Hamartomas of the spleen have been associated with hamartomas in other areas of the body and can be seen in patients with tuberous sclerosis [41, 42].

On MR imaging, splenic hamartomas are isointense to normal splenic parenchyma on T1-weighted images and

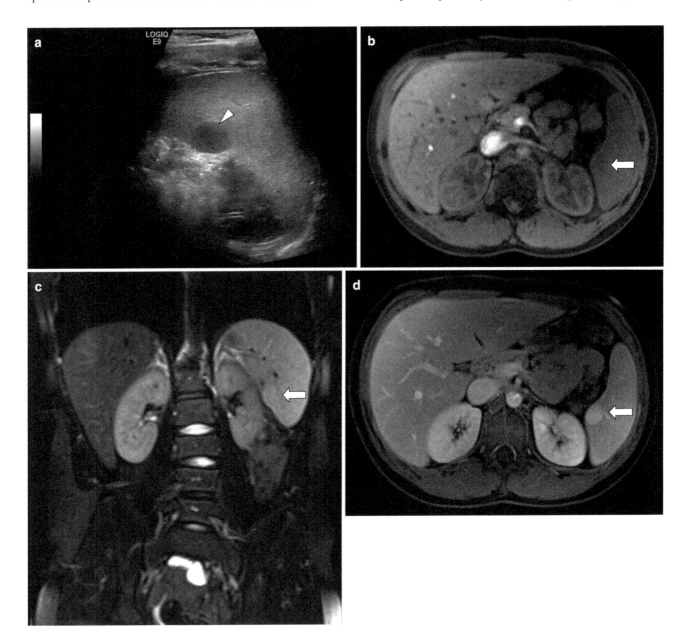

Fig. 10.14 Splenic hemangioma in a 9-year-old boy with incidentally identified hypoechoic lesion within the periphery of the spleen on renal ultrasound performed for evaluation of nephrolithiasis. (**a**) Transverse grayscale ultrasound image of the spleen demonstrates a hypoechoic lesion (*white arrowhead*) adjacent to the splenic hilum. (**b**) Axial unenhanced T1-weighted fat-suppressed, (**c**) coronal T2-weighted fat-suppressed, and (**d**) axial T1-weighted fat-suppressed contrast-enhanced MR images demonstrate a mildly T1-weighted hypointense, T2-weighted hyperintense, and homogeneously enhancing lesion (*white arrows*) within the spleen compatible with a hemangioma. Histology confirmed diagnosis of hemangioma on biopsy

heterogeneously hyperintense to normal splenic tissue on T2-weighted images. Immediately after administration of IV contrast material, splenic hamartomas tend to show heterogeneous hypoenhancement compared with normal parenchyma on arterial and portal venous phase images, with more uniform enhancement typically observed on delayed MR images [39] (Fig. 10.15). While MR imaging characteristics often are suggestive of splenic hamartoma, distinction from malignant splenic lesions on the basis of imaging alone may be difficult and require biopsy.

Angiosarcoma Angiosarcoma is the most common primary nonhematologic malignant splenic tumor, arising from the endothelial lining of splenic blood vessels [27, 37]. Although very rare and most commonly seen in adults over the age of 40, splenic angiosarcoma has been described in pediatric patients [43]. Affected pediatric patients typically have massive splenomegaly and may present with abdominal pain, fever, fatigue, weight loss, and signs and symptoms of hemoperitoneum in the setting of spontaneous tumor rupture [37, 44]. Metastatic disease is common and typically involves the liver, lungs, bone marrow, bone, and lymph nodes [37].

The MR imaging appearance of splenic angiosarcoma reflects the hemorrhagic nature of the tumor and is characterized by mixed areas of high and low signal on T1- and T2-weighted images corresponding to the presence of blood products and necrosis [27, 40]. Low signal intensity foci of susceptibility on GRE images have been shown to correlate with siderotic nodules [45]. Contrast-enhanced MR images typically show heterogenous enhancement with multiple nodular-enhancing foci throughout the tumor, and washout can be seen on delayed phase images [46].

Leukemia Leukemia is the most common childhood malignancy, and nearly all cases are the acute form – including acute lymphoblastic leukemia (ALL) and acute myeloid leukemia (AML) [47]. Leukemic involvement of the solid viscera is common, especially the spleen. Splenomegaly is the most consistent finding, resulting from diffuse infiltration or less likely one or more focal lesions [47, 48] (Fig. 10.16). Splenic manifestations of infection in the immunocompromised pediatric patient, described earlier, may also be seen in the pediatric patient with leukemia and may be difficult to differentiate from leukemic involvement.

Lymphoma Lymphoma, including Hodgkin lymphoma and non-Hodgkin lymphoma, is the third most common malignant neoplasm in pediatric patients and is the commonest malignant tumor of the spleen [13, 47]. The spleen is the largest lymphoid organ in the body and is involved in one-third of

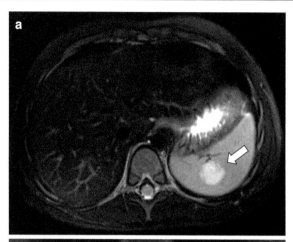

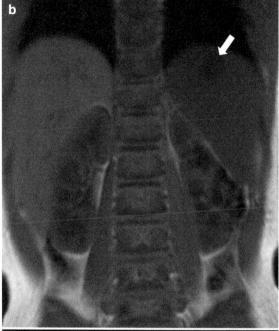

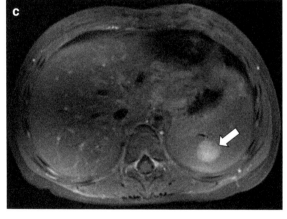

Fig. 10.15 Splenic hamartoma in a 4-year-old boy with incidentally noted splenic lesion on prior renal ultrasound for hematuria. (**a**) Axial T2-weighted fat-suppressed MR image demonstrates a well-circumscribed lesion (*white arrow*) heterogeneously hyperintense to normal splenic tissue. (**b**) Coronal T1-weighted MR image demonstrates the lesion (*white arrow*) is mildly hypointense to normal splenic tissue. (**c**) Axial T1-weighted fat-suppressed contrast-enhanced MR image demonstrates mildly heterogeneous enhancement of the lesion (*white arrow*). The constellation of MR imaging findings is most consistent with splenic hamartoma which was confirmed histologically upon surgical excision

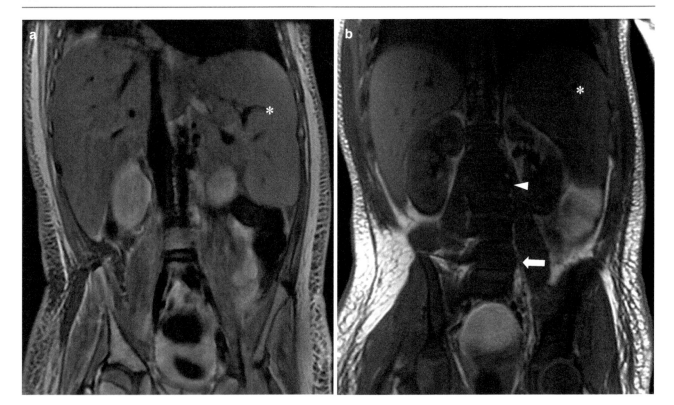

Fig. 10.16 Splenomegaly in a 10-year-old boy with acute lymphoblastic leukemia and abnormal bone marrow who presented with fever, bone pain, and labile blood pressure. High-risk B-cell acute lymphoblastic leukemia confirmed on bone marrow aspirate. (**a**) Coronal T2-weighted MR image demonstrates mild splenic enlargement (*aster-*isk). (**b**) Coronal T1-weighted MR image demonstrates diffusely abnormal marrow hypointensity throughout the spine and pelvis. Vertebral bone marrow signal (*white arrow*) is darker than adjacent disc (*arrowhead*). Splenomegaly (*asterisk*) is also seen.

all Hodgkin lymphoma and approximately one-third of non-Hodgkin lymphoma cases at presentation [49]. Splenic infiltration is considered nodal in Hodgkin lymphoma and extra-nodal disease in non-Hodgkin lymphoma [48].

Splenic involvement in lymphoma can be either primary or much more commonly secondary. Primary splenic lymphoma is defined as lymphomatous involvement of the spleen with or without splenic hilar lymphadenopathy. Secondary lymphoma is defined as lymphomatous involvement of the spleen and nodes other than those in the splenic hilum. Four imaging patterns of splenic lymphoma have been described: (1) splenomegaly without a focal lesion, (2) diffuse infiltration with innumerable small miliary lesions, (3) multiple discrete focal nodular lesions, and (4) single solitary mass [48, 50, 51] (Fig. 10.17). On MR imaging, lymphomatous splenic lesions show low to intermediate signal intensity on T1-weighted images, mild to moderate hyperintensity on T2-weighted images, and hypoenhancing compared to the normal splenic tissue on contrast-enhanced T1-weighted images [13, 52] (see Table 10.1).

Metastasis In pediatric patients, overt metastatic disease to the spleen is uncommon and, when present, is most likely due to aggressive neoplasms with hematogenous dissemination [30, 53]. On MR imaging, metastatic lesions are usually iso- or hypointense compared to the normal splenic parenchyma on T1-weighted images and hyperintense compared to the normal splenic parenchyma on T2-weighted images. Splenic metastases show variable enhancement but are often hypoenhancing compared to the normal splenic parenchyma on contrast-enhanced T1-weighted fat-suppressed images [27, 40] (Fig. 10.18).

Posttransplant Lymphoproliferative Disorder Posttransplant lymphoproliferative disorder (PTLD) refers to a variety of abnormal lymphoid proliferative disorders that occur in the posttransplant setting. The majority of PTLDs are B-lymphocyte proliferations related to EBV infection [54]. PTLD is most common in patients requiring high levels of immunosuppression and in those patients who were EBV-seronegative prior to transplantation [55]. PTLD can affect any organ system, though there appears to be an association between the allograft type and the location of PTLD after solid organ transplantation [56, 57]. Splenic involvement in PTLD occurs with a greater prevalence in liver transplant patients than in patients with other solid organ transplantation [54].

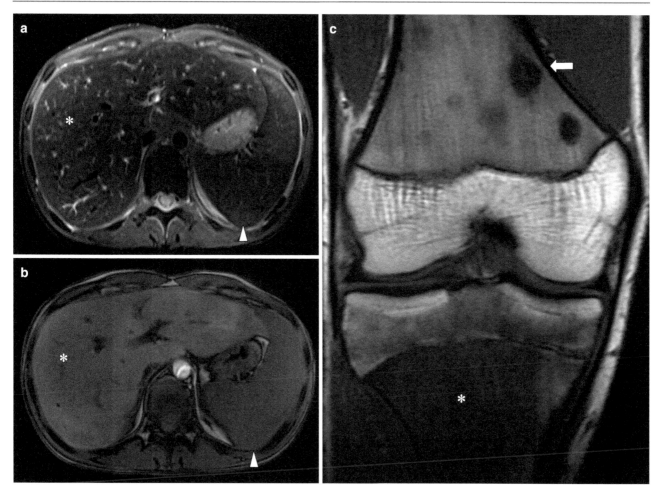

Fig. 10.17 Splenomegaly in a 13-year-old boy with history of Crohn disease on adalimumab and oral methotrexate who presented with right knee pain found to have multiple osseous lesions. Biopsy consistent with diffuse large B-cell lymphoma with renal involvement and hepatosplenomegaly. (a) Axial T2-weighted fat-suppressed and (b) axial T1-weighted fat-suppressed post-contrast MR images demonstrate hepatomegaly (*asterisks*) and splenomegaly (*white arrowheads*). (c) Coronal T1-weighted MR image demonstrates multiple low signal intensity lesions (*white arrow*) compatible with lymphoma involvement within the femoral metaphysis manifesting as abnormal marrow signal (*asterisk*) within the proximal tibial epiphysis and metaphysis

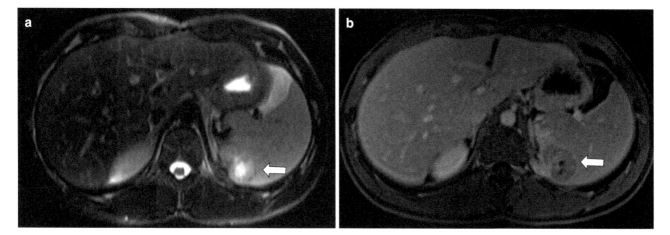

Fig. 10.18 Metastatic renal cell carcinoma within the spleen in a 17-year-old boy with history of recurrent left renal cell carcinoma status post nephrectomy with palpable abnormality in the left upper quadrant. Patient underwent splenectomy which confirmed metastatic deposit within the spleen. (a) Axial T2-weighted fat-suppressed MR image demonstrates a centrally hyperintense lesion with irregular margins (*white arrow*) within the medial aspect of the spleen adjacent to left nephrectomy bed. (b) Axial T1-weighted fat-suppressed contrast-enhanced MR image demonstrates hypoenhancement of the lesion (*white arrow*) relative to the normal splenic tissue

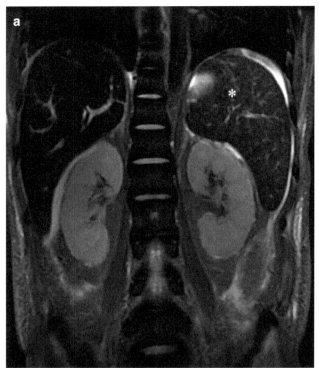

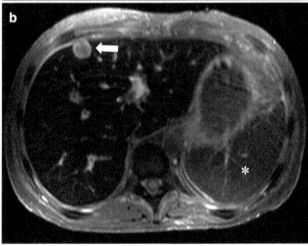

Fig. 10.19 Splenomegaly in a 17-year-old boy with Philadelphia chromosome positive acute myelogenous leukemia and posttransplant lymphoproliferative disorder (PTLD) who presented with fever after bone marrow transplant. Patient was found to have mild splenomegaly and multiple liver lesions. (**a**) Coronal T2-weighted fat-suppressed MR image demonstrates mild splenomegaly (*asterisk*). (**b**) Axial T2-weighted fat-suppressed MR image demonstrates a well-circumscribed, hyperintense lesion (*white arrow*) within the liver. PTLD was diagnosed histologically on hepatic biopsy. Mild splenomegaly (*asterisk*) is also seen

The most common imaging finding in the spleen in patients with PTLD is splenomegaly (Fig. 10.19). Less commonly, multiple small lesions may be identified. PTLD lesions are typically isointense on T1-weighted images and iso- to hypointense on T2-weighted images relative to the normal spleen. Importantly, in this immunosuppressed

patient population, opportunistic infections are also common and may affect the spleen – rendering MR imaging assessment important in distinguishing lesions of PTLD from those of infection that are typically markedly T2 hyperintense relative to the normal spleen and demonstrate peripheral enhancement [54].

Traumatic Splenic Disorder

Blunt Traumatic Injury The spleen is the most commonly injured organ during blunt abdominal trauma in pediatric patients. Motor vehicle collisions are the most frequent cause of splenic injury in children, with injuries often more severe than those in adults due to seat belt position and decreased abdominal coverage by the ribs and bony pelvis [58]. Splenic injuries most often present with left upper quadrant or generalized abdominal pain, occasionally with pain radiating to the left shoulder. Symptoms may be related to peritoneal inflammation or signs of hypovolemia from hemorrhage. The spleen may be injured during difficult childbirth or cardiopulmonary resuscitation in neonates, and shock or abdominal rigidity may be the only presenting symptoms [26].

In the setting of blunt traumatic injury, there are variable patterns of splenic injury including subcapsular and intraparenchymal hematomas, lacerations, infarction, and vascular injury. Ultrasound and contrast-enhanced CT are the standard imaging modalities for patients with a history of blunt abdominal trauma who are hemodynamically stable and suspected of having intra-abdominal injury. Injuries on CT may be graded by the standardized organ injury scale from the American Association for the Surgery of Trauma (AAST) [59].

Injuries observed at MR imaging in the subacute or chronic phase of injury may include any of the above injury patterns. Lacerations appear as linear areas of signal abnormality on both T1- and T2-weighted images and may be associated with subcapsular or perisplenic hematoma with signal that is variable on T1- and T2-weighted images, reflecting the chemical state of hemoglobin at the time of imaging (Fig. 10.20). Injury to splenic vascular structures may result in partial or complete devascularization of the spleen as well as splenic artery pseudoaneurysm [13, 26]. MR imaging may serve a secondary role, offering further and perhaps more conclusive evaluation of indeterminate splenic lesions identified on CT for evaluation of blunt abdominal trauma [60].

Miscellaneous Splenic Disorders

Splenic Infarction Splenic infarction can occur in a variety of settings in pediatric patients, including entities that pre-

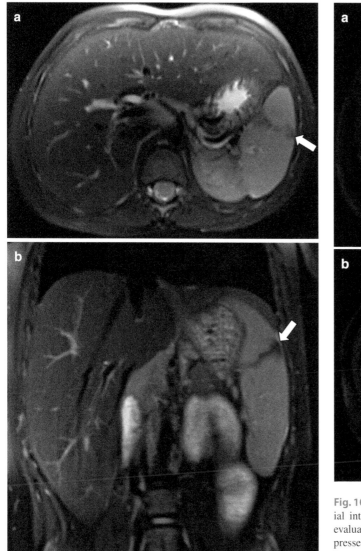

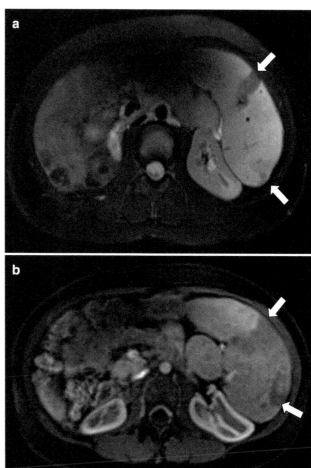

Fig. 10.20 Splenic laceration in a 5-year-old boy who presented with left upper quadrant pain following a motor vehicle accident. (**a**) Axial T2-weighted fat-suppressed and (**b**) coronal T2-weighted fat-suppressed MR images demonstrate a linear area of decreased T2-weighted signal intensity compatible with splenic laceration (*white arrows*)

Fig. 10.21 Splenic infarct in a 10-year-old girl with progressive familial intrahepatic cholestasis type III who presented for MR imaging evaluation of multiple hepatic nodules. (**a**) Axial T2-weighted fat-suppressed and (**b**) axial T1-weighted fat-suppressed post-contrast MR images demonstrate multiple peripheral, wedge-shaped areas of decreased T2-weighted signal intensity and hypoenhancement relative to the normal splenic parenchyma on post-contrast imaging compatible with splenic infarcts (*white arrows*)

dispose to splenic torsion, splenomegaly, sickle cell disease, storage disorders, embolic disease, portal hypertension, traumatic injury, and therapy-related vascular occlusion. Affected pediatric patients may be either asymptomatic (in the setting of smaller infarcts) or have abdominal pain and fever.

When only involving a portion of the spleen, infarcts may appear as peripheral wedge-shaped or round/irregular areas of variable signal on T1- and T2-weighted images, likely reflecting variable degrees of internal hemorrhage and necrosis. Contrast-enhanced images show a lack of enhancement

in the infarcted regions of the spleen (Fig. 10.21). When the entire spleen is acutely infarcted, there may be heterogenous signal intensity throughout with only a rim of capsular enhancement on contrast-enhanced images. Chronic infarction may result in irregularity of the splenic margin, calcification, and decreased signal intensity on T1- and T2-weighted images [17, 30].

Sickle Cell Disease Sickle cell disease is one of the most common monogenetic diseases in the world, caused by the mutation in the β-globin gene, resulting in abnormal polymerization within the nucleus that disrupts the normal red blood cell architecture, flexibility, and cellular dehydration. Affected patients may inherit hemoglobin SS, hemoglobin

SC, or hemoglobin S/β-thalassemia with variable degrees of resultant disease severity. Two main pathophysiological processes result from the abnormal red blood cell characteristics with polymerization of the hemoglobin molecules: vaso-occlusion with ischemia-reperfusion injury and hemolytic anemia [61].

The splenic complications of sickle cell disease may occur as early as 5 months of age [50]. Sequestration is one complication that may be observed in younger patients with either homozygous or heterozygous forms of the disease. Acute episodes are caused by rapid congestion of the splenic red pulp by sickled red blood cells, resulting in rapid enlargement of the spleen that causes substantial pain and may lead to rapid decline in hematocrit, thrombocytopenia, hypotension, and shock. On MR imaging, the spleen is enlarged with areas of heterogenous internal signal intensity and focal T2-weighted hyperintense regions relative to the normal spleen corresponding to areas of hemorrhage [62].

Patients with sickle cell disease may have functional asplenia where the spleen is anatomically present but nonfunctional due to multiple prior infarctions. They may also infarct the entire spleen, with imaging appearances as previously described with infarction. The spleen may ultimately end up as small, densely calcified mass that is low in signal on all MR sequences (Fig. 10.22). As a result of their pervasive anemia and transfusions, affected pediatric patients may have iron deposition (hemosiderosis) in the reticuloendothelial system that results in diffusely diminished splenic signal intensity on T1- and T2-weighted (especially GRE) images [11, 63] (Fig. 10.23).

Storage Disorders Gaucher disease is a lysosomal storage disorder caused by the lack of the enzyme glucocerebrosidase. While there are multiple types of Gaucher disease, all cases result in the accumulation of glucocerebroside in the cells of the reticuloendothelial system and hepatosplenomegaly. On MR imaging, T1-weighted signal intensity in patients with Gaucher disease is lower than in the normal spleen due to the accumulation of glucocerebroside. T2-weighted signal intensity is normal. Focal splenic nodules that are hypo- to isointense to normal splenic parenchyma on T1-weighted images and hypointense on T2-weighted images may be seen in some patients, typically those with markedly enlarged spleens (Fig. 10.24). Patients with Gaucher disease may also exhibit splenic infarcts [17, 64–66].

Peliosis Peliosis is a rare disease characterized by multiple blood-filled cavities within the spleen, most commonly seen in conjunction with hepatic peliosis. Isolated splenic peliosis

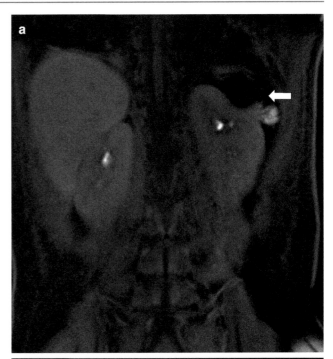

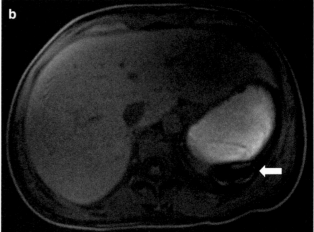

Fig. 10.22 Splenic atrophy in a 17-year-old girl with history of sickle cell disease. (**a**) Coronal and (**b**) axial T1-weighted volumetric GRE fat-suppressed contrast-enhanced MR images demonstrate marked splenic atrophy (*white arrows*). There is also blooming artifact (**b**; *white arrow*) compatible with a diffuse splenic calcification

is rare [67]. Peliosis has been associated with disseminated tuberculosis, hematological malignancies, and steroids [68]. While peliosis is usually discovered incidentally, one of the main risks of the disease process lies in the potential for splenic rupture, which may lead to life-threatening intraperitoneal hemorrhage [37, 69]. On MR imaging, lesions related to peliosis are usually numerous and have mixed signal intensity owing to the variable state of hemoglobin contained within the blood-filled spaces. Similar to hepatic peliosis, splenic peliosis may demonstrate a characteristic

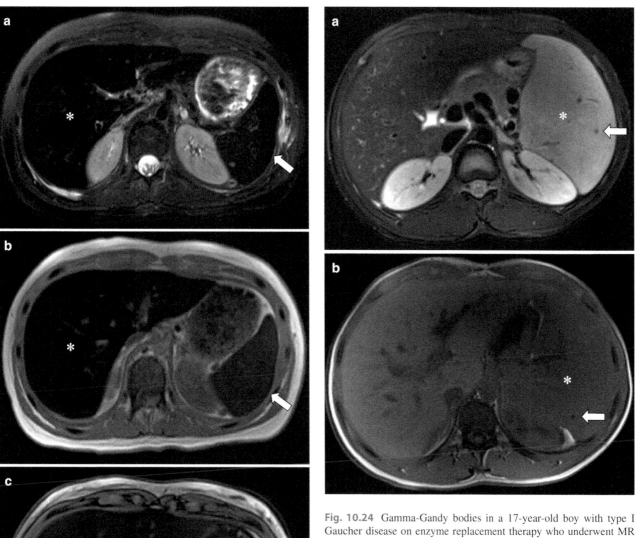

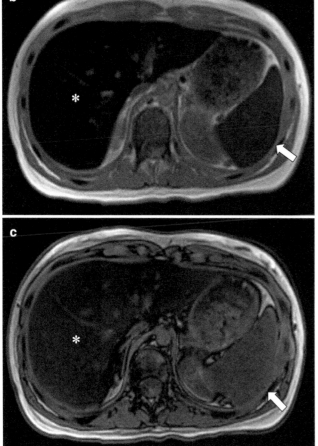

Fig. 10.24 Gamma-Gandy bodies in a 17-year-old boy with type I Gaucher disease on enzyme replacement therapy who underwent MR imaging to evaluate liver and spleen volume. (**a**) Axial T2-weighted fat-suppressed and (**b**) axial T1-weighted MR images demonstrate marked splenomegaly (*asterisks*). Note the relative decreased signal of the spleen on the T1-weighted image. Multiple, scattered, subcentimeter low T1-weighted and T2-weighted signal intensity nodules (*white arrows*) are visualized within the spleen consistent with Gamna-Gandy bodies

Fig. 10.23 Splenic iron deposition in a 17-year-old girl with multiple prior blood transfusions. (**a**) Axial T2-weighted fat-suppressed MR image demonstrates diffusely decreased signal intensity within the liver (*asterisk*) and spleen (*white arrow*). Axial GRE T1-weighted (**b**) in-phase and (**c**) out-of-phase MR images demonstrate diffusely decreased signal intensity within the liver (*asterisks*) and spleen (*white arrows*) on the longer TE in-phase image as compared to the out-of-phase image secondary to iron deposition from secondary hemosiderosis

centrifugal pattern of enhancement (starting at the center and progressing peripherally). Siderotic nodules form at the periphery of the lesions and result in characteristic low sig-nal intensity from susceptibility artifact, most apparent on GRE images [17, 67].

Lymphatic Malformation Splenic lymphatic malforma-tions are benign lesions more commonly identified in chil-dren than adults [37]. Lesions may be single, multiple, or part of a generalized lymphangiomatosis, where multiple organs are involved and the spleen is partly or completely replaced by lymphatic malformations. Generally, lesions are slow growing and remain asymptomatic unless they reach a large size, or the spleen enlarges, resulting in com-pression of adjacent structures. Lymphatic malformations may develop internal hemorrhage and result in consump-tive coagulopathy, hypersplenism, and portal hypertension

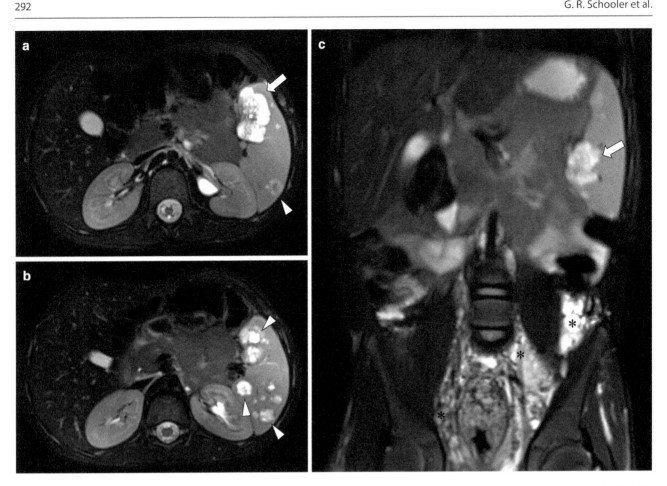

Fig. 10.25 Splenic lymphatic malformation in a 7-year-old boy with Klippel-Trenaunay syndrome (KTS) who presented for further evaluation of known intra-abdominal and lower extremity lymphatic malformations (**a**). (**b**) Axial T2-weighted fat-suppressed MR images demonstrate numerous hyperintense lesions (*white arrowheads*) within the spleen. The largest lesion (*arrow*) is noted in the anterior inferior aspect of the spleen and demonstrates thin internal septations. (**c**) Coronal T2-weighted fat-suppressed MR image shows the largest splenic lymphatic malformation (*white arrow*) and partially visualized pelvic lymphatic malformation (*asterisks*)

[70]. By histology, lymphatic malformations are closely related to hemangiomas, although the endothelium-lined spaces within lymphatic malformations are filled with proteinaceous material rather than blood [37].

Lymphatic malformations within the spleen are usually microcystic or solid. On MR imaging, the lesions are generally hypointense on T1-weighted images though high amounts of internal hemorrhage or protein may result in higher signal intensity. T2-weighted images generally show hyperintense signal within multilocular cysts, although this signal may be affected by the presence of internal hemorrhage as well [71] (Fig. 10.25).

Portal Hypertension Portal hypertension has a variety of etiologies in pediatric patients including extrahepatic portal vein thrombosis and intrinsic liver disease [30]. The increased resistance to portal venous flow into the liver results in flow reversal and splenomegaly. Portal hypertension is the most common cause of splenomegaly in pediatric patients [17]. When splenomegaly second-

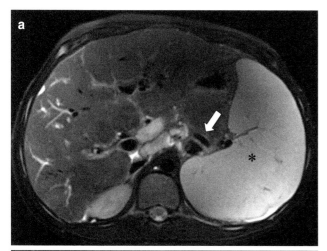

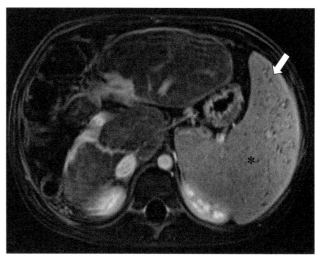

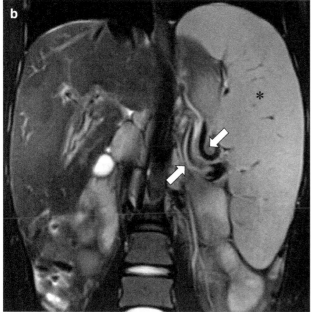

Fig. 10.26 Splenomegaly secondary to portal hypertension in a 13-year-old boy with type 1 diabetes, celiac disease, and primary sclerosing cholangitis. Axial (**a**) and coronal (**b**) T2-weighted fat-suppressed MR images demonstrate marked enlargement of the spleen (*asterisks*). Multiple varices (*white arrows*) are demonstrated at the porta hepatis and splenic hilum. Findings are consistent with splenomegaly secondary to portal hypertension

Fig. 10.27 Gamma-Gandy bodies and splenomegaly in a 12-year-old boy with common variable immune deficiency and portal hypertension. Axial T2-weighted fat-suppressed MR image demonstrates marked enlargement of the spleen (*asterisk*). Multiple subcentimeter foci (*white arrow*) of hypointense signal are demonstrated throughout the spleen compatible with foci of hemosiderin deposition within the spleen called Gamna-Gandy bodies (siderotic nodules) resulting from splenic microhemorrhages. The constellation of findings is most in keeping with splenomegaly secondary to portal hypertension

ary to portal hypertension is seen on MR imaging, there may be signs of liver disease or portal venous occlusion. Perisplenic and splenorenal varices may be evident near the splenic hilum (Fig. 10.26). There may be foci of hemosiderin deposition within the spleen called Gamna-

Gandy bodies (siderotic nodules) that result from splenic microhemorrhages. These nodules are best detected on MR imaging. They are usually less than 1 cm in diameter and hypointense on all sequences, especially GRE sequences [72, 73] (Fig. 10.27).

Conclusion

A wide variety of disorders may affect the pediatric spleen either singularly or as part of a systemic disease process. MR imaging can yield useful diagnostic information about many of these disorders and help to guide clinical management in the pediatric population.

References

1. Varga I, Babala J, Kachlik D. Anatomic variations of the spleen: current state of terminology, classification, and embryological background. Surg Radiol Anat. 2018;40(1):21–9.

2. Courtier J, Rao AG, Anupindi SA. Advanced imaging techniques in pediatric body MRI. Pediatr Radiol. 2017;47(5):522–33.

3. Jaimes C, Kirsch JE, Gee MS. Fast, free-breathing and motion-minimized techniques for pediatric body magnetic resonance imaging. Pediatr Radiol. 2018;48(9):1197–208.

4. Chavhan GB, Babyn PS, Vasanawala SS. Abdominal MR imaging in children: motion compensation, sequence optimization, and protocol organization. Radiographics. 2013;33(3):703–19.

5. Antonov NK, Ruzal-Shapiro CB, Morel KD, Millar WS, Kashyap S, Lauren CT, et al. Feed and wrap MRI technique in infants. Clin Pediatr (Phila). 2017;56(12):1095–103.

6. Mirowitz SA, Brown JJ, Lee JK, Heiken JP. Dynamic gadolinium-enhanced MR imaging of the spleen: normal enhancement patterns and evaluation of splenic lesions. Radiology. 1991;179(3):681–6.

7. Soares BP, Lequin MH, Huisman T. Safety of contrast material use in children. Magn Reson Imaging Clin N Am. 2017;25(4):779–85.

8. Jaspan ON, Fleysher R, Lipton ML. Compressed sensing MRI: a review of the clinical literature. Br J Radiol. 2015;88(1056):20150487.

9. Vasanawala SS, Alley MT, Hargreaves BA, Barth RA, Pauly JM, Lustig M. Improved pediatric MR imaging with compressed sensing. Radiology. 2010;256(2):607–16.

10. Varga I, Galfiova P, Adamkov M, Danisovic L, Polak S, Kubikova E, et al. Congenital anomalies of the spleen from an embryological point of view. Med Sci Monit. 2009;15(12):RA269–76.

11. Adler DD, Glazer GM, Aisen AM. MRI of the spleen: normal appearance and findings in sickle-cell anemia. AJR Am J Roentgenol. 1986;147(4):843–5.

12. Donnelly LF, Emery KH, Bove KE, Bissett GS. Normal changes in the MR appearance of the spleen during early childhood. AJR Am J Roentgenol. 1996;166(3):635–9.

13. Elsayes KM, Narra VR, Mukundan G, James S, Lewis J, Menias CO, Heiken JP. MR imaging of the spleen: spectrum of abnormalities. Radiographics. 2005;25(4):967–82.

14. Chavhan GB, AlSabban Z, Babyn PS. Diffusion-weighted imaging in pediatric body mr imaging: principles, technique, and emerging applications. Radiographics. 2014;34(3):E73–88.

15. Gayer G, Hertz M, Strauss S, Zissin R. Congenital anomalies of the spleen. Semin Ultrasound CT MR. 2006;27(5):358–69.

16. Klingler PJ, Tsiotos GG, Glaser KS, Hinder RA. Laparoscopic splenectomy: evolution and current status. Surg Laparosc Endosc. 1999;9(1):1–8.

17. Paterson A, Frush DP, Donnelly LF, Foss JN, O'Hara SM, George S, Bisset IA. Pattern-oriented approach to splenic imaging in infants and children. Radiographics. 1999;19(6):1465–85.

18. Reisner DC, Burgan CM. Wandering spleen: an overview. Curr Probl Diagn Radiol. 2018;47(1):68–70.

19. Richman M, Hiyama DT, Wasson E. Wandering spleen. Surgery. 2014;155(4):728.

20. Perrotta S, Gallagher PG, Mohandas N. Hereditary spherocytosis. Lancet. 2008;372(9647):1411–26.

21. Manciu S, Matei E, Trandafir B. Hereditary spherocytosis–diagnosis, surgical treatment and outcomes. A literature review. Chirurgia (Bucur). 2017;112(2):110–6.

22. Gungor A, Yarali N, Fettah A, Ok-Bozkaya I, Ozbek N, Kara A. Hereditary spherocytosis: retrospective evaluation of 65 children. Turk J Pediatr. 2018;60(3):264–9.

23. Gaetke-Udager K, Wasnik AP, Kaza RK, Al-Hawary MM, Maturen KE, Udager AM, et al. Multimodality imaging of splenic lesions and the role of non-vascular, image-guided intervention. Abdom Imaging. 2014;39(3):570–87.

24. Ranganath SH, Lee EY, Eisenberg RL. Focal cystic abdominal masses in pediatric patients. AJR Am J Roentgenol. 2012;199(1):W1–W16.

25. Ito K, Mitchell DG, Honjo K, Fujita T, Uchisako H, Matsumoto T, et al. MR imaging of acquired abnormalities of the spleen. AJR Am J Roentgenol. 1997;168(3):697–702.

26. Lynn KN, Werder GM, Callaghan RM, Sullivan AN, Jafri ZH, Bloom DA. Pediatric blunt splenic trauma: a comprehensive review. Pediatr Radiol. 2009;39(9):904–16.. quiz 1029-30

27. Thipphavong S, Duigenan S, Schindera ST, Gee MS, Philips S. Nonneoplastic, benign, and malignant splenic diseases: cross-sectional imaging findings and rare disease entities. AJR Am J Roentgenol. 2014;203(2):315–22.

28. Lennon P, Crotty M, Fenton JE. Infectious mononucleosis. BMJ. 2015;350:h1825.

29. Jenson HB. Acute complications of Epstein-Barr virus infectious mononucleosis. Curr Opin Pediatr. 2000;12(3):263–8.

30. Hilmes MA, Strouse PJ. The pediatric spleen. Semin Ultrasound CT MR. 2007;28(1):3–11.

31. Luna A, Ribes R, Caro P, Luna L, Aumente E, Ros PR. MRI of focal splenic lesions without and with dynamic gadolinium enhancement. AJR Am J Roentgenol. 2006;186(6):1533–47.

32. Kamaya A, Weinstein S, Desser TS. Multiple lesions of the spleen: differential diagnosis of cystic and solid lesions. Semin Ultrasound CT MR. 2006;27(5):389–403.

33. Semelka RC, Kelekis NL, Sallah S, Worawattanakul S, Ascher SM. Hepatosplenic fungal disease: diagnostic accuracy and spectrum of appearances on MR imaging. AJR Am J Roentgenol. 1997;169(5):1311–6.

34. Harisinghani MG, McLoud TC, Shepard JA, Ko JP, Shroff MM, Mueller PR. Tuberculosis from head to toe. Radiographics. 2000;20(2):449–70; quiz 528–9, 32

35. De Backer AI, Vanhoenacker FM, Mortele KJ, Vanschoubroeck IJ, De Keulenaer BL, Parizel PM. MRI features of focal splenic lesions in patients with disseminated tuberculosis. AJR Am J Roentgenol. 2006;186(4):1097–102.

36. Polat P, Kantarci M, Alper F, Suma S, Koruyucu MB, Okur A. Hydatid disease from head to toe. Radiographics. 2003;23(2):475–94.. quiz 536-7

37. Abbott RM, Levy AD, Aguilera NS, Gorospe L, Thompson WM. From the archives of the AFIP. Radiographics. 2004;24(4):1137–63.

38. Dufau JP, le Tourneau A, Audouin J, Delmer A, Diebold J. Isolated diffuse hemangiomatosis of the spleen with Kasabach-Merritt-like syndrome. Histopathology. 1999;35(4):337–44.

39. Ramani M, Reinhold C, Semelka RC, Siegelman ES, Liang L, Ascher SM, et al. Splenic hemangiomas and hamartomas: MR imaging characteristics of 28 lesions. Radiology. 1997;202(1):166–72.

40. Kaza RK, Azar S, Al-Hawary MM, Francis IR. Primary and secondary neoplasms of the spleen. Cancer Imaging. 2010;10:173–82.

41. Darden JW, Teeslink R, Parrish A. Hamartoma of the spleen: a manfestation of tuberous sclerosis. Am Surg. 1975;41(9):564–6.

42. Morgenstern L, McCafferty L, Rosenberg J, Michel SL. Hamartomas of the spleen. Arch Surg. 1984;119(11):1291–3.

43. Chen G, Li M, Wu D, Tang H, Tang D. Primary splenic angiosarcoma in a 2.5-year-old boy with hepatic metastasis. Pediatr Surg Int. 2012;28(11):1147–50.

44. Winde G, Sprakel B, Bosse A, Reers B, Wendt M. Rupture of the spleen caused by primary angiosarcoma. Case report. Eur J Surg. 1991;157(3):215–7.

45. Kaneko K, Onitsuka H, Murakami J, Honda H, Kimura M, Shiraishi N, et al. MRI of primary spleen angiosarcoma with iron accumulation. J Comput Assist Tomogr. 1992;16(2):298–300.

46. Karakas HM, Demir M, Ozyilmaz F, Cakir B. Primary angiosarcoma of the spleen: in vivo and in vitro MRI findings. Clin Imag. 2001;25(3):192–6.

47. Guillerman RP, Voss SD, Parker BR. Leukemia and lymphoma. Radiol Clin N Am. 2011;49(4):767–97.. vii

48. Saboo SS, Krajewski KM, O'Regan KN, Giardino A, Brown JR, Ramaiya N, et al. Spleen in haematological malignancies: spectrum of imaging findings. Br J Radiol. 2012;85(1009):81–92.

49. Paes FM, Kalkanis DG, Sideras PA, Serafini AN. FDG PET/CT of extranodal involvement in non-Hodgkin lymphoma and Hodgkin disease. Radiographics. 2010;30(1):269–91.

50. Rabushka LS, Kawashima A, Fishman EK. Imaging of the spleen: CT with supplemental MR examination. Radiographics. 1994;14(2):307–32.

51. Bhatia K, Sahdev A, Reznek RH. Lymphoma of the spleen. Semin Ultrasound CT MR. 2007;28(1):12–20.

52. Punwani S, Cheung KK, Skipper N, Bell N, Bainbridge A, Taylor SA, et al. Dynamic contrast-enhanced MRI improves accuracy for detecting focal splenic involvement in children and adolescents with Hodgkin disease. Pediatr Radiol. 2013;43(8):941–9.

53. Lam KY, Tang V. Metastatic tumors to the spleen: a 25-year clinicopathologic study. Arch Pathol Lab Med. 2000;124(4):526–30.

54. Borhani AA, Hosseinzadeh K, Almusa O, Furlan A, Nalesnik M. Imaging of posttransplantation lymphoproliferative disorder after solid organ transplantation. Radiographics. 2009;29(4):981–1000; discussion -2

55. Wilde GE, Moore DJ, Bellah RD. Posttransplantation lymphoproliferative disorder in pediatric recipients of solid organ transplants: timing and location of disease. AJR Am J Roentgenol. 2005;185(5):1335–41.

56. Donnelly LF, Frush DP, Marshall KW, White KS. Lymphoproliferative disorders: CT findings in immunocompromised children. AJR Am J Roentgenol. 1998;171(3):725–31.

57. Pickhardt PJ, Siegel MJ. Posttransplantation lymphoproliferative disorder of the abdomen: CT evaluation in 51 patients. Radiology. 1999;213(1):73–8.

58. Santschi M, Echave V, Laflamme S, McFadden N, Cyr C. Seat-belt injuries in children involved in motor vehicle crashes. Can J Surg. 2005;48(5):373–6.

59. Tinkoff G, Esposito TJ, Reed J, Kilgo P, Fildes J, Pasquale M, et al. American Association for the Surgery of Trauma Organ Injury Scale I: spleen, liver, and kidney, validation based on the national trauma data bank. J Am Coll Surg. 2008;207(5):646–55.

60. Gordic S, Alkadhi H, Simmen HP, Wanner G, Cadosch D. Characterization of indeterminate spleen lesions in primary CT after blunt abdominal trauma: potential role of MR imaging. Emerg Radiol. 2014;21(5):491–8.

61. Rees DC, Williams TN, Gladwin MT. Sickle-cell disease. Lancet. 2010;376(9757):2018–31.

62. Roshkow JE, Sanders LM. Acute splenic sequestration crisis in two adults with sickle cell disease: US, CT, and MR imaging findings. Radiology. 1990;177(3):723–5.

63. Wood JC, Cohen AR, Pressel SL, Aygun B, Imran H, Luchtman-Jones L, et al. Organ iron accumulation in chronically transfused children with sickle cell anaemia: baseline results from the TWiTCH trial. Br J Haematol. 2016;172(1):122–30.

64. Hill SC, Damaska BM, Ling A, Patterson K, Di Bisceglie AM, Brady RO, et al. Gaucher disease: abdominal MR imaging findings in 46 patients. Radiology. 1992;184(2):561–6.

65. Lanir A, Hadar H, Cohen I, Tal Y, Benmair J, Schreiber R, et al. Gaucher disease: assessment with MR imaging. Radiology. 1986;161(1):239–44.

66. Regenboog M, Bohte AE, Somers I, van Delden OM, Maas M, Hollak CE. Imaging characteristics of focal splenic and hepatic lesions in type 1 Gaucher disease. Blood Cells Mol Dis. 2016;60:49–57.

67. Tsokos M, Erbersdobler A. Pathology of peliosis. Forensic Sci Int. 2005;149(1):25–33.

68. Urrutia M, Mergo PJ, Ros LH, Torres GM, Ros PR. Cystic masses of the spleen: radiologic-pathologic correlation. Radiographics. 1996;16(1):107–29.

69. Lashbrook DJ, James RW, Phillips AJ, Holbrook AG, Agombar AC. Splenic peliosis with spontaneous splenic rupture: report of two cases. BMC Surg. 2006;6:9.

70. Dietz WH Jr, Stuart MJ. Splenic consumptive coagulopathy in a patient with disseminated lymphangiomatosis. J Pediatr. 1977;90(3):421–3.

71. Ito K, Murata T, Nakanishi T. Cystic lymphangioma of the spleen: MR findings with pathologic correlation. Abdom Imaging. 1995;20(1):82–4.

72. Dobritz M, Nomayr A, Bautz W, Fellner FA. Gamna-Gandy bodies of the spleen detected with MR imaging: a case report. Magn Reson Imaging. 2001;19(9):1249–51.

73. Sagoh T, Itoh K, Togashi K, Shibata T, Nishimura K, Minami S, et al. Gamna-Gandy bodies of the spleen: evaluation with MR imaging. Radiology. 1989;172(3):685–7.

Adrenal Glands

James M. Brian, Anil G. Rao, and Michael M. Moore

Introduction

MR imaging is well suited for viewing adrenal gland pathology in the pediatric population. While requesting clinicians often choose ultrasound for the initial evaluation of a suspected adrenal lesion, MR imaging offers unique tissue characterization and the ability to evaluate for evidence of metastatic or remote disease.

This chapter briefly reviews the anatomy and embryology of the adrenal gland as well as the physics underlying MR imaging sequences most useful in evaluating pediatric adrenal lesions. Congenital and acquired disorders of the adrenal gland commonly affecting infants and children are reviewed including clinical features, characteristic MR imaging findings, and treatment approaches.

Magnetic Resonance Imaging Techniques

A comprehensive review of magnetic resonance physics is not within the scope of this chapter. However, a focused discussion of several points to augment understanding of adrenal lesions is helpful, particularly fat-suppression techniques and how they pertain to adrenal adenomas. It should be noted that, in contradistinction to adult imaging, myelolipomas are exceedingly rare in children.

J. M. Brian · M. M. Moore (✉)
Department of Radiology, Penn State Hershey Children's Hospital, Penn State College of Medicine, Hershey, PA, USA
e-mail: mmoore5@pennstatehealth.psu.edu

A. G. Rao
Desert Radiology, Las Vegas, NV, USA

MR Imaging Pulse Sequences and Protocols

MR fat-suppression methods include chemical shift imaging, frequency-selective fat-suppression, and inversion recovery-based techniques. Chemical shift techniques are based on differential precession frequency of protons associated with fat and water; specifically, fat protons precess at 3.5 parts per million slower than water protons in a 1.5 Tesla magnet. This difference in precessional frequency allows for the determination of intravoxel lipid content when signal acquisition occurs at different echo times (TE) corresponding to in-phase and opposed-phase imaging. For a 1.5 Tesla MR scanner, in-phase imaging occurs at 4.4 milliseconds and opposed-phase imaging at either 2.2 or 6.6 milliseconds. When opposed-phase imaging occurs, the fat and water protons demonstrate a 180-degree difference in transverse magnetization resulting in signal loss. Voxels that contain significant amounts of both fat and water lose signal intensity on opposed-phase imaging [1].

An important point is that both fat and water protons need to be present to observe signal intensity change on chemical shift imaging. If lesions contain nearly all lipid or adipose tissue elements, other fat-suppression techniques are needed for visualization. These include frequency-selective fat suppression (also known as chemical saturation or simply "fat sat"), in which a radio-frequency (RF) pulse selective for fat protons is used in combination with a spoiler gradient to null fat signal. Another commonly utilized abdominal fat-suppression technique is inversion recovery, in which an inversion RF pulse is used to invert the longitudinal magnetization, followed by an inversion time interval (TI) chosen to null fat signal prior to standard RF excitation. There are also hybrid chemical saturation-inversion recovery techniques including spectral adiabatic inversion recovery (SPAIR) [2]. In clinical practice, chemical shift in- and opposed-phase imaging as well as chemical saturation are the most common fat-suppression techniques used for routine adrenal MR imaging protocols.

Anatomy

Embryology

The adrenal glands have two tissue precursors. At about 6 weeks gestational age, the cortex of the adrenal gland arises from mesenchymal cells in the region of the developing gonads. During the seventh week, ectodermal neural crest cells migrating to form adjacent sympathetic ganglia develop into the medulla of the adrenal gland. The medulla abuts and is surrounded by cortex during the eighth week of gestation. During gestation and infancy, the adrenal glands contain fetal cortex. As a result, the adrenal gland of a newborn is 10 to 20 times larger relative to other abdominal organs compared to an adult adrenal gland. The fetal cortex regresses during the first year of life and is often not visible outside of infancy.

By the end of the third year of life, the adrenal cortex has three layers: the superficial zona glomerulosa, the zona fasciculata, and the innermost zona reticularis. These zones are responsible for the production of mineralocorticoids (aldosterone), glucocorticoids, and androgens, respectively. The individual cortical layers cannot be distinguished on MR imaging. Adrenocortical carcinoma and adrenal adenomas arise from the adrenal cortex and are collectively called adrenocortical tumors. The adrenal medulla lies in the center of the adrenal gland and produces catecholamines. Neuroblastic tumors arise from the adrenal medulla or its neural crest cell precursors. Pheochromocytomas are tumors of the chromaffin cells of the adrenal medulla [3, 4].

The triangular or crescent shape of the adrenal gland derives from the upward pressure of the developing ipsilateral kidney. In the event of the congenital absence of the ipsilateral kidney from the renal fossa, the adrenal gland may take on a flattened, rounded shape, sometimes referred to as a pancake or discoid adrenal gland [5, 6]. Identification of the pancake adrenal gland should result in a search for an associated congenital renal anomaly such as renal agenesis, pelvic kidney, or cross-fused renal ectopia.

Normal Development and Anatomy

The adrenal glands are paired suprarenal endocrine organs located in the retroperitoneal space. The triangular right adrenal gland sits superior to the right kidney, while the more crescent-shaped left adrenal gland is found anterior and superior to the left kidney. The adrenal glands are found within the renal fascia and are surrounded by perirenal fat. The adrenal anatomy is readily visible with MR imaging.

Although the vascular supply to the adrenal gland is typically below the resolution of MR imaging, the gland is a vascular organ and demonstrates contrast enhancement [7]. The adrenal gland receives arterial blood from the inferior phrenic artery superiorly, the adrenal arterial branch of the aorta

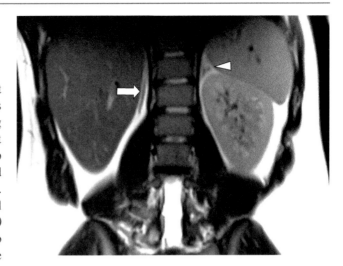

Fig. 11.1 Discoid or pancake right adrenal gland and congenitally absent ipsilateral kidney incidentally found in a 13-year-old boy who presented with suspected appendicitis. Coronal single-shot T2-weighted MR image shows discoid or pancake right adrenal gland (*arrow*) and the normal-appearing left adrenal gland (*arrowhead*) for comparison

medially, and branches from the renal arteries inferiorly. The right adrenal vein empties directly into the inferior vena cava, while the left adrenal vein drains into the left renal vein via the inferior phrenic vein. Multiple accessory adrenal veins exist and can be the source of collateral blood flow in the case of large tumors [3].

Anatomic Variants

Discoid Adrenal As noted above, in order for a developing adrenal gland to form a proper Y-shaped configuration, ipsilateral renal tissue must be present within the renal fossa. In the setting of renal agenesis, the shape of the adrenal gland is abnormal. Most commonly, the shape is referred to as a discoid adrenal gland. Alternatively, the morphology may also be referred to as pancake or straight adrenal gland. While the morphology is abnormal on imaging, adrenal gland function is not affected, and the finding of a discoid adrenal gland is otherwise without clinical significance [7]. Figure 11.1 demonstrates a discoid adrenal gland as an incidental finding during MR imaging appendicitis evaluation in a patient with renal agenesis.

Spectrum of Adrenal Gland Disorders

Congenital Adrenal Gland Disorders

Congenital Adrenal Hyperplasia Congenital adrenal hyperplasia results from a complex biochemically mediated increase in adrenal cortex cellularity. There is a defect in enzymes involved in cortisol or aldosterone production, which results in increased output of adrenocorticotropin from the anterior pituitary. This pathologic negative feedback induces overproduction of androgens and adrenal cortical enlargement. While there are several enzymatic deficiencies that can result in congenital adrenal hyperplasia, 21-hydroxylase deficiency is the most common cause.

Female infants with congenital adrenal hyperplasia often demonstrate virilization of their external genitalia leading to early diagnosis of congenital adrenal hyperplasia. Affected male infants may not demonstrate early clinical signs of congenital adrenal hyperplasia and, if undiagnosed, are affected by rapid growth and precocious maturation later in childhood. Fortunately, mandatory newborn screening includes tests for the most common causes of congenital adrenal hyperplasia, thereby limiting the cases of undiagnosed or poorly controlled disease [8].

MR imaging of poorly controlled congenital adrenal hyperplasia reveals an enlarged, nodular adrenal gland possibly containing adrenal tumors such as myelolipomas or adenomas [4, 9]. An adrenal limb length of 20 mm or greater and a limb width of greater than 4 mm is indicative of enlargement due to congenital adrenal hyperplasia [5]. In Fig. 11.2 an enlarged adrenal gland is noted in a 16-year-old girl undergoing work-up for clitoromegaly and excessive facial hair. She was diagnosed with congenital adrenal hyperplasia secondary to 21-hydroxylase deficiency.

Testicular Adrenal Rest Tumor Noting that adrenal cortical tissue arises from mesenchymal cells near the developing gonads, it is not surprising that adrenal rest tissue can be found along the path of gonadal descent, including the celiac plexus, broad ligament of the uterus, ovaries, inguinal canals, epididymides, and testes. Testicular adrenal rest tumors may be seen in prepubertal male patients with poorly controlled congenital adrenal hyperplasia. While these lesions are readily identified with ultrasound, they can also be seen with MR imaging.

Testicular adrenal rest tumor lesions appear isointense to the testicle on T1-weighted sequences but are hypointense relative to the surrounding hyperintense testicular tissue on T2-weighted images regardless of whether or not fat suppression is used. Testicular adrenal rest lesions enhance strongly after gadolinium administration [5, 10]. Fig. 11.3 demonstrates testicular adrenal rest lesions in a 16-year-old boy with congenital adrenal hyperplasia.

Neoplastic Adrenal Gland Disorders

Neuroblastic Tumors

Neuroblastoma, ganglioneuroblastoma, and ganglioneuroma (collectively called neuroblastic tumors) are tumors that arise from ectodermal neural crest cells destined to form sympathetic ganglion cells and the medulla of the adrenal glands. Neuroblastic tumors may appear along the pathway of these migrating neural crest cells. As such, neuroblastic tumors may be seen in the neck, posterior mediastinum, adrenal gland, retroperitoneum, and pelvis.

Neuroblastoma, ganglioneuroblastoma, and ganglioneuroma tumors each differ in the degree of cellular and extracellular maturation, with immature tumors having more aggressive behavior and mature tumors being more benign. Neuroblastomas have immature, undifferentiated cells. They are the most malignant of the neuroblastic tumors and typically appear in younger children. Neuroblastomas are sporadic in occurrence, with only about 1% being familial [11–13]. Conversely, ganglioneuromas have mature gangliocytes and stroma and are typically considered benign. They are commonly diagnosed in older children and adolescents. Ganglioneuroblastoma tumors contain both mature gangliocytes and immature neuroblasts and, as such, demonstrate intermediate malignant potential [11].

In rare cases, neuroblastic tumors may occur in patients with other congenital disorders, including neurofibromatosis type 1, Beckwith-Wiedemann syndrome, Hirschsprung disease, and DiGeorge syndrome [11].

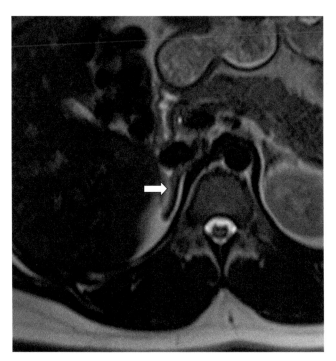

Fig. 11.2 Enlarged right adrenal gland in a 16-year-old girl who presented with androgen excess manifested by clitoromegaly and facial hair. The patient was diagnosed with congenital adrenal hyperplasia secondary to 21-hydroxylase deficiency. Axial single-shot T2-weighted MR image shows enlarged right adrenal gland (*arrow*). The right adrenal gland medial limb measured 4.2 cm in length by 0.6 cm. The left adrenal gland is incompletely visualized on this axial single-shot T2-weighted MR image but was also enlarged

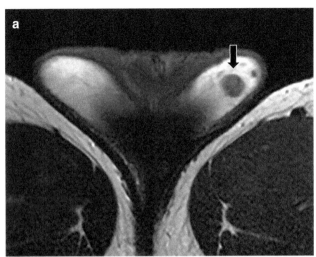

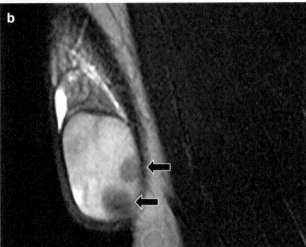

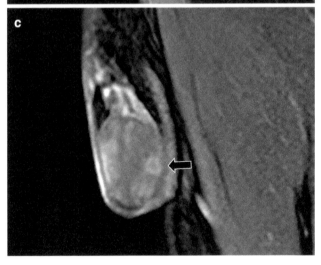

Fig. 11.3 Testicular adrenal rest tumors in a 16-year-old boy with congenital adrenal hyperplasia. (a) Axial and sagittal (b) T2-weighted MR images demonstrate the testicular adrenal rest tumors (*arrows*) that are hypointense on T2-weighted MR imaging. (c) Sagittal T1-weighted fat-suppressed post-contrast MR image demonstrates that the testicular adrenal rest tumors (*arrow*) enhance after contrast administration. (Images courtesy of Michael S. Gee, MD, PhD, Massachusetts General Hospital)

Neuroblastoma and Ganglioneuroblastoma Neuroblastomas and ganglioneuroblastomas both share a higher malignant potential than ganglioneuromas and are grouped together for purposes of cancer reporting, staging, and survival statistics. The majority of neuroblastomas and ganglioneuroblastomas are found in the abdomen and to a lesser degree the chest. Within the abdomen, half of these tumors arise from the adrenal medulla, and half are found in the extra-adrenal retroperitoneum. Within the chest, neuroblastomas and ganglioneuroblastomas are seen in the posterior mediastinum. Other less common sites include the neck, pelvis, thymus, lung, kidney, anterior mediastinum, stomach, and cauda equina [11].

Neuroblastomas are far more common than ganglioneuroblastoma or ganglioneuroma, making up 97% of neuroblastic tumors. Neuroblastomas are also the most commonly diagnosed cancer in infancy and the third most common childhood cancer, comprising approximately 10% of all childhood cancers but accounting for 15% of childhood cancer fatalities. Nearly 40% of the patients with neuroblastoma are diagnosed by 3 months of age, and 95% of them are diagnosed by 10 years of age [11, 12].

Clinical symptoms of neuroblastoma are varied and can include constipation, abdominal distension, hypertension from compression of renal vessels, and neurologic symptoms if there is spinal canal extension from paravertebral sympathetic ganglia involvement. Less commonly, paraneoplastic syndromes such as opsoclonus-myoclonus syndrome can be caused by an autoimmune response to neurologic tissues. Watery diarrhea and electrolyte imbalances may arise from autonomous secretion of vasoactive intestinal peptide.

Diagnosis of neuroblastoma is made by either surgical biopsy of the tumor demonstrating neuroblastoma cells or a combination of positive bone marrow aspirate and increased urinary catecholamine metabolites – vanillylmandelic acid and homovanillic acid [13]. Neuroblastoma cells are small round relatively undifferentiated cells with large hyperchromatic nuclei with a blue appearance and thin cytoplasmic rim and as such fall under the category of small, round blue cell tumors.

The International Neuroblastoma Staging System (INSS) was devised in 1986 based on clinical, radiologic, and surgical features. The International Neuroblastoma Risk Group (INRG) staging system was published in 2008 to stratify and stage patients prior to surgery, as the INSS was a postsurgical staging. INRG staging provides a pre-treatment risk stratification using clinical criteria and image-defined risk factors (IDRFs) [14]. Brisse et al. published a consensus report in 2011 from the International Neuroblastoma Risk Group Project with the guidelines for imaging and staging of neuroblastic tumors [15] and defined various terms for assessing IDRFs such as "encasement," "contact," and "flattening" to assess tumor relationship with adjacent blood vessels. In this paper, Brisse et al. also described the rationale for using different imaging modalities such as US, CT, and MR imaging including technical guidelines.

The International Neuroblastoma Pathology Classification (the Shimada system) published in 1999 [16] categorizes patients with neuroblastic tumors into two groups having either favorable histology or unfavorable histology. This classification considers the amount of Schwannian stroma, the degree of nodularity, the degree of neuroblastic differentiation, the mitosis-karyorrhexis index (MKI), and the presence or absence of calcification along with the patient's age. Patients are grouped as less than 1.5 years, 1.5–5 years, and greater than 5 years of age. A *favorable* histologic result is given to children less than 1.5 years old with a low or intermediate MKI having a differentiating or a partially differentiating tumor and to children 1.5–5 years of age with a low MKI having a differentiating tumor. Other combinations are considered to have *unfavorable* histologic characteristics. Genetic analysis of the tumor is also an important part of risk stratification

and can help determine the prognosis of the tumor, including presence or absence of N-myc amplification or ALK activation. By combining INSS/INRG staging with the patient's age at diagnosis, tumor histology, and the biology and genetics of the tumor, the patient is assigned to a low-, intermediate-, or high-risk group and treated accordingly.

Imaging has a role in determining the site of origin, characteristics and extent of these tumors, and the presence or absence of metastatic disease. Abdominal neuroblastic tumors often arise either from the adrenal glands or a paraspinal location. These tumors are iso- to hypointense to adjacent soft tissues on T1-weighted images and hyperintense on T2-weighted images. There is variable enhancement following intravenous gadolinium contrast administration. The tumor margins may be smooth, lobulated, or irregular. There is heterogeneity in the tumor due to necrosis, hemorrhage, and calcification. Necrotic areas are T1-weighted hypointense and T2-weighted hyperintense and do not demonstrate contrast enhancement (Figs. 11.4, 11.5, and 11.6). Areas of

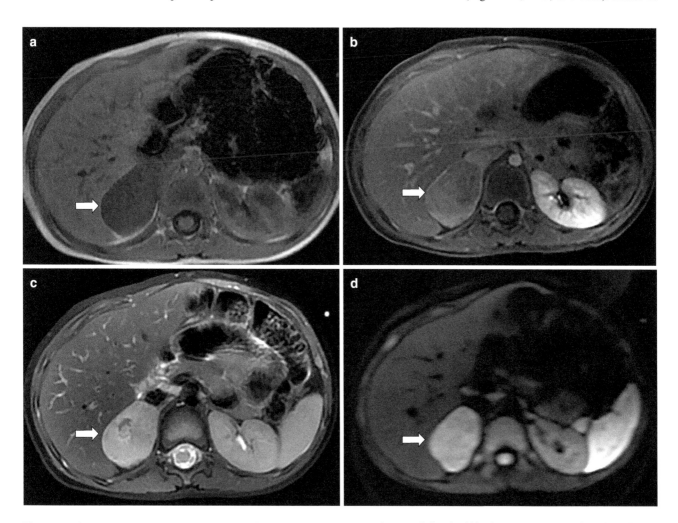

Fig. 11.4 Right adrenal ganglioneuroblastoma in a 3-year-old boy. (**a**) Axial T1-weighted MR image demonstrates a large hypointense right suprarenal mass (*arrow*). (**b**) Axial T1-weighted fat-suppressed postcontrast MR image demonstrates inhomogeneous tumor enhancement (*arrow*). (**c**) Axial T2-weighted MR image with fat suppression demonstrates increased signal within the tumor (*arrow*). (**d**) Axial diffusion weighted MR image (*b* = 800) demonstrates increased signal (*arrow*) indicating restricted diffusion within the tumor. (**e**) Corresponding axial apparent diffusion coefficient (ADC) map demonstrates low ADC values (*arrow*) confirming restricted diffusion within the tumor

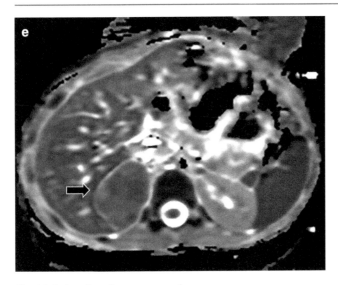

Fig. 11.4 (continued)

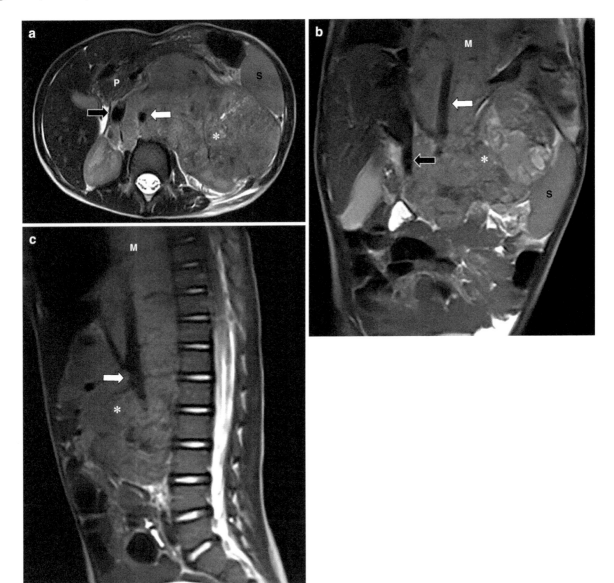

Fig. 11.5 Left adrenal neuroblastoma in a 3-year-old boy. Axial (**a**), coronal (**b**), and sagittal (**c**) single-shot T2-weighted MR images demonstrate a large left adrenal mass (*asterisk*) that encases the aorta (*white arrows*) and renal vessels but displaces the inferior vena cava (*black arrows*), spleen (S), pancreas (P), and left kidney (*not shown*). The tumor extends cranially into the mediastinum (M)

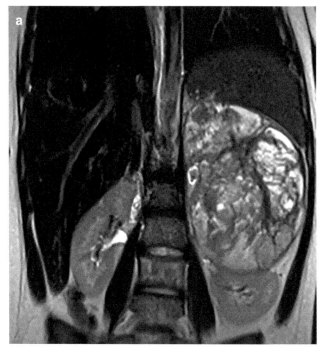

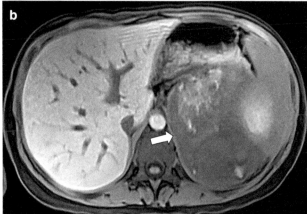

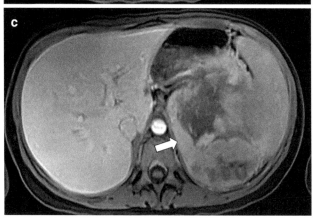

Fig. 11.6 Left adrenal neuroblastoma in a 15-year-old girl. Coronal single-shot T2-weighted MR image (**a**) demonstrates a large left adrenal lesion hyperintense to muscle that is inferiorly displacing the left kidney. Axial T1-weighted fat-suppressed MR images before (**b**) and after (**c**) contrast administration show that mass to have internal regions of T1-weighted hyperintense hemorrhage (**b**) and heterogeneous enhancement (**b** and **c**; *arrows*)

calcification have low signal intensity on T1- and T2-weighted images, whereas hemorrhagic areas can have variable T1- and T2-weighted signal characteristics based on the stage of degradation of hemoglobin.

Neuroblastic tumors typically encase or displace blood vessels in the abdomen instead of directly invading them (see Fig. 11.5). This can be seen on the T1-weighted fat-suppressed pre-contrast and post-contrast images. Adrenal masses typically displace the kidney inferiorly and laterally (see Fig. 11.6). Paraspinal neuroblastic tumors displace the kidney superiorly and laterally. Invasion of the kidney can be present. Renal atrophy could be due to several factors such as encasement and compression of the renal vessels or could be the result of surgery, chemotherapy, or radiation therapy [13]. Extension of the tumor across the midline, regional lymph node involvement, or intraspinal extension may be seen. Intraspinal extension of a paraspinal neuroblastic tumor is better seen on MR imaging than CT (Fig. 11.7). Metastases to the skin, liver, distant lymph nodes, cortical bone, and bone marrow that may be present can also be seen on MR imaging (Fig. 11.8). Neuroblastoma and ganglioneuroblastoma tumors often show restricted diffusion on DWI (see Fig. 11.4d, e). Whole-body MR imaging from the vertex to the toes can be helpful to assess for metastatic disease.

Congenital Neuroblastoma Congenital neuroblastoma is a tumor detected within 1 month of birth. Neuroblastoma is the most common malignancy in the first month of life and accounts for 30% to 50% of all malignant tumors at this age. Neuroblastoma occurring the perinatal timeframe may be categorized as fetal or neonatal neuroblastoma, based on the patient's age at presentation. Both types have very good prognoses but differ somewhat in their patterns of metastatic spread and organ of origin.

Neonatal neuroblastoma has an adrenal origin in 45% of patients. Like older children with neuroblastoma, about 60% of neonates have metastatic disease at the time of diagnosis. Metastases are often found in the liver, bone cortex, marrow, and skin, although any site may be affected. Neonatal neuroblastoma usually has a favorable tumor biologic behavior, and the survival rate is greater than 90% [11, 17].

Fetal neuroblastoma arises from the adrenal glands in approximately 90% of the cases. Fetal neuroblastoma may be seen on obstetric ultrasound with a mean age of discovery at 36 weeks gestation but has been seen as early as 19 weeks gestation. Fetal neuroblastoma is associated with hepatic and bone marrow metastases. Metastases to the bone cortex are extremely rare. Fetal neuroblastomas are usually stage 1, 2, or 4S at presentation based on the International Neuroblastoma Staging System. Placental metastases are typically limited to the placental vasculature but rarely may involve the placental parenchyma. Fetal hydrops can result from placental vascular metastases. Catecholamines released from these tumors

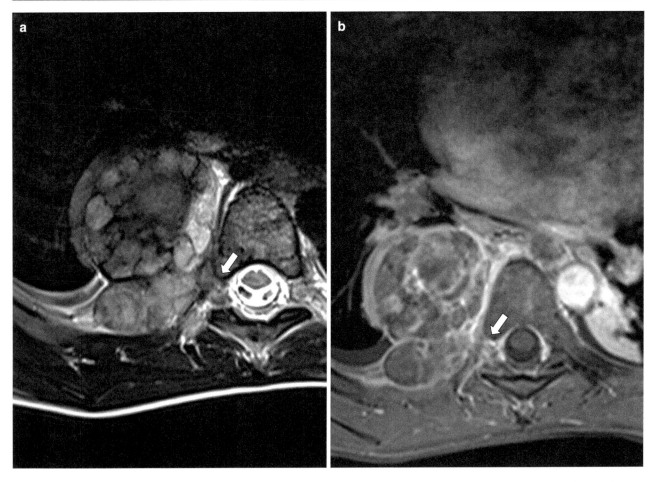

Fig. 11.7 Paraspinal neuroblastoma with intraspinal extension in a 5-year-old boy. (a) Axial T2-weighted MR image demonstrates intraspinal extension (*arrow*) of the paraspinal mass. (b) Axial T1-weighted fat-suppressed post-contrast MR image confirms neuroforaminal extension (*arrow*) of the mass as well as variable enhancement

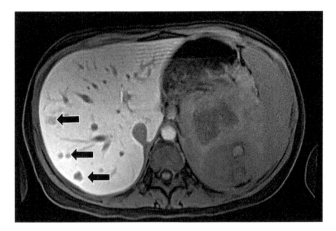

Fig. 11.8 Neuroblastoma metastatic to the liver in the same 15-year-old girl seen in Fig. 11.6. Axial T1-weighted fat-suppressed MR image obtained 20 minutes post-contrast (gadoxetate) in the hepatobiliary phase demonstrates multiple hypointense hepatic metastases (*black arrows*)

have been implicated in the development of maternal pre-eclampsia. The prognosis for patients with fetal neuroblas-

toma is excellent, and conservative approach to management is recommended [11].

Ganglioneuroma Ganglioneuroma is a rare tumor. As previously discussed, ganglioneuroma, being a mature neuroblastic tumor, presents later in life (median age of 7 years). It can occur along the location of the sympathetic ganglia but most commonly occur in the posterior mediastinum, retroperitoneum, adrenal gland, and neck in descending order. Elevated levels of catecholamine metabolites in the urine such as vanillylmandelic acid and homovanillic acid may be present in 37% of patients compared to around 90% of neuroblastomas and ganglioneuroblastomas. These tumors are comprised entirely of mature gangliocytes and Schwannian stroma and do not contain immature elements and are considered benign. The MR imaging features are similar to neuroblastoma and ganglioneuroblastoma; however, they typically do not demonstrate aggressive invasion or metastatic disease [11]. Figure 11.9 demonstrates a left adrenal ganglioneuroma in a 16-year-old boy who had a right ganglioneuroma resected at age 9.

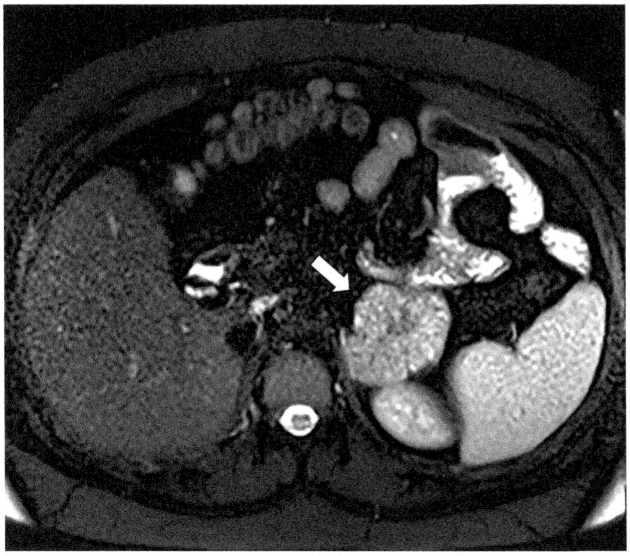

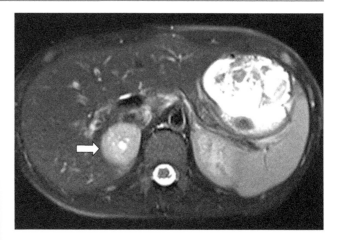

Fig. 11.9 Left adrenal ganglioneuroma in a 16-year-old boy with a history of prior right adrenal ganglioneuroma removed at 9 years of age. Axial T2-weighted fat-suppressed MR image shows a hyperintense left adrenal lesion (*arrow*), unchanged in size over the previous 7 years, consistent with ganglioneuroma

Fig. 11.10 Right adrenal pheochromocytoma discovered on screening ultrasound in a 12-year-old girl with von Hippel-Lindau syndrome. Axial T2-weighted fat-suppressed MR image demonstrates an adrenal mass (*arrow*) with characteristically marked T2-weighted hyperintensity. Small cystic areas within the mass are also present

Pheochromocytoma

Pheochromocytomas, although rare in the pediatric population compared to adults, are the most common endocrine neoplasm in children. They can arise from chromaffin cells both within and external to the adrenal gland [18]. The majority of pediatric pheochromocytomas arise from the adrenal medulla. Extra-adrenal pheochromocytomas, also called extra-axial paragangliomas, commonly occur along the great vessels of the abdomen, including the upper retroperitoneum and the organ of Zuckerkandl near the origin of the inferior mesenteric artery [18–20]. However, extra-adrenal pheochromocytomas can also be found in the head and neck, chest, and pelvis. Children are more likely than adults to have bilateral or extra-adrenal lesions [21].

Pediatric pheochromocytomas are twice as common in boys and typically appear in young adolescents, with an average age of presentation of 11 years [18]. Nearly 40% of pheochromocytomas are associated with known genetic mutations such as multiple endocrine neoplasia type 2, von Hippel-Lindau syndrome, neurofibromatosis type 1, and familial paraganglioma syndromes [20]. Adrenal pheochromocytomas often are hormonally active and result in excessive production and secretion of catecholamines such as epinephrine and norepinephrine as well as vasoactive intestinal peptides. Symptoms associated with the catecholamine excess in hormonally active pediatric pheochromocytomas include hypertension, headaches, sweating, anxiety, pallor, and weight loss [20].

Diagnosis of pheochromocytoma includes both biochemical testing for evidence of excess catecholamines followed by imaging to localize the tumor. MR imaging is an ideal modality to evaluate children with suspected pheochromocytoma and, when compared to CT and nuclear medicine metaiodobenzylguanidine (MIBG) scanning, has been shown to be more sensitive in the detection of adrenal pheochromocytomas [22]. The tumors are typically round to oval solid lesions that measure 2 to 5 cm in diameter but may be larger [19]. Pheochromocytomas are isointense on T1-weighted sequences and are characteristically markedly hyperintense on T2-weighted sequences (known as the "light bulb" sign; Fig. 11.10). Larger tumors may demonstrate intermediate or low intensity on T2-weighted sequences secondary to necrosis or internal hemorrhage. Most pheochromocytomas avidly and homogeneously enhance after contrast administration [20]. There is no signal loss with T1-weighted chemical shift opposed-phase imaging. Although the majority of pediatric pheochromocytomas are benign, malignant lesions can demonstrate local invasion or metastatic spread to bones, lungs, liver, and lymph nodes [21].

Surgical excision is the treatment of choice for solitary benign pheochromocytomas. The high incidence of associated genetic mutations requires genetic screening in children with pheochromocytomas.

Adrenocortical Tumors

Adrenocortical tumors are rare in children. They typically are seen in children under the age of 5 years. In this young age group, there is a 2:1 female predominance that is not present in older children. There is an association with congenital syndromes including Li-Fraumeni syndrome, Beckwith-Wiedemann syndrome, and multiple endocrine neoplasia type 1. These tumors are often hormonally active. As the cortex of the adrenal gland produces miner-alocorticoids, glucocorticoids, and androgens, the clinical presentation of adrenocortical tumors often involves endocrine abnormalities related to the excess hormone. Laboratory evaluation for excess hormones is helpful for both the diagnosis of adrenocortical tumors and monitoring for tumor recurrence. Most commonly, adrenocortical tumors manifest with excessive androgens, leading to virilization of girls and premature puberty in boys. Less commonly, younger children present with symptoms of Cushing syndrome, although this is a more common presentation in older children. Hypertension is a common presenting symptom and is thought to be due to either excessive mineralocorticoid or glucocorticoid production or, like neuroblastic tumors, tumor mass effect on the renal artery.

It can be difficult to distinguish whether an adrenocortical tumor is malignant (adrenocortical carcinoma) or benign (adenoma) based on imaging and histology alone. Increased size, invasion of adjacent organs and vessels, and regional lymph node involvement are indicative of malignancy [23]. The majority of adrenocortical tumors in children are thought to be malignant on pathologic analysis [24, 25].

On MR imaging, adrenocortical carcinoma appears as large (greater than 4 centimeter) suprarenal masses that demonstrate heterogeneous T1-weighted isointensity and T2-weighted hyperintensity relative to the liver. The heterogeneity often reflects areas of central necrosis and hemorrhage. The lesion does not demonstrate uniform signal loss on in- and opposed-phase imaging. Adrenocortical carcinoma avidly enhances after gadolinium administration and shows slow contrast washout (Fig. 11.11). There may be focal areas of central calcification which are better appreciated on CT. MR imaging is useful for the detection of local metastatic invasion [26].

Treatment of both benign and malignant adrenocortical neoplasms relies upon surgical excision with close clinical and diagnostic follow-up for evidence of recurrence.

Adrenal Adenoma

Adrenal adenomas are benign lesions that arise from the zona fasciculata in the adrenal cortex. In an adult-focused radiology practice, there is substantial discussion on how to detect adrenal adenoma fat by MR imaging as they are common incidental findings often without clinical significance. Most commonly, radiologists assess adrenal signal loss on opposed-phase imaging qualitatively. Quantitative assessment of signal intensity may also be performed using (in-phase signal intensity – opposed-phase signal intensity)/(in-phase signal intensity) × 100% greater than 16.5% indicating a lipid-rich adrenal adenoma. Adrenal adenoma

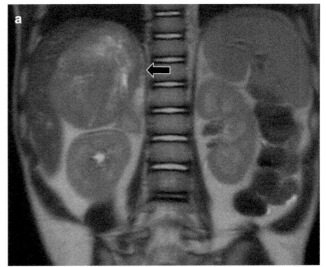
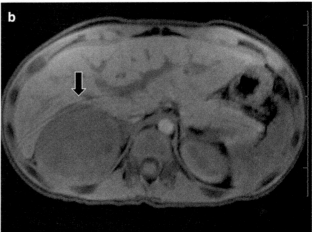
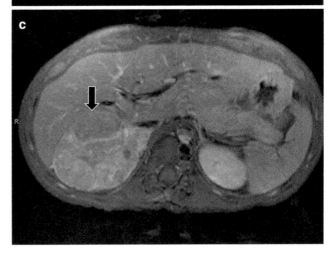

Fig. 11.11 Adrenocortical carcinoma in a 3-year-old boy who presented with precocious puberty. Coronal T2-weighted MR image (**a**) demonstrates a large right adrenal mass (*arrow*) with heterogeneous signal intensity causing inferior displacement of the right kidney. Axial T1-weighted fat-suppressed MR images obtained before (**b**) and after (**c**) contrast administration show the mass (*arrows*) to demonstrate avid enhancement. (Case courtesy of Nancy A. Chauvin, MD, Penn State College of Medicine, and Asef Khwaja, MD, Children's Hospital of Philadelphia, Philadelphia, Pennsylvania, USA)

MR imaging characterization sensitivity and specificity are reported at 81% to 100% and 94% to 100%, respectively [27]. In adults, pathologic distinction is often not warranted given the high sensitivity and specificity of MR imaging. Like much of pediatric care, children are different than adults – even for adrenal adenomas. In contradistinction to adults, adrenal adenomas are quite rare in children and more common in girls. Also in pediatrics, adrenal adenomas are often either hormonally active or with potential endocrine manifestations such as precocious puberty.

While suspected adrenal adenomas in adults are often characterized by either multiphase CT or MR imaging, MR imaging is the modality of choice in children. Adrenal ade-

nomas with "lipid-rich" content demonstrate signal loss on opposed-phase imaging, as demonstrated in Fig. 11.12. However, "lipid-poor" adenomas (Fig. 11.13) without obvious fat elements are also seen but do not have any distinguishing imaging features from other adrenal lesions such as metastases, adrenocortical carcinoma, or neurogenic tumors [7]. One advantage of CT over MR imaging for adrenal adenoma characterization is its ability to diagnose lipid-poor adenomas on the basis of enhancement kinetics.

Given that childhood adrenal adenomas are often hormonally active as well as the potential overlap of "lipid-poor" adenomas with adrenocortical carcinomas, biopsy or surgical resection is typically performed unless there is

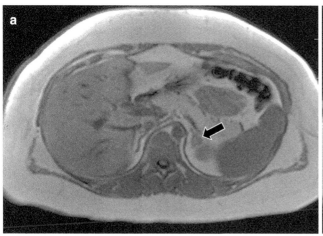
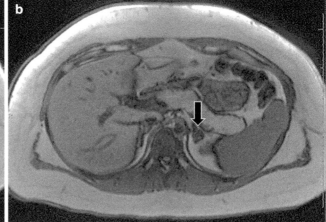

Fig. 11.12 Lipid-rich adrenal adenoma in a 16-year-old obese girl being evaluated for an elevated serum DHEA. Axial T1-weighted in-phase (**a**) and opposed-phase (**b**) MR images demonstrate a left adrenal nodule with intrinsic T1-weighted signal intensity (**a**; *arrow*) and signal loss on opposed-phase imaging (**b**; *arrow*) consistent with intracellular fat within an adenoma. (Case courtesy of Nancy A. Chauvin, MD, Penn State College of Medicine, and Asef Khwaja, MD, Children's Hospital of Philadelphia, Philadelphia, Pennsylvania, USA)

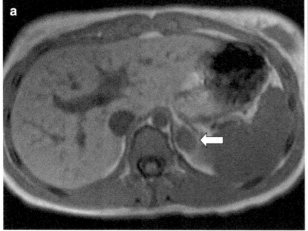
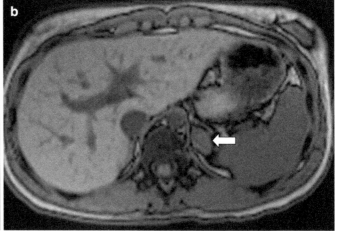

Fig. 11.13 Lipid-poor adenoma in a 14-year-old girl with an incidental discovered left adrenal lesion during imaging evaluation for appendicitis. Axial T1-weighted in-phase (**a**) and opposed-phase (**b**) MR images demonstrate a small T1-weighted hypointense left adrenal lesion (**a**; *arrow*) with no signal loss on opposed-phase imaging (**b**; *arrow*) indicating an absence of detectable intracellular fat. This was confirmed histologically to be an adrenal adenoma

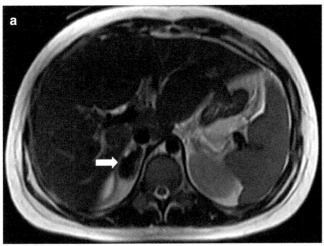

Fig. 11.14 Subacute right adrenal hemorrhage in a 16-year-old girl 6 days after a motor vehicle collision, seen on MR imaging performed to evaluate a pancreatic duct injury. Axial single-shot T2-weighted image (**a**) shows a predominantly hypointense right adrenal lesion (*arrow*) with peripheral areas of increased signal intensity. Axial T1-weighted fat-suppressed image (**b**) shows the lesion (*arrow*) to have high intrinsic T1-weighted signal intensity suggestive of subacute adrenal hemorrhage in the setting of recent trauma

clear imaging evidence of adenoma and the patient is asymptomatic.

Traumatic Adrenal Gland Disorder

Adrenal Hemorrhage There is rarely a primary indication for requesting MR imaging in the setting of adrenal hemorrhage in children although understanding its imaging characteristics remains important. The most common cause of adrenal hemorrhage is neonatal adrenal hemorrhage, which occurs in approximately 1/500 births. The etiology of neonatal adrenal hemorrhage is variable but is most commonly associated with birth trauma, sepsis, hypoxia as well as renal vein thrombosis [7]. This occurs much more commonly than neonatal neuroblastoma although the distinction is important. The critical imaging feature is evolution and resolution from imaging at multiple points over a time period of weeks to several months.

Serial ultrasound is the best imaging modality in the neonatal period to follow adrenal lesions. In addition to becoming smaller over time, another important distinguishing feature of adrenal hemorrhage is its lack of internal Doppler vascularity. Although uncommon, the other cause of adrenal hemorrhage in children is severe blunt abdominal trauma, which typically occurs outside the neonatal period and is imaged by CT in the acute setting. The evaluation of adrenal hemorrhage is rarely the primary cause for abdominal imaging, but adrenal hemorrhage can still be encountered during neuroblastoma evaluation or unrelated examination such as MR cholangiopancreatography following blunt trauma and pancreatic duct injury. In Fig. 11.14, a known adrenal hemorrhage is demonstrated by MR imaging during evaluation for

traumatic pancreatic duct injury in this 16-year-old girl, 6 days after she was injured as an unrestrained passenger in a motor vehicle collision.

The appearance of adrenal hemorrhage on MR imaging can be quite variable and in part depends on the age of the adrenal hemorrhage. In the acute phase, the paramagnetic effect of deoxyhemoglobin results in isointense to hypointense signal on T1-weighted images and hypointense signal on T2-weighted images. In the subacute phase, the paramagnetic effects of methemoglobin result in hyperintensity on T1-weighted images and variable signal on T2-weighted images. Eventually, the hemorrhage transforms into cystic changes with low signal intensity at the margins due to peripheral hemosiderin deposition. Overall, an "ideal" picture of adrenal hemorrhage would be a T1-weighted hyperintense lesion with hyperintense T2-weighted fluid with peripheral and layering hypointense blood products. On postgadolinium images, hemorrhage should be without enhancement, although an associated mass lesion may show a solid enhancing portion [7, 27].

Conclusion

MR imaging is useful in evaluating congenital and acquired pediatric adrenal gland abnormalities. The comprehensive view of the abdomen and pelvis allows for characterization of congenital adrenal abnormalities in the context of adjacent organs that may also be involved, such as renal agenesis associated with a discoid adrenal gland and testicular adrenal rest tumors in the setting of congenital adrenal hyperplasia. While there are MR imaging features of adrenal tumors that are similar, specific MR imaging features, such as opposed-phase T1-weighted signal loss in adrenal adenomas or marked

T2-weighted hyperintensity in pheochromocytomas, can be quite helpful in lesion diagnosis. Additionally, MR imaging provides evidence of metastatic or local spread of malignant adrenal lesions such as neuroblastic or adrenocortical tumors. MR imaging also permits repeat follow-up imaging for the assessment of tumor response to treatment without exposure to ionizing radiation. In conclusion, utilization of MR imaging of the adrenal gland in children provides great value by identifying and characterizing adrenal lesions and providing critical information to facilitate both surgical planning and response to medical treatment.

References

1. Shetty AS, Sipe AL, Zulfiqar M, Tsai R, Raptis DA, Raptis CA, et al. In-phase and opposed-phase imaging: applications of chemical shift and magnetic susceptibility in the chest and abdomen. Radiogaphics. 2019;39(1):115–35.
2. Moore MM, Chung T. Review of key concepts in magnetic resonance physics. Pediatr Radiol. 2017;47(5):497–506.
3. Avisse C, Marcus C, Patey M, Ladam-Marcus V, Delattre JF, Flament JB. Surgical anatomy and embryology of the adrenal glands. Surg Clin North Am. 2000;80(1):403–15.
4. Moore K, TVN P, Torchia MG. The developing human. Clinically oriented embryology. 10th ed. Philadelphia: Elsevier; 2016.
5. Sargar KM, Khanna G, Hulett Bowling R. Imaging of nonmalignant adrenal lesions in children. Radiographics. 2017;37(6):1648–64.
6. Planz VB, Dyer RB. The "pancake" adrenal. Abdom Imaging. 2015;40(6):2041–3.
7. Sargar KM, Khanna G, Bowling RH. Imaging of nonmalignant adrenal lesions in children. Radiographics. 2017;37(6):1648–64.
8. Weismiller DG. Expanded newborn screening: information and resources for the family physician. Am Family Physician. 2017;95(11):703–9.
9. Kok HK, Sherlock M, Healy NA, Doody O, Govender P, Torreggiani WC. Imaging features of poorly controlled congenital adrenal hyperplasia in adults. Br J Radiol. 2015;88(1053):20150352.
10. Stikkelbroeck NM, Suliman HM, Otten BJ, Hermus AR, Blickman JG, Jager GJ. Testicular adrenal rest tumours in postpubertal males with congenital adrenal hyperplasia: sonographic and MR features. Eur Radiol. 2003;13(7):1597–603.
11. Lonergan GJ, Schwab CM, Suarez ES, Carlson CL. Neuroblastoma, ganglioneuroblastoma, and ganglioneuroma: radiologic-pathologic correlation. Radiographics. 2002;22(4):911–34.
12. Swift CC, Eklund MJ, Kraveka JM, Alazraki AL. Updates in diagnosis, management, and treatment of neuroblastoma. Radiographics. 2018;38(2):566–80.
13. Siegel MJ, Jaju A. MR imaging of neuroblastic masses. Magn Reson Imaging Clin N Am. 2008;16(3):499–513.. vi
14. Monclair T, Brodeur GM, Ambros PF, Brisse HJ, Cecchetto G, Holmes K, et al. The International Neuroblastoma Risk Group (INRG) staging system: an INRG Task Force report. J Clin Oncol. 2009;27(2):298–303.
15. Brisse HJ, McCarville MB, Granata C, Krug KB, Wootton-Gorges SL, Kanegawa K, et al. Guidelines for imaging and staging of neuroblastic tumors: consensus report from the International Neuroblastoma Risk Group Project. Radiology. 2011;261(1):243–57.
16. Shimada H, Ambros IM, Dehner LP, Hata J, Joshi VV, Roald B, et al. The international neuroblastoma pathology classification (the Shimada system). Cancer. 1999;86(2):364–72.
17. Hwang SM, Yoo SY, Kim JH, Jeon TY. Congenital adrenal neuroblastoma with and without cystic change: differentiating features with an emphasis on the of value of ultrasound. AJR Am J Roentgenol. 2016;207(5):1105–11.
18. Ross JH. Pheochromocytoma. Special considerations in children. Urol Clin North Am. 2000;27(3):393–402.
19. Balassy C, Navarro OM, Daneman A. Adrenal masses in children. Radiol Clin N Am. 2011;49(4):711–27.. vi
20. Havekes B, Romijn JA, Eisenhofer G, Adams K, Pacak K. Update on pediatric pheochromocytoma. Pediatr Nephrol. 2009;24(5):943–50.
21. Paterson A. Adrenal pathology in childhood: a spectrum of disease. Eur Radiol. 2002;12(10):2491–508.
22. Jalil ND, Pattou FN, Combemale F, Chapuis Y, Henry JF, Peix JL, et al. Effectiveness and limits of preoperative imaging studies for the localisation of pheochromocytomas and paragangliomas: a review of 282 cases. French Association of Surgery (AFC), and The French Association of Endocrine Surgeons (AFCE). Eur J Surg. 1998;164(1):23–8.
23. McHugh K. Renal and adrenal tumours in children. Cancer Imaging. 2007;7(1):41–51.
24. Dehner LP. Pediatric adrenocortical neoplasms: on the road to some clarity. Am J Surg Pathol. 2003;27(7):1005–7.
25. Wieneke JA, Thompson LD, Heffess CS. Adrenal cortical neoplasms in the pediatric population: a clinicopathologic and immunophenotypic analysis of 83 patients. Am J Surg Pathol. 2003;27(7):867–81.
26. Bharwani N, Rockall AG, Sahdev A, Gueorguiev M, Drake W, Grossman AB, et al. Adrenocortical carcinoma: the range of appearances on CT and MRI. AJR Am J Roentgenol. 2011;196(6):W706–14.
27. Kilcoyne AMS, Blake MA. MR imaging of adrenal lesions. Appl Radiol. 2017;46(4):18–24.

Gastrointestinal Tract

12

Samantha G. Harrington, Katherine Nimkin, and Michael S. Gee

Introduction

Magnetic resonance (MR) imaging is an excellent modality for the evaluation of bowel pathology and adjacent perienteric changes. The lack of ionizing radiation means that MR imaging can be performed serially in pediatric patients with conditions that often require multiple imaging studies over time, such as inflammatory bowel disease. In addition, MR imaging allows multiple acquisitions of the same body part in one examination, which is ideally suited for cinematic evaluation of bowel peristalsis and multiphase assessment of bowel enhancement. The superior soft tissue contrast of MR imaging is well suited to evaluate spaces associated with the gastrointestinal (GI) tract, such as the small bowel mesentery, greater omentum, and anal sphincter complex, which can be sites of associated GI tract pathology. Lastly, gastrointestinal abnormalities seen on other imaging modalities may be further evaluated with MR imaging to aid with lesion localization and tissue characterization.

This chapter reviews up-to-date MR protocols to evaluate the GI tract (Table 12.1); the embryology and normal development of the esophagus, stomach, small bowel, and large bowel; as well as imaging findings of various congenital, infectious/inflammatory, and neoplastic processes in the pediatric population (Table 12.2).

Table 12.1 Typical pulse sequences in pediatric gastrointestinal tract MR protocols

Protocol	Sequence	Planes
Fetal	SST2W	Axial, sagittal, coronal
	bSSFP	Axial, sagittal, coronal
	T1W GRE	Axial, sagittal, coronal
Enterography	SST2W	Axial, coronal
	bSSFP	Coronal
	SS or FSE T2W FS	Axial
	Thick-slab cinematic bSSFP	Coronal
	DWI	Axial
	Multiphase T1W FS GRE pre- and post-contrast images (including 55–70 second enteric phase)	Coronal (multiphase), axial (delayed)
Perianal fistula	Large FOV T2W	Axial, coronal
	Small FOV (16–20 cm) T2W FS or short tau inversion recovery (STIR)	Axial, coronal
	T1W FS GRE pre- and post-contrast	Axial, coronal
	DWI	Axial
Appendicitis	SST2W	Axial, coronal
	SST2W FS	Axial, coronal
	Radial FSE T2W FS (optional)	Axial

SS single-shot, *bSSFP* balanced steady-state free precession, *T1* T1-weighted, *T2W* T2-weighted, *FSE* fast spin echo, *GRE* gradient-recalled echo, *DWI* diffusion-weighted imaging, *FOV* field of view

Table 12.2 Spectrum of pediatric gastrointestinal tract pathologies seen on MR imaging

Congenital disorders	Infectious and inflammatory disorders	Neoplastic disorders
Congenital diaphragmatic hernia	Inflammatory bowel disease	Gastrointestinal stromal tumors
Gastrointestinal atresias	Appendicitis	Lymphoma
Other bowel malformations (e.g., duodenal web)	Meckel diverticulum	
Foregut duplication cysts	Typhlitis	
Anorectal malformation	Pneumatosis intestinalis	

S. G. Harrington (✉)
Department of Radiology, Massachusetts General Hospital, Boston, MA, USA
e-mail: sgharrington@partners.org

K. Nimkin · M. S. Gee
Division of Pediatric Imaging, Department of Radiology, Massachusetts General Hospital, Harvard Medical School, Boston, MA, USA

© Springer Nature Switzerland AG 2020
E. Y. Lee et al. (eds.), *Pediatric Body MRI*, https://doi.org/10.1007/978-3-030-31989-2_12

Magnetic Resonance Imaging Techniques

MR Imaging Pulse Sequences and Protocols

Fetal MR Gastrointestinal Tract Imaging Protocol

Fetal MR imaging can be used to diagnose *in utero* bowel abnormalities detected on prenatal ultrasound. Protocols for fetal MR bowel imaging vary depending on the suspected abnormality. Ultimately, the protocol is tailored to help answer questions that impact prenatal and antenatal management of the fetus. Single-shot T2-weighted and balanced steady-state free precession sequences are primarily used for fetal anatomic evaluation due to their fast imaging time and minimal motion artifact. In addition, fast gradient-recalled echo (GRE) T1-weighted sequences are helpful for colonic evaluation due to the high T1-weighted signal intensity of meconium, which is seen in the colon at approximately 20 weeks' gestation [1]. Given the frequent movement of the fetus *in utero*, acquisition of the sequences is typically monitored by radiologists to optimize acquiring axial, sagittal, and coronal planes relative to the fetus.

MR Enterography Protocol

MR enterography has become the preferred imaging modality for evaluating pediatric patients with inflammatory bowel disease (IBD) [2]. The protocol is optimized to evaluate the bowel wall (e.g., thickness, enhancement, edema, and narrowing) and mesentery (e.g., lymphadenopathy, stranding, fistulous tracts, and fluid) [3, 4]. Extraintestinal manifestations, such as sclerosing cholangitis or sacroiliitis, can also be seen incidentally. MR enterography protocol requires both large-volume oral contrast (nonabsorbable biphasic contrast demonstrating low signal intensity on T1-weighted images and high signal on T2-weighted images) and intravenous contrast. Enteric contrast is given over a period of 45–60 minutes prior to imaging, to optimize distention of small bowel loops inaccessible to optical endoscopy. Typical sequences acquired include T2-weighted single-shot fast spin echo (ssFSE), balanced steady-state free procession (bSSFP), thick-slab cinematic bSSFP, diffusion-weighted imaging (DWI), and multiphase 3D T1-weighted fat-suppressed GRE post-contrast imaging, including images obtained during the enteric phase (55–70 seconds) [5].

Perianal Fistula Protocol

Fistulizing perianal disease is a common complication of Crohn disease. MR imaging provides detailed anatomic evaluation of the anal sphincter complex and the perianal soft tissues, which is critical for fistula visualization and planning medical and/or surgical therapy [6]. The protocol is tailored to evaluate for fistulous tracks and abscesses and their relationship to the anal sphincter complex. Typical sequences acquired include small field of view (16–20 cm) T2-weighted fat-suppressed or short tau inversion recovery (STIR) images, 3D T1-weighted fat-suppressed GRE post-contrast images in the axial and coronal planes, and diffusion-weighted imaging (DWI) [7].

Appendicitis Protocol

There is growing evidence that MRI has similar sensitivity and specificity to computed tomography (CT) for the detection of acute appendicitis in the pediatric population, without ionizing radiation exposure [8–11]. A rapid appendicitis protocol with four sequences (axial and coronal single-shot T2-weighted images with and without fat suppression) can be acquired in under 5 minutes and does not require oral or intravenous contrast, thereby obviating the need for sedation for children 5 years of age and older. Additional fast spin echo T2-weighted images can be obtained, if the patient is able to tolerate, which are longer but have higher image contrast for detecting subtle appendiceal tip inflammation and assessing for appendix perforation [8].

Anatomy

Embryology

Esophagus The folding of the embryo during the 4th week of gestation results in the primitive gut, which can be divided into the foregut, midgut, and hindgut (Fig. 12.1). The foregut includes the pharynx to the proximal duodenum. The esophagus arises from the foregut. The tracheoesophageal septum develops during the 4th week, separating the respiratory and digestive tracts. Errors in the development of the tracheoesophageal septum result in tracheoesophageal fistulas or esophageal atresias. The esophagus elongates rapidly and eventually occludes by the 5th week due to proliferation of epithelium. The esophagus recanalizes by the 9th week. Esophageal stenosis occurs with errors in recanalization.

Stomach The stomach also arises from the foregut. Although initially a fusiform tube, asymmetric growth of the dorsal side of the stomach produces the greater curvature, while the ventral side develops into the lesser curvature. The stomach undergoes 90° rotation along the craniocaudal (longitudinal) axis, which results in the greater curvature being located to the left and the lesser curvature located to the right.

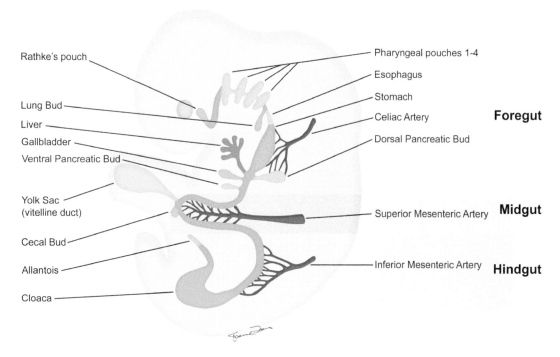

Fig. 12.1 Embryonic divisions of the gastrointestinal tract. The primitive gut is divided into the foregut, midgut, and hindgut. The foregut includes the trachea, respiratory tract, esophagus, stomach, liver, gallbladder, pancreas, and the first two portions of the duodenum. The midgut includes the remaining duodenum, jejunum, ileum, cecum, ascending colon, and proximal two-thirds of the transverse colon. The hindgut includes the distal one-third of the transverse colon, descending colon, rectum, upper anal canal, and urogenital sinus. (Image: Susanne L. Loomis, MS, FBCA; Department of Radiology, Massachusetts General Hospital, Boston, Massachusetts, USA)

Small Bowel and Large Bowel The small and large bowel arise from all three portions of the primitive gut. The foregut includes the first and second portions of the duodenum. The midgut includes the third and fourth parts of the duodenum, jejunum, ileum, cecum, ascending colon, and proximal transverse colon. The hindgut includes the distal transverse colon, descending colon, sigmoid colon, and rectum. The midgut loop herniates out of the umbilicus, rotates 270° counterclockwise, and retracts by the 10th week (Fig. 12.2). Errors in rotation result in malrotation. Failure of retraction produces an omphalocele. Persistence of the vitelline duct (connection between the ileum and yolk sac) results in a Meckel diverticulum.

Normal Development and Anatomy

Esophagus The esophagus extends from the hypopharynx to the gastroesophageal junction. The esophageal wall is composed of four layers: (1) mucosa, (2) submucosa, (3) muscularis externa, and (4) adventitia (or serosa in the abdominal portion). The Z-line marks the transition of the mucosa from stratified squamous epithelium to simple columnar epithelium. The upper third muscularis is striated muscle, while the inferior third is composed of smooth muscle. The arterial supply includes the inferior thyroid artery (upper third), esophageal branches of the thoracic aorta (middle third), and esophageal branches of the left gastric artery (lower third). The venous drainage is generally divided into the systemic system, while the abdominal portion has a component of portal drainage via the gastric veins.

Stomach The stomach extends from the gastroesophageal junction to the pyloric sphincter and is composed of the cardia, fundus, body, and pylorus (Fig. 12.3). Similar to the esophagus, the stomach contains mucosa, submucosa, muscularis externa, and serosa. The arterial supply of the stomach comes from the celiac trunk, while the venous drainage includes the portal, splenic, and superior mesenteric veins.

Small Intestines The small intestines include the duodenum, jejunum, and ileum and run from the pylorus to the

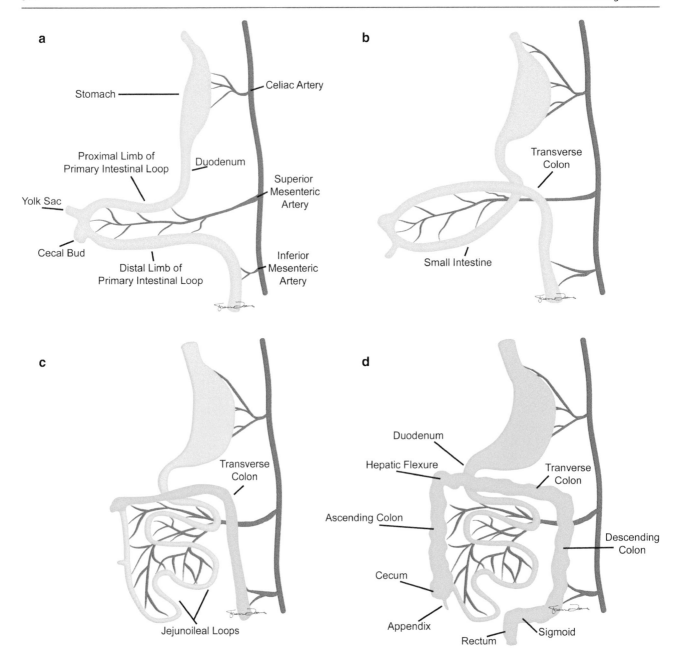

Fig 12.2 Embryonic folding of the gastrointestinal tract. (a) At approximately 6 weeks' gestation, (b) the midgut herniates out of the umbilicus, (c) rotates 270°, and (d) eventually retracts by 10 weeks' gestation. (Image: Susanne L. Loomis, MS, FBCA; Department of Radiology, Massachusetts General Hospital, Boston, Massachusetts, USA)

ileocecal valve (see Fig. 12.3). The duodenum is categorized into four parts based primarily on location. The arterial supply of the small bowel primarily comes from the superior mesenteric artery. However, there is a small portion that arises from the celiac trunk (gastroduodenal and pancreaticoduodenal arteries supply the duodenum). While

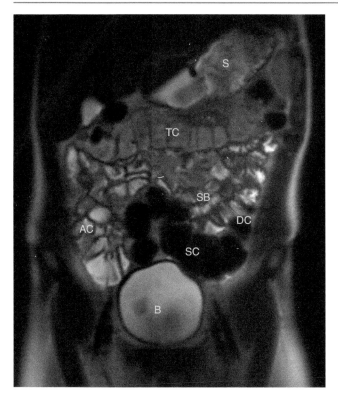

Fig 12.3 A normal MRE exam in a 10-year-old boy shows the typical appearance of the stomach (S), small bowel (SB), ascending colon (AC), transverse colon (TC), descending colon (DC), sigmoid colon (SC), and bladder (B) on a coronal single-shot T2-weighted image

some duodenal veins drain directly to the portal vein, venous drainage is mostly via the superior mesenteric vein.

Large Bowel The large bowel includes the cecum, colon (ascending, transverse, descending, and sigmoid), rectum, and anus (see Fig. 12.3). The arterial supply is via the superior mesenteric artery and the inferior mesenteric artery. The venous drainage is primarily through the inferior mesenteric and superior mesenteric veins.

Anatomic Variants

Although anatomic variants often present with symptoms (e.g., malrotation with volvulus), other variants are asymptomatic. For example, a duodenal diverticulum is an outpouching of all three layers of the duodenal wall, usually located in the second or third part of the duodenum. The prevalence of duodenal diverticulum is up to 23% [12, 13]. Although duodenal diverticula are often asymptomatic, affected pediatric patients can present with chronic abdominal pain, bloating, or vomiting (Fig. 12.4). A potential complication of duodenal diverticulum is duodenal diverticulitis.

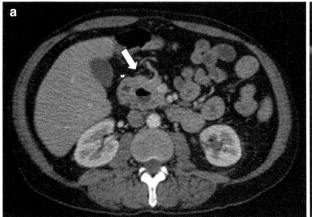
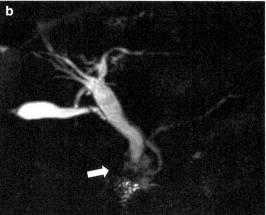

Fig 12.4 Duodenal diverticulum in an 18-year-old boy with epigastric pain. Axial contrast-enhanced CT image (**a**) demonstrates a diverticulum (*arrow*) of the second portion of the duodenum. Magnetic resonance cholangiopancreatography (MRCP) (**b**) demonstrates common bile duct (CBD) dilation with a transition at the level of the diverticulum (*arrow*). Axial T2-weighted fat-suppressed MR images (**c**, **d**) demonstrate a dilated CBD above the diverticulum (*arrows*), which is narrowed and displaced by the diverticulum

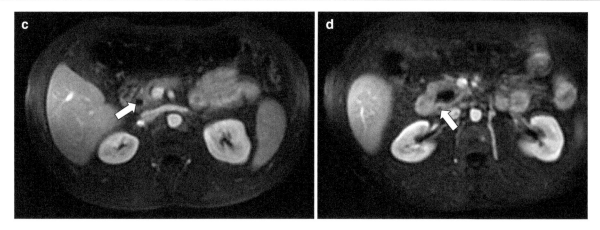

Fig. 12.4 (continued)

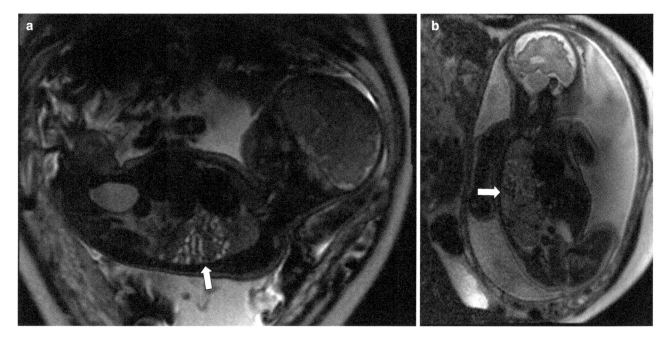

Fig. 12.5 Congenital diaphragmatic hernia in a fetus. Sagittal (**a**) and coronal (**b**) single-shot T2-weighted MR images demonstrate a large left posterior congenital diaphragmatic hernia containing loops of bowel (*arrows*) resulting in contralateral mediastinal shift in a 22-week fetus

Spectrum of Gastrointestinal Tract Disorders

Congenital Gastrointestinal Tract Disorders

Abnormalities Diagnosed *In Utero*

Congenital Diaphragmatic Hernia Fetal MR imaging is useful for the assessment of congenital diaphragmatic hernias (CDH), particularly for anatomic evaluation, as well as for screening for associated malformations. Anatomic assess-ment is essential for surgical management, including location of the diaphragmatic defect and hernia contents. CDH can be classified as intrapleural (left lateral) or mediastinal (ventral, Morgagni, or hiatal) [14]. The most common type of dia-phragmatic hernia is intrapleural [14, 15] (Fig. 12.5). There are a wide range of associated malformations, including tetralogy of Fallot, Beckwith-Wiedemann, Fryns syndrome, and holoprosencephaly. Fetal lung volumes and the presence of herniated visceral organs can be readily assessed using MR imaging and are used to predict patient outcomes.

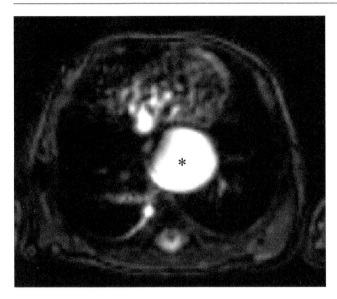

Fig. 12.6 Esophageal atresia in a fetus. Axial T2-weighted GRE fat-suppressed MR image demonstrates a dilated esophagus (*asterisk*) in esophageal atresia at 24 weeks gestation

Gastrointestinal Atresias Fetal MR imaging can be used to assess bowel atresias, including esophageal, duodenal, and jejunal/ileal small bowel atresias. Anal atresia is difficult to assess on MR imaging because colon caliber can be normal [1]. Typical findings of atresias include upstream dilation and downstream collapse. For example, esophageal atresia demonstrates a dilated esophageal pouch with contracted stomach (Fig. 12.6). Duodenal atresia classically demonstrates the "double bubble" sign of distended stomach and duodenal bulb (Fig. 12.7). Jejunal and ileal atresias are the most common intestinal atresias [16]. In these cases, dilated small bowel is associated with a microcolon containing meconium that demonstrates T1-weighted hyperintensity (Fig. 12.8). Fetal MR imaging can be particularly useful for differentiating meconium ileus from ileal atresia [17, 18]. Diagnoses of esophageal or duodenal atresia should prompt evaluation for associated disorders, such as VACTERL (vertebral anomalies, anal atresia, cardiac defects, tracheoesophageal fistula, renal anomalies, and limb defects) or trisomy 21.

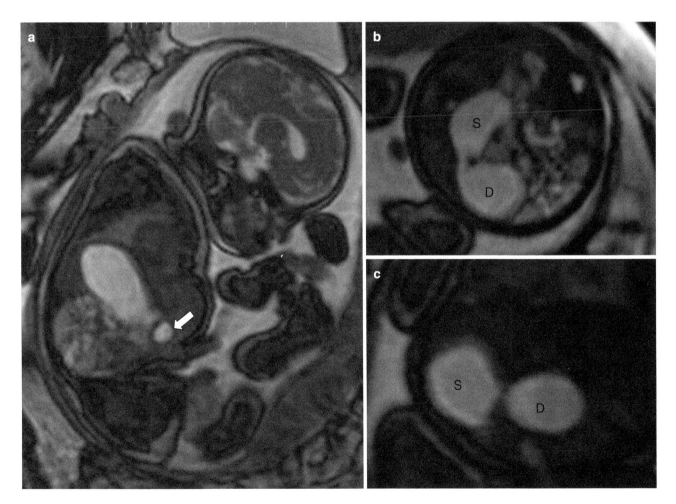

Fig. 12.7 Duodenal atresia in a fetus. Sagittal (**a**), axial (**b**), and coronal (**c**) SSFP MR images demonstrate a blind-ending duodenum (*arrow*) with a "double bubble" sign, with distension of the stomach (S) and proximal duodenum (D) at 23 weeks gestation

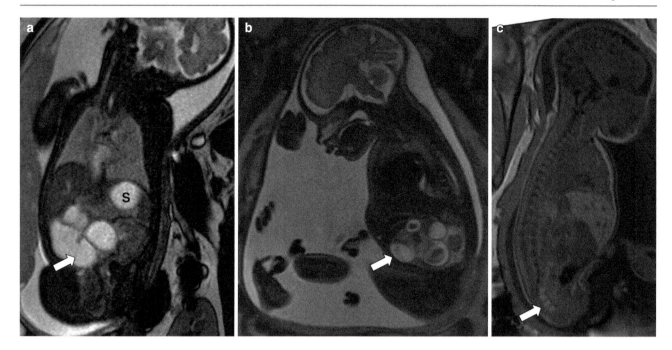

Fig. 12.8 Jejunal atresia in a fetus. Coronal (**a**) and sagittal (**b**) single-shot T2-weighted as well as sagittal (**c**) T1-weighted images demonstrate multiple dilated small bowel loops (**a** and **b**; *arrows*) consistent with jejunal atresia in a 22-week fetus. T1-weighted MR images show meconium in the microcolon (**c**; *arrow*), S = stomach. (Case courtesy of Teresa Victoria, MD, PhD, Children's Hospital of Philadelphia, Philadelphia, Pennsylvania, USA)

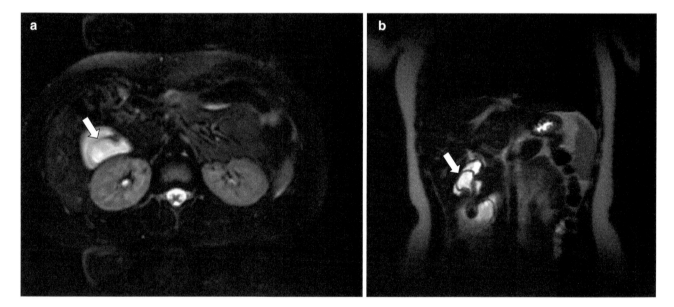

Fig. 12.9 Duodenal web in a 15-year-old girl who presented with abdominal pain. Axial single-shot T2-weighted (**a**) and coronal single-shot T2-weighted fat-suppressed (**b**) MR images demonstrate a curvilinear intraluminal structure (*arrows*) in the second portion of the duodenum associated with duodenal dilation. Surgical pathology confirmed diagnosis of a duodenal web

Other Bowel Malformations Bowel malformations may be found incidentally on MR imaging. For example, a duodenal web is an incomplete obstruction of the duodenum, which can have a variety of clinical presentations. Duodenal webs are often detected on fluoroscopy with a classic "windsock" sign [19]. However, duodenal webs can be incidentally found on MR imaging (Fig. 12.9).

Foregut Duplication Cysts Foregut duplication cysts encompass a variety of anomalies including bronchogenic, neurenteric, esophageal, lingual, and gastric duplication cysts [20, 21]. Pediatric patients with foregut duplication cysts are often asymptomatic. However, they may present with vague symptoms, such as chest pain, dysphagia, or cough. MR imaging is useful for distinguishing the anatomy of

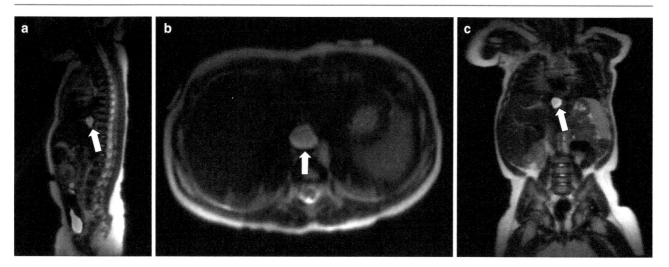

Fig. 12.10 (**a**) Esophageal duplication cyst in a 7-month-old girl with a cystic lesion noted on prenatal ultrasound. Sagittal (**a**), axial (**b**), and coronal (**c**) single-shot T2-weighted MR images demonstrate a well-defined simple cystic lesion (*arrows*) adjacent to the gastroesophageal junction consistent with an esophageal duplication cyst

the cyst, as well as excluding other diagnoses such as neoplasms (Fig. 12.10).

Anorectal Malformations MR imaging is increasingly utilized for preoperative evaluation of anorectal malformations (ARMs); associated spinal and genitourinary anomalies are also well delineated. MR imaging is useful in delineating the position of the rectum relative to the levator ani and sphincter complex, which guides surgical management. The classification of ARMs has evolved over time with the most recent categorization divided by gender, as well as malformations that share common features. Male ARMs include rectovesical (bladder neck) fistula, rectourethral (prostatic) fistula (Fig. 12.11), rectourethral (bulbar) fistula, rectoperineal fistula, imperforate anus without fistula, and rectal atresia. Female ARMs include rectoperineal fistula, rectovestibular fistula, cloaca with short common channel (<3 cm), cloaca with long common channel (>3 cm), imperforate anus without fistula, and rectal atresia [22]. Postoperatively, MR imaging is particularly useful to evaluate the position of the rectum relative to the levator ani and anal sphincter complex.

Infectious and Inflammatory Gastrointestinal Tract Disorders

Inflammatory Bowel Disease MR enterography and pelvic fistula protocol MR imaging have become the gold standard for imaging of pediatric inflammatory bowel disease, particularly Crohn disease [23]. MR enterography is useful for characterizing both active and chronic Crohn disease, which guides medical and surgical management of the disease (Fig. 12.12). As previously described, MR

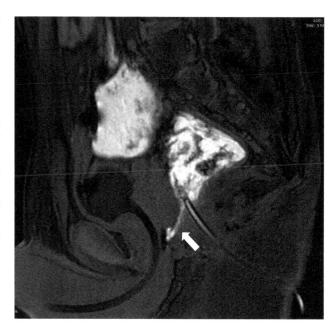

Fig. 12.11 Recurrent anorectal malformation with a rectourethral fistula in a 16-year-old boy. A sagittal T1-weighted fat-suppressed GRE MR image following rectal contrast instillation demonstrates a fistulous tract (*arrow*) between the rectum and urethra. Catheters are present in both the bladder and rectum. (Case courtesy of Daniel J. Podberesky, MD, Nemours Children's Hospital, Orlando, Florida, USA)

enterography can characterize bowel wall and mesenteric involvement. Disease activity can be quantified in terms of scoring systems, such as the magnetic resonance index of activity (MaRIA), which includes bowel wall thickness, contrast enhancement, edema, and ulcerations [5]. Additionally, MR imaging can be used to assess penetrating complications including fistulae and abscesses, which are an important complication of Crohn disease that may require urgent intervention (Fig. 12.13).

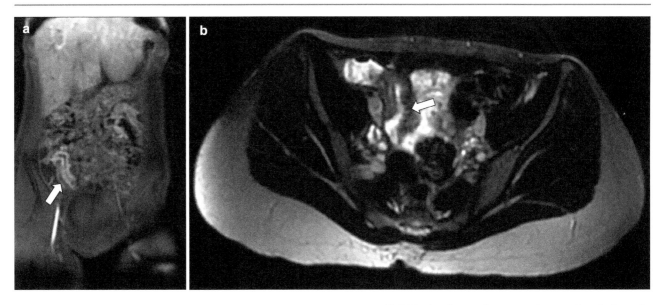

Fig. 12.12 Active Crohn disease in a 17-year-old girl who presented with abdominal pain. Coronal T1-weighted fat-suppressed GRE post-contrast (**a**) and axial non-enhanced T2-weighted (**b**) MR images dem-onstrate wall thickening, hyperenhancement (**a**, *arrow*), and edema (**b**, *arrow*) of the terminal ileum consistent with active Crohn disease

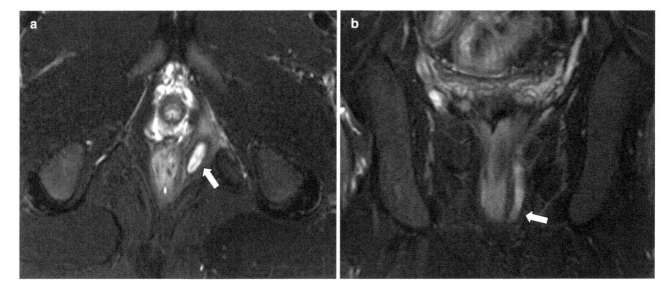

Fig. 12.13 Perianal fistula in a 15-year-old boy with known Crohn disease who presented with perianal discomfort. Axial (**a**) and coronal (**b**) STIR MR images demonstrate an intersphincteric perianal fistula containing fluid (*arrows*)

Appendicitis Although ultrasound is usually the first step for the assessment of acute appendicitis in children, MR imaging is an excellent modality for equivocal ultrasound findings, particularly in cases of a nonvisualized retrocecal appendix. Findings of acute appendicitis on MR imaging include enlarged appendix (greater than 7 mm in caliber) and periappendiceal fluid or inflammatory stranding (Fig. 12.14). MR imaging is also helpful for visualizing appendicoliths (which demonstrate low signal intensity on T1-weighted and T2-weighted images) as well as evidence of appendiceal perforation. One poten-tial issue for appendiceal MR imaging at some centers is scanner availability after-hours, in which case low-dose CT with intravenous contrast can be considered [24].

Meckel Diverticulum A Meckel diverticulum is a blind-ending structure along the antimesenteric side of the distal ileum, which represents persistence of the vitelline duct. The prevalence of a Meckel diverticulum is 2%, making it the most common congenital anomaly of the GI tract [25, 26]. Although a Meckel diverticulum can be asymptomatic, it can present with bleeding, infection, or obstruction (Fig. 12.15). Usually a

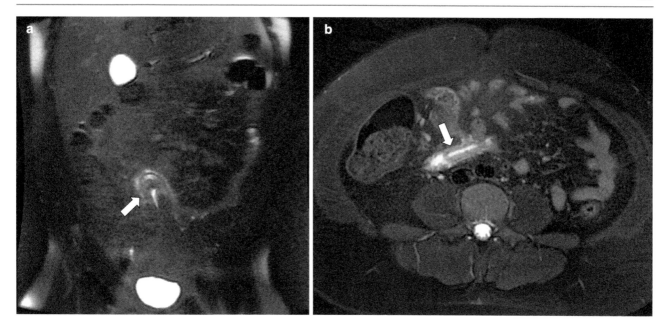

Fig. 12.14 Acute appendicitis in a 14-year-old boy who presented with right lower quadrant pain. Coronal (**a**) and axial (**b**) single-shot T2-weighted fat-suppressed MR images demonstrate a distended appendix with wall edema (*arrows*) and periappendiceal fluid consistent with acute appendicitis

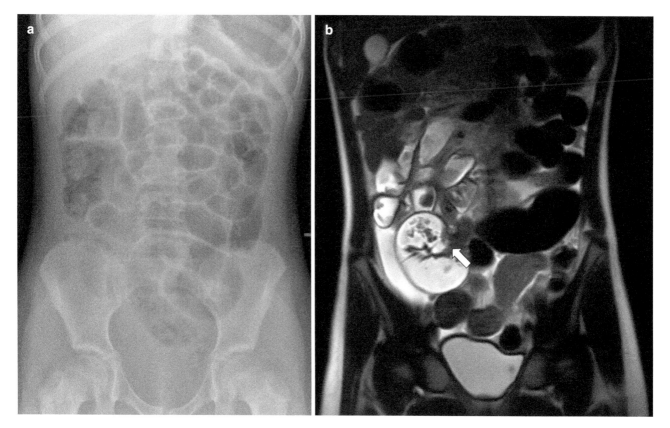

Fig. 12.15 Closed-loop bowel obstruction from a Meckel diverticulum in an 11-year-old girl who presented with acute abdominal pain. Abdominal radiograph (**a**) demonstrates multiple loops of dilated bowel. Coronal single-shot T2-weighted MR image (**b**) demonstrates a blinded-ending diverticulum (*arrow*) with associated dilated loops of small bowel and free fluid consistent with an inflamed Meckel diverticulum causing obstruction

Meckel diverticulum can be diagnosed on ultrasound, CT or with a ⁹⁹ᵐTc-Na-pertechnetate scintigraphy. Although MR imaging is not first-line imaging modality of choice, it can be helpful in making the diagnosis, particularly in cases associated with perforation to distinguish from perforated appendicitis (Fig. 12.16). The soft tissue contrast of MR imaging can help to distinguish abscess from diverticulum and also establish a site of origin in the distal small bowel rather than the cecum.

Typhlitis MR imaging can be used to assess for less common GI pathologies such as typhlitis (also known as neutropenic enterocolitis). Typhlitis is characterized by necrotizing inflammation of the bowel, usually the cecum, in immuno-compromised patients [27]. In the pediatric population, typh-

litis is often associated with patients with malignancy and neutropenia secondary to cytotoxic therapy. Although not typically first-line imaging study for evaluating acute abdominal pain, MR imaging can be used to diagnose typhlitis incidentally in patients undergoing MR imaging for appendicitis or inflammatory bowel disease evaluation (Fig. 12.17).

Pneumatosis Intestinalis Pneumatosis intestinalis refers to gas within the bowel wall and is considered a sign of bowel ischemia. In infants, it is most commonly associated with necrotizing enterocolitis, which is usually evaluated by radiographs or ultrasound [28]. However, pneumatosis intestinalis can be seen on MR imaging as punctate intramural foci of low signal intensity on T1-weighted and T2-weighted images (Fig. 12.18).

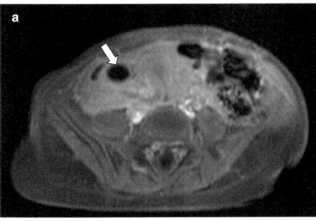
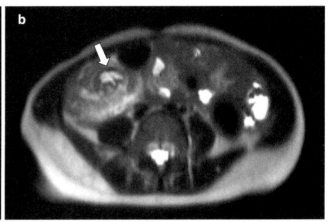

Fig. 12.16 Perforated Meckel diverticulum in a 20-month-old boy who presented with multiple episodes of abdominal pain and vomiting. Axial T1-weighted fat-suppressed post-contrast (**a**) and axial non-enhanced single-shot T2-weighted (**b**) MR images demonstrate a com-

plex, enhancing mass (*arrows*) with central non-enhancing cystic components in the right lower quadrant adjacent to the distal ileum. Surgical pathology revealed a perforated Meckel diverticulum

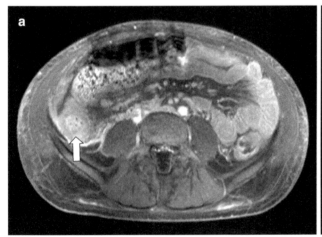
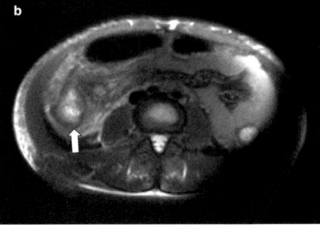

Fig. 12.17 Typhlitis in an 18-year-old male with a history of ulcerative colitis, primary sclerosing cholangitis and lymphoma who presented with abdominal pain. Axial T1-weighted fat-suppressed post-contrast (**a**) and

axial unenhanced T2-weighted fat-suppressed (**b**) MR images demonstrate cecal bowel wall thickening and pericolonic inflammatory changes (*arrows*) consistent with typhlitis in an immunosuppressed patient

If pneumatosis is present, close attention should be paid to other signs of bowel ischemia including bowel wall thickening and air in the portal venous system or in the peritoneum. Two general patterns of pneumatosis are recognized on the basis of the morphology of the air foci: cystic or bubbly pneumatosis with large air foci that is more often chronic and benign and linear pneumatosis with smaller dots of air that is more suspicious for acute ischemia [29].

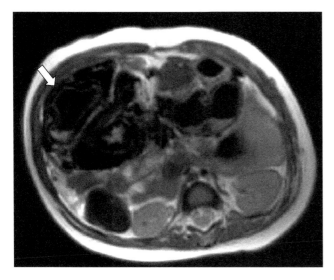

Fig. 12.18 Pneumatosis intestinalis in a 3-year-old girl. Axial T2-weighted MR image demonstrates extensive pneumatosis involving partially imaged colon (*arrow*). Given lack of symptoms, the pneumatosis was thought to be benign cystic pneumatosis secondary to prior steroid use

Neoplastic Gastrointestinal Tract Disorders

Gastrointestinal Stromal Tumors Gastrointestinal stromal tumors (GISTs) are significantly more common in adults than in children [30]. These tumors arise from the interstitial cells of Cajal and are commonly associated with an activating mutation in the KIT receptor tyrosine kinase [31], although the mutation frequency is much lower in pediatric patients compared with adults [32]. A number of congenital syndromes are associated with increased risk of GIST development, including neurofibromatosis type 1 and the Carney triad (pulmonary chondroma, GIST, paraganglioma) [32]. In the adult population, GISTs are typically evaluated by CT or PET-CT. However, MR imaging can be used for anatomic assessment, as well as for surveillance of disease in the pediatric population [32] (Fig. 12.19).

Lymphoma Lymphoma is not commonly evaluated with MR imaging, with few exceptions (e.g., head and neck imaging of CNS lymphoma or whole-body MR imaging surveillance of Hodgkin lymphoma) [33]. However, non-CNS lymphoma may be incidentally found on MR imaging. Primary gastrointestinal tract lymphoma is usually non-Hodgkin's B-cell lymphoma [34]. Lymphoma of the bowel can appear as either a focal mural mass or circumferential wall thickening, with associated aneurysmal luminal dilation present if there is lymphomatous involvement of the bowel wall autonomic plexus (Fig. 12.20). Bowel lymphoma can

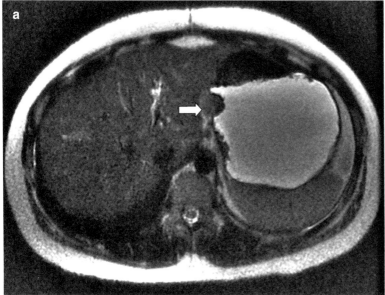
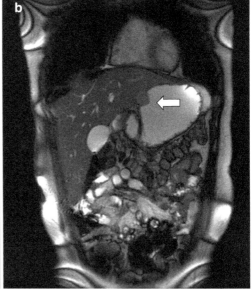

Fig. 12.19 Gastrointestinal stromal tumor in a 17-year-old boy who initially presented with gastrointestinal bleed and was found to have a mass on endoscopy. Axial single-shot T2-weighted (**a**) and coronal SSFP (**b**) MR images demonstrate a well-circumscribed mass (*arrows*) in the anterior wall of the gastric antrum. Surgical pathology of the mass revealed a gastrointestinal stromal tumor

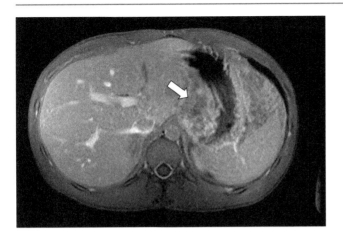

Fig. 12.20 Burkitt lymphoma in a 17-year-old boy who presented with abdominal pain, constipation, and weight loss. Axial T1-weighted fat-suppressed post-contrast MR image demonstrates an irregular enhancing mass (*arrow*) along the lesser curvature of the stomach. Surgical pathology confirmed Burkitt lymphoma

either be the primary site of lymphoma or secondary to lymphatic involvement. Burkitt lymphoma is a highly aggressive variant of B-cell lymphoma that often presents with other abdominal visceral organ involvement [35]. Lymphoma often demonstrates marked diffusion restriction on DWI due to the high nucleus/cytoplasm ratio associated with the tumor cells.

Conclusion

MR imaging is useful for the evaluation of both acute and chronic conditions of the GI tract in children. Given the lack of ionizing radiation, MR imaging is particularly well suited for the pediatric population. Continued refinement of MR protocols has increased the feasibility of MR imaging use, including reducing the need for sedation in infants and young children [36]. The radiologist should also be aware of incidental or unexpected pediatric GI findings on MR imaging.

References

1. Furey EA, Bailey AA, Twickler DM. Fetal MR imaging of gastrointestinal abnormalities. Radiographics. 2016;36(3):904–17.
2. Kordbacheh H, Baliyan V, Serrao J, Gee MS, Yajnik V, Sahani DV, et al. Imaging in patients with Crohn's disease: trends in abdominal CT/MRI utilization and radiation exposure considerations over a 10-year period. Inflamm Bowel Dis. 2017;23(6):1025–33.
3. Mollard BJ, Smith EA, Dillman JR. Pediatric MR enterography: technique and approach to interpretation—how we do it. Radiology. 2015;274(1):29–43.
4. Chalian M, Ozturk A, Oliva-Hemker M, Pryde S, Huisman TAGM. MR enterography findings of inflammatory bowel disease in pediatric patients. AJR Am J Roentgenol. 2011;196(6):W810–6.
5. Mojtahed A, Gee MS. Magnetic resonance enterography evaluation of Crohn disease activity and mucosal healing in young patients. Pediatr Radiol. 2018;48(9):1273–9.
6. de Miguel Criado J, del Salto LG, Rivas PF, del Hoyo LF, Velasco LG, de las Vacas MI, et al. MR imaging evaluation of perianal fistulas: spectrum of imaging features. Radiographics. 2012;32(1):175–94.
7. Shenoy-Bhangle A, Gee MS. Magnetic resonance imaging of perianal Crohn disease in children. Pediatr Radiol. 2016;46(6):838–46.
8. Dillman JR, Gadepalli S, Sroufe NS, Davenport MS, Smith EA, Chong ST, et al. Equivocal pediatric appendicitis: unenhanced MR imaging protocol for nonsedated children—a clinical effectiveness study. Radiology. 2016;279(1):216–25.
9. Duke E, Kalb B, Arif-Tiwari H, Daye ZJ, Gilbertson-Dahdal D, Keim SM, et al. A systematic review and meta-analysis of diagnostic performance of MRI for evaluation of acute appendicitis. AJR Am J Roentgenol. 2016;206(3):508–17.
10. Dibble EH, Swenson DW, Cartagena C, Baird GL, Herliczek TW. Effectiveness of a staged US and unenhanced MR imaging algorithm in the diagnosis of pediatric appendicitis. Radiology. 2018;286(3):1022–9.
11. Mushtaq R, Desoky SM, Morello F, Gilbertson-Dahdal D, Gopalakrishnan G, Leetch A, et al. First-line diagnostic evaluation with MRI of children suspected of having acute appendicitis. Radiology. 2019;291(1):170–7.
12. Pearl MS, Hill MC, Zeman RK. CT findings in duodenal diverticulitis. AJR Am J Roentgenol. 2006;187(4):W392–5.
13. Bittle MM, Gunn ML, Gross JA, Rohrmann CA. Imaging of duodenal diverticula and their complications. Curr Probl Diagn Radiol. 2012;41(1):20–9.
14. Mehollin-Ray AR, Cassady CI, Cass DL, Olutoye OO. Fetal MR imaging of congenital diaphragmatic hernia. Radiographics. 2012;32(4):1067–84.
15. Pober BR, Russell MK, Ackerman KG. Congenital diaphragmatic hernia overview. In: Adam MP, Ardinger HH, Pagon RA, Wallace SE, Bean LJ, Stephens K, et al., editors. GeneReviews®. [Internet]. Seattle: University of Washington; 1993.
16. Best KE, Tennant PWG, Addor MC, Bianchi F, Boyd P, Calzolari E, et al. Epidemiology of small intestinal atresia in Europe: a register-based study. Arch Dis Child Fetal Neonatal Ed. 2012;97(5):F353–8.
17. Carcopino X, Chaumoitre K, Shojai R, Panuel M, Boubli L, D'Ercole C. Use of fetal magnetic resonance imaging in differentiating ileal atresia from meconium ileus. Ultrasound Obstet Gynecol. 2006;28(7):976–7.
18. Rubio EI, Blask AR, Badillo AT, Bulas DI. Prenatal magnetic resonance and ultrasonographic findings in small-bowel obstruction: imaging clues and postnatal outcomes. Pediatr Radiol. 2017;47(4):411–21.
19. Materne R. The duodenal wind sock sign. Radiology. 2001;218(3):749–50.
20. Fitch SJ, Tonkin IL, Tonkin AK. Imaging of foregut duplication cysts. Radiographics. 1986;6(2):189–201.
21. Jeung MY, Gasser B, Gangi A, Bogorin A, Charneau D, Wihlm JM, et al. Imaging of cystic masses of the mediastinum. Radiographics. 2002;22(suppl_1):S79–93.
22. Podberesky DJ, Towbin AJ, Eltomey MA, Levitt MA. Magnetic resonance imaging of anorectal malformations. Magn Reson Imaging Clin N Am. 2013;21(4):791–812.
23. Kim DH, Carucci LR, Baker ME, Cash BD, Dillman JR, Feig BW, et al. ACR appropriateness criteria Crohn disease. J Am Coll Radiol. 2015;12(10):1048–1057.e4.
24. Swenson DW, Ayyala RS, Sams C, Lee EY. Practical imaging strategies for acute appendicitis in children. AJR Am J Roentgenol. 2018;211(4):901–9.

25. Lee NK, Kim S, Jeon TY, Kim HS, Kim DH, Seo HI, et al. Complications of congenital and developmental abnormalities of the gastrointestinal tract in adolescents and adults: evaluation with multimodality imaging. Radiographics. 2010;30(6):1489–507.

26. Elsayes KM, Menias CO, Harvin HJ, Francis IR. Imaging manifestations of Meckel's diverticulum. AJR Am J Roentgenol. 2007;189(1):81–8.

27. Hoeffel C, Crema MD, Belkacem A, Azizi L, Lewin M, Arrivé L, et al. Multi–detector row CT: spectrum of diseases involving the ileocecal area. Radiographics. 2006;26(5):1373–90.

28. Epelman M, Daneman A, Navarro OM, Morag I, Moore AM, Kim JH, et al. Necrotizing enterocolitis: review of state-of-the-art imaging findings with pathologic correlation. Radiographics. 2007;27(2):285–305.

29. Soyer P, Martin-Grivaud S, Boudiaf M, Malzy P, Duchat F, Hamzi L, et al. Linear or bubbly: a pictorial review of CT features of intestinal pneumatosis in adults. J Radiol. 2008;89(12):1907–20. [Article in French].

30. Benesch M, Wardelmann E, Ferrari A, Brennan B, Verschuur A. Gastrointestinal stromal tumors (GIST) in children and adolescents: a comprehensive review of the current literature. Pediatr Blood Cancer. 2009;53(7):1171–9.

31. Hirota S, Isozaki K, Moriyama Y, Hashimoto K, Nishida T, Ishiguro S, et al. Gain-of-function mutations of c-kit in human gastrointestinal stromal tumors. Science. 1998;279(5350):577–80.

32. Herzberg M, Beer M, Anupindi S, Vollert K, Kröncke T. Imaging pediatric gastrointestinal stromal tumor (GIST). J Pediatr Surg. 2018;53(9):1862–70.

33. Toma P, Granata C, Rossi A, Garaventa A. Multimodality imaging of Hodgkin disease and non-Hodgkin lymphomas in children. Radiographics. 2007;27(5):1335–54.

34. d'Almeida M, Jose J, Oneto J, Restrepo R. Bowel wall thickening in children: CT findings. Radiographics. 2008;28(3):727–46.

35. Harris AC, MacLean KA, Grunau GL, Chang SD, Martin N. Imaging intra-abdominal Burkitt's lymphoma: from discrete bowel wall thickening to diffuse soft tissue infiltration. Can Assoc Radiol J. 2017;68(3):286–92.

36. Jaimes C, Gee MS. Strategies to minimize sedation in pediatric body magnetic resonance imaging. Pediatr Radiol. 2016;46(6):916–27.

Kidney, Ureter, and Bladder

13

Jeffrey J. Tutman, Edward Y. Lee, Abdusamea Shabani, and Harriet J. Paltiel

Introduction

Disorders of the urinary tract are common in children and have been traditionally evaluated with a combination of sonographic, fluoroscopic, and scintigraphic imaging. Recent advances in MR imaging techniques that permit motion reduction and limited use of sedation and anesthesia have made the routine incorporation of this powerful technique a feasible option in pediatric imaging.

In this chapter, up-to-date MR imaging techniques for evaluating the kidney, ureter, and bladder in pediatric patients are discussed. The pertinent embryology and common anatomic variants are reviewed. The clinical features, characteristic MR imaging findings, and current treatment approaches to congenital, infectious, neoplastic, and traumatic urinary tract disorders affecting infants and children are discussed.

Magnetic Resonance Imaging Techniques

Patient Preparation

Patient cooperation varies by age. A "feed and wrap" protocol is generally successful in the evaluation of young infants, precluding the need for sedation. Most children 8 years of age and older are able to cooperate with the MR imaging examination. For pediatric patients falling between these two age groups, sedation is frequently necessary. Many children are more comfortable when allowed to use MR-compatible music or video systems during their imaging examinations.

MR Imaging Pulse Sequences and Protocols

MR imaging of the pediatric urinary tract may be performed on either 1.5 T or 3.0 T magnets, with each having advantages and disadvantages. The benefits of 3.0 T imaging include high signal-to-noise and contrast-to-noise ratios, resulting in better image resolution and shorter imaging times. Disadvantages include increased energy deposition that may prevent the performance of some pulse sequences and exacerbation of magnetic susceptibility and chemical shift artifacts [1].

An adult head coil usually fits well for abdominal imaging of infants and small children, while a phased array or whole-body coil is usually required for larger children [2]. For evaluation of renal parenchymal abnormalities or masses, the examination should include T1-weighted, T2-weighted, Dixon in-phase and out-of-phase, and T1-weighted fat-suppressed post-contrast MR images [2]. Gadolinium chelate contrast agents are administered at a dose of 0.1 mmol/kg [3]. Our current preferred protocol for evaluation of renal masses includes axial, coronal, and sagittal T2-weighted fat-suppressed fast spin echo, axial T1-weighted Dixon (in-phase and out-of-phase), and axial and coronal volumetric T1-weighted fat-suppressed post-contrast MR images (Table 13.1).

MR Urography

MR urography is particularly useful when evaluation of parenchymal function is desired. In the authors' department, patients are asked to void prior to the study. A Foley catheter is placed in infants as well as in those children with suspected vesico-

J. J. Tutman
Division of Pediatric Radiology, Department of Radiology, Children's Hospital of Colorado, University of Colorado School of Medicine, Aurora, CO, USA

E. Y. Lee
Division of Thoracic Imaging, Department of Radiology, Boston Children's Hospital, Harvard Medical School, Boston, MA, USA

A. Shabani
Division of Body and Diagnostic Imaging, Sidra Medicine, Doha, Qatar

H. J. Paltiel (✉)
Department of Radiology, Boston Children's Hospital, Harvard Medical School, Boston, MA, USA
e-mail: harriet.paltiel@childrens.harvard.edu

© Springer Nature Switzerland AG 2020
E. Y. Lee et al. (eds.), *Pediatric Body MRI*, https://doi.org/10.1007/978-3-030-31989-2_13

Table 13.1 Essential MR imaging protocol for evaluation of a renal mass

Body coil
Coronal T2-weighted FSE
Sagittal T2-weighted FSE
Axial T1-weighted Dixon
Axial DWI
Coronal 3D GRE T1-weighted fat-suppressed post-contrast
Axial 3D GRE T1-weighted fat-suppressed post-contrast

FSE Fast spin echo, *DWI* Diffusion-weighted imaging, *GRE* Gradient-recalled echo

Table 13.2 Essential MR imaging protocol for MR urography

Body coil
Dynamic oblique coronal 3D GRE T1-weighted fat-suppressed post-contrast
Sagittal T2-weighted FSE
Axial T2-weighted FSE
Coronal T2-weighted FSE
Coronal T2-weighted 3D high TE
Axial FS VIBE

FSE Fast spin echo, *TE* Echo time, *GRE* Gradient-recalled echo

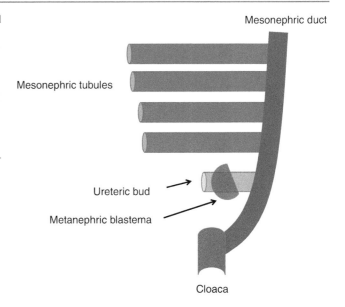

Fig. 13.1 Embryonic development of the metanephros, the precursor to the permanent kidney and collecting system. The mesonephric tubules regress as the metanephros forms. The ureteric bud arises from the caudal mesonephric duct and in combination with the metanephric blastema leads to development of the permanent kidney (*arrows*)

ureteral reflux (VUR). They are hydrated with intravenous fluid over 20 minutes (10 mg/kg NS up to 500 mL) followed by administration of 1.0 mg/kg intravenous (IV) furosemide (up to 20 mg). The diuretic assists in distribution of the contrast agent and prevents the loss of signal from T2* effects that may occur from concentrated gadolinium [4]. After contrast administration, coronal radial stack of stars 3D T1-weighted fat-suppressed images are obtained every 3 seconds over a period of 6 minutes. Continuous imaging allows assessment of renal perfusion and also permits post-processing for calculation of data such as split renal function and glomerular filtration rate (GFR). Multiplanar T2-weighted fat-suppressed or heavily T2-weighted (such as a 3D magnetic resonance cholangiopancreatography) images and delayed axial T1-weighted fat-suppressed images are then obtained (Table 13.2).

Anatomy

Embryology

Development of the urinary tract begins in the fourth week of gestation. It arises from a ridge of mesodermal tissue, the intermediate mesoderm, which is located along the posterior wall of the abdominal cavity. The urogenital ridge, a longitudinal elevation of the mesoderm, forms along both sides of the abdominal aorta. A portion of the urogenital ridge develops into the nephrogenic cord that ultimately forms the urinary system. A separate portion develops into the gonadal ridge that ultimately forms the genital system.

Three pairs of excretory organs develop in the human embryo, the pronephros, the mesonephros, and the meta-

nephros. These embryonic kidneys appear sequentially from cranial to caudal in position. The pronephros and mesonephros arise from the nephrogenic cord. They both eventually regress in utero, while the metanephros develops into the permanent kidney.

The mesonephros contains glomeruli and mesonephric tubules. The mesonephric tubules drain into the mesonephric (Wolffian) duct which in turn opens into the cloaca, the common embryonic excretory cavity. The mesonephros regresses toward the end of the first trimester. In the fifth week of gestation, the metanephros begins to develop in the sacral region from the ureteric bud, a diverticulum of the mesonephric duct, and from the metanephric blastema, which arises from the nephrogenic cord (Fig. 13.1). The stalk of the ureteric bud becomes the ureter. The ureteric bud grows into the metanephric blastema, with each component exerting an inductive effect on the other. Branching of the ureteric bud leads to formation of the renal pelvis, calyces, and collecting tubules. Nephron formation occurs in the metanephric blastema and includes the glomerulus, proximal tubule, loop of Henle, and distal tubule.

In the 4th to 6th weeks of gestation, the urorectal septum develops and separates the cloaca into the urogenital sinus anteriorly and the rectum posteriorly. The superior portion of the urogenital sinus develops into the bladder. The ureterovesical junction (UVJ) develops as the distal portions of the mesonephric duct are incorporated into the enlarging bladder. Development of the ureters and bladder is complete by the fourth gestational month.

The inferior portion of the urogenital sinus develops into the membranous urethra in both males and females. The distal male urethra is derived from a cord of ectoderm that grows from the tip of the glans penis to meet the spongy portion of the urethra derived from the caudal portion of the urogenital sinus.

Congenital anomalies of the urinary tract are frequent. Early degeneration of a ureteric bud or involution of the metanephros leads to regression of the metanephric blastema and renal agenesis. If the ureteric bud and metanephric blastema do not join normally, abnormal induction of the blastemal elements may result in a multicystic dysplastic kidney. Bifurcation of the ureteric buds results in partial duplication of the collecting system. Maldevelopment or an abnormal location of the origin of the ureteric bud may lead to the development of VUR and/or ureteral ectopia [5, 6].

Early in embryonic life, two pairs of genital ducts develop from mesodermal tissue in males and females: the mesonephric (Wolffian) ducts described above and the paramesonephric (Müllerian) ducts. The paramesonephric ducts are present in both sexes at 6 weeks. In males, regression of the paramesonephric ducts begins at 8 weeks and is almost complete by 10 weeks. In females, the paramesonephric ducts extend caudally, reaching the urogenital sinus by 9 weeks. By the 12th week, the two ducts fuse into a single tube, the uterovaginal canal, which terminates at the Müllerian tubercle, an elevation on the posterior wall of the urogenital sinus. The unfused upper portions of the paramesonephric ducts form the fallopian tubes, while the lower fused portions form the uterus. The vaginal plate develops from outgrowths of the distal paramesonephric ducts. The upper vagina forms from vacuolization of the vaginal plate, while the lower vagina forms from vacuolization of paired outgrowths from the Müllerian tubercle. Canalization begins caudally and proceeds proximally and is complete by the fifth month of gestation.

The germ cell layers involved in the formation of the reproductive tract in males and females include the mesoderm, endoderm, and ectoderm. An insult to or defect in the mesodermally derived mesonephros or metanephros may lead to congenital anomalies of the kidneys, gonads, and associated ducts. Fusion of endoderm and ectoderm is involved in the canalization process of the genital tract in both males and females. Defects in this process lead to fusion failure or obstructive lesions.

Normal Development and Anatomy

The structure of the kidney is complete by 32–36 weeks of gestation, although nephron maturation continues after birth. The permanent kidneys are initially located in the pelvis. As the embryo grows, the kidneys ascend to a lumbar position and undergo a 90-degree rotation so that their convex borders are directed laterally. The ureters course inferiorly through the retroperitoneum along the psoas muscles and into the pelvis, crossing anteriorly to the iliac vessels and connecting to the bladder. The normal ureter inserts along the posterolateral aspect of the bladder trigone.

On MR imaging the normal renal cortex is hyperintense to the medulla on both T1- and T2- weighted images [7]. Distinct corticomedullary differentiation should be seen. Normal fetal lobulations may be seen early in life, and while these usually regress, they may persist into adulthood as a normal variant (Fig. 13.2).

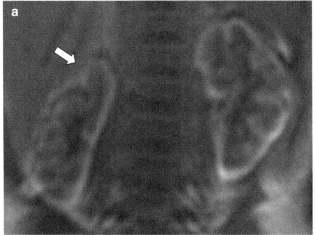
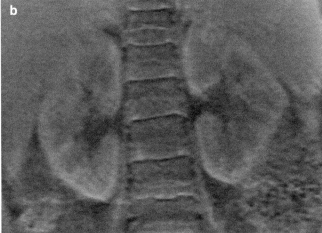

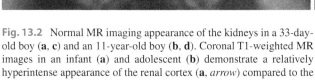

Fig. 13.2 Normal MR imaging appearance of the kidneys in a 33-day-old boy (**a**, **c**) and an 11-year-old boy (**b**, **d**). Coronal T1-weighted MR images in an infant (**a**) and adolescent (**b**) demonstrate a relatively hyperintense appearance of the renal cortex (**a**, *arrow*) compared to the medulla. Coronal T2-weighted MR images in an infant (**c**) and adolescent (**d**) also demonstrate relative hyperintensity of the cortex compared to the medulla. Fetal lobulations (**c**, *arrow*) are present in the infant

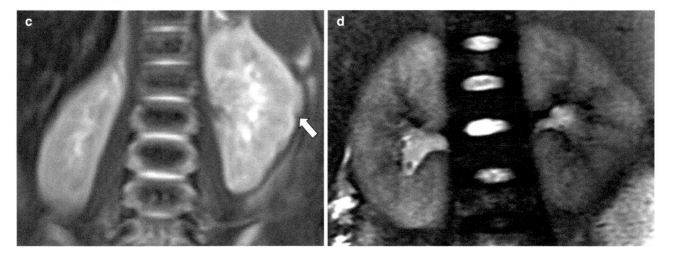

Fig. 13.2 (continued)

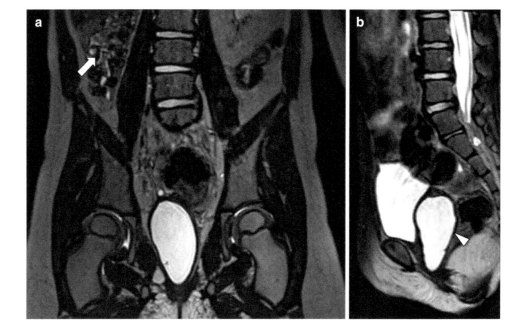

Fig. 13.3 Renal agenesis in a 3-year-old girl. Coronal (**a**) T2-weighted fat-suppressed MR image demonstrates absence of renal parenchyma in the right renal fossa (*arrow*). Sagittal (**b**) T2-weighted fat-suppressed MR image demonstrates distal vaginal agenesis with dilation of the proximal vagina (*arrowhead*) and absence of the uterus

Anatomic Variants

Renal Agenesis

Renal agenesis denotes a complete absence of one or both kidneys. There is a strong association with anomalies of the associated mesonephric (Wolffian) duct derivatives in the male (seminal vesicles, vas deferens, and epididymis) and paramesonephric (Müllerian) duct derivatives in the female (uterus, cervix, fallopian tubes, upper vagina). The incidence of associated reproductive tract anomalies is estimated at 20% in males and 30% in females [8]. Bilateral renal agenesis is incompatible with life. The absence of renal tissue and of urine in the bladder is an important diagnostic feature of bilateral renal agenesis on fetal MR imaging. Children with unilateral renal agenesis may present with a wide range of symptoms. Long-term consequences include proteinuria, hypertension, and/or renal insufficiency [9].

MR imaging typically demonstrates complete unilateral absence of renal tissue anywhere from the pelvis to the renal fossa and exquisitely depicts any associated genitourinary anomalies (Fig. 13.3).

Treatment of unilateral renal agenesis is primarily supportive. The remaining kidney usually undergoes compensatory hypertrophy, and survival rates are similar to those of age- and sex-matched controls [9].

Renal Ectopia

Renal ectopia is characterized by an abnormal location of one or both kidneys and results from abnormal migration of the kidney during embryological development. The ectopic kidney may be located anywhere from the pelvis to the thorax. The majority of patients with renal ectopia are asymptomatic, and the diagnosis is usually made incidentally. The term "crossed renal ectopia" refers to the location of both kidneys on the same side of the spine. The crossed ectopic kidney may be fused to the ipsilateral kidney or unfused. Crossed renal ectopia represents a more severe migration anomaly than simple ectopia, and up to half of affected patients have additional associated congenital anomalies and develop complications such as urinary tract infection, obstruction, or renal calculi [10].

MR imaging demonstrates the ectopic kidney and its relationship to adjacent structures (Figs. 13.4 and 13.5). Associated abnormalities are common, with VUR identified in 30% of patients with simple renal ectopia. In addition, there is a high incidence of VUR in the contralateral orthotopic kidney, and therefore evaluation with voiding cystourethrography (VCUG) is warranted [11].

Patient management is focused on treatment of associated abnormalities. Overall prognosis is excellent for both simple ectopia and crossed ectopia, without demonstrable long-term adverse effects on blood pressure or renal function [12].

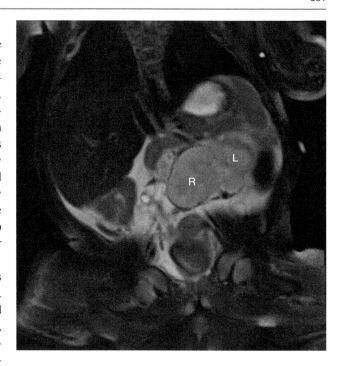

Fig. 13.5 Crossed renal ectopia in a 60-day-old girl with multiple congenital anomalies. Coronal T2-weighted fat-suppressed MR image demonstrates the right kidney (R) in the left hemiabdomen, fused to the lower pole of the orthotopic left kidney (L)

Horseshoe Kidney

Horseshoe kidney represents the most common fusion anomaly, where kidneys located on both sides of the spine are fused together by an isthmus of fibrous tissue or renal parenchyma. Fusion may be symmetric, with the connecting tissue located in the midline, or asymmetric, with the connecting tissue located laterally. Although no clear genetic predisposition has been elucidated, the incidence of horseshoe kidney is higher in several chromosomal disorders than in the general population, including Down syndrome (trisomy 21), Turner syndrome, and Edward syndrome (trisomy 18) [13]. Affected children are commonly asymptomatic, with 1/3 remaining asymptomatic throughout their lives. Horseshoe kidneys are characterized by abnormalities of position, rotation, and vascular supply and are predisposed to ureteropelvic junction obstruction (UPJO) and its associated complications of hydronephrosis, infection, and stone formation. Affected pediatric patients are susceptible to blunt trauma due to the location of the isthmus in relation to the spine and are at increased risk for numerous malignancies, including Wilms tumor and transitional cell carcinoma [14].

MR imaging readily demonstrates fusion of the right- and left-sided kidneys (Fig. 13.6) and is useful for depicting complications such as sequelae of infection, UPJO, and tumor.

Treatment of pediatric patients with horseshoe kidney is primarily supportive [14]. If a diagnosis is made prenatally, a postnatal ultrasound study should be performed to delineate renal anatomy and to evaluate for obstruction. Pediatric patients with associated urinary tract infection should

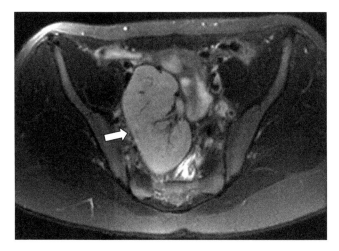

Fig. 13.4 Renal ectopia in a 12-year-old girl with a known uterine anomaly. Axial T2-weighted fat-suppressed MR image demonstrates an ectopic kidney (*arrow*) located within the right hemipelvis

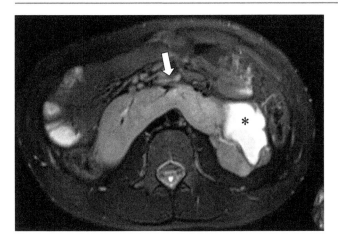

Fig. 13.6 Horseshoe kidney in a 6-year-old boy who presented for evaluation of hydronephrosis. Axial T2-weighted fat-suppressed MR image demonstrates midline fusion (*arrow*) of the lower poles of both renal moieties. There is hydronephrosis (*asterisk*) on the left

undergo a VCUG. Lithotripsy is less effective for treatment of stones in patients with horseshoe kidney, and percutaneous removal may be necessary [15].

Duplex Kidney and Ureteral Duplication

Duplex kidney results from anomalies in development of the ureteric bud and may be partial or complete. Ureteral duplication is the most common anomaly of the urinary tract, with incomplete duplication being far more common than complete duplication [16]. The overall estimated incidence ranges from 0.8% to 5% [17]. Affected pediatric patients may be asymptomatic, particularly in the case of incomplete duplication, and no further investigation is warranted. However, symptoms of reflux or obstruction may occur.

MR imaging, and in particular MR urography, is useful in depicting pelvic and ureteral duplication. In complete duplication, the lower pole ureter inserts orthotopically and is prone to reflux, while the upper pole ureter inserts ectopically and is prone to obstruction and ureterocele formation (Fig. 13.7). In females, the ectopic upper pole ureter may insert below the urethral sphincter, resulting in urinary incontinence. MR urography is particularly useful when the anatomy is complex (e.g., when the site of ectopic ureteral insertion is unclear by ultrasound and/or fluoroscopy) or when functional evaluation is required.

The vast majority of duplex kidneys require no intervention. Depending on the function of the upper moiety, a duplex system with an ectopic ureter may be treated surgically with reimplantation or with resection of the dysplastic renal segment and proximal ureter [18].

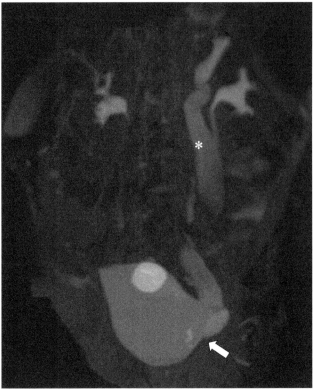

Fig. 13.7 Duplex left kidney in a 4-year-old girl. Coronal 3D T2-weighted sequence with high TE MR image demonstrates a dilated left upper pole ureter (*asterisk*) with an ectopic ureteral insertion (*arrow*) near the bladder base

Urinary Tract Disorders

Congenital Urinary Tract Abnormalities

Ureteropelvic Junction Obstruction

Ureteropelvic junction obstruction (UPJO) is the most common cause of urinary tract obstruction in children. Various theories regarding pathogenesis have been proposed, such as abnormal smooth muscle or abnormal innervation at the UPJ [19]. The most common associated anomaly is contralateral multicystic dysplastic kidney (MCDK). The diagnosis is frequently made prenatally. Affected individuals are typically asymptomatic [20]. Previously undiagnosed patients may present later in life with infection, pain, or hematuria.

The classic imaging appearance of UPJO is dilation of the renal pelvis and calyces with abrupt transition to a normal caliber ureter at the UPJ (Fig. 13.8). Ultrasound is the initial imaging examination of choice, while MR imaging and MR urography are particularly helpful for identifying associated crossing vessels and providing functional information [21].

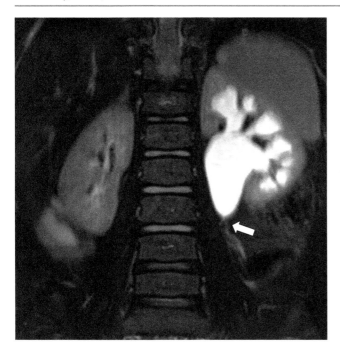

Fig. 13.8 Ureteropelvic junction obstruction in a 4-year-old boy who presented with flank pain. Coronal T2-weighted fat-suppressed MR image demonstrates dilation of the left renal pelvis and calyces, with an abrupt transition at the ureteropelvic junction (*arrow*) to a normal caliber ureter

Treatment is based on the severity of obstruction and its effect on kidney function. The obstruction often resolves spontaneously, with excellent long-term outcomes provided that renal function is preserved. In patients with compromised renal function, surgical intervention is frequently required [22].

Primary Megaureter

Primary megaureter is the sequela of a functional or anatomic abnormality at the UVJ. It is the second most common cause of neonatal hydronephrosis after UPJO, accounting for approximately 20% of cases [23]. It occurs bilaterally approximately 30–40% of the time [24]. Primary megaureter is classified into several types based on the presence of reflux and/or obstruction, as their presence or absence affects patient management. Affected patients are usually diagnosed by antenatal ultrasound. If not detected prenatally, affected children may present with urinary tract infection (UTI), hematuria, or abdominal pain [25].

On MR imaging, and in particular MR urography, the obstructive site is well demonstrated, with a narrowed, aperi-staltic segment of distal ureter (Fig. 13.9). MR imaging also demonstrates the degree of hydronephrosis and can be useful to evaluate for concomitant UPJO or congenital megacalyces [26, 27]. Renal parenchymal abnormalities such as cortical thinning and scarring are also readily depicted [28].

Asymptomatic pediatric patients are typically monitored conservatively with serial ultrasound studies and diuretic renography, as spontaneous resolution of the obstruction may occur. Surgical intervention is warranted when patients become symptomatic or when there is evidence of progressive hydronephrosis or a decrease in renal function [25].

Ureterocele

Ureterocele represents a cystic dilation of the submucosal segment of the distal ureter. It may be associated with an ectopic or orthotopic ureteral insertion and with single or duplicated ureter(s). The ureterocele may be intravesical or may insert into the bladder neck or urethra [29]. In children, ureterocele generally presents as a congenital obstruction of the ureteral orifice [30], manifesting as urinary tract infection in infancy, or with the sequelae of stasis, including infection and/or stone formation in older children [31].

MR urography is particularly useful in the diagnosis of ureterocele, with a sensitivity of 89%, compared to 31% for ultrasound and 74% for VCUG [32]. The ureterocele usually appears as a cystic outpouching of the distal ureter that protrudes into the urinary bladder (Fig. 13.10). MR urography can also evaluate function of the affected kidney and provide anatomic information regarding associated gynecologic abnormalities in girls.

Treatment of ureterocele varies widely and depends on patient age, mode of presentation, ureterocele type, and renal function. Management is largely dictated by the need to preserve renal function, including relief of associated obstruction and treatment of associated VUR. In the neonatal period, endoscopic incision is frequently performed, particularly with intravesical ureteroceles. In children with duplex systems and a poorly functioning upper pole moiety, upper pole heminephrectomy with or without lower tract reconstruction may be the treatment of choice [33].

Multicystic Dysplastic Kidney

MCDK represents the most severe form of cystic renal dysplasia. Numerous non-communicating cysts are present with dysplastic intervening tissue and pelviureteral or ureteral atresia. The affected kidney is generally nonfunctional. Abnormalities of the contralateral kidney occur up to 25% of the time with the most common anomalies being VUR and

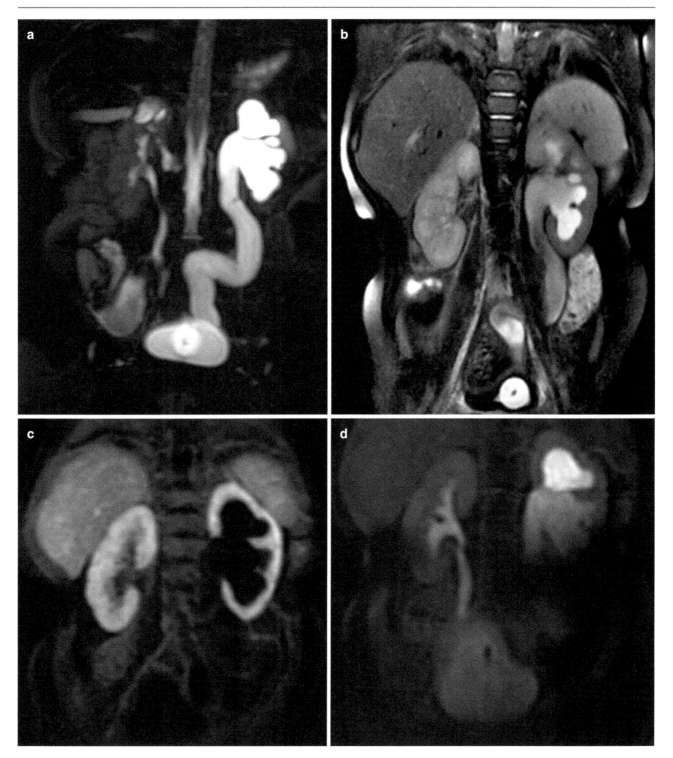

Fig. 13.9 Primary megaureter in a 65-day-old boy with prenatal hydronephrosis. Coronal 3D T2-weighted sequence with high TE MIP image (**a**) and coronal T2-weighted fat-suppressed MR image (**b**) demonstrate moderate-to-severe left-sided hydroureteronephrosis. The right kidney is normal. Dynamic early (**c**) and late (**d**) coronal 3D T1-weighted fat-suppressed post-contrast MR images from MR urography demonstrate symmetric cortical transit time, parenchymal enhancement, and excretion of contrast material

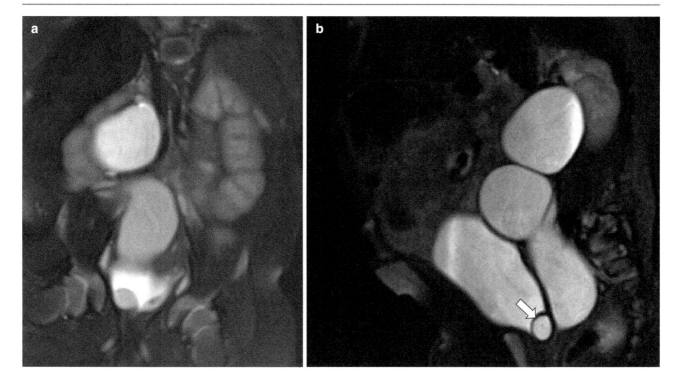

Fig. 13.10 Ectopic ureterocele in a 28-day-old girl who presented with prenatal hydronephrosis. Coronal T2-weighted fat-suppressed MR image (**a**) demonstrates severe hydroureteronephrosis of the upper pole collecting system and ureter of a duplex right kidney. Sagittal T2-weighted fat-suppressed MR image (**b**) demonstrates the upper pole ureter terminating in a cystic structure (*arrow*) located close to the bladder neck consistent with a ureterocele

UPJO [34]. The affected kidney commonly involutes, and the contralateral kidney usually undergoes compensatory hypertrophy. Inheritance is considered sporadic, although some genetic mutations have been implicated in the etiology of MCDK [35]. Affected children are commonly diagnosed prenatally but are usually asymptomatic. If the patient is not diagnosed prenatally, a bulging flank mass may occasionally be detected on physical examination.

MR imaging typically plays a complementary role to ultrasound in the diagnosis and follow-up of MCDK. If the sonographic appearance is typical, no additional imaging is needed. If there are atypical features, there may be overlap with other cystic renal pathology, and MR imaging may be useful in better characterizing the renal abnormality [36]. A reniform mass in the renal fossa with numerous non-communicating cysts replacing normal renal parenchyma is a characteristic of MCDK (Fig. 13.11). No renal function is demonstrated by MR urography.

Patients with simple MCDK should undergo a repeat ultrasound study at 1–2 years to document compensatory hypertrophy of the contralateral kidney. Historically, it was

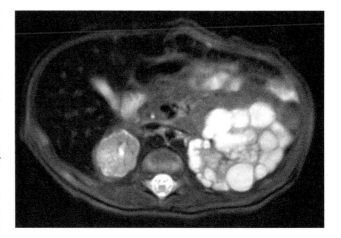

Fig. 13.11 Multicystic dysplastic kidney in a 10-day-old boy. Axial T2-weighted fat-suppressed MR image demonstrates multiple hyperintense, non-communicating cysts replacing the left kidney, with no identifiable normal renal parenchyma

thought that patients with MCDK were at increased risk of Wilms tumor, although more recent studies do not support this claim. Patients with complex MCDK, such as those with identifiable abnormalities of the contralateral kidney, warrant further urological or nephrology follow-up [37].

Autosomal Recessive Polycystic Kidney Disease

Autosomal recessive polycystic kidney disease (ARPKD) is a hereditary cystic condition resulting from mutations of the polycystic kidney and hepatic disease 1 gene (*PKHD1*). Mutation of this gene results in ectasia of the tubules and collecting ducts of the kidney [38]. Pulmonary and musculoskeletal abnormalities may develop in tandem due to associated oligohydramnios. The clinical course of affected patients varies according to the degree of renal and hepatic involvement. The diagnosis can usually be made prenatally by 24–26 weeks of gestation, although occasionally the prenatal appearance may be normal and the child may not present until later in life. Associated conditions related to renal and hepatic impairment, such as systemic hypertension and portal hypertension, occur frequently in these patients [39].

MR imaging demonstrates nephromegaly with diffuse intermediate to low signal intensity on T1-weighted images and high signal intensity on T2-weighted images, likely a reflection of the innumerable tiny, fluid-filled parenchymal cysts (Fig. 13.12). A linear radial pattern of enhancement has been described that is related to microcystic dilation of the collecting ducts [40]. Macrocysts are not usually identified at birth but may be seen in later childhood.

Treatment varies based on disease severity. Renal transplantation is frequently required, with dialysis as a bridge to transplant. Nephrectomy is performed when mass effect from the kidney(s) impairs respiratory function. Hepatic transplantation may also be necessary due to progressive hepatic fibrosis.

Autosomal Dominant Polycystic Kidney Disease

Autosomal dominant polycystic kidney disease (ADPKD) represents the other major hereditary cystic renal disease. Resulting from a mutation in the *PKD1* or *PKD2* gene, the disease manifests as cystic dilation in all parts of the neph-

ron. The overall prevalence of ADPKD is greater than that of ARPKD and is the most common hereditary kidney disease, although it is not usually manifested until adulthood [41]. Pancreatic and hepatic cysts may also be present, although they are much rarer in children than in adults. Affected children may present with a range of symptoms, including hematuria, proteinuria, hypertension, or pain. Renal insufficiency is uncommon before adulthood [42].

MR imaging depicts renal cysts with intervening normal renal parenchyma (Fig. 13.13). A single cyst is adequate to

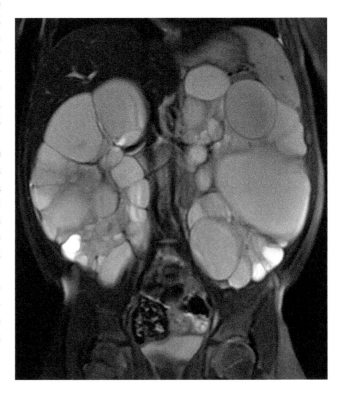

Fig. 13.13 Autosomal dominant polycystic kidney disease in a 33-month-old girl with a palpable abdominal mass. Coronal T2-weighted fat-suppressed MR image demonstrates numerous well-circumscribed cysts replacing most of the renal parenchyma, with marked renal enlargement

Fig. 13.12 Autosomal recessive polycystic kidney disease in a 4-year-old boy. Axial T1-weighted MR image (**a**) of the kidneys demonstrates bilateral renal enlargement with symmetric, diffusely decreased T1-weighted parenchymal signal. Coronal T2-weighted fat-suppressed MR image (**b**) demonstrates diffusely increased T2-weighted signal intensity in both kidneys. Multiple tiny, discrete bilateral parenchymal cysts are also depicted

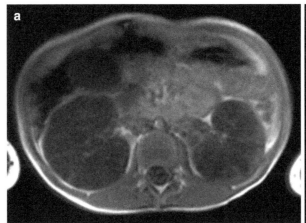
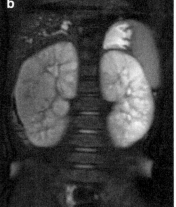

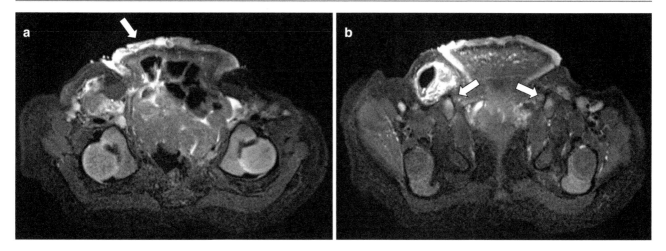

Fig. 13.14 Bladder exstrophy in a 38-day-old boy. Axial T2-weighted fat-suppressed MR image (**a**) demonstrates an anterior abdominal wall defect with an extruded, open bladder (*arrow*). Axial T2-weighted fat-suppressed MR image (**b**) shows the marked pubic symphyseal diastasis (*arrows*)

make the diagnosis in at-risk individuals with a positive family history [43]. The cysts are hypointense on T1-weighted images and hyperintense on T2-weighted images and demonstrate no contrast enhancement. MR imaging has high sensitivity for cyst detection and allows concurrent detection of hepatic and pancreatic cysts. Nephromegaly may be present, even in the absence of a significant cyst burden [44, 45].

The course of the disease in children is usually benign with a good prognosis, and specific interventions are not performed in the absence of symptoms. Therefore, screening is not recommended in asymptomatic children with a positive family history. Targeted imaging evaluation may be performed for evaluation of specific symptoms such as hypertension, pain, or infection [43].

Bladder Exstrophy

Bladder exstrophy is a rare malformation characterized by an infra-abdominal wall defect, incomplete closure of the bladder with mucosa continuous with the anterior abdominal wall, epispadias, diastasis of the pubic symphysis, and abnormal pelvic floor musculature [46]. Bladder exstrophy is the most common disorder of the exstrophy-epispadias complex, with cloacal exstrophy representing the most severe end of the spectrum and epispadias the mildest abnormality. It has an incidence of approximately 1 in 10,000–50,000 live births and is more frequently seen in males. Most cases are sporadic [47]. Affected patients are commonly diagnosed prenatally. After birth the anomaly is readily apparent, with a low umbilicus; extruding, open bladder; epispadias; short penis in males with wide separation of the corporal attachments; bifid clitoris in females; and anterior displacement of the anus [46, 48].

Prenatal MR imaging may demonstrate a low abdominal mass below the cord insertion, absence of a normal urinary bladder, and normal amniotic fluid volume. Although these findings may be seen on ultrasound, fetal MR imaging pro-

vides greater anatomic detail with higher sensitivity. Fetal MR imaging also allows ease of differentiation of classic bladder exstrophy and the more complex abnormalities associated with cloacal exstrophy [49]. On MR imaging done postnatally, the abdominal wall defect, symphyseal diastasis, and open bladder are readily apparent (Fig. 13.14). MR imaging is also useful for preoperative evaluation of the pelvic floor musculature [50, 51].

Treatment involves surgical repair of the bladder exstrophy and associated anomalies. Two approaches have been described. In modern staged repair of bladder exstrophy, the patient undergoes closure of the bladder, posterior urethra, and abdominal wall defect as well as epispadias repair in the newborn period. Concurrent pelvic osteotomy may also be performed depending on the degree of diastasis. At 4–5 years of age, bladder neck reconstruction and ureteral reimplantation are performed with the goal of achieving urinary continence. Alternatively, complete primary repair of bladder exstrophy, epispadias repair, and ureteral reimplantation may be combined into a single operation [52, 53]. It is currently undetermined as to which approach results in better long-term outcomes.

Prune-Belly Syndrome

Prune-belly syndrome, also known as Eagle-Barrett syndrome, is characterized by urinary tract malformations, bilateral cryptorchidism, and abdominal wall muscle deficiency. It has an estimated incidence of 1 in 30,000–50,000 live births. Nearly all affected patients are male (95–99%). Although its etiology and pathogenesis are currently unknown, theories include early in utero bladder outlet obstruction and a primary mesodermal defect [54]. Nearly all affected patients present with hydroureteronephrosis, and a large number have VUR. Chronic kidney disease is relatively common, with many affected children ultimately requiring kidney transplant [55]. Nearly half of all patients have additional congenital anomalies, most commonly of the cardiac or musculoskeletal systems.

MR imaging plays a valuable role in the evaluation of these patients, particularly MR urography which permits both anatomical and functional evaluation. There is usually some degree of bilateral hydroureteronephrosis (Fig. 13.15a). Other frequently seen abnormalities include renal dysplasia, scarring, and/or calyceal diverticula [56]. The abdominal wall musculature and location of the testes can also be evaluated (Fig. 13.15b).

The main prognostic factor is the degree of renal dysplasia, and approximately 15% of patients ultimately require renal transplantation [55]. Surgery is frequently required and may include upper urinary tract reconstruction, ureteral reimplantation, abdominoplasty, orchiopexy, and vesicostomy [57]. Outcomes depend on the comorbidities, ranging from perinatal death to a relatively normal quality of life. Many of these patients can be successfully treated despite severe malformations, and aggressive intervention is frequently warranted [58].

Megacystis-Microcolon-Intestinal Hypoperistalsis Syndrome

Megacystis-microcolon-intestinal hypoperistalsis syndrome (MMIHS) is a disease affecting smooth muscle function in the genitourinary and gastrointestinal tracts. It is inherited in an autosomal recessive fashion and is much more common in females, with fewer than 30% of reported cases occurring in males [59, 60]. It is one of a group of conditions caused by mutations in the ACTG2 gene and is either inherited in an autosomal dominant manner or as a result of de novo mutations in the ACTG2 gene. Presentation usually occurs in the neonatal period, with abdominal distension or an inability to void. The symptoms may mimic other more common neonatal disorders such as bladder outlet obstruction and proximal bowel obstruction (e.g., bilious emesis, abdominal distension) [61].

The most common imaging findings include hydroureteronephrosis, megacystis, microcolon, and small bowel dilation related to hypoperistalsis (Fig. 13.16) [62]. Due to the rarity of the disease, the MR imaging features of MMIHS are not well described in the literature. The diagnosis may be suggested on prenatal MR imaging when a combination of megacystis, microcolon, and/or sparse meconium is demonstrated in a female fetus [62]. T2-weighted images are useful for evaluation of the renal collecting systems and ureters, while T1-weighted images best demonstrate the fetal microcolon and absence of hyperintense meconium.

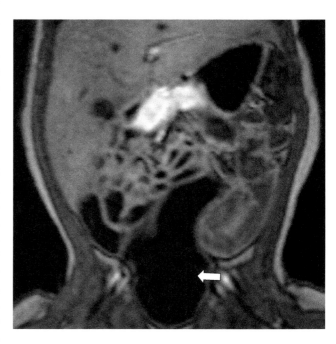

Fig. 13.16 Megacystis-microcolon-intestinal hypoperistalsis syndrome in a 5-month-old girl. Coronal T1-weighted MR image of the abdomen demonstrates a dilated urinary bladder (*arrow*). (Case courtesy of Beth M. Kline-Fath, MD, Cincinnati Children's Hospital Medical Center, Cincinnati, Ohio, USA)

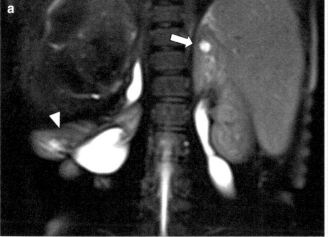
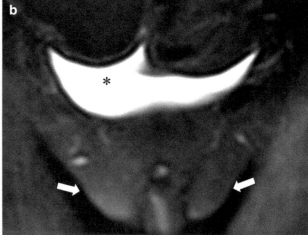

Fig. 13.15 Prune-belly syndrome in a 10-year-old boy with bowel pseudo-obstruction. Coronal T2-weighted fat-suppressed MR image (**a**) of the kidneys demonstrates malrotation of the right kidney (*arrowhead*) and bilateral collecting system dilation. A simple cyst (*arrow*) is also present in the upper pole of the left kidney. Coronal T2-weighted fat-suppressed MR image of the pelvis (**b**) demonstrates an irregular bladder contour (*asterisk*) and absence of testes within the scrotum (*arrows*)

Management of these patients is complex and generally futile, with most infants dying within a year of birth. Surgical intervention and prokinetic drugs are not effective at restoring intestinal function. Children who survive beyond the first few months of life inevitably require long-term total parenteral nutrition. Multiorgan transplantation is currently the only intervention that has been somewhat effective in prolonging the lives of these patients [63].

Infectious Urinary Tract Disorders

Pyelonephritis

Pyelonephritis is an acute infection of the renal parenchyma which may result from hematogenous seeding or via ascent from the lower urinary tract, with the majority of cases occurring via the latter mechanism [64]. While many risk factors exist for UTI, including anatomical abnormalities, functional disorders, and immunosuppression, a secondary mechanism for ascent to the kidney needs to be present in order for pyelonephritis to develop [65]. Approximately 25–40% of cases

are associated with VUR which is more common in females, and therefore pyelonephritis is also more frequent in girls [66]. Affected children present with a variety of symptoms, which vary based on age of presentation. Younger children usually present with non-specific symptoms such as malaise, fever, and abdominal pain, while children older than 5 years of age present with more classic symptoms such as dysuria, urgency, urinary frequency, and flank pain [64].

Pyelonephritis is primarily a clinical diagnosis, with imaging performed to evaluate for predisposing factors such as reflux or for complicating features such as abscess. If imaged in the acute phase, T1-weighted images of an affected kidney demonstrate loss of normal corticomedullary differentiation, while T2-weighted images show hyperintense signal in the regions of the affected parenchyma, with corresponding areas of decreased contrast enhancement related to hypoperfusion. Diffusion-weighted images depict diffusion restriction corresponding to areas of nephritis or abscess formation, with a similar sensitivity to perfusion defects demonstrated on contrast-enhanced T1-weighted sequences (Fig. 13.17) [67].

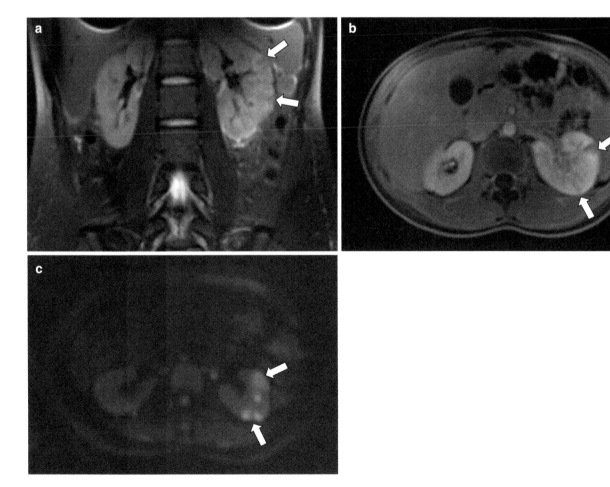

Fig. 13.17 Pyelonephritis in a 17-year-old girl with fever and left flank pain. Coronal T2-weighted fat-suppressed MR image (**a**) demonstrates peripheral foci of striated signal abnormality (*arrows*) within the left kidney. Axial T1-weighted fat-suppressed contrast-enhanced MR image (**b**) demonstrates corresponding areas of decreased enhancement (*arrows*). Axial diffusion-weighted MR image (**c**) demonstrates zones of restricted diffusion (*arrows*) in the left kidney in the same distribution as the abnormalities depicted in (**a**) and (**b**)

Treatment of pyelonephritis includes prompt initiation of antibiotic therapy. Fluids and other supportive measures may be required depending on the clinical course [64]. Renal scarring often occurs regardless of the rapidity of disease detection and treatment, and therefore diagnosis and management of VUR and other predisposing factors in the development of pyelonephritis are of paramount importance [68].

Xanthogranulomatous Pyelonephritis

Xanthogranulomatous pyelonephritis is a chronic kidney infection characterized by a destructive granulomatous inflammatory infiltrate that contains lipid-laden macrophages. Predominantly occurring in adults, it develops in association with long-term urinary tract obstruction and infection. The disease may rarely be seen in children who are usually less than 5 years of age [69]. Both diffuse and focal forms of xanthogranulomatous pyelonephritis have been described, with the latter form being less frequent overall but more commonly seen in children. Affected children present with non-specific findings including abdominal pain, fever, weight loss, anorexia, or a palpable abdominal mass [70].

Imaging findings are non-specific and frequently overlap with other entities, making the diagnosis challenging. The diffuse form demonstrates global renal enlargement with multiple collections of intermediate to high T1-weighted and T2-weighted signal intensity and associated diffusion restriction related to internal debris and/or purulent material

(Fig. 13.18). Peripheral contrast enhancement is seen, and a staghorn calculus is frequently present. Local extension into the perinephric fat or psoas muscle is possible, and the diagnosis should be considered in children presenting with a perirenal or psoas abscess. The focal form shows similar imaging characteristics but does not involve the entire kidney, and focal calcification is seen rather than a staghorn calculus [71]. The focal form may mimic many different neoplastic entities.

In the diffuse form of xanthogranulomatous pyelonephritis, antibiotics are a temporizing measure, with effective treatment ultimately requiring nephrectomy. Antibiotics may be effective in treating focal xanthogranulomatous pyelonephritis, assuming the diagnosis can be confidently made by imaging and histologic sampling. Patients with the focal form also frequently require at least partial nephrectomy [72].

Neoplastic Urinary Tract Disorders

MR imaging evaluation of renal neoplasms in children provides valuable information that can aid in initial diagnosis, surgical planning, and follow-up (Table 13.3).

Benign Urinary Tract Neoplasms

Mesoblastic Nephroma Mesoblastic nephroma is a benign tumor usually diagnosed in the first 3 months of life and is the

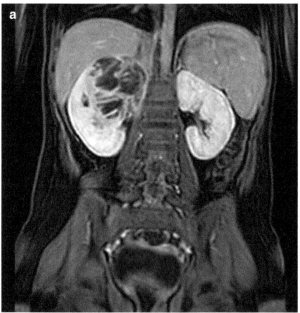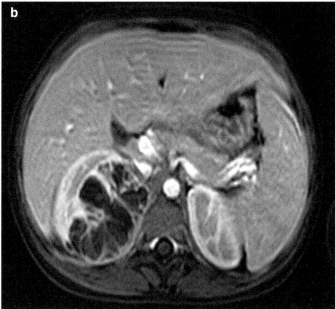

Fig. 13.18 Xanthogranulomatous pyelonephritis in a 14-year-old boy who presented with a 4-month history of low grade fever and weight loss. Contrast-enhanced coronal (**a**) and axial (**b**) T1-weighted fat-suppressed MR images demonstrate a heterogeneous cystic and solid mass in the upper pole of the right kidney. Axial diffusion-weighted (**c**) and (**d**) apparent diffusion coefficient (ADC) MR images show corresponding diffusion restriction within the mass

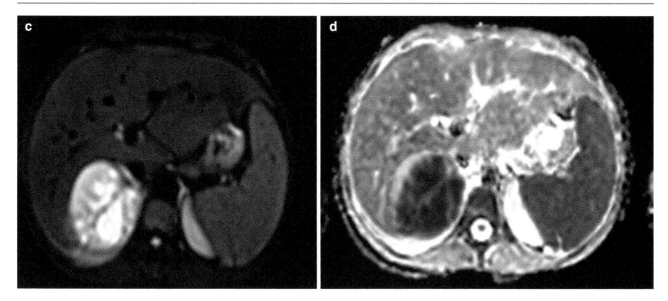

Fig. 13.18 (continued)

Table 13.3 Characteristic MR imaging findings of pediatric renal neoplasms

Renal neoplasms	Characteristic MR imaging findings
Benign urinary tract neoplasms	
Mesoblastic nephroma	Mass involving the renal sinus, with variable cystic and solid components
Multilocular cystic renal tumor	Solitary multicystic lesion with thin enhancing septations
Angiomyolipoma	Mass containing varying degrees of internal fat
Malignant urinary tract neoplasms	
Wilms tumor	Large homogenous mass that may contain focal areas of necrosis or hemorrhage
Nephroblastomatosis	Focal or diffuse T1-weighted hypointense and T2-weighted hyperintense nodules
Renal cell carcinoma	Heterogeneous mass with variable necrosis, hemorrhage, and calcification
Clear cell sarcoma	Non-specific and often indistinguishable from Wilms. Mass with variable calcification and necrosis and heterogeneous enhancement
Rhabdoid tumor	Heterogeneous, lobulated mass with central hilar location and curvilinear calcifications outlining tumor lobules. May have a crescentic subcapsular fluid collection
Medullary carcinoma	Infiltrative, heterogeneous mass with extensive hemorrhage and necrosis
Lymphoma	Homogenous, T1- and T2-weighted hypointense mass that enhances less than renal parenchyma

most common solid renal tumor of infancy [73]. It is composed of spindle cells and is divided into classic and cellular types, with the cellular type being the more common and aggressive variant [74]. Affected patients most commonly present with a palpable abdominal mass, with less common presentations including hypertension, vomiting, or anemia [75].

Congenital mesoblastic nephroma may be diagnosed with prenatal ultrasound. The tumor is usually large with involvement of the renal sinus. On MR imaging, its appearance varies, depending on the extent of internal cystic components and of hemorrhage (Fig. 13.19). The classic type typically presents earlier and usually includes a prominent solid component. The cellular type usually presents later, is larger, and more frequently demonstrates T2-weighted hyperintense cystic components or necrosis and T1-weighted hyperintense internal hemorrhage. Both types are generally heterogeneous in appearance with varying enhancement of the solid and septal components [74].

Wide resection of mesoblastic nephroma is almost always curative. Disease recurrence or metastases are extremely rare but have been reported, with metastatic sites including the lung, heart, and liver [76].

Multilocular Cystic Renal Tumor Multilocular cystic renal tumor (MCRT) is a benign neoplasm arising from the metanephric blastema. This term actually encompasses two separate pathologic entities, cystic nephroma and cystic partially differentiated nephroblastoma, which are indistinguishable by imaging and gross pathologic appearance [77]. MCRT demonstrates a bimodal age and sex distribution, most commonly occurring in young males aged 3 months to 4 years and older females aged 40–60 years [78]. Affected pediatric patients most commonly present with a painless abdominal mass, although hematuria and UTI may also occur [79].

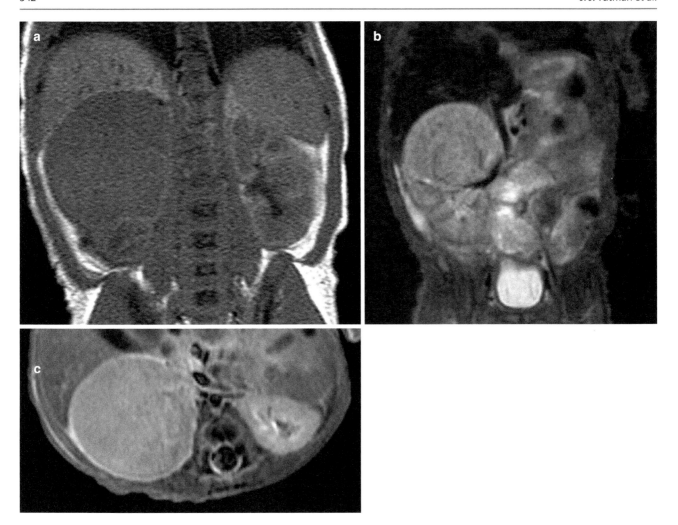

Fig. 13.19 Mesoblastic nephroma in a 7-day-old boy with a prenatally detected abdominal mass. Coronal T1-weighted (**a**) and inversion recovery (**b**) MR images demonstrate a round, well-circumscribed mass in the upper pole of the right kidney. Axial enhanced T1-weighted fat-suppressed MR image (**c**) demonstrates homogeneous enhancement of the tumor

On MR imaging, the most commonly demonstrated features are a solitary multicystic lesion with thin internal, enhancing septations (Fig. 13.20). The signal intensity of the cystic spaces most commonly follows fluid signal but may vary depending on the degree of internal hemorrhage or proteinaceous material. Herniation of the tumor into the renal collecting system is commonly seen [80].

Although considered benign, MCRT cannot be differentiated with certainty from other malignant tumors such as cystic Wilms tumor or cystic renal cell carcinoma on the basis of imaging features, and therefore partial or complete nephrectomy is the treatment of choice. Removal of the tumor with clear margins is curative [81].

Angiomyolipoma Angiomyolipoma is a benign tumor composed of varying amounts of smooth muscle, vessels, and adipose tissue. While most commonly occurring as an isolated, sporadic lesion (80% of the time), there is also a strong syndromic association with tuberous sclerosis complex and pulmonary lymphangioleiomyomatosis [82]. Angiomyolipomas occur in approximately 80% of patients with tuberous sclerosis [83]. Affected children are most commonly asymptomatic but can also present with flank pain, hematuria, or hemorrhage.

On imaging, angiomyolipomas are readily diagnosed if they contain fat. The fatty portion of the tumor classically displays high T1- and T2-weighted signal intensity and signal loss on fat-suppressed MR images (Fig. 13.21). Opposed-phase images can demonstrate loss of signal due to microscopic fat in lipid-poor angiomyolipomas but is not diagnostic. Contrast administration does not contribute to the diagnosis and is not necessary in evaluating patients with known tuberous sclerosis. Contrast administration may be necessary in the evaluation of indeterminate or growing

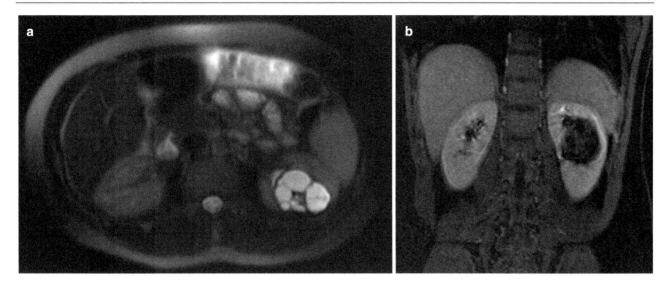

Fig. 13.20 Multilocular cystic renal tumor in an 11-year-old boy who presented with flank pain. Axial balanced steady-state free precession fat-suppressed MR image (**a**) demonstrates a multiloculated cystic mass in the mid-left kidney. Contrast-enhanced coronal T1-weighted fat-suppressed MR image (**b**) demonstrates no internal enhancement of the lesion

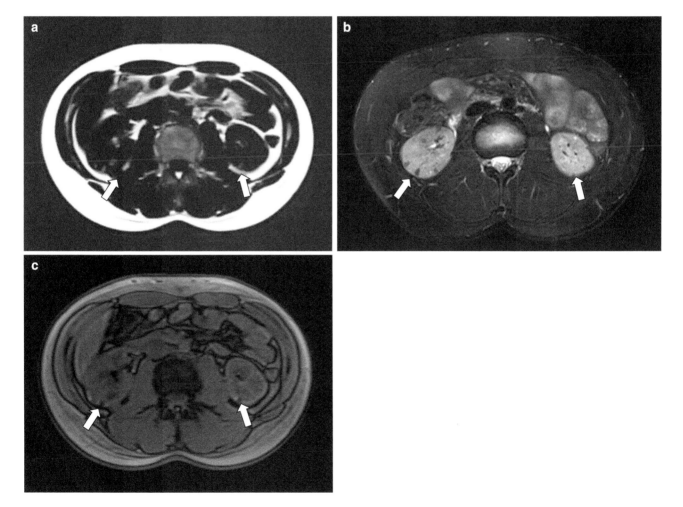

Fig. 13.21 Angiomyolipomas in a 16-year-old boy with tuberous sclerosis. Axial T1-weigthted Dixon fat only MR image (**a**) demonstrates multiple fatty lesions (*arrows*) in both kidneys. Axial T2-weighted fat-suppressed MR image (**b**) shows corresponding signal loss within the lesions (*arrows*). Axial T1-weighted out-of-phase MR image (**c**) demonstrates signal loss within the lesions (*arrows*) in keeping with fat

lesions. The primary diagnostic dilemma is in the evaluation of lipid-poor angiomyolipomas, which cannot always be differentiated from renal cell carcinoma. In this situation, percutaneous biopsy may be necessary [84].

Conservative management is the management approach of choice. MR imaging should be done at the time of diagnosis, and surveillance should be performed at 1- to 3-year intervals [85]. Treatment involves prophylaxis of hemorrhage, with an increase in risk associated with an increase in tumor size. Historically, lesions less than 4 cm in diameter have been followed, while those greater than 4 cm in diameter were considered for partial nephrectomy or embolization. These recommendations have recently come under scrutiny, with active surveillance being preferred in select patients [86]. For tumors more than 3 cm in diameter, treatment with mTOR inhibitors such as sirolimus or everolimus is often recommended [85].

Malignant Urinary Tract Neoplasms

Wilms Tumor and Nephroblastomatosis Wilms tumor is the second most common pediatric solid tumor and the most common renal tumor of childhood, accounting for greater than 90% of renal tumors in this population [87]. It arises from metanephric rests, considered to be a precursor lesion to Wilms tumor. These rests are termed "nephroblastomatosis" after 36 weeks of gestation. Although the majority of these tumors are sporadic, several conditions have a known association with Wilms tumor, including hemihypertrophy, Beckwith-Wiedemann syndrome, and WAGR syndrome [88]. Affected children are usually asymptomatic, although

20–30% of patients may present with malaise, abdominal pain, hematuria, or hypertension [89].

On MR imaging, Wilms tumor appears as a large, usually homogenous mass with a claw of surrounding renal parenchyma (Fig. 13.22). Focal areas of necrosis, hemorrhage, or cystic degeneration may be present, with fat and calcification less commonly seen. Tumors are T1-weighted hypointense and T2-weighted hyperintense and demonstrate heterogeneous contrast enhancement [90]. The primary utility of MR imaging compared to other imaging modalities lies in its ability to better define disease extent. Particular attention should be paid to the contralateral kidney to assess for bilateral involvement, and the renal vein should also be examined closely for invasion, as both of these findings affect patient management [3]. Nephroblastomatosis may be multifocal or diffuse and appears as multiple T1 hypointense and T2 hyperintense nodules without significant contrast enhancement [78].

Nephrectomy followed by chemotherapy is the mainstay of treatment for Wilms tumor, with radiation being used in some cases. For bilateral disease, preoperative chemotherapy is given followed by nephron-sparing surgery [91]. Currently, the approach to treatment of nephroblastomatosis is varied and may consist of observation, chemotherapy, and/or surgery. Close surveillance is necessary to detect progression to Wilms tumor.

Renal Cell Carcinoma Renal cell carcinoma (RCC) is a rare, malignant tumor of childhood, accounting for approximately 2–3% of all pediatric renal tumors [92]. The incidence increases with age, with a median age at diagnosis of

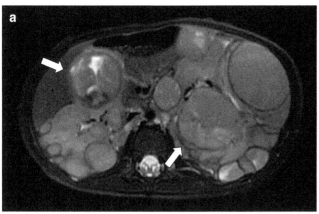
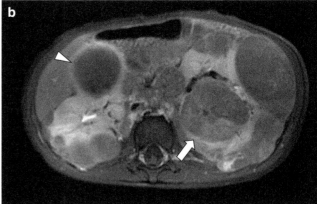

Fig. 13.22 Wilms tumor and nephroblastomatosis in a 33-month-old girl who presented with abdominal pain. Axial T2-weighted fat-suppressed MR image (**a**) demonstrates multiple homogeneous, round masses throughout both kidneys in keeping with nephroblastomatosis. In addition, heterogeneous lesions (*arrows*) are seen in the anterior right kidney and mid-left kidney. Contrast-enhanced axial T1-weighted fat-suppressed MR image (**b**) demonstrates a necrotic, non-enhancing lesion (*arrowhead*) within the anterior right kidney and a heterogeneously enhancing lesion (*arrow*) in the mid-left kidney consistent with focal bilateral progression to Wilms tumor

9 years [93]. The relative prevalence also increases with age, with renal cell carcinoma accounting for 32% of all primary renal tumors in children between the ages of 10 and 14 years and 63% of all primary renal tumors in patients between the ages of 15 and 19 years [94]. The incidence of RCC in the second decade of life is similar to that of Wilms tumor [95]. It has been suggested that pediatric RCC is a separate entity compared to adult RCC, based on differences in clinical behavior, genetics, and pathologic characteristics of the tumor in these two different populations [96]. Several subtypes exist, with translocation RCC and papillary RCC being the most common in the pediatric population [97]. The clear cell subtype has an association with von Hippel-Lindau disease [94]. Affected patients most commonly present with macroscopic hematuria or flank pain but can also present with a palpable abdominal mass, anemia, or fever [92].

On MR imaging, pediatric RCC has a variable appearance. It is usually unilateral and solitary, although multifocal or bilateral disease can occasionally occur. The mass is most often T1-weighted hypointense and T2-weighted hyperintense (Fig. 13.23), although it may be heterogeneous in appearance due to necrosis, hemorrhage, or calcification [3]. Internal or perilesional hemorrhage has been reported in 50% of tumors and internal calcification in up to 40% of tumors [94]. The greatest utility of cross-sectional imaging is in tumor staging. Extracapsular or vascular extension, nodal spread, and metastatic disease are readily evaluated by MR imaging. It is frequently not possible to confidently distinguish RCC from other renal neoplasms such as Wilms tumor [91].

Treatment and prognosis depend on tumor staging. Survival rate ranges from greater than 90% for stage I dis-

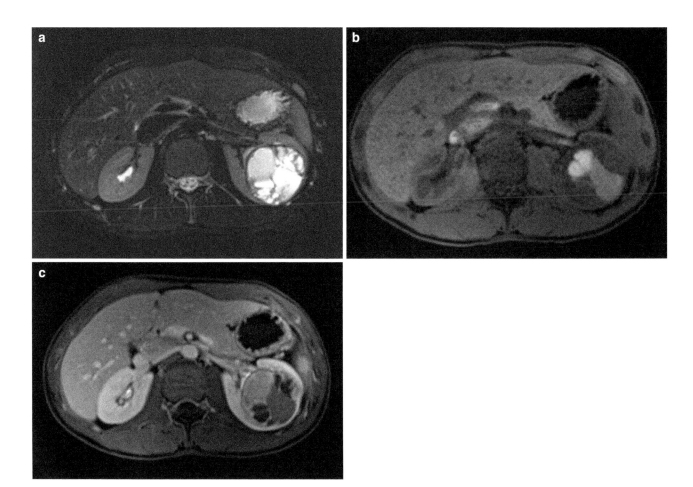

Fig. 13.23 Renal cell carcinoma in a 14-year-old boy who presented with decreased appetite and fatigue. Axial T2-weighted fat-suppressed MR image (**a**) demonstrates a heterogeneous, multiseptated mass in the mid-left kidney. Axial T1-weighted fat-suppressed MR image (**b**) shows a predominantly hypointense mass within the mid-left kidney that contains foci of intermediate and hyperintense signal. Contrast-enhanced axial T1-weighted, fat-suppressed MR image (**c**) demonstrates heterogeneous enhancement of the mass

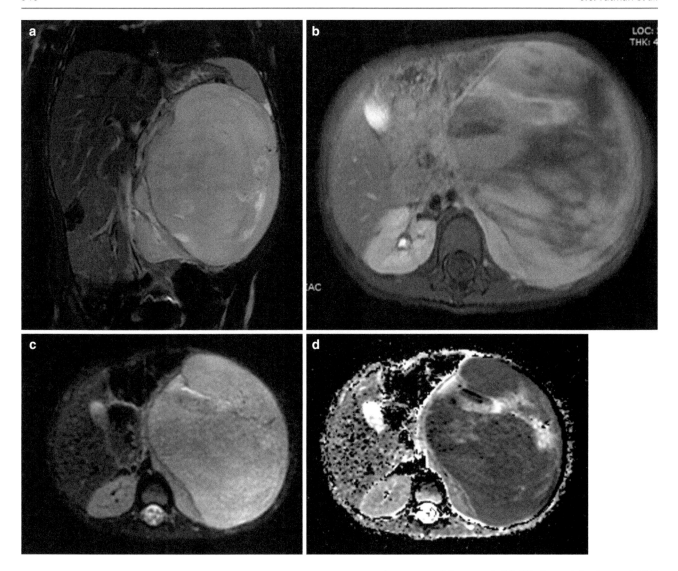

Fig. 13.24 Clear cell sarcoma in a 2-year-old girl who presented with a palpable abdominal mass. Coronal T2-weighted fat-suppressed MR image (**a**) demonstrates a large mass arising from the left kidney, with predominantly intermediate signal. Axial contrast-enhanced T1-weighted fat-suppressed MR image (**b**) demonstrates heteroge- neous enhancement of the mass. Axial diffusion weighted (**c**) and ADC map (**d**) MR images demonstrate restricted diffusion throughout most of the mass. (Case courtesy of Narendra Shet, MD, Children's National Health System, the George Washington University School of Medicine and Health Sciences, Washington, DC, USA)

ease to less than 15% for stage IV disease, with an overall survival rate of 63%. In contrast to adults, the presence of local lymph node involvement is associated with a relatively favorable prognosis. All patients receive radical nephrec- tomy, and consideration may be given to interleukin-2 ther- apy in patients with metastatic disease. Chemotherapy and radiotherapy have not been shown to influence outcome [93].

Clear Cell Sarcoma Clear cell sarcoma is a rare, malignant tumor accounting for approximately 4–5% of pediatric renal tumors. The incidence peaks between 1 and 4 years of age and occurs predominantly in males. It has a unique propen- sity for bone metastases, although other renal tumors, includ- ing Wilms tumor, can also metastasize to bone. Affected

pediatric patients typically present with a painless abdominal mass; rarely they may present with pain related to bone involvement [91].

MR imaging features are non-specific and indistin- guishable from Wilms tumor. There is typically a large, heterogeneous, T1-weighted hypointense and T2-weighted hyperintense mass with heterogeneous enhancement (Fig. 13.24). Calcification, vascular invasion, and cystic or necrotic foci may be present [3]. Metastatic lesions may occur to the lymph nodes, lungs, bone, liver, and brain [98].

Clear cell sarcoma of the kidney is aggressive and dif- ficult to treat. Current management consists of radical nephrectomy followed by radiotherapy and chemotherapy.

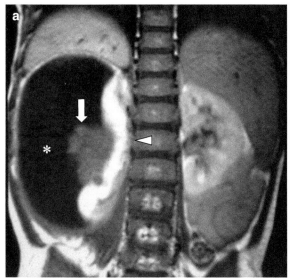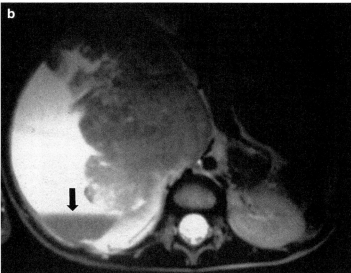

Fig. 13.25 Rhabdoid tumor in a 3-year-old boy who presented with vomiting and abdominal distension. Coronal contrast-enhanced T1-weighted fat-suppressed MR image (**a**) demonstrates a solid mass (*arrow*) in the mid-right kidney with a large subcapsular fluid collection (*asterisk*). The right kidney (*arrowhead*) is compressed against the spine. Axial T2-weighted fat-suppressed MR image (**b**) shows the large, lobulated mass with a fluid-fluid level (*arrow*) in the subcapsular collection in keeping with hematoma

Late relapse frequently occurs, with 30% of relapses occurring at least 2 years after diagnosis. Long-term surveillance is therefore necessary [99]. Despite its aggressive nature, with recent advances in therapy, disease-free survival rates of up to 80% have been reported [100].

Rhabdoid Tumor Rhabdoid tumor is a rare, aggressive childhood tumor that accounts for approximately 2% of all pediatric renal malignancies [101]. Most are diagnosed within the first year of life and have a uniformly poor prognosis [102]. There is a unique association of rhabdoid tumors of the kidney with central nervous system (CNS) malignancies, both primary and metastatic, particularly atypical teratoid rhabdoid tumor which is seen in up to 10–15% of patients with rhabdoid tumor of the kidney [103]. Affected pediatric patients typically present with hematuria or a palpable abdominal mass or may present secondarily with neurologic symptoms attributable to CNS or other metastatic lesions [102].

On MR imaging, the most typical feature is an eccentric, crescentic subcapsular fluid collection attributable to either hemorrhage or necrosis, occurring as often as 50–70% of the time (Fig. 13.25). Other tumor pathologies may uncommonly show a similar peripheral subcapsular fluid collection, and therefore this finding is non-specific [104]. Other common imaging features include a lobulated mass with a central hilar location and the presence of curvilinear calcifications outlining tumor lobules [102].

The prognosis of rhabdoid tumor of the kidney is poor, with overall survival rates of 20–25%. Younger patients and those with metastatic disease or CNS tumors have a worse

outcome [103]. Treatment includes a combination of surgical resection, radiation, and chemotherapy.

Medullary Carcinoma Renal medullary carcinoma is a highly aggressive tumor uniquely occurring in young African-American males with sickle cell trait, but not sickle cell disease [105]. It is a tumor of adolescence and young adulthood, with a mean age of diagnosis of 20 years. Most tumors are large, and metastases are usually present at the time of diagnosis. Affected patients most frequently present with gross hematuria or flank pain and less commonly with a palpable mass or weight loss [106].

The tumor typically originates in the renal medulla and extends into the renal sinus, resulting in caliectasis and renal enlargement. On MR imaging, it typically appears as an infiltrative, heterogeneous mass with extensive hemorrhage and central necrosis (Fig. 13.26). Local invasion into the renal vein and IVC frequently occur. The most common sites of metastatic disease are the lung and liver [90]. While MR imaging and CT are similar in their ability to depict the borders of the mass and to detect lymphadenopathy, MR imaging is superior for evaluation of intratumoral hemorrhage and better demonstrates liver metastases [107].

Treatment of this aggressive tumor is difficult, with most patients presenting with advanced disease at the time of diagnosis. Despite chemotherapy and radiotherapy, the mean survival from the time of diagnosis is approximately 15 weeks [91].

Lymphoma Lymphoma comprises a large group of malignant neoplasms of the lymphoid tissues, broadly categorized

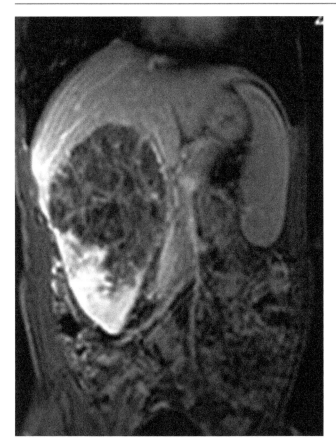

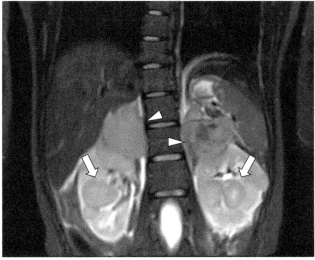

Fig. 13.27 Lymphoma in a 16-year-old boy who presented with weight loss. Coronal STIR MR image demonstrates multiple bilateral, homogeneous, round renal masses (*arrows*) of intermediate signal intensity. Bilateral adrenal masses (*arrowheads*) demonstrate signal characteristics, similar to the renal tumors

Fig. 13.26 Medullary carcinoma in a 17-year-old boy who presented with right flank pain. Coronal contrast-enhanced T1-weighted fat-suppressed MR image demonstrates an infiltrative, predominantly necrotic mass in the upper pole of the right kidney. (Case courtesy of Netta M. Blitman, MD, NYU Langone Health, New York, New York, USA)

into Hodgkin's and non-Hodgkin's types. Renal involvement occurs in approximately 8% of all cases of lymphoma [108] and is usually secondary, developing as a consequence of hematogenous or retroperitoneal spread [3]. It occurs more frequently with non-Hodgkin's lymphoma. Primary renal lymphoma is exceedingly rare due to the absence of intrinsic renal lymphoid tissue [109]. Affected patients present with a wide range of symptoms, usually attributable to the systemic manifestations of lymphoma. Specific renal symptoms include obstructive uropathy and renal insufficiency [108].

MR imaging of renal lymphoma is sparsely described in the literature. Three patterns of involvement have been described on CT, including unilateral solitary or bilateral masses, multiple bilateral masses, or diffuse infiltration of the affected kidney. The masses enhance less than the renal parenchyma [108]. Small series of adult patients have sug-

gested that MR imaging is as accurate as CT in the detection of renal lymphoma. The renal lesions are hypointense on T1-weighted images, hypointense to isointense on T2-weighted images, and enhance less than normal renal parenchyma after contrast administration (Fig. 13.27) [110]. Lymphomatous renal lesions can also demonstrate diffusion restriction on diffusion-weighted imaging due to the low nucleus: cytoplasm of the tumor cells. The imaging features are often non-specific, and attention should be paid to the extrarenal tissues to detect additional sites of lymphoma.

Management of secondary renal lymphoma involves treatment of the primary disease, including chemotherapy and radiation. Any renal dysfunction typically resolves rapidly after the initiation of treatment. Primary renal lymphoma is associated with a poor prognosis. Affected patients have been treated with chemotherapy, but no consensus treatment regimen exists due to the rarity of this diagnosis [108].

Traumatic Urinary Tract Injury

Blunt abdominal trauma in the pediatric patient most frequently occurs as a result of motor vehicle collisions, auto-pedestrian accidents, and falls. Children are at increased risk of solid organ injury compared to adults due to their comparative lack of abdominal fat, underdeveloped muscu-

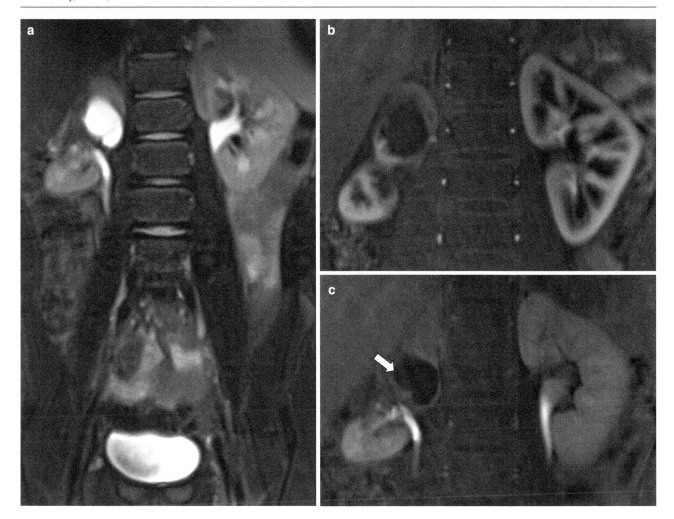

Fig. 13.28 Renal trauma in a 13-year-old boy who presented 3 months following grade V renal injury with transection of the interpolar region of the right kidney. Coronal T2-weighted fat-suppressed MR image (**a**) demonstrates dilation of the right upper renal pole collecting system. The left kidney is normal. Coronal early contrast-enhanced radial stack of stars T1-weighted fat-suppressed MR image (**b**) shows relatively delayed enhancement of the right upper pole renal parenchyma compared to the right lower pole parenchyma and left renal parenchyma. Coronal delayed contrast-enhanced radial stack of stars T1-weighted fat-suppressed MR image (**c**) demonstrates delayed excretion into the right upper pole collecting system (*arrow*), with normal excretion into the right lower pole and left renal collecting systems

lature, and relatively larger abdominal viscera. Renal injury occurs in approximately 25–30% of cases of pediatric blunt abdominal trauma [111]. Affected children most commonly present with microscopic or macroscopic hematuria.

MR imaging does not play a primary role in the evaluation of traumatic urinary tract disorders, related to its limited availability and slow scan time. The primary utility of MR imaging is in the acute setting of a patient with suspected renal injury with a contraindication to iodinated contrast and with a negative or equivocal ultrasound study. MR imaging has been shown to be similar to CT in terms of its depiction of renal parenchymal perfusion and in the evaluation of contrast extravasation, particularly when delayed images are obtained [112, 113]. MR urography also plays a role in the evaluation of renal parenchymal function in patients with high-grade injuries (Fig. 13.28).

Treatment of children with traumatic renal injury is generally conservative, even with higher-grade injuries. However, surgical intervention may be required in a hemodynamically unstable patient or in the setting of arterial injury [114].

Urinary Tract Calcification

Nephrocalcinosis
Nephrocalcinosis is generally defined as increased calcium content in the kidneys, related to deposition of calcium within the renal cortex or medulla at either the microscopic

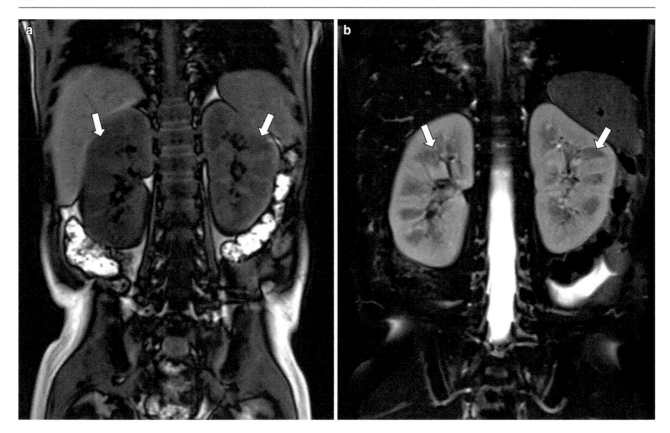

Fig. 13.29 Nephrocalcinosis in a 6-year-old boy with a history of renal tubular acidosis. Coronal T1-weighted MR image (**a**) and coronal T2-weighted fat-suppressed MR image (**b**) demonstrate diffusely hypointense signal within the renal medullary pyramids (*arrows*)

or macroscopic level [115]. The medullary subtype is much more common than the cortical subtype. As compared to urolithiasis, nephrocalcinosis tends to occur earlier in life, as it is more frequently associated with renal tubulopathies or inborn errors of metabolism. Prematurity is also a known risk factor, related to the immaturity of the kidney and medication use (particularly furosemide) [116]. Affected children are usually asymptomatic, and the diagnosis is made when imaging is performed for other reasons [116].

MR imaging is not a primary tool for the diagnosis of nephrocalcinosis, due to the relatively poor visualization of calcium [117]. However, when detectable, it manifests as low signal on both T1- and T2-weighted images and does not demonstrate enhancement (Fig. 13.29).

Treatment consists of correction of the underlying cause of the nephrocalcinosis. Prognosis is variable and dependent on etiology. The majority of patients do not progress to end-stage renal disease. Most affected neonates with nephrocalcinosis who do not have an underlying genetic defect demonstrate spontaneous resolution within the first years of life. Surveillance US imaging should be performed to document resolution or progression [118].

Urolithiasis

Urolithiasis is the formation of stones within the urinary tract. The etiology of stone formation is broad and includes dietary, genetic, metabolic, climatic, infectious, and anatomic influences. The frequency of stone formation in the pediatric population has been increasing in recent years. The majority of patients with urinary tract stones have an underlying metabolic abnormality, most frequently hypercalciuria or hypocitraturia. Bladder stones develop most often in patients with a history of urinary tract reconstruction. Affected children typically present with hematuria, flank pain, or abdominal pain. Patients may also have recurrent UTI or urinary tract dysfunction such as enuresis or incontinence [119].

MR imaging does not play a primary role in the evaluation of the pediatric patient with suspected urolithiasis. Although its sensitivity for stone detection is similar to that of ultrasound, it is not routinely used due to its low specificity, high cost, limited availability, and associated time constraints. A urinary tract stone appears as a signal void on all imaging sequences [120]. Due to its lack of signal, the stone usually requires adjacent contrasting urine or renal parenchyma in order to be visible and is best depicted on T2-weighted images (Fig. 13.30). MR imaging has limited sensitivity for the detection of stones smaller than 1 cm, with a lower limit of detectable size of about 4–5 mm [121, 122].

Treatment depends on the size of the stone. Most stones less than 5 mm in diameter typically pass spontaneously, and treatment is expectant, including pain control and hydration [123]. Surgical intervention may be warranted

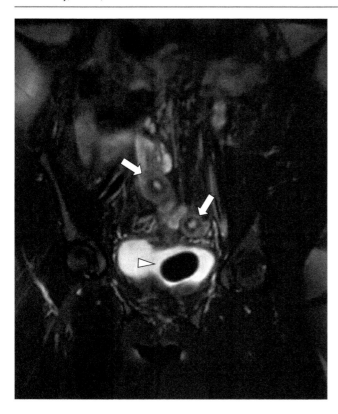

Fig. 13.30 Urolithiasis in a 17-year-old girl with a cloacal malformation. Coronal T2-weighted fat-suppressed MR image shows a large hypointense bladder calculus (*arrowhead*). A didelphys uterus (*arrows*) is partially seen

for small stones that do not pass within 2–4 weeks or for larger stones that are unlikely to pass spontaneously. Bladder calculi necessitate surgical intervention, with percutaneous cystolithotomy currently favored over open procedures [124].

Conclusion

MR imaging offers a valuable adjunct to the more traditional imaging modalities in the evaluation of the pediatric genitourinary tract. It has the capability of providing useful anatomic information without the risks associated with ionizing radiation and can also supply useful functional information with MR urography. Familiarity with the techniques and capabilities of MR imaging can therefore be a boon to the provider in the evaluation of the pediatric patient.

References

1. Chang KJ, Kamel IR, Macura KJ, Bluemke DA. 3.0-T MR imaging of the abdomen: comparison with 1.5 T. Radiographics. 2008;28(7):1983–98.
2. Stanescu AL, Acharya PT, Lee EY, Phillips GS. Pediatric renal neoplasms: MR imaging-based practical diagnostic approach. Magn Reson Imaging Clin N Am. 2019;27(2):279–90.
3. Gee MS, Bittman M, Epelman M, Vargas SO, Lee EY. Magnetic resonance imaging of the pediatric kidney: benign and malignant masses. Magn Reson Imaging Clin N Am. 2013;21(4):697–715.
4. Dillman JR, Darge K. Kidneys and urinary tract. In: Lee EY, editor. Pediatric radiology—practical imaging evaluation of infants and children. Philadelphia: Wolters Kluwer; 2018. p. 881–943.
5. Bedard MP, Wildman S, Dillman JR. Embryology, anatomy, and variants of the genitourinary tract. In: Coley BD, editor. Caffey's pediatric diagnostic imaging. 12th ed. Philadelphia: Elsevier; 2013. p. 1163–73.
6. Zweyer M. Embryology of the kidney. In: Quaia E, editor. Radiological imaging of the kidney. 2nd ed. Berlin Heidelberg: Springer-Verlag; 2014. p. 3–15.
7. Leung AW, Bydder GM, Steiner RE, Bryant DJ, Young IR. Magnetic resonance imaging of the kidneys. AJR Am J Roentgenol. 1984;143(6):1215–27.
8. Shapiro E, Goldfarb DA, Ritchey ML. The congenital and acquired solitary kidney. Rev Urol. 2003;5(1):2–8.
9. Argueso LR, Ritchey ML, Boyle ET Jr, Milliner DS, Bergstralh EJ, Kramer SA. Prognosis of patients with unilateral renal agenesis. Pediatr Nephrol. 1992;6(5):412–6.
10. Solanki S, Bhatnagar V, Gupta AK, Kumar R. Crossed fused renal ectopia: challenges in diagnosis and management. J Indian Assoc Pediatr Surg. 2013;18(1):7–10.
11. Guarino N, Tadini B, Camardi P, Silvestro L, Lace R, Bianchi M. The incidence of associated urological abnormalities in children with renal ectopia. J Urol. 2004;172(4 Pt 2):1757–9.
12. van den Bosch CM, van Wijk JA, Beckers GM, van der Horst HJ, Schreuder MF, Bokenkamp A. Urological and nephrological findings of renal ectopia. J Urol. 2010;183(4):1574–8.
13. Taghavi K, Kirkpatrick J, Mirjalili SA. The horseshoe kidney: surgical anatomy and embryology. J Pediatr Urol. 2016;12(5):275–80.
14. Lee SH, Bae MH, Choi SH, Lee JS, Cho YS, Joo KJ, et al. Wilms' tumor in a horseshoe kidney. Korean J Urol. 2012;53(8):577–80.
15. Kirkpatrick JJ, Leslie SW. Horseshoe kidney. In: StatPearls. Treasure Island: StatPearls Publishing; 2019.
16. Fernbach SK, Feinstein KA, Spencer K, Lindstrom CA. Ureteral duplication and its complications. Radiographics. 1997;17(1):109–27.
17. Williams H. Renal revision: from lobulation to duplication--what is normal? Arch Dis Child Educ Pract Ed. 2007;92(5):ep152–8.
18. Thomas JC. Vesicoureteral reflux and duplex systems. Adv Urol. 2008:651891.
19. Senol C, Onaran M, Gurocak S, Gonul II, Tan MO. Changes in Cajal cell density in ureteropelvic junction obstruction in children. J Pediatr Urol. 2016;12(2):89.
20. Nguyen HT, Benson CB, Bromley B, Campbell JB, Chow J, Coleman B, et al. Multidisciplinary consensus on the classification of prenatal and postnatal urinary tract dilation (UTD classification system). J Pediatr Urol. 2014;10(6):982–98.
21. Parikh KR, Hammer MR, Kraft KH, Ivancic V, Smith EA, Dillman JR. Pediatric ureteropelvic junction obstruction: can magnetic resonance urography identify crossing vessels? Pediatr Radiol. 2015;45(12):1788–95.
22. Mei H, Pu J, Yang C, Zhang H, Zheng L, Tong Q. Laparoscopic versus open pyeloplasty for ureteropelvic junction obstruction in children: a systematic review and meta-analysis. J Endourol. 2011;25(5):727–36.
23. Stoll C, Alembik Y, Roth MP, Dott B, Sauvage P. Risk factors in internal urinary system malformations. Pediatr Nephrol. 1990;4(4):319–23.

24. Shukla AR, Cooper J, Patel RP, Carr MC, Canning DA, Zderic SA, et al. Prenatally detected primary megaureter: a role for extended followup. J Urol. 2005;173(4):1353–6.

25. Farrugia M-K, Hitchcock R, Radford A, Burki T, Robb A, Murphy F. British Association of Paediatric Urologists consensus statement on the management of the primary obstructive megaureter. J Pediatr Urol. 2014;10(1):26–33.

26. McGrath MA, Estroff J, Lebowitz RL. The coexistence of obstruction at the ureteropelvic and ureterovesical junctions. AJR Am J Roentgenol. 1987;149(2):403–6.

27. Vargas B, Lebowitz RL. The coexistence of congenital megacalyces and primary megaureter. AJR Am J Roentgenol. 1986;147(2): 313–6.

28. Dickerson EC, Dillman JR, Smith EA, DiPietro MA, Lebowitz RL, Darge K. Pediatric MR urography: indications, techniques, and approach to review. Radiographics. 2015;35(4):1208–30.

29. Glassberg KI, Braren V, Duckett JW, Jacobs EC, King LR, Lebowitz RL, et al. Suggested terminology for duplex systems, ectopic ureters and ureteroceles. J Urol. 1984;132(6):1153–4.

30. Berrocal T, Lopez-Pereira P, Arjonilla A, Gutierrez J. Anomalies of the distal ureter, bladder, and urethra in children: embryologic, radiologic, and pathologic features. Radiographics. 2002;22(5):1139–64.

31. Coplen DE, Duckett JW. The modern approach to ureteroceles. J Urol. 1995;153(1):166–71.

32. Payabvash S, Kajbafzadeh AM, Saeedi P, Sadeghi Z, Elmi A, Mehdizadeh M. Application of magnetic resonance urography in diagnosis of congenital urogenital anomalies in children. Pediatr Surg Int. 2008;24(9):979–86.

33. Shokeir AA, Nijman RJ. Ureterocele: an ongoing challenge in infancy and childhood. BJU Int. 2002;90(8):777–83.

34. Ismaili K, Avni FE, Alexander M, Schulman C, Collier F, Hall M. Routine voiding cystourethrography is of no value in neonates with unilateral multicystic dysplastic kidney. J Pediatr. 2005;146(6):759–63.

35. Hwang DY, Dworschak GC, Kohl S, Saisawat P, Vivante A, Hilger AC, et al. Mutations in 12 known dominant disease-causing genes clarify many congenital anomalies of the kidney and urinary tract. Kidney Int. 2014;85(6):1429–33.

36. Avni FE, Garel C, Cassart M, D'Haene N, Hall M, Riccabona M. Imaging and classification of congenital cystic renal diseases. AJR Am J Roentgenol. 2012;198(5):1004–13.

37. Psooy K. Multicystic dysplastic kidney (MCDK) in the neonate: the role of the urologist. Can Urol Assoc J. 2016;10(1–2):18–24.

38. Onuchic LF, Furu L, Nagasawa Y, Hou X, Eggermann T, Ren Z, et al. PKHD1, the polycystic kidney and hepatic disease 1 gene, encodes a novel large protein containing multiple immunoglobulin-like plexin-transcription-factor domains and parallel beta-helix 1 repeats. Am J Hum Genet. 2002;70(5):1305–17.

39. Bergmann C, Senderek J, Windelen E, Kupper F, Middeldorf I, Schneider F, et al. Clinical consequences of PKHD1 mutations in 164 patients with autosomal-recessive polycystic kidney disease (ARPKD). Kidney Int. 2005;67(3):829–48.

40. Kern S, Zimmerhackl LB, Hildebrandt F, Ermisch-Omran B, Uhl M. Appearance of autosomal recessive polycystic kidney disease in magnetic resonance imaging and RARE-MR-urography. Pediatr Radiol. 2000;30(3):156–60.

41. Niemczyk M, Niemczyk S, Paczek L. Autosomal dominant polycystic kidney disease and transplantation. Ann Transplant. 2009;14(4):86–90.

42. Tee JB, Acott PD, McLellan DH, Crocker JF. Phenotypic heterogeneity in pediatric autosomal dominant polycystic kidney disease at first presentation: a single-center, 20-year review. Am J Kidney Dis. 2004;43(2):296–303.

43. Chapman AB, Devuyst O, Eckardt KU, Gansevoort RT, Harris T, Horie S, et al. Autosomal-dominant polycystic kidney disease (ADPKD): executive summary from a Kidney Disease: Improving Global Outcomes (KDIGO) controversies conference. Kidney Int. 2015;88(1):17–27.

44. Chapman AB. Autosomal dominant polycystic kidney disease: time for a change? J Am Soc Nephrol. 2007;18(5):1399–407.

45. Gradzik M, Niemczyk M, Gołębiowski M, Pączek L. Diagnostic imaging of autosomal dominant polycystic kidney disease. Pol J Radiol. 2016;81:441–53.

46. Pierre K, Borer J, Phelps A, Chow JS. Bladder exstrophy: current management and postoperative imaging. Pediatr Radiol. 2014;44(7):768–86.

47. Yiee J, Wilcox D. Abnormalities of the fetal bladder. Semin Fetal Neonatal Med. 2008;13(3):164–70.

48. Ebert AK, Zwink N, Jenetzky E, Stein R, Boemers TM, Lacher M, et al. Association between exstrophy-epispadias complex and congenital anomalies: a German multicenter study. Urology. 2019;123:210–20.

49. Goldman S, Szejnfeld PO, Rondon A, Francisco VV, Bacelar H, Leslie B, et al. Prenatal diagnosis of bladder exstrophy by fetal MRI. J Pediatr Urol. 2013;9(1):3–6.

50. Tekes A, Ertan G, Solaiyappan M, Stec AA, Sponseller PD, Huisman TA, et al. 2D and 3D MRI features of classic bladder exstrophy. Clin Radiol. 2014;69(5):e223–9.

51. Gargollo PC, Borer JG, Retik AB, Peters CA, Diamond DA, Atala A, et al. Magnetic resonance imaging of pelvic musculoskeletal and genitourinary anatomy in patients before and after complete primary repair of bladder exstrophy. J Urol. 2005;174(4 Pt 2): 1559–66.

52. Grady RW, Mitchell ME. Newborn exstrophy closure and epispadias repair. World J Urol. 1998;16(3):200–4.

53. Ansell JS. Surgical treatment of exstrophy of the bladder with emphasis on neonatal primary closure: personal experience with 28 consecutive cases treated at the University of Washington Hospitals from 1962 to 1977: techniques and results. 1979. J Urol. 2002;168(1):214–7.

54. Tonni G, Ida V, Alessandro V, Bonasoni MP. Prune-belly syndrome: case series and review of the literature regarding early prenatal diagnosis, epidemiology, genetic factors, treatment, and prognosis. Fetal Pediatr Pathol. 2013;31(1):13–24.

55. Seidel NE, Arlen AM, Smith EA, Kirsch AJ. Clinical manifestations and management of prune-belly syndrome in a large contemporary pediatric population. Urology. 2015;85(1):211–5.

56. Garcia-Roig ML, Grattan-Smith JD, Arlen AM, Smith EA, Kirsch AJ. Detailed evaluation of the upper urinary tract in patients with prune belly syndrome using magnetic resonance urography. J Pediatr Urol. 2016;12(2):122.e1–7.

57. Lopes RI, Tavares A, Srougi M, Denes FT. 27 years of experience with the comprehensive surgical treatment of prune belly syndrome. J Pediatr Urol. 2015;11(5):276.e1–7.

58. Zugor V, Schott GE, Labanaris AP. The Prune belly syndrome: urological aspects and long-term outcomes of a rare disease. Pediatr Rep. 2012;4(2):e20.

59. Winter RM, Knowles SA. Megacystis-microcolon-intestinal hypoperistalsis syndrome: confirmation of autosomal recessive inheritance. J Med Genet. 1986;23(4):360–2.

60. Gosemann JH, Puri P. Megacystis microcolon intestinal hypoperistalsis syndrome: systematic review of outcome. Pediatr Surg Int. 2011;27(10):1041–6.

61. Ballisty MM, Braithwaite KA, Shehata BM, Dickson PN. Imaging findings in megacystis-microcolon-intestinal hypoperistalsis syndrome. Pediatr Radiol. 2013;43(4):454–9.

62. Furey EA, Bailey AA, Twickler DM. Fetal MR imaging of gastrointestinal abnormalities. Radiographics. 2016;36(3):904–17.

63. Masetti M, Rodriguez MM, Thompson JF, Pinna AD, Kato T, Romaguera RL, et al. Multivisceral transplantation for megacystis microcolon intestinal hypoperistalsis syndrome. Transplantation. 1999;68(2):228–32.

64. Chishti AS, Maul EC, Nazario RJ, Bennett JS, Kiessling SG. A guideline for the inpatient care of children with pyelonephritis. Ann Saudi Med. 2010;30(5):341–9.

65. Chang SL, Shortliffe LD. Pediatric urinary tract infections. Pediatr Clin North Am. 2006;53(3):379–400.

66. Morello W, La Scola C, Alberici I, Montini G. Acute pyelonephritis in children. Pediatr Nephrol. 2016;31(8):1253–65.

67. Vivier PH, Sallem A, Beurdeley M, Lim RP, Leroux J, Caudron J, et al. MRI and suspected acute pyelonephritis in children: comparison of diffusion-weighted imaging with gadolinium-enhanced T1-weighted imaging. Eur Radiol. 2014;24(1):19–25.

68. Hewitt IK, Zucchetta P, Rigon L, Maschio F, Molinari PP, Tomasi L, et al. Early treatment of acute pyelonephritis in children fails to reduce renal scarring: data from the Italian Renal Infection Study Trials. Pediatrics. 2008;122(3):486–90.

69. Shah K, Parikh M, Gharia P, Modi PR. Xanthogranulomatous pyelonephritis-mimicking renal mass in 5-month-old child. Urology. 2012;79(6):1360–2.

70. Bingol-Kologlu M, Ciftci AO, Senocak ME, Tanyel FC, Karnak I, Buyukpamukcu N. Xanthogranulomatous pyelonephritis in children: diagnostic and therapeutic aspects. Eur J Pediatr Surg. 2002;12(1):42–8.

71. Verswijvel G, Oyen R, Van Poppel H, Roskams T. Xanthogranulomatous pyelonephritis: MRI findings in the diffuse and the focal type. Eur Radiol. 2000;10(4):586–9.

72. Gupta S, Araya CE, Dharnidharka VR. Xanthogranulomatous pyelonephritis in pediatric patients: case report and review of literature. J Pediatr Urol. 2010;6(4):355–8.

73. Glick RD, Hicks MJ, Nuchtern JG, Wesson DE, Olutoye OO, Cass DL. Renal tumors in infants less than 6 months of age. J Pediatr Surg. 2004;39(4):522–5.

74. Chaudry G, Perez-Atayde AR, Ngan BY, Gundogan M, Daneman A. Imaging of congenital mesoblastic nephroma with pathological correlation. Pediatr Radiol. 2009;39(10):1080–6.

75. Sheth MM, Cai G, Goodman TR. AIRP best cases in radiologic-pathologic correlation: congenital mesoblastic nephroma. Radiographics. 2012;32(1):99–103.

76. Do AY, Kim JS, Choi SJ, Oh SY, Roh CR, Kim JH. Prenatal diagnosis of congenital mesoblastic nephroma. Obstet Gynecol Sci. 2015;58(5):405–8.

77. Silver IMF, Boag AH, Soboleski DA. Multilocular cystic renal tumor: cystic nephroma. Radiographics. 2008;28(4):1221–5.

78. Lonergan GJ, Martínez-León MI, Agrons GA, Montemarano H, Suarez ES. Nephrogenic rests, nephroblastomatosis, and associated lesions of the kidney. Radiographics. 1998;18(4):947–68.

79. Madewell JE, Goldman SM, Davis CJ, Hartman DS, Feigin DS, Lichtenstein JE. Multilocular cystic nephroma: a radiographic-pathologic correlation of 58 patients. Radiology. 1983;146(2):309–21.

80. Kettritz U, Semelka RC, Siegelman ES, Shoenut JP, Mitchell DG. Multilocular cystic nephroma: MR imaging appearance with current techniques, including gadolinium enhancement. J Magn Reson Imaging. 1996;6(1):145–8.

81. Agrons GA, Wagner BJ, Davidson AJ, Suarez ES. Multilocular cystic renal tumor in children: radiologic-pathologic correlation. Radiographics. 1995;15(3):653–69.

82. Fittschen A, Wendlik I, Oeztuerk S, Kratzer W, Akinli AS, Haenle MM, et al. Prevalence of sporadic renal angiomyolipoma: a retrospective analysis of 61,389 in- and out-patients. Abdom Imaging. 2014;39(5):1009–13.

83. Ewalt DH, Sheffield E, Sparagana SP, Delgado MR, Roach ES. Renal lesion growth in children with tuberous sclerosis complex. J Urol. 1998;160(1):141–5.

84. Park BK. Renal angiomyolipoma: radiologic classification and imaging features according to the amount of fat. AJR Am J Roentgenol. 2017;209(4):826–35.

85. Krueger DA, Northrup H. Tuberous sclerosis complex surveillance and management: recommendations of the 2012 International Tuberous Sclerosis Complex Consensus Conference. Pediatr Neurol. 2013;49(4):255–65.

86. Flum AS, Hamoui N, Said MA, Yang XJ, Casalino DD, McGuire BB, et al. Update on the diagnosis and management of renal angiomyolipoma. J Urol. 2016;195(4 Pt 1):834–46.

87. Pastore G, Znaor A, Spreafico F, Graf N, Pritchard-Jones K, Steliarova-Foucher E. Malignant renal tumours incidence and survival in European children (1978–1997): report from the Automated Childhood Cancer Information System project. Eur J Cancer. 2006;42(13):2103–14.

88. Scott RH, Stiller CA, Walker L, Rahman N. Syndromes and constitutional chromosomal abnormalities associated with Wilms tumour. J Med Genet. 2006;43(9):705–15.

89. Davidoff AM. Wilms tumor. Adv Pediatr Infect Dis. 2012;59(1):247–67.

90. Siegel MJ, Chung EM. Wilms' tumor and other pediatric renal masses. Magn Reson Imaging Clin N Am. 2008;16(3):479–97, vi.

91. Lowe LH, Isuani BH, Heller RM, Stein SM, Johnson JE, Navarro OM, et al. Pediatric renal masses: Wilms tumor and beyond. Radiographics. 2000;20(6):1585–603.

92. Abdellah A, Selma K, Elamin M, Asmae T, Lamia R, Abderrahmane M, et al. Renal cell carcinoma in children: case report and literature review. Pan Afr Med J. 2015;20:84.

93. Geller JI, Dome JS. Local lymph node involvement does not predict poor outcome in pediatric renal cell carcinoma. Cancer. 2004;101(7):1575–83.

94. Downey RT, Dillman JR, Ladino-Torres MF, McHugh JB, Ehrlich PF, Strouse PJ. CT and MRI appearances and radiologic staging of pediatric renal cell carcinoma. Pediatr Radiol. 2012;42(4):410–7.

95. Hartman DS, Davis CJ Jr, Madewell JE, Friedman AC. Primary malignant renal tumors in the second decade of life: Wilms tumor versus renal cell carcinoma. J Urol. 1982;127(5):888–91.

96. Estrada CR, Suthar AM, Eaton SH, Cilento BG Jr. Renal cell carcinoma: Children's Hospital Boston experience. Urology. 2005;66(6):1296–300.

97. Chung EM, Lattin GE Jr, Fagen KE, Kim AM, Pavio MA, Fehringer AJ, et al. Renal tumors of childhood: radiologic-pathologic correlation part 2. The 2nd decade: from the radiologic pathology archives. Radiographics. 2017;37(5):1538–58.

98. Kusumakumary P, Mathews A, James FV, Chellam VG, Harihara S, Varma RR, et al. Clear cell sarcoma kidney: clinical features and outcome. Pediatr Hematol Oncol. 1999;16(2):169–74.

99. Green DM, Breslow NE, Beckwith JB, Moksness J, Finklestein JZ, D'Angio GJ. Treatment of children with clear-cell sarcoma of the kidney: a report from the National Wilms' Tumor Study Group. J Clin Oncol. 1994;12(10):2132–7.

100. Spreafico F, Gandola L, Melchionda F. Stage I clear cell sarcoma of the kidney: is it the time for a less intensive adjuvant treatment? Transl Pediatr. 2014;3(1):1–3.

101. Charles AK, Vujanić GM, Berry PJ. Renal tumours of childhood. Histopathology. 1998;32(4):293–309.

102. Chung CJ, Lorenzo R, Rayder S, Schemankewitz E, Guy CD, Cutting J, et al. Rhabdoid tumors of the kidney in children: CT findings. AJR Am J Roentgenol. 1995;164(3):697–700.

103. Tomlinson GE, Breslow NE, Dome J, Guthrie KA, Norkool P, Li S, et al. Rhabdoid tumor of the kidney in the National Wilms' Tumor Study: age at diagnosis as a prognostic factor. J Clin Oncol. 2005;23(30):7641–5.

104. Agrons GA, Kingsman KD, Wagner BJ, Sotelo-Avila C. Rhabdoid tumor of the kidney in children: a comparative study of 21 cases. AJR Am J Roentgenol. 1997;168(2):447–51.

105. Davidson AJ, Choyke PL, Hartman DS, Davis CJ Jr. Renal medullary carcinoma associated with sickle cell trait: radiologic findings. Radiology. 1995;195(1):83–5.

106. Davis CJ Jr, Mostofi FK, Sesterhenn IA. Renal medullary carcinoma. The seventh sickle cell nephropathy. Am J Surg Pathol. 1995;19(1):1–11.

107. Blitman NM, Berkenblit RG, Rozenblit AM, Levin TL. Renal medullary carcinoma: CT and MRI features. AJR Am J Roentgenol. 2005;185(1):268–72.

108. Chepuri NB, Strouse PJ, Yanik GA. CT of renal lymphoma in children. AJR Am J Roentgenol. 2003;180(2):429–31.

109. Coca P, Linga VG, Gundeti S, Tandon A. Renal lymphoma: primary or first manifestation of aggressive pediatric B-cell lymphoma. Indian J Med Paediatr Oncol. 2017;38(4):538–41.

110. Sheth S, Ali S, Fishman E. Imaging of renal lymphoma: patterns of disease with pathologic correlation. Radiographics. 2006;26(4):1151–68.

111. Cooper A, Barlow B, DiScala C, String D. Mortality and truncal injury: the pediatric perspective. J Pediatr Surg. 1994;29(1):33–8.

112. Ku JH, Jeon YS, Kim ME, Lee NK, Park YH. Is there a role for magnetic resonance imaging in renal trauma? Int J Urol. 2001;8(6):261–7.

113. Marcos HB, Noone TC, Semelka RC. MRI evaluation of acute renal trauma. J Magn Reson Imaging. 1998;8(4):989–90.

114. Fernandez-Ibieta M. Renal trauma in pediatrics: a current review. Urology. 2018;113:171–8.

115. Sayer JA, Carr G, Simmons NL. Nephrocalcinosis: molecular insights into calcium precipitation within the kidney. Clin Sci (Lond). 2004;106(6):549–61.

116. Habbig S, Beck BB, Hoppe B. Nephrocalcinosis and urolithiasis in children. Kidney Int. 2011;80(12):1278–91.

117. Hiorns MP. Imaging of the urinary tract: the role of CT and MRI. Pediatr Nephrol. 2011;26(1):59–68.

118. Hoppe B, Duran I, Martin A, Kribs A, Benz-Bohm G, Michalk DV, et al. Nephrocalcinosis in preterm infants: a single center experience. Pediatr Nephrol. 2002;17(4):264–8.

119. Penido MG, de Sousa Tavares M. Pediatric primary urolithiasis: symptoms, medical management and prevention strategies. World J Nephrol. 2015;4(4):444–54.

120. Brisbane W, Bailey MR, Sorensen MD. An overview of kidney stone imaging techniques. Nat Rev Urol. 2016;13(11):654–62.

121. Ibrahim E-SH, Cernigliaro JG, Bridges MD, Pooley RA, Haley WE. The capabilities and limitations of clinical magnetic resonance imaging for detecting kidney stones: a retrospective study. Int J Biomed Imaging. 2016;2016:article ID 4935656:6 pages.

122. Kalb B, Sharma P, Salman K, Ogan K, Pattaras JG, Martin DR. Acute abdominal pain: is there a potential role for MRI in the setting of the emergency department in a patient with renal calculi? J Magn Reson Imaging. 2010;32(5):1012–23.

123. Pietrow PK, Pope JC 4th, Adams MC, Shyr Y, Brock JW 3rd. Clinical outcome of pediatric stone disease. J Urol. 2002;167(2 Pt 1):670–3.

124. Docimo SG, Orth CR, Schulam PG. Percutaneous cystolithotomy after augmentation cystoplasty: comparison with open procedures. Tech Urol. 1998;4(1):43–5.

Male Genital Tract

14

Gerald Behr, Jennifer K. Son, Ricardo Restrepo, and Edward Y. Lee

Introduction

The male genital tract is a complex set of pelvic anatomic structures. A clear understanding of its development and the various disease entities that affect it is needed for prompt diagnosis of male genital pathology in pediatric patients. Traditionally, the genital tract has been imaged primarily with fluoroscopy and ultrasound. However, the complex relationship of the multiple soft tissue structures, which may be obscured by surrounding bowel, requires an imaging modality with multiplanar capability, excellent soft tissue contrast, and an ability to image anatomically deeply situated structures. MR imaging is well suited for this task. MR imaging in some cases is the preferred imaging modality for male genital tract pathology evaluation, while in others, it serves as a second-line tool to characterize abnormalities initially seen on other imaging studies.

This chapter reviews up-to-date MR imaging techniques, including pediatric patient preparation as well as MR imaging pulse sequences and protocols. In addition, male genital tract anatomy including embryology, normal development, and anatomic variants is discussed. Finally, clinically relevant male genital disorders, which are encountered in daily clinical practice in the pediatric population, are reviewed.

G. Behr (✉)
Department of Radiology, Memorial Sloan Kettering Cancer Center, New York, NY, USA
e-mail: behrg@mskcc.org

J. K. Son
Division of Pediatric Radiology, Russell H. Morgan Department of Radiology and Radiological Sciences, Johns Hopkins University School of Medicine, Baltimore, MD, USA

R. Restrepo
Department of Interventional Radiology and Body Imaging, Nicklaus Children's Hospital, Miami, FL, USA

E. Y. Lee
Division of Thoracic Imaging, Department of Radiology, Boston Children's Hospital, Harvard Medical School, Boston, MA, USA

Magnetic Resonance Imaging Techniques

Patient Preparation

As with all MR imaging, patient comfort is of paramount importance in order to minimize motion artifact and optimize patient experience, particularly for young children. If detailed images of the bladder are to be performed, a moderately full bladder may be useful although this should be balanced against the patient's potential discomfort in the non-sedated patient. If the patient is not undergoing sedation, fasting is not necessary.

Male pelvic MR imaging studies are usually obtained with phased array coils and with the patient in supine position. If dedicated scrotal imaging is desired in the older child, a folded towel placed between the legs can serve to elevate the scrotum out of the plane of the upper thighs. In the older child, the penis may be secured to the anterior abdominal wall with tape, depending on the desired anatomy to be imaged. Endorectal coils – often used in adult prostate imaging – are not utilized in the pediatric population.

MR Imaging Pulse Sequences and Protocols

Ideally, the MR imaging strategy should be tailored to the anatomy of interest and to the relevant clinical question. Nonetheless, there are some general guidelines that apply to most MR imaging studies of the male genital tract (Table 14.1). For example, a high-resolution T2-weighted fast spin-echo sequence is recommended for nearly all MR imaging of the male genital tract (Fig. 14.1). At least one fluid-sensitive sequence with preserved visualization of the normal pelvic fat (i.e., without fat suppression) is essential because it provides anatomic contrast for depiction of disease margins, lymph nodes, and anatomy (Fig. 14.2). A single fluid-sensitive sequence with fat suppression can often render the pathology itself more conspicuous and may be achieved by either inversion recovery (e.g., STIR) or spectral fat suppression (Fig. 14.3).

As some of the relevant anatomy is near an air interface, the resultant inhomogeneous magnetic field can render

Table 14.1 Suggested male genital tract MR imaging protocols

General	Bladder	Notes
3-plane localizer	3-plane localizer	
Cor T2 single-shot spin-echo technique. Wide FOV to include kidneys	Cor T2 single-shot spin-echo technique. Wide FOV to include kidneys	Some institutions use an MRCP with reconstructed maximal intensity projection (MIP) as an overview of the collecting system
Axial T2 FSE (preferably high resolution)	Axial T2 FSE with fat suppression	1. The fat suppression technique is optional for tumors isolated to the bladder. Many such pediatric tumors exhibit a higher signal intensity than muscle but considerably lower than urine 2. Add coronal FSE for scrotal imaging (without fat suppression) to assess integrity of tunica albuginea (in the setting of trauma or tumor)
Axial T2 FSE with spectral fat suppression or short tau inversion recovery (STIR)	High resolution Sagittal T2 FSE and T1 FSE	
Axial diffusion-weighted images (or coronal if unclear location of testes)	Axial or sagittal diffusion-weighted sequence	This is a key sequence when searching for a "missing" testicle
Axial T1 FSE with spectral fat suppression before and after IV gadolinium-based contrast	Gradient echo-based dynamic contrast sequence (e.g., LAVA, VIBE, THRIVE, FLASH) in axial or sagittal planes	Administration of gadolinium-based contrast agent is optional, depending on study indication

MRCP magnetic resonance cholangiopancreatography, *FSE* fast spin echo, *LAVA* liver acquisition with volume acquisition, *VIBE* volumetric interpolated breath-hold examination, *THRIVE* T1W high resolution isotropic volume examination, *FLASH* fast low angle shot

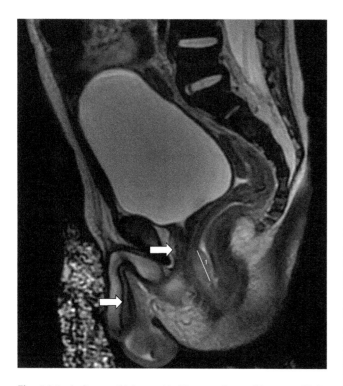

Fig. 14.1 A 2-year-old boy with history of neuroblastoma. High-resolution three-dimensional sagittal T2-weighted MR image (CUBE, General Electric) demonstrates the normal appearance of the male urethra (*arrows*). The penile urethra demonstrates low signal as it is void of urine. Calipers delineate a rectal wall abscess

spectral fat suppression techniques incomplete. The suppression of the fat signal in a STIR sequence, however, is less sensitive to field heterogeneity, and thus this sequence may be more effective in the pelvis. The trade-off is lower signal-to-noise ratios using inversion recovery technique as compared with spectral fat suppression techniques.

For T1-weighted images, a spin-echo sequence offers excellent signal and depiction of anatomy. If gadolinium contrast is used (such as for assessment of neoplasms or infection),

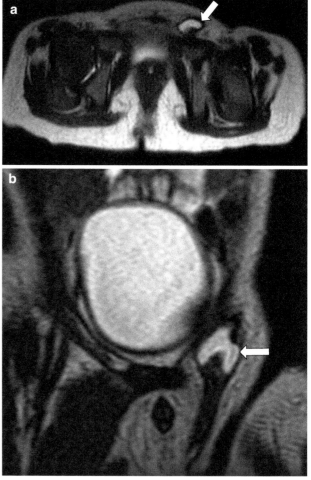

Fig. 14.2 Hydrocele of the spermatid cord in a 17-month-old boy. Axial T2-weighted MR image (**a**) shows a well-defined fluid collection (*arrow*) with similar signal intensity to the urinary bladder. Coronal T2-weighted MR image (**b**) demonstrates a well-defined fluid collection (*arrow*) in the left inguinal canal with similar signal intensity to the urinary bladder. Note that the left inguinal canal can be seen further caudally on the coronal plane due to the background contrast from the adjacent fat

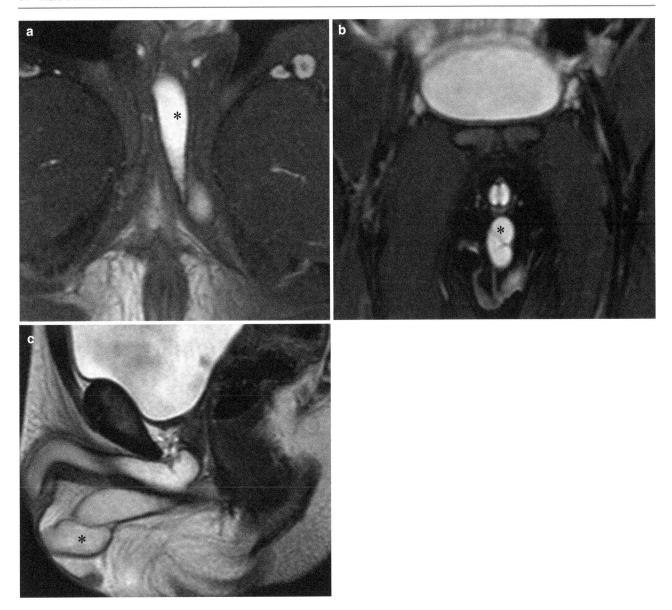

Fig. 14.3 Cowper gland syringocele in a 13-year-old boy who presented with perineal pain and gross hematuria. Axial T2-weighted fat-suppressed MR image (**a**) shows an oblong cystic structure (*asterisk*). Coronal T2-weighted fat-suppressed MR image (**b**) shows that the cystic structure (*asterisk*) is located just ventral to the urethra. Note improved conspicuity of the lesion with the use of fat suppression technique (compare with **c**). Sagittal T2-weighted MR image (**c**) demonstrates a syringocele (*asterisk*) ventral to the urethra

three-dimensional gradient recalled echo (GRE) T1-weighted fat-suppressed sequences such as T1-weighted high-resolution isotropic volume excitation (THRIVE; Philips, Amsterdam, Netherlands), liver acquisition with volume acquisition (LAVA; General Electric, Boston, Massachusetts), or volumetric interpolated breath-hold examination (VIBE; Siemens, Munich, Germany) are generally acquired before and after intravenous (IV) contrast administration. Alternatively, T1-weighted fast spin-echo sequences can be used before and after contrast, although with longer acquisition times compared with GRE sequences. The use of spin-echo post-contrast imaging is possible in the lower pelvis because there is less respiratory and peristaltic motion degradation compared with imaging of the upper abdomen, and spin-echo sequences are less prone to susceptibility artifact from air within the colon or lesion calcifications.

One caveat involves post-contrast imaging of the bladder post-contrast. Imaging of the ureters and bladder can be difficult on excretory phase MR imaging post-contrast because of the relative delay in bladder excretion of contrast compared with the ureters. A single, wide field of view MR urography sequence that is heavily T2-weighted using a long echo time (TE) may provide a better overall view of the entire urinary collecting system without reliance on IV contrast.

Motion artifact is particularly problematic in infants and young children. This includes both bulk motion (in the younger or noncooperative child) and physiologic motion from respiration and bowel peristalsis. Supportive techniques, including involvement of a child life specialist, can be of benefit although in many cases, including younger children, sedation is required. Peristaltic motion is less problematic in lower pelvic imaging than abdominal imaging. In children, antiperistalsis agents (glucagon or Buscopan, IV or intramuscular [IM]) have been advocated for bowel imaging although there is a paucity of literature advocating its use for genital tract MR imaging in children [1]. In adult pelvic imaging, use of pharmacologic peristalsis suppressants is more commonly employed [2]. Respiratory motion is also relatively less problematic in lower pelvic imaging compared with abdominal imaging. There are several techniques to minimize this including different forms of respiratory gating and non-Cartesian filling of k-space strategies that are beyond the scope of this chapter. Addition of a pre-saturation pulse ("saturation band") over the anterior abdominal wall can often mitigate this artifact by nulling the signal from tissues outside the area of interest, particularly on MR imaging sequences where the signal from the anterior abdominal wall fat is not suppressed.

Anatomy

Embryology

Both the urinary and genital system develop from the intermediate mesoderm which arises from the urogenital ridge on either side of the primitive abdominal aorta [3]. The urogenital ridge gives rise to the gonadal ridge, the embryologic precursor to the genital system. The nephrogenic cord also arises from the urogenital ridge to give rise to the urinary system. This process is further explored in Chap. 14.

At about 7 weeks gestation, the genital ridge differentiates into either a testis or an ovary, contingent on the presence of the sex-determining region (SYR gene) that is present on the Y chromosome (Fig. 14.4). The SYR gene encodes for testis-determining factor. Together with H-Y antigens

Fig. 14.4 Embryologic development of the testis. The gonadal ridge, derived from the medial portion of the urogenital ridge, is shown where primordial germ cells have migrated from the hindgut. The cortical tissue (*shown in pink*) involutes, and the medullary tissue develops into the testis, the seminiferous tubules, and Sertoli cells. The male genital ductal system develops from the mesonephric tubules

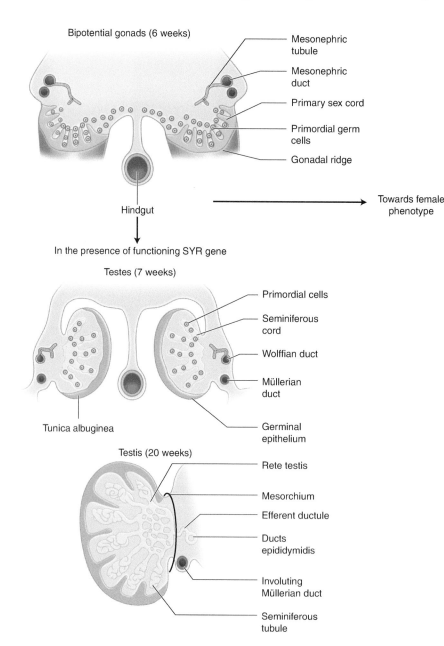

expressed on cells of the XY genotype, testis-determining factor directs both testicular differentiation and germ cells to differentiate into Sertoli and Leydig cells. A cascade of downstream cellular and biochemical events, which include secretion of Müllerian inhibiting substance and production of dihydrotestosterone (DHT), results in the Wolffian duct system to develop into the epididymis, vas deferens, seminal vesicles, penis, and scrotum. In the absence of the SYR gene or in the event of its abnormal encoding, the gonad defaults to ovarian differentiation (passive differentiation).

Male/female differentiation

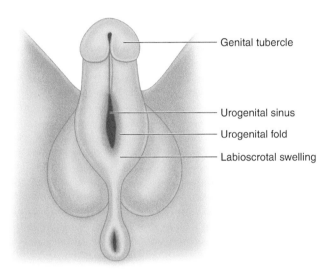

Fig. 14.5 Schematic of the genital system from the cloaca at the junction of differentiation toward the male or female phenotype. The urogenital sinus arises from the ventral portion of the cloaca. The caudal extent of the cloaca meets and opens through the genital tubercle

Normal Development and Anatomy

The ventral portion of the cloaca, a common cavity at the end of the digestive tract for the release of both excretory and genital products in vertebrates, is the urogenital sinus (Fig. 14.5). Its superior portion gives rise to the posterior urethra and bladder. Initially, the bladder is contiguous along its superior margin with the allantois. The lumen of the allantois obliterates, forming the urachus which persists and connects the bladder apex to the umbilicus. The caudal extent of the cloaca (phallic cloaca) opens through the genital tubercle, exiting just caudal to the glans. The distal cloaca fuses, forming the urethral plate and further directing urethral opening caudally. The most distal urethra in the male is formed by way of fusion of folds from the glans and the urethral plate.

The middle segment of the urogenital sinus gives rise to the prostate gland in males, through which the posterior urethra passes. The posterior (proximal urethra) is anatomically divided into prostatic and membranous segments (Fig. 14.6). The anterior urethra (distal urethra) is divided into the bulbous urethra and the longer, penile urethra.

During infancy, much of the body of the bladder and its dome occupy the lower abdomen. During bladder filling, it can often demonstrate mass-like impressions from adjacent bowel on contrast fluoroscopic or radiographic studies. Although this seldomly presents a diagnostic dilemma for the experienced radiologist, a cross-sectional study, such as MR imaging, can demonstrate the benign nature of the finding. In fact, a coronal single-shot T2-weighted sequence, in which all of k-space is filled in one "shot" (TR interval), might best demonstrate the finding because the technique is fast and consequently far less sensitive to artifact from bowel peristalsis.

Fig. 14.6 The urethral segments in males, consisting of the prostatic, membranous, bulbar, and penile portions of the urethra

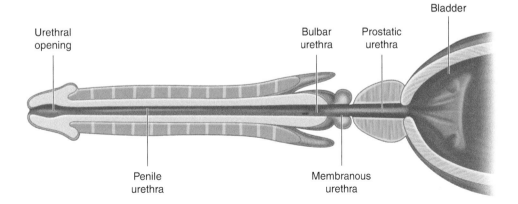

Anatomic Variants

There are several anatomic variants that can be understood in the context of the relevant embryology. For example, incomplete or failure of obliteration of the allantois lumen above the bladder dome results in a persistent patent ura-

chus (urachal fistula), urachal cyst, sinus, or diverticulum (Fig. 14.7) [4]. Distally, failure of the proliferating mesoderm to properly direct the distal urethra to the glans may result in epispadias [3]. Discontinuity in the urethral plate or abnormality of fusion of the urethral folds can result in hypospadias.

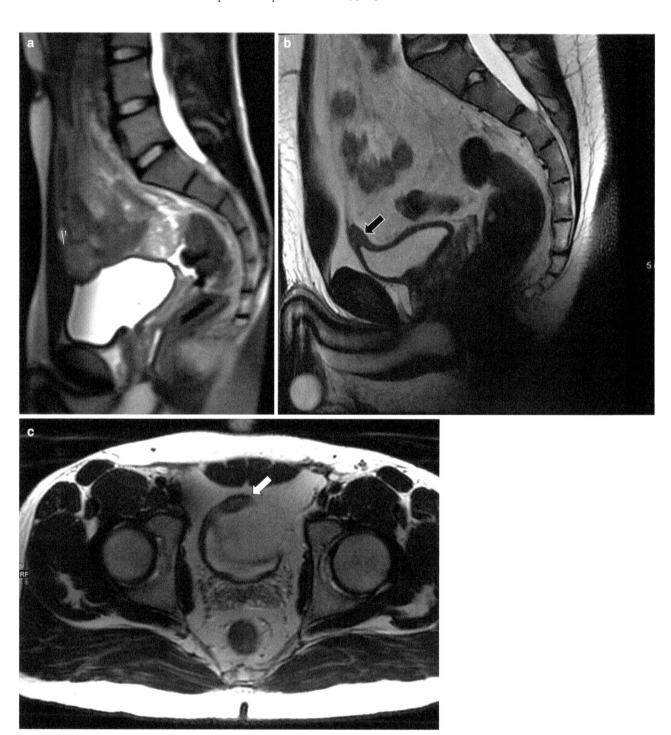

Fig. 14.7 Urachal cyst in a 16-year-old asymptomatic boy. Sagittal T2-weighted MR image (**a**) demonstrates a urachal cyst (**calipers**) along the expected course of the median umbilical ligament (urachus). Sagittal T2-weighted MR image (**b**) demonstrates a normal urachal remnant (*arrow*). Axial T2-weighted MR image (**c**) demonstrates a normal urachal remnant (*arrow*)

If, in early fetal life, mesenchymal cells between the ectoderm and cloaca fail to migrate, the bladder does not fuse and instead gives rise to bladder exstrophy, in which the entire bladder mucosa is externally exposed and is contiguous with the anterior abdominal wall (Fig. 14.8). Cloacal exstrophy, a more complex disorder, is characterized by two hemi-bladders separated by externally exposed ileocecal bowel mucosa. The terminal ileum pro-

lapses through the exposed cecum in what is known as an "elephant trunk" deformity. Affected patients may have a two-vessel cord, omphalocele, abnormal genitalia, spinal defects, and renal abnormalities. Maldevelopment of the cloacal membrane during development underlies this constellation of abnormalities.

The common origin of the renal and genital system from the intermediate mesoderm underlies the association of

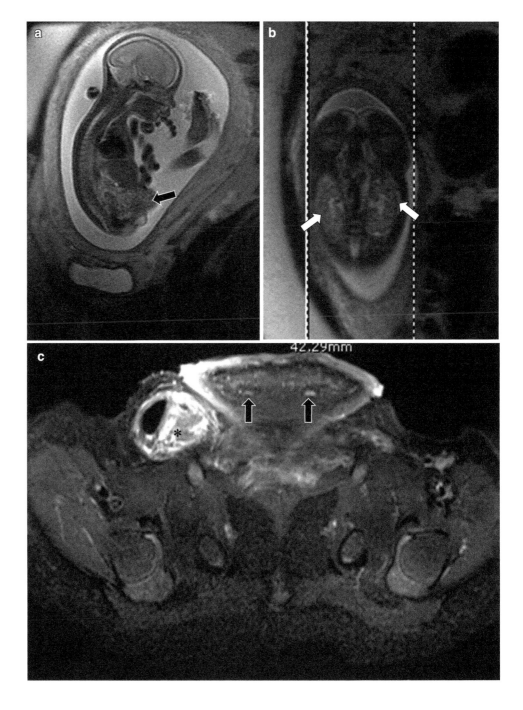

Fig. 14.8 Bladder exstrophy in a 32-week gestational age fetus. Sagittal (with respect to the fetus) T2-weighted fetal MR image (**a**) shows exstrophy of the bladder (*arrow*). Coronal T2-weighted fetal MR image (**b**) demonstrates presence of both kidneys (*arrows*). Postnatal axial T2-weighted fat-suppressed MR image (**c**) demonstrates high signal mucosal bladder plate which is externalized. The ureters (*arrows*) course toward the anterior wall. There is also a large bowel containing right inguinal hernia (*asterisk*) (different patient than in Fig. 14.8a, b)

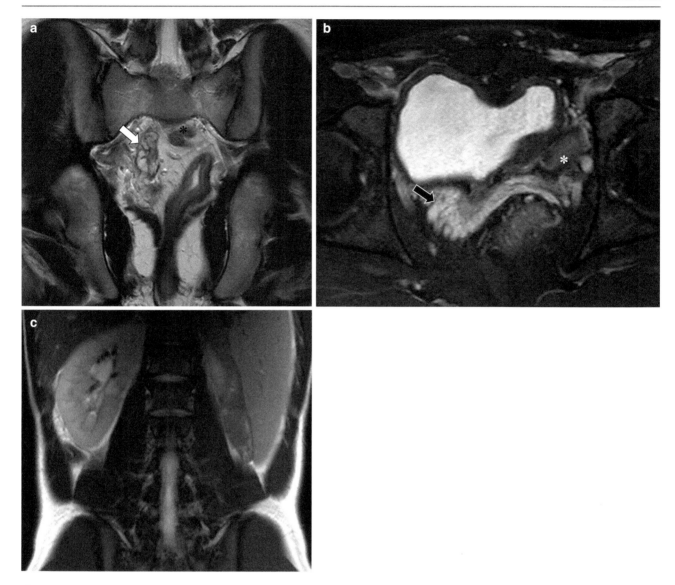

Fig. 14.9 Association of agenesis of the seminal vesicles and kidney in a 14-year-old boy. Coronal T2-weighted MR image (**a**) shows normal right-sided seminal vesicles (*arrow*) with absent seminal vesicles on the left (*asterisk*). Axial T2-weighted fat-suppressed MR image (**b**) shows normal right-sided seminal vesicles (*arrow*) with absent seminal vesicles on the left (*asterisk*). Coronal T2-weighted MR image (**c**) shows a normal right kidney and agenesis of the left kidney

renal agenesis and deficient Wolffian duct structures such as agenesis of the seminal vesicles or dysplastic seminal vesicle with cyst [5, 6] (Figs. 14.9 and 14.10). Seminal vesicle agenesis or hypoplasia is also associated with the cystic fibrosis transmembrane regulator (CFTR) gene mutations [7] (Fig. 14.11).

MR imaging is ideal for evaluation of disorders of sex differentiation [8–10], which often presents at birth with ambiguous genitalia. For example, in a genetic female (46, XX) with virilization from exposure to androids, there is no testicular tissue nor presence of Wolffian duct derivatives. Ovaries and uterus should be visible. Adrenal glands

may be imaged most efficiently with a coronal single-shot T2-weighted sequence without fat suppression because they may be enlarged in the setting of 21-hydroxylase deficiency. Hyperintense urine can be seen in the bladder and often in the uterus due to communication from persistence of the urogenital sinus.

The spectrum of male (46, XY) disorder of sex differentiation includes the family of androgen hormonal abnormalities, partial or complete androgen receptor insensitivity, and gonadal dysgenesis/agenesis. In the latter case, there is no Müllerian inhibiting factor. Thus, MR imaging may reveal Müllerian derivatives such as a dysplastic uterus and/

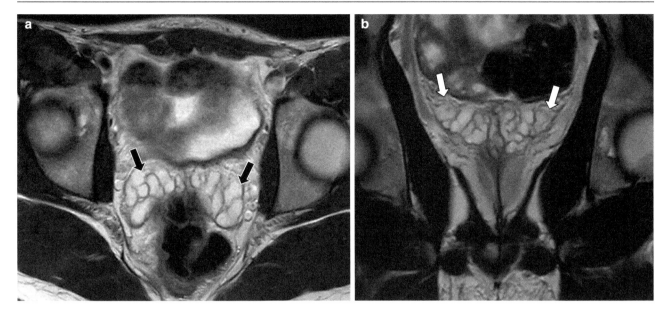

Fig. 14.10 Normal seminal vesicle in a 15-year-old boy who underwent MR imaging for evaluation of appendicitis. Axial T2-weighted MR image (**a**) demonstrates the normal MR imaging appearance of the seminal vesicles (*arrows*). Coronal T2-weighted MR image (**b**) demonstrates the normal MR imaging appearance of the seminal vesicles (*arrows*)

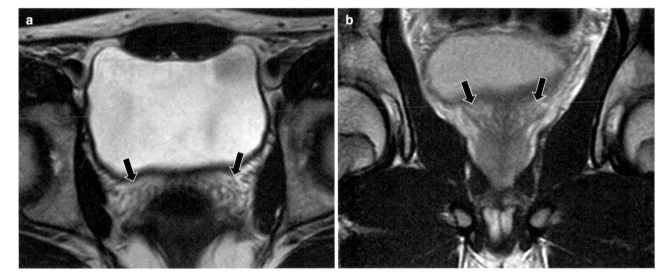

Fig. 14.11 Azoospermia and cystic fibrosis in a 15-year-old boy. Axial T2-weighted MR image (**a**) demonstrates small and dysplastic bilateral seminal vesicles (*arrows*). Coronal T2-weighted MR image (**b**) demonstrates small and dysplastic bilateral seminal vesicles (*arrows*)

or a pseudo-vagina, unilateral fallopian tube, and urogenital sinus in addition to the presence of testes (Fig. 14.12). The testis has varying appearances due to fibrous stroma and may appear streak-like with lower signal on T2-weighted MR imaging sequences than normal. Signal and morphologic atypia suggest dysgenesis, but diagnosis still needs histologic confirmation. Notably, the uterus is present; however, it may be difficult to visualize because there is loss of the typical uterine zonal anatomy seen on T2-weighted MR imaging sequences, instead demonstrating uniform low

myometrial MR imaging signal [8]. Patients with complete androgen receptor insensitivity, also referred to as "testicular feminization syndrome" (Fig. 14.13), have external female genitalia, absent uterus but often presence of undescended testes.

Gender assignment may or may not be completed in childhood. It is a complex process that includes radiologic anatomy and chromosomal makeup, as well as patient and environmental considerations. Gender decisions also encompass psychosocial considerations and thus include input from

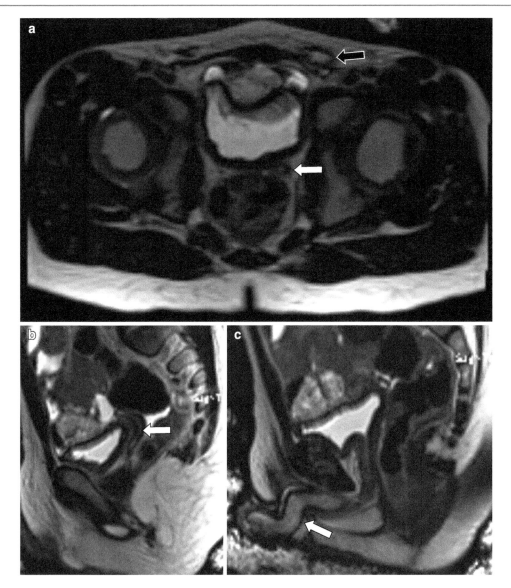

Fig. 14.12 Ambiguous genitalia in a 3-year-old with genotype 46, XY with SRY mutation. Axial T2-weighted MR image during infancy (**a**) demonstrates a vagina, left-sided uterus (*white arrow*), and some portions of the fallopian tube. Single, left-sided gonad (*black arrow*) within the left inguinal canal is also seen. Sagittal T2-weighted MR image (**b**) after first stage of bilateral orchiopexy. There is a left-sided uterus (*arrow*) with suspected left fallopian tube (*not shown*). Sagittal T2-weighted MR image in the midline (**c**) demonstrates a penis (*arrow*) with hypospadias

multiple specialities including psychiatry and other mental health counsellors. After gender determination is made, treatment is aimed at surgically fashioning the appropriate genitalia. In the event of gonadal dysgenesis, gonadectomy is performed due to eliminate potentially increased risk of neoplasia [8].

Polyorchidism, or presence of more than two testes, is a developmental anomaly of uncertain etiology but generally believed to be related to peritoneal bands dividing the embryologic genital ridge. There is increased risk of testicular torsion and cryptorchidism associated with polyorchidism [11].

Fig. 14.13 Androgen insensitivity disorder in a 15-year-old with genotype 46, XY. Axial T2-weighted fat-suppressed MR image (**a**) demonstrates absence of the uterus. Dysplastic undescended small testes were found during surgical exploration. Sagittal T2-weighted fat-suppressed MR image (**b**) demonstrates absence of the uterus. Axial T2-weighted MR image (**c**) shows female external genitalia. Axial T2-weighted fat-suppressed MR image (**d**) shows female external genitalia

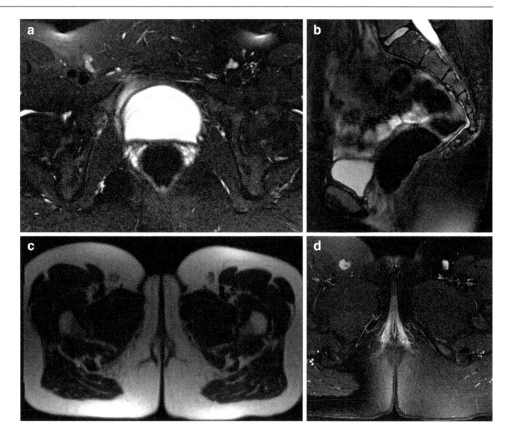

Spectrum of Male Genital Tract Disorders

Congenital Male Genital Tract Disorders

Posterior Urethral Valves Posterior urethral "valves" (PUV) are thought to be due to a remnant Wolffian duct membrane which originates in the region of the verumontanum. The luminal narrowing can cause severe obstruction resulting in bladder muscular wall hypertrophy, bladder trabeculation, vesicoureteral reflux, and renal damage although in practice, there is a wide spectrum of disease severity. Unilateral vesicoureteral reflux occurs in 50% of patients with PUV and can mitigate bladder pressures by acting as a "pop-off" valve [12]. This often results in asymmetric kidney function in which the kidney receiving the refluxate becomes hypofunctional, while the contralateral kidney without reflux has preserved function.

Renal/bladder ultrasound and voiding cystourethrogram are the mainstays of diagnosing posterior urethral valves, including assessment of the upper urinary tract. In the postnatal setting, MR imaging plays a lesser role. However, since the advent and developing popularity of functional MR

urography, the bladder and urethra are often included in the field of view or partially depicted on localizer sequences. A dilated prostatic urethra with high T2-weighted urine signal delineating the lumen may be seen. Sequelae of bladder outlet obstruction, including bladder muscular wall thickening, diverticula, and trabeculation, may be apparent as well. These studies are typically performed with the bladder decompressed via bladder catheterization. To optimize visualization of the bladder, including muscular wall thickening and diverticula, the catheter can be clamped. However, it should be remembered that, although controversial, several authors believe an indwelling catheter can stent open a narrowed prostatic urethra, potentially obscuring PUV [13–15]. This is not an issue during fluoroscopic voiding cystourethrograms in which images are acquired both with the urethral catheter in place and removed. There are few data to support or refute this claim in the context of MR imaging. As such, exclusion of PUV with an indwelling catheter on MR imaging is not advised. On prenatal MR imaging, the generic term "lower urinary tract obstruction", which is often used as the specific site of obstruction, is not always discernible [16]. Hydronephrosis, urinomas, and urinary ascites may be seen with lower urinary tract obstruction (Fig. 14.14).

A multidisciplinary effort is often needed in boys with posterior urethral valves. This includes a nephrologist to manage associated metabolic derangements. Relief of the obstructed urinary tract in boys with posterior urethral valves should occur as early as possible in order to preserve both bladder and renal function and to promote growth of the child. Most patients undergo a primary endoscopic ablation of the valves with the minority needing preoperative urinary diversion [17].

Utricle Cyst An utricle cyst is thought to represent the remnant of the fused caudal ends of the Müllerian ducts. It

is, in effect, the male homologue to the vagina and uterus [18]. Although the terms Müllerian cyst and utricle cyst are often applied arbitrarily, it seems still clear that the utricle cyst in the pediatric population is a distinct entity because it is associated with hypospadias and disorders of sex differentiation. In general, increasing utricle cyst size is associated with greater severity of hypospadias.

On MR imaging, the utricle cyst appears in the midline, posterior to the prostatic urethra, and is of variable size (Fig. 14.15). It is often more tubular than spherical because it communicates with the adjacent urethra. The utricle cyst may cause mass effect on the bladder or, if large enough, on the ureters. MR imaging signal characteristics follow

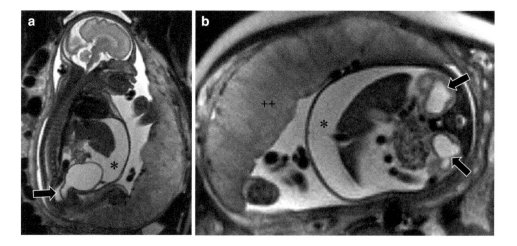

Fig. 14.14 Posterior urethral valves in a 30-week gestational age fetus. Sagittal (with respect to fetus) T2-weighted prenatal MR image (**a**) demonstrates a dilated posterior urethra (*arrow*) and ascites (*asterisk*). Axial (with respect to fetus) T2-weighted prenatal MR image (**b**) demonstrates bilateral hydronephrosis (*arrows*) with forniceal rupture and urinary ascites (*asterisk*). Maternal placenta (++) is also seen

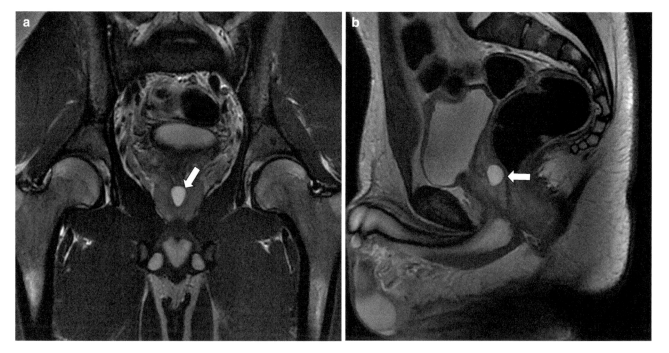

Fig. 14.15 Utricle cyst in a 16-year-old boy. Coronal (**a**), sagittal (**b**) and axial (**c**) T2-weighted MR images demonstrate a midline cyst in the prostate consistent with utricle cyst (*arrows*)

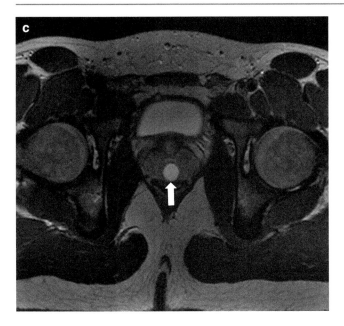

Fig. 14.15 (continued)

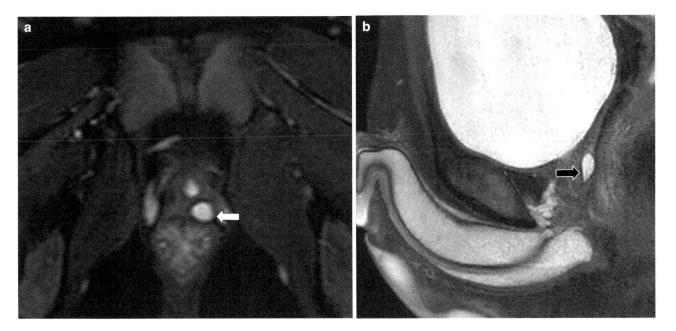

Fig. 14.16 Müllerian duct cyst in a 5-year-old boy. Axial T2-weighted fat-suppressed MR image (**a**) demonstrates a high signal cyst (*arrow*) located posterior to the urethra. Sagittal T2-weighted MR image (**b**) demonstrates the posterior position of the periprostatic cyst (*arrow*)

that of urine on all MR imaging sequences. There should be no internal enhancement after contrast administration.

Utricle cysts are most often small and require no treatment [19]. They are surgically resected when large or symptomatic, or if associated with infertility later in life. This is often performed via a transvesical approach. More recently, laparoscopic excision has been advocated [19, 20].

Müllerian Duct Cyst Müllerian duct cyst typically presents later in childhood or in the adult and may not communicate with the urethra. More recent work has suggested that the term might be a misnomer because there is no histologic evidence that the structure actually arises from the Müllerian duct, at least in the adult population [21].

Müllerian duct cysts are midline cysts in the prostatic region and are most commonly low signal on T1-weighted and high signal on T2-weighted MR imaging (Fig. 14.16); however, this can be altered in the occasional setting of hemorrhage or pus [22]. Management of Müllerian duct cysts is similar to that of utricle cysts.

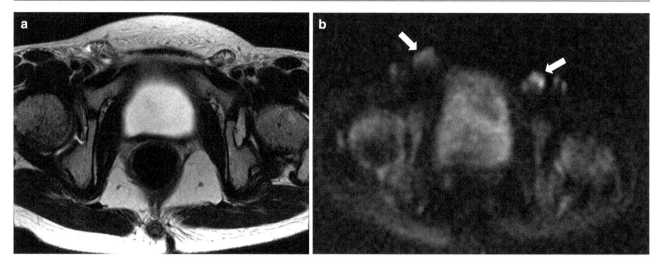

Fig. 14.17 Undescended testes in a 13-year-old boy. Axial T2-weighted MR image (**a**) shows incompletely descended testis (calipers) in each inguinal canal, associated with small size and low T2-weighted signal intensity. Axial diffusion-weighted MR image (**b**) demonstrates high signal in the undescended testes (*arrows*) consistent with diffusion restriction

Cryptorchidism Cryptorchidism is defined as one or both testicles not positioned within the scrotal sac and the inability to manually relocate [23]. It is much more common in premature infants. 70% of affected infants self-correct during the first year of life [23]. Persistent cryptorchidism is a risk factor for both infertility and neoplastic transformation. Associated syndromes include prune belly syndrome, PUV, abdominal wall defects, spinal dysraphism, cloacal exstrophy, and disorders of sex differentiation (see Fig. 14.12). Most cases, however, are isolated and the underlying etiology remains uncertain.

Although widely used, presurgical evaluation with ultrasound has not been shown effective due to poor sensitivity and specificity in localization of the testis, albeit its performance is adequate when the testis is in the groin and not intra-abdominal [24]. It is the intra-abdominal position that is of most interest to the surgeon. Several investigators have assessed the performance of MR imaging in evaluation of cryptorchidism. Historically, MR imaging and ultrasound have both shown only modest ability to locate undescended testes, particularly in localization of intra-abdominal testes [23]. However, recent work has shown an advantage of MR imaging over ultrasound when high b-value ($\geq$800 s/mm^2) diffusion-weighted imaging was added to conventional sequences [23, 25]. DWI often highlights a "hidden" testicle because it uniquely restricts diffusion compared with the normal structures in the lower pelvis (see Figs. 14.17 and 14.18). Still, there are pitfalls for testicular DWI to be aware of; for example, a nonviable testis often does not restrict diffusion, while enlarged retroperitoneal or pelvic sidewall lymph nodes may show restricted diffusion. Finally, higher b values can cause anatomic distortion, especially when there is nearby air-filled bowel. Nonetheless, in the majority of patients, DWI can be of great value in confidently localizing undescended testes to the abdomen, inguinal canal, or scrotum.

Because DWI does not offer optimal anatomy, conventional MR imaging sequences should be obtained as well for evaluation of cryptorchidism. STIR may be a complementary MR imaging sequence. The appearance of undescended testes on conventional MR imaging sequences is that of a homogenous signal which is moderately low on T1-weighted MR imaging sequences and moderately high on T2-weighted MR imaging sequences (Figs. 14.17 and 14.18). Ectopic or transposed but otherwise normal testes have similar MR imaging signal characteristics to intrascrotal testes (see Fig. 14.18). The coronal plane has been shown to add particular value in its detection although we recommend both axial and coronal plane acquisitions [26]. Contrast-enhanced MR angiography has been shown to be of added value in testicular localization [27]; however, gadolinium is not typically used for this indication.

If the testis fails to descend, orchiopexy is performed. Orchiopexy, if performed before puberty, can mitigate risk of malignancy [24]. Earlier intervention can also decrease the risk of infertility. The optimal age at which the procedure is performed, however, remains a matter of some debate.

Infectious Male Genital Tract Disorders

Orchitis Inflammation, including infection, of the testes is known as "orchitis" and is most typically seen in the context of epididymitis (epididymo-orchitis). In this context, inciting agents are often bacterial in the setting of sexual activity.

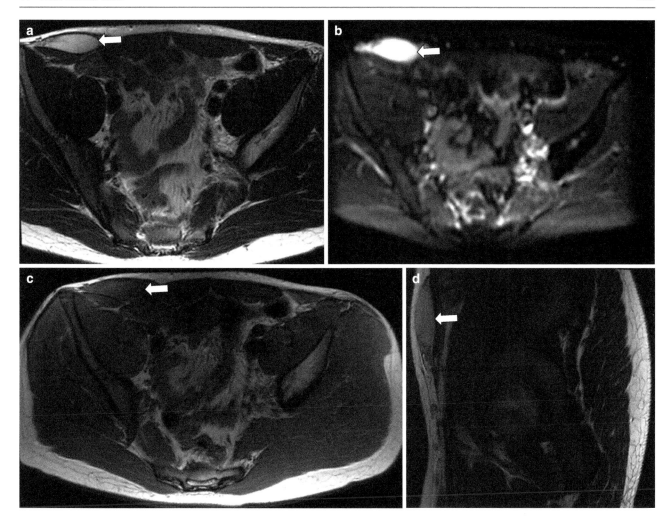

Fig. 14.18 A 16-year-old boy with rhabdomyosarcoma who has undergone temporary transposition of the testis for planned radiation therapy. Axial T2-weighted MR image (**a**) shows an ovoid structure (*arrow*) in the anterior abdominal wall. Without the proper history, this could easily be interpreted as a soft tissue neoplasm. Axial diffusion-weighted MR image (**b**) demonstrates high signal in the ovoid structure (*arrow*), normal for a testis. Axial T1-weighted MR image (**c**) shows normal low signal of the transposed testis (*arrow*). Sagittal T2-weighted MR image (**d**) demonstrates the transposed testis (*arrow*)

In isolated orchitis, multiple viruses can be responsible, most commonly mumps virus. It should be noted that mumps-associated orchitis is only seen in postpubescent males [11].

On MR imaging, the normal testes show a homogeneous, T1-weighted isointense, T2-weighted hyperintense (relative to muscle) MR imaging signal. The more fibrous albuginea and mediastinum testis are depicted as low-signal bands. When inflamed, testes show a lower T1-weighted and increased T2-weighted MR imaging signal. After administration of a gadolinium-based contrast agent, there is either homogeneous enhancement or a more characteristic "tiger skin" pattern due to the presence of non-enhancing, intervening septa [28]. Focal or diffuse orchitis can mimic neoplasia although there is little sign of mass effect in the former. Most commonly, the clinical history and laboratory abnormalities would confirm suspicion of infection.

In adolescent boys, antimicrobial therapy is usually initiated empirically after urinalysis and culture. This can later be tailored based on the results of culture. In the setting of mumps orchitis, treatment is conservative unless there is a secondary bacterial infection. In prepubertal children, orchitis is typically idiopathic and treatment is conservative.

Epididymitis In prepubescent boys, common etiologies of epididymal inflammation are not well-established although probably involve trauma, viruses, or other causes of inflammation [29, 30]. In the postpubescent male, epididymitis is the most common cause of an acute, painful scrotum. Most often in the young adult, it is due to a bacterial infection such as *Chlamydia trachomatis* or *Neisseria gonorrhoeae.* The affected pediatric patient is often febrile with a unilaterally painful scrotum and may report dysuria or even pyuria [31]. Risk factors include urinary tract infection, distal urethral obstruction, neurogenic bladder, or voiding dysfunction. Occasionally, epididymitis can be related to an enlarged seminal vesicle cyst; however, this is more commonly discovered in young adults [22]. Although typically discovered only incidently in children, seminal vesicle cysts can also be related to urinary tract infections [6, 32] (Fig. 14.19).

In infants and young children, established etiologies of epididymitis include ectopic ureter draining into the vas deferens, anorectal malformation, ectopic vas deferens, or a congenitally patulous seminal duct orifice allowing urine to reflux from the urethra [22, 33]. Iatrogenic causes in all ages include urethral instrumentation and indwelling urethral catheters.

Typically, the imaging diagnosis of epididymitis is based on ultrasound. When imaged by MR imaging, the affected epididymis appears enlarged and demonstrates increased and/or heterogeneous T2-weighted MR imaging signal intensity with hyperemia (Figs. 14.20, 14.21, and 14.22). There is often associated engorgement of the vessels, depicted as flow voids on T2-weighted fast spin-echo MR imaging sequences. There may be an associated hydrocele.

Treatment is aimed at the underlying cause, which, in the case of a bacterial agent, warrants antimicrobial therapy. However, establishing a causative agent in children is more challenging, and there is strong evidence that antibiotics have been overprescribed in this population [29].

Fig. 14.19 Seminal vesicle cyst in a 1-year-old boy who presented with a history of multiple urinary tract infections. Sagittal T2-weighted MR image (**a**) demonstrates a large cyst (*asterisk*) posterior to the bladder (labelled B). Coronal thick slab reconstruction of a heavily T2-weighted MR image (**b**) shows the cyst (*asterisk*) just off of the midline

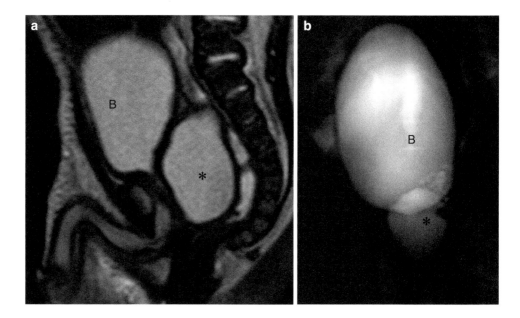

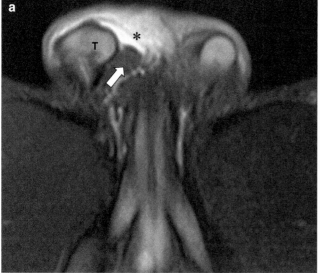

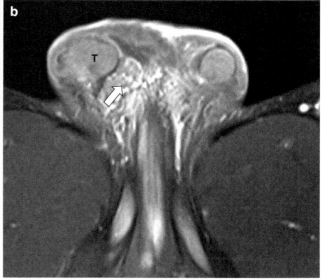

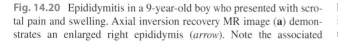

Fig. 14.20 Epididymitis in a 9-year-old boy who presented with scrotal pain and swelling. Axial inversion recovery MR image (**a**) demonstrates an enlarged right epididymis (*arrow*). Note the associated hydrocele (*asterisk*). Axial enhanced T1-weighted fat-suppressed MR image (**b**) shows an enlarged, enhancing right epididymis (*arrow*). The testicle is also visualized (T)

Fig. 14.21 Epididymitis in an 8-year-old boy with a neurogenic bladder. Coronal T2-weighted fat-suppressed MR image shows an enlarged, edematous epididymis (*arrow*). Note the trabeculations in the urinary bladder (UB) in this patient with neurogenic bladder

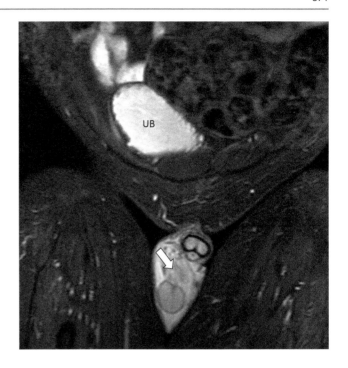

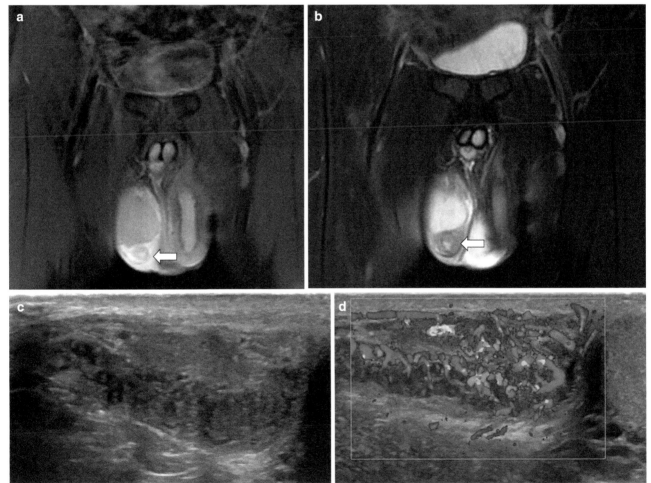

Fig. 14.22 Epididymitis in a 16-year-old boy who presented with a right scrotal lump. Coronal T2-weighted fat-suppressed MR image (**a**) demonstrates enlargement and edema of the right epididymis (*arrow*). Coronal T1-weighted fat-suppressed post-contrast MR image (**b**) shows avid enhancement of the right epididymis (*arrow*). Longitudinal gray-scale ultrasound image (**c**) demonstrates a markedly enlarged body and tail of epididymis. Longitudinal Doppler ultrasound image (**d**) shows marked epididymal hyperemia

Fournier Gangrene An acute, necrotizing infection of the soft tissues involving the penis, scrotum, or perineum is known as Fournier gangrene. The infection is usually polymicrobial and often caused by inoculation from the skin, from the adjacent colon/rectum, or directly from the genita tract [34]. Although more common in adults, specific etiologies of Fournier gangrene in the pediatric population include omphalitis, diaper rash, burns, insect bites, anorectal trauma, abscess, recent circumcision, or herniorrhaphy [35, 36]. Children with hematologic malignancies or other causes of compromised immune function are at elevated risk of developing Fournier gangrene.

The diagnosis of Fournier gangrene is typically clinical. Imaging is reserved for cases that are clinically uncertain or for evaluation of extent of infection. On CT, findings of Fournier gangrene include asymmetric soft tissue thickening and fat stranding associated with air and fluid. There is a paucity of data on the use of MR imaging in the workup of Fournier gangrene, as its rapidly progressive nature often leads to surgical debridement before MR imaging. However, given its superior soft tissue contrast, it is likely that MR imaging reliably demonstrates its findings at least as well as CT, including fascial involvement (Fig. 14.23). In addi-

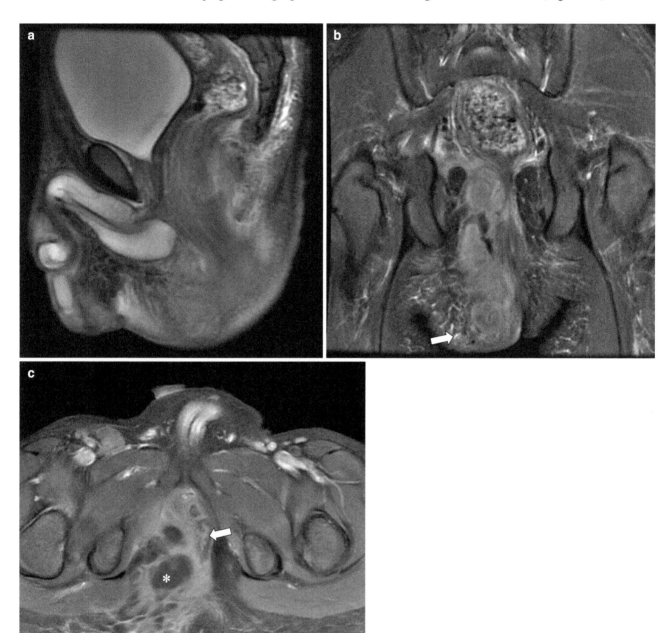

Fig. 14.23 Fournier gangrene in a 2-year-old boy with a history of immunodeficiency who presented with perineal swelling, erythema, and sepsis. Sagittal T2-weighted fat-suppressed MR image (**a**) shows ill-defined edematous soft tissues of the perineum. Coronal T2-weighted fat-suppressed MR image (**b**) demonstrates ill-defined edematous soft tissues of the perineum and scrotum. Note the subcutaneous reticulations from scrotal skin thickening and edema (*arrow*). (**c**) Axial enhanced T1-weighted fat-suppressed MR image shows perineal abscesses (*asterisk*) with rectal displacement (*arrow*)

tion, MR imaging is particularly useful to assess the soft tissue anatomic extent of Fournier gangrene. For example, extension into the retroperitoneal planes is not uncommon, and MR imaging can provide precise anatomic information that could be helpful for potential surgical planning [34]. However, disadvantages of MR imaging in comparison with CT include inferior sensitivity to detection of soft tissue emphysema and longer time of image acquisition. These are relevant factors when the diagnosis of Fournier gangrene is under consideration because necrotizing fasciitis often manifests early with crepitus and soft tissue gas, warranting rapid treatment.

Fluid resuscitation and broad-spectrum antimicrobial therapy are standard initial treatments in the child with suspected Fournier gangrene, with surgical debridement reserved for rapidly progressive or medically refractory cases [36].

Neoplastic Male Genital Tract Disorders

Testicular Germ Cell Tumor Testicular germ cell tumors can be divided into non-seminomatous and seminomatous type. The non-seminomatous germ cell tumors are a heterogeneous group comprised of embryonal carcinoma, teratoma, choriocarcinoma, and yolk sac carcinoma (endodermal sinus tumor). Approximately 95% of all newly diagnosed testicular malignant neoplasms in all patients are germ cell tumors, of which about half are of the seminomatous type [37]. In the prepubescent population, the proportion of malignant tumors is much lower although there is wide variation in reported incidence, probably due to selection bias [38–40]. In contradistinction to the adult population, teratomas are most often benign in this young population. Most prepubescent testicular tumors include teratomas and malignant yolk sac tumor. Seminomas occur nearly exclusively in postpubescent patients except in the setting of cryptorchidism [9].

Ultrasound is the primary imaging modality used to diagnose intratesticular masses. The role of MR imaging in the setting of an intratesticular tumor has not been clearly established, and its use is not widely adopted. However, in recent years, there has been growing interest in replacing the abdominal screening for retroperitoneal metastasis with MR imaging. This is particularly true in the setting of testicular malignancies because most affected patients have excellent long-term outcomes, along with the potential long-term ionizing radiation risk associated with annual CT imaging. There are data suggesting that the sensitivity of detection of metastatic retroperitoneal lymph nodes by experienced radiologists using MR imaging in patients with testicular tumors is comparable to that of CT [41, 42].

Despite the advances in using MR imaging in detection of metastatic disease, it is generally reserved for post-operative surveillance and not routinely used for initial diagnosis of suspected testicular tumors, due to the high performance and low cost of ultrasound. It is possible that this may change in the future as there is now early evidence that seminomatous tumors can be differentiated from non-seminomatous tumors using MR imaging [43, 44]. For example, seminomatous tumors have been reported to demonstrate homogeneous, low T2-weighted signal and septal enhancement after the administration of intravenous contrast. Conversely, it is reported that non-seminomatous testicular tumors tend to have more heterogeneous signal and demonstrate cystic and necrotic elements [45] (Fig. 14.24).

Differentiating benign from malignant testicular tumors also would be useful because this can potentially obviate the need for, or reduce the extent of, surgery (e.g., enucleation rather than orchiectomy). Although there is currently not enough data to prove the ability of MR imaging to reliably and consistently differentiate between the two, recent work has suggested enhancement kinetics may play a role. It has been shown that, in an adult population, malignant lesions demonstrate early enhancement and rapid washout of intravenous contrast on MR imaging [46]. However, these MR imaging findings should not automatically be extrapolated to the pediatric population because the preponderance of intratesticular tumors in the adult population is seminomas. Nonetheless, MR imaging is likely to be at least as accurate as ultrasound in the diagnosis of intratesticular tumors and can render a specific diagnosis in some cases, such as a testicular teratoma [47].

Among the non-seminomatous germ cell tumors, teratomas may have specific features such as fatty elements that MR imaging excels at displaying. A sequence performed both with and without spectral fat suppression is ideal. An alternative is to use an inversion recovery technique (i.e., STIR). One potential pitfall with inversion recovery, however, is the occasional loss of signal in a hemorrhagic tumor where methemoglobin may be confused for fat [48]. Teratomas are typically well circumscribed [49].

Epidermoid cysts, or keratocysts, are benign, squamous cell-lined lesions of germ cell origin [50]. They usually lie just deep to the tunica albuginea and contain keratin. On MR imaging, they are hyperintense on T2-weighted and hypointense on T1-weighted MR imaging sequences [51]. Concentric rings may be seen, mirroring the well-known "onion skin" appearance on ultrasound. Additionally, these lesions show restricted diffusion [44].

For the overwhelming majority of childhood intratesticular tumors, including malignant tumors, the prognosis is very good [52]. Orchiectomy has historically been the mainstay of management for most intratesticular neoplasms. However, recent recognition of the high proportion of benign tumors in children coupled with better pretreatment imaging has resulted

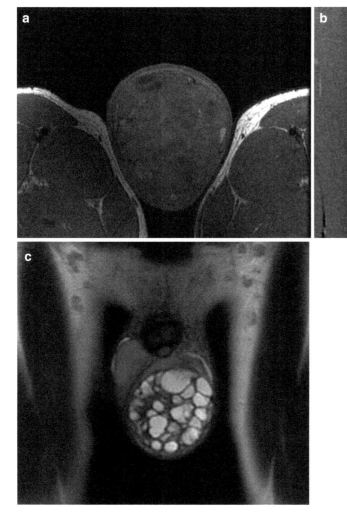

Fig. 14.24 A 17-year-old boy with a non-seminomatous testicular tumor (teratoma). (**a**) Axial T1-weighted MR image demonstrates a predominantly low signal, heterogeneous testicular mass with internal hyperintense areas. (**b**) Coronal T1-weighted, contrast-enhanced, fat-suppressed MR image demonstrates a heterogeneously enhancing multilocular cystic mass arising from the left testis. (**c**) Coronal T2-weighted MR image demonstrates the cystic locules and heterogeneity. (Case courtesy of Paul G. Thacker, Jr., MD, MHA, Mayo Clinic, Rochester, Minnesota, USA)

in a more conservative surgical approach which includes testis-sparing surgery in select cases [53]. Further treatment, including retroperitoneal lymph node dissection, chemotherapy, and/or chemoradiation, is based on tumor type and staging [54].

Testicular Non-germ Cell Tumors Testicular sex cord-stromal tumors in children are uncommon and usually benign, accounting for 25–30% of testicular tumors in the pediatric population [55]. They include juvenile granulosa cell tumors, Sertoli and Leydig tumors, and thecoma/fibroma.

Juvenile granulosa cell tumors typically present before 6 months of age [56, 57]. Based on their appearance on ultrasound and one case report in the literature, these tumors are expected to demonstrate numerous low T1-weighted and high T2-weighted MR imaging areas, demarcated by intervening septa [57]. Testicular Leydig cell tumors have a peak incidence of 4 years of age and often present with precocious puberty as they are hormonally active [9, 55]. On MR imag-

ing, testicular Leydig cell tumors show a homogeneously low signal on T2-weighted MR imaging, often with a high signal rim [58]. Beyond such generalizations, there are currently no known reliable discriminating MR imaging features among the family of testicular sex cord-stromal tumors in the pediatric population. The differential diagnosis for infiltrative testicular and epididymal involvement is listed in Table 14.2.

Table 14.2 Differential diagnosis for infiltrative processes for testicle and epididymis

Entity	Characteristic features
Epididymo-orchitis	Diagnosis supported by the clinical history such as pain, tenderness, and fever
Lymphoma	Usually diffuse enlargement but may be multifocal discrete lesions
Leukemia	Historically, often a site of disease relapse in children with acute lymphoblastic leukemia
Sarcoma	Rare in childhood (except for rhabdomyosarcoma, which is typically extratesticular)

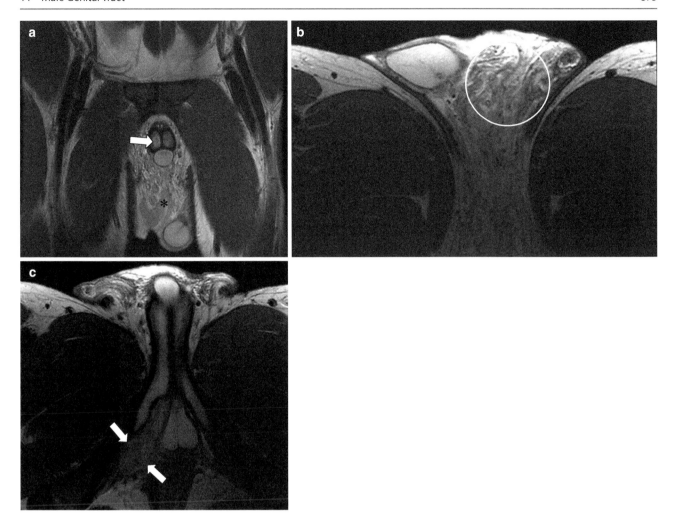

Fig. 14.25 Rhabdomyosarcoma of the perineum and scrotum in a 16-year-old boy. Coronal T2-weighted MR image (**a**) shows a focal tumor in the right corpus cavernosum (*arrow*) as well as extensive infiltration of the soft tissues (*asterisk*) of the perineum and lower scrotum. Axial T2-weighted MR image (**b**) demonstrates extensive infiltration of the soft tissue of the scrotum (*circle*). Axial T2-weighted MR image (**c**) shows the mass (*arrow*s) displacing the right ischiocavernosus muscle

Genital Rhabdomyosarcoma Rhabdomyosarcoma is a mesenchymal-derived tumor and is the most common soft tissue mass arising from the genital tract in the pediatric population. It is categorized as either alveolar, embryonal, or pleomorphic. Botryoid is a subtype of embryonal rhabdomyosarcoma. In the child, the pleomorphic subtype is rare. In the genital tract, the embryonal type is much more common than the alveolar subtype and is comparatively less aggressive. However, the bladder and prostate are considered "unfavorable" anatomic sites with an overall worse prognosis. If the tumor involves the genital tract but arises from the perineum, it is usually of the alveolar, more aggressive subtype – particularly in older children [59] (Fig. 14.25).

Before tissue sampling is performed, imaging is central to the diagnostic workup in a child suspected of genital tract rhabdomyosarcoma. There are no circulating tumor markers to assist in diagnosis. Most often, the initial imaging examination of choice is ultrasound. If a genital mass is seen or suspected, MR imaging is obtained (1) to confirm the presence of the mass, (2) to localize the site of origin (e.g., bladder, urethra, or prostate), (3) to establish the extent of local invasion, and (4) to evaluate regional node involvement.

Rhabdomyosarcoma arising from the urinary bladder often involves the trigone and/or bladder neck and occurs in younger children during the first 3 years of life [60, 61]. On MR imaging, it is usually low signal on T1-weighted MR imaging with heterogeneously high signal on T2-weighted MR imaging with variable contrast enhancement. A bulky, polypoid intraluminal mass is characteristic (Fig. 14.26). However, in contradistinction to the common bladder masses in the adult which arise from the epithelium, rhabdomyosarcomas of the bladder

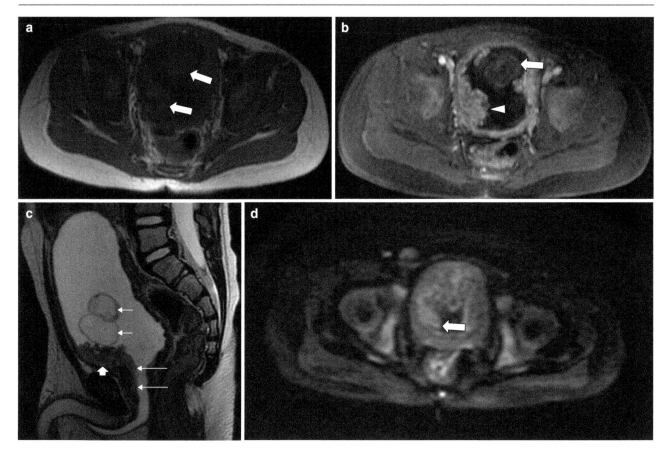

Fig. 14.26 Rhabdomyosarcoma of the bladder in a 2-year-old boy. Axial T1-weighted MR image (**a**) shows lobular intraluminal masses (*arrows*) in the bladder with mild hyperintensity. Axial enhanced T1-weighted fat-suppressed MR image (**b**) demonstrates an intraluminal, partially necrotic mass (*arrow*) as well as a plaque-like mass (*arrowhead*) along the mucosa. Sagittal T2-weighted MR image (**c**) shows lobular intraluminal, masses (*short arrows*) and a plaque-like mass (*wide arrow*) along the mucosa with soft tissue extending toward the prostatic urethra (*long arrows*). Of note, the high signal urine renders the low signal mass highly conspicuous. This is particularly helpful for outlining submucosal tunnelling of the tumor. Axial diffusion-weighted MR image (**d**) shows lobular intraluminal masses (*arrow*) with restricted diffusion

can "tunnel" within the submucosa, even into the proximal urethra (see Fig. 14.26). Other than primary location, there are no known unique MR imaging signal characteristics that can differentiate between the embryonal and alveolar histologic subtypes. Occasionally, other soft tissue bladder masses may present with a suggestive clinical history for an alternative, specific diagnosis. For example, bladder paragangliomas (*aka* extra-adrenal pheochromocytoma), although rare, can present with hypertension in children. On MR, paragangliomas are often mildly hyperintense on T1-weighted imaging and avidly enhance [62] (Fig. 14.27).

Optimal bladder imaging presents unique trade-offs in the selection of MR imaging sequences in order to maximize signal contrast between a mural mass and the intraluminal urine contents. For example, MR imaging assessment of enhancement may be obscured by uri-

nary excretion of contrast. As such, care must be taken to ensure adequate post-contrast images are acquired before the excretory phase [62]. Further, a high-resolution T2-weighted MR imaging sequence can be invaluable in the detection of focal bladder lesions, particularly the lower signal masses [63] (see Figs. 14.1 and 14.26c). However, this must be complemented by T1-weighted MR imaging sequence because the high signal from the urine can potentially obscure mural lesions with prolonged T2 relaxation time. In fact, the margins of mural bladder tumors are often most conspicuous against the dark intraluminal urine signal on T1-weighted MR imaging sequences. This differs from tumors located outside the bladder that are typically more reliably seen on fluid-sensitive sequences (STIR or T2-weighted). The addition of a diffusion-weighted MR imaging sequence can be of benefit. Importantly, the urine is "suppressed" on

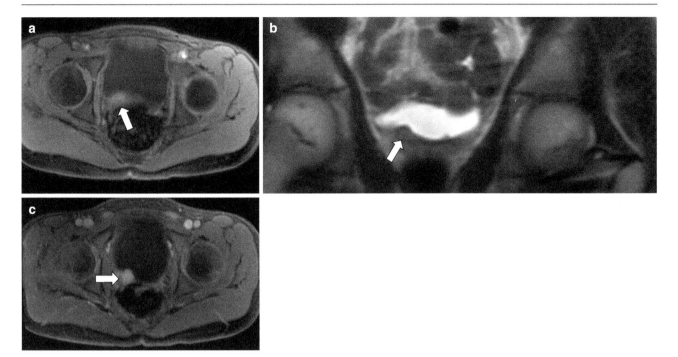

Fig. 14.27 Bladder pheochromocytoma in a 13-year-old boy who presented with hypertension and elevated catecholamines. Axial T1-weighted fat-suppressed MR image (**a**) shows a small, moderately hyperintense soft tissue tumor (*arrow*) involving the posterior bladder wall. Coronal T2-weighted MR image (**b**) demonstrates a soft tissue mass (*arrow*) seen as a "filling defect" along the right inferior wall of the bladder. Axial enhanced T1-weighted fat-suppressed MR image (**c**) shows avid mass enhancement (*arrow*)

this sequence, rendering bladder lesions more visible (see Fig. 14.26d). Its utility, however, has not yet been empirically validated in the evaluation of childhood bladder masses. In the posttreatment state, however, the finding of focal bladder wall thickening can be difficult to interpret because this can represent recurrent tumor or represent nonviable, treated disease or even focal cystitis [62].

Tumors that arise from the prostate often are larger and present with urinary retention and/or constipation [64] (Fig. 14.28). Often, the tumor involves both the urinary bladder and the prostate giving rise to the catch-all term "bladder-prostate rhabdomyosarcoma" [61].

Beside the description of the primary mass, cross-sectional imaging should assess for local and regional lymph nodes including pelvic or retroperitoneal nodes at or below the level of the renal vessels. Lymph node involvement beyond these sites is considered distant metastasis [65]. Involvement of vascular structures should be noted in the radiology report as well. To facilitate clear communication with the surgeon, the interpreting radiologist should adhere to standard lexicon. For example, the term vessel "encasement" is used to describe a 180^0 or greater of circumferential contact without intervening normal tissue planes [65]. Cross-sectional images of the chest (with CT) and the remainder of the abdomen (either MR imaging or CT) are essential to search for distant disease which is present in 10–20% of presenting cases [62]. Complementary imaging with bone scintigraphy or PET is also warranted in the initial workup [66]. Metastasis from rhabdomyosarcoma has a predilection for the lungs and cortical bone.

Paratesticular Rhabdomyosarcoma In contrast to the adult in whom extratesticular masses are usually benign, childhood findings of a painless extratesticular mass have a 50% chance of malignancy, most of which are rhabdomyosarcomas of the embryonal histologic subtype [67, 68]. The paratesticular location is considered a "favorable" site because it is associated with better prognosis.

Although ultrasound is currently considered the imaging modality of choice for evaluation of pediatric patients suspected of having paratesticular rhabdomyosarcoma, MR imaging offers superior tumor localization and evaluation for involvement of surrounding soft tissues [69, 70]. Paratesticular rhabdomyosarcomas often involve or arise from the epididymis or spermatic cord. They can involve the ipsilateral testis but rarely primarily arise from it. MR imaging signal and enhancement characteristics are similar to bladder-prostate rhabdomyosarcomatous masses. However, the surrounding structures render each sequence

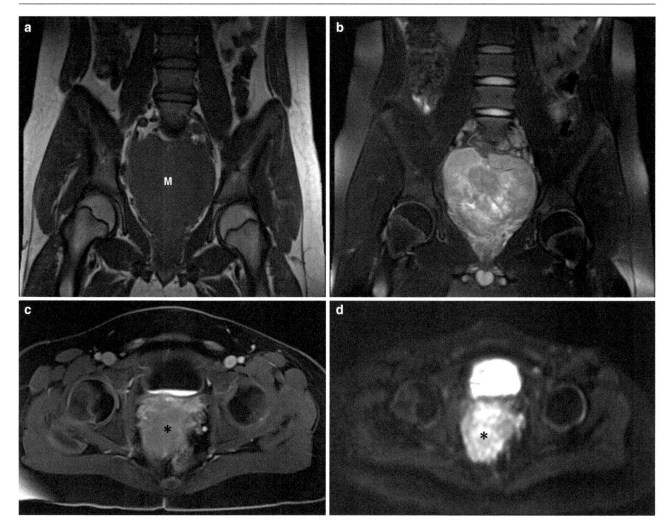

Fig. 14.28 Prostate rhabdomyosarcoma in a 14-year-old boy who presented with pelvic pain and constipation. Coronal T1-weighted MR image (**a**) shows a large hypointense mass (M) in the region of the prostate gland. Coronal T2-weighted MR image (**b**) demonstrates the mass to be hyperintense compared with normal bladder parenchyma. Axial enhanced T1-weighted fat-suppressed MR image (**c**) shows an enhancing mass (*asterisk*) arising from the prostate. Axial diffusion-weighted MR image (**d**) demonstrates restricted diffusion in the mass (*asterisk*). Pathology revealed embryonal rhabdomyosarcoma

to be of different value when compared with bladder masses. For example, on T1-weighted MR images, the homogeneous low signal from the mass may be indistinguishable from the adjacent testis (Fig. 14.29a). However, on fluid-sensitive sequences, a sharp low signal from the tunica albuginea may be seen separating the two structures [71] (Fig. 14.29b). DWI may be useful but it should be remembered that the normal testis restricts diffusion. Other, mostly benign, extratesticular entities can potentially mimic rhabdomyosarcoma on imaging. These are listed in Table 14.3 [68].

Most cases of suspected paratesticular rhabdomyosarcoma undergo chemotherapy and radical orchiectomy via an inguinal approach [69]. Retroperitoneal lymph node dissection is often performed although there is some controversy surrounding patient selection. Radiation therapy is often used for local control unless there has been complete primary resection with clear margins.

Metastatic Disease The testis can also be a site for secondary malignancies, most commonly leukemia and lymphoma. The lesions are often bilateral and may be the first sign of disease relapse after bone marrow remission. In males with leukemia, the testicle is the most common extramedullary site of recurrence, and affected testes are usually enlarged [72]. There is little experience with scrotal MR imaging in the setting of lymphoma although it has been observed that there is a diffuse parenchymal infiltrating appearance but, in contrast to the germ cell tumors, the architecture is preserved [73]. Although to date there has

Fig. 14.29 Paratesticular rhabdomyosarcoma in a 15-year-old boy who presented with a palpable scrotal mass. Axial T1-weighted fat-suppressed MR image (**a**) shows a paratesticular mass (*arrow*) that is not well-differentiated from the testicle. Coronal T2-weighted MR image (**b**) demonstrates the mass (*asterisk*), which is more conspicuous than in Fig. 14.29a. Coronal enhanced T1-weighted fat-suppressed MR image (**c**) shows the heterogeneously enhancing paratesticular mass (*asterisk*)

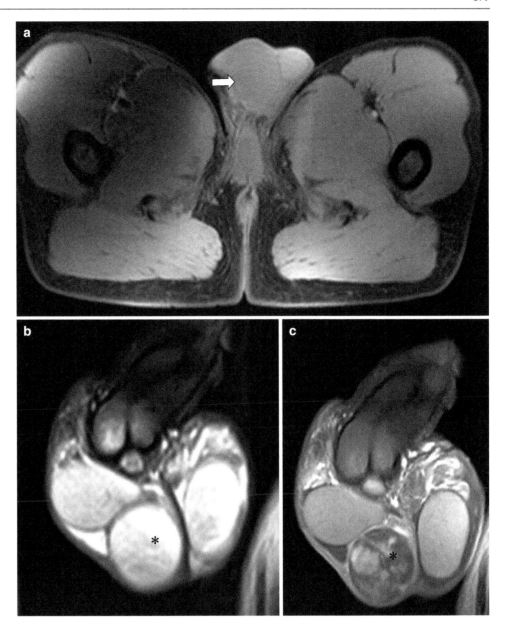

Table 14.3 Differential diagnosis of paratesticular masses in children [68]

Entity	Malignant or benign
Rhabdomyosarcoma	Malignant
Metastasis	Malignant
Pheochromocytoma/paraganglioma	Benign; occasionally malignant
Neurofibroma	Usually benign
Hemangiomas and vascular malformations of the scrotum	Usually benign
Inflammatory myofibroblastic tumor (*aka* fibrous pseudotumor, pseudotumor)	Benign
Meconium periorchitis (from in utero bowel perforation with patent process vaginalis)	Benign
Torsion of the appendix testis or appendix epididymis	Benign
Epididymitis	Benign

been a dearth of data, this description is in keeping with the usual ultrasound appearance which may be diffusely hypoechoic and even normal on grayscale ultrasound but with increased blood flow seen with the use of Doppler. Others have reported multiple well-defined lesions in testicular lymphoma. Multiple lesions can also be seen in systemic illnesses such as sarcoidosis or lymphoma with testicular involvement [11] (Figs. 14.30 and 14.31). The differential diagnosis for infiltrative testicular and epididymal involvement is listed in Table 14.2.

Extratesticular malignancies other than rhabdomyosarcoma are uncommon. Occasionally, however, metastatic disease can present in this space (Figs. 14.32 and 14.33). Although rare, neuroblastoma is among the more commonly reported pediatric malignancies with metastatic disease to the scrotum (see Fig. 14.33). Evidence suggests that this

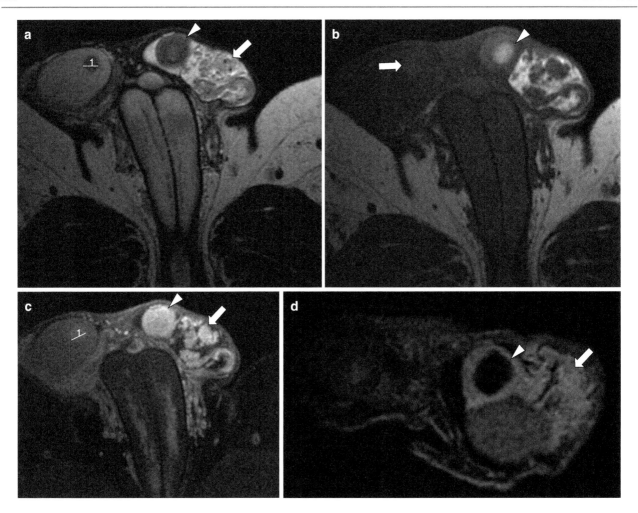

Fig. 14.30 Sarcoid involvement of the scrotum in a 16-year-old boy who presented with a scrotal mass. Axial T2-weighted MR image (**a**) shows an intratesticular hypointense granuloma (caliper in the right testicle). The left epididymis is enlarged (*arrow*). The patient also has an epididymal cyst (*arrowhead*) with low signal intensity likely from proteinaceous content. Axial T1-weighted MR image (**b**) demonstrates the granuloma to have low signal intensity (*arrow*), in contrast to the hyperintense proteinaceous epididymal cyst (*arrowhead*). Axial enhanced T1-weighted fat-suppressed MR image (**c**) shows low signal intensity (caliper) in the right testicular granuloma with high signal intensity in the epididymal cyst (*arrowhead*) and epididymis (*arrow*). Axial digital subtraction MR image (**d**) shows non-enhancement in the right testicular granuloma and non-enhancement of the epididymal cyst (*arrowhead*). The enlarged epididymis (*arrow*) does enhance, demonstrating the value of digital subtraction imaging for evaluation of lesions with high T1-weighted signal intensity on pre-contrast MR imaging

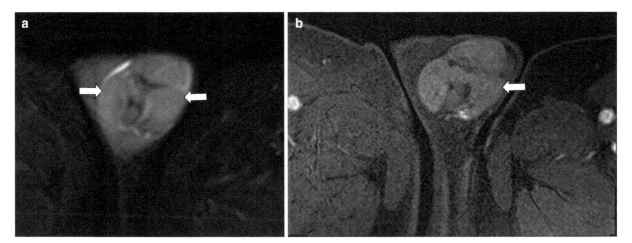

Fig. 14.31 Testicular metastasis from non-Hodgkin lymphoma in a 17-year-old boy. Axial T2-weighted MR image (**a**) demonstrates testicular replacement by multilobulated, mildly hyperintense masses (*arrows*). Axial enhanced T1-weighted fat-suppressed MR image (**b**) shows lesion enhancement (*arrow*)

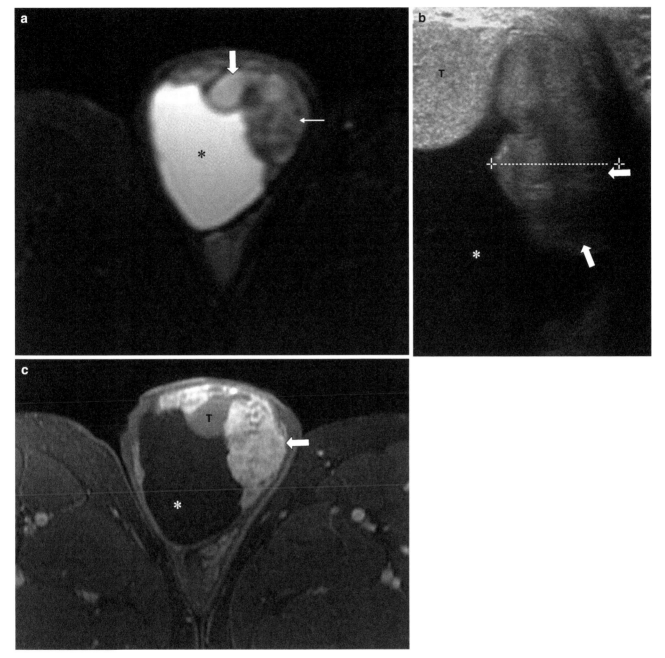

Fig. 14.32 Metastatic desmoplastic small round cell tumor to the scrotum in a 17-year-old boy who presented with a rapidly growing and painful scrotal mass. Axial T2-weighted fat-suppressed MR image (**a**) shows metastatic tumor implants (*thin arrow*) and a right-sided hydrocele (*asterisk*). Note the displaced right testis (*thick arrow*) with normal signal intensity. Transverse grayscale ultrasound image (**b**) demonstrates metastatic soft tissue intrascrotal deposits (*arrows*). Note the hydrocele (*asterisk*). Axial enhanced T1-weighted fat-suppressed MR image (**c**) shows the enhancing scrotal masses (*arrow*). The testicle (T) and a hydrocele (*asterisk*) are also visible

occurs by malignant cells travelling from the adjacent retroperitoneum rather than hematogenous spread [74].

Other Male Genital Tract Disorders

Testicular Torsion Ultrasound remains the imaging test of choice in the diagnosis of complete testicular torsion because it is highly sensitive, specific, and more widely available compared with MR imaging [75]. However, in the setting of incomplete torsion, the sonographic findings can be subtle [76]. One retrospective study showed disappointing performance of MR imaging in diagnosing incomplete torsion [77]. Other authors suggest true added value of MR imaging in suspected incomplete torsion based on case reports. Both the twisting of the cord itself and relative decreased enhancement of the affected testis in the setting of surgically confirmed cases

Fig. 14.33 Intrascrotal metastasis from neuroblastoma in a 2-year-old boy who presented with a painful and hard scrotal mass. Axial T2-weighted MR image (**a**) shows lobular, intermediate signal masses in the scrotum bilaterally. Metaiodobenzylguanidine (MIBG) planar scintigraphic image (**b**) demonstrates widespread metastasis, including bone marrow and scrotal disease (*arrows*)

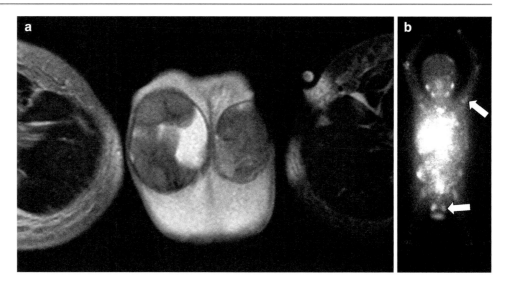

have been described on MR imaging [78, 79]. Diffusion-weighted MR imaging has been studied and shows decreased ADC values in the affected testis compared with the contralateral control, consistent with ischemia-associated cytotoxic edema during the torsion process [80]. The acute nature of testicular torsion and time sensitivity of detorsion often preclude the use of MR imaging because of its relatively long wait and image acquisition times compared with ultrasound.

Testicular torsion is considered a genital surgical emergency with the goal of timely restoration of blood flow to the ischemic testicle. In the case of surgical delay or during surgical preparation of the patient, manual detorsion is sometimes attempted. This does not replace surgery as an orchiopexy is still required if the testicle is salvageable. If infarcted, orchiectomy is performed.

Testicular and Epididymal Appendage Torsion Both the appendix epididymis and the appendix testis are embryologic remnants of the mesonephric ducts [81]. Torsion of either of these structures presents with acute scrotal pain and typically occurs between 6 and 12 years of age, somewhat younger than the expected occurrence of testicular torsion. Clinically, this entity can mimic acute testicular torsion. On physical examination, a characteristic focal bluish hue over the affected area on the scrotal skin, the so-called "blue-dot" sign, may be present.

There is a paucity of literature describing MR imaging features of torsion of these embryologic remnants. The imaging strategy, rather, should be focused primarily on excluding a urologic surgical emergency, namely, testicular torsion. Although intuitively appealing, it should not currently be assumed that an MR imaging diagnosis can be made based on diminished appendageal enhancement in combination with normal testis and epididymis. In fact, ultra-

sound Doppler studies often show reactive hyperemia in the adjacent epididymis or testis [82], which may be difficult to distinguish from infection.

Treatment is generally conservative and is centered on pain management.

Vascular Anomalies Affecting the Genitalia The spectrum of vascular anomalies in children is grouped into either vascular tumors or vascular malformations [83, 84]. Depending on the type and severity, they can be associated with bleeding, ulceration, pain, infection, or thrombocytopenia. The perineal area is particularly prone to ulceration [85]. Vascular tumors involving the perineum, such as the infantile hemangioma, are associated with spinal dysraphism and tethered cord. As such, MR imaging of the spine is recommended when such a lesion is discovered in the child [86]. Vascular malformations, such as venous or lymphatic malformations, can cause significant disfigurement, resulting in psychological distress.

On MR imaging, lymphatic malformations usually appear cystic (Fig. 14.34). On T1-weighted imaging, they have variable appearance depending on the presence of internal proteinaceous debris and hemorrhage. Lymphatic malformations are typically high signal on T2-weighted imaging. After the administration of gadolinium-based contrast agent, there is a lack of internal enhancement; however, their walls and intervening septa may enhance. In contradistinction, venous malformations enhance but in a delayed fashion after the administration of gadolinium contrast.

Treatment is aimed at the nature of the underlying biology. Infantile hemangiomas most often regress during childhood. Vascular malformations are sometimes managed conservatively or may undergo sclerotherapy or even surgical resection [87]. Surgical management of lymphatic

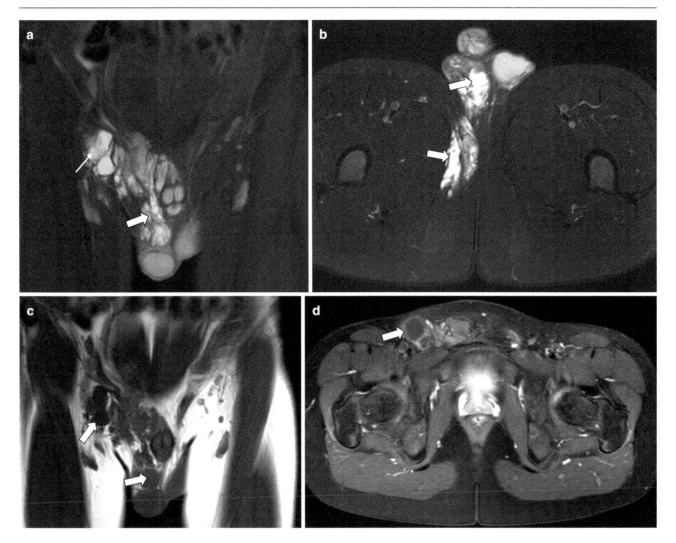

Fig. 14.34 Scrotal lymphatic malformation in a 9-year-old boy who presented with intermittent right inguinal swelling. Coronal T2-weighted fat-suppressed MR image (**a**) shows a multilobulated, high signal cystic collection (*thin arrow*). Note the involvement of the spermatic cord (*thick arrow*). Axial T2-weighted fat-suppressed MR image (**b**) demonstrates a multilobulated, high signal cystic collection (*arrows*) in the scrotum and perineum. Coronal T1-weighted MR image (**c**) shows a multilobulated, low signal cystic collection (*arrows*). Axial enhanced T1-weighted fat-suppressed MR image (**d**) demonstrates the cysts (*arrow*) to have peripheral but not central enhancement

malformations of the male genitalia is often uniquely complicated as they are inclined to intertwine around the spermatic cord [85].

Conclusion

There are several primary modalities for the imaging evaluation of the male genital tract in the pediatric population. These include ultrasound, vesicourethrography, and retrograde urethrography. MR imaging has been used primarily as a complimentary modality. However, in recent years, it is rapidly gaining popularity. Besides its widely recognized role as a "problem-solving" technique when there are equivocal findings on another examination, it has been shown in many instances to be the superior imaging modality due to its superb soft tissue contrast. The soft tissues of the pelvis particularly lend themselves to evaluation by MR imaging. MR imaging has proven most valuable when detailed mapping of anatomy or extent of disease evaluation is called for. The unique advantages of MR imaging over alternative modalities for evaluating male genital tract disorders need to be weighed against its costs. These include financial cost, limited availability, potential need for sedation, and the small but present risks associated with gadolinium contrast material.

References

1. Darge K, Anupindi SA, Jaramillo D. MR imaging of the abdomen and pelvis in infants, children, and adolescents. Radiology. 2011;261(1):12–29.
2. Raza SA, Jhaveri KS. MR imaging of urinary bladder carcinoma and beyond. Radiol Clin N Am. 2012;50(6):1085–110.
3. Levin TL, Han B, Little BP. Congenital anomalies of the male urethra. Pediatr Radiol. 2007;37(9):851–62; quiz 945
4. Berrocal T, Lopez-Pereira P, Arjonilla A, Gutierrez J. Anomalies of the distal ureter, bladder, and urethra in children: embryologic, radiologic, and pathologic features. Radiographics. 2002;22(5):1139–64.
5. Pichler R, Oswald J, Glodny B, Skradski V, Aigner F, Rehder P. Unilateral renal agenesis with absent ductus deferens, epididymis and seminal vesicle: incidental finding in a 22-year-old patient with maldevelopment of the mesonephric duct. Urol Int. 2011;86(3):365–9.
6. Kim B, Kawashima A, Ryu JA, Takahashi N, Hartman RP, King BF Jr. Imaging of the seminal vesicle and vas deferens. Radiographics. 2009;29(4):1105–21.
7. Bouzouita A, Kerkeni W, Abouda H, Khrouf M, Elloumi H, Mnif N, et al. Seminal vesicle agenesis: an uncommon cause of azoospermia. Can Urol Assoc J. 2014;8(3–4):E266–9.
8. Choi HK, Cho KS, Lee HW, Kim KS. MR imaging of intersexuality. Radiographics. 1998;18(1):83–96.
9. Riccabona M. Pediatric urogenital radiology: Springer International Publishing. Switzerland: Cham; 2018.
10. Epelman M, Dinan D, Gee MS, Servaes S, Lee EY, Darge K. Müllerian duct and related anomalies in children and adolescents. Magn Reson Imaging Clin N Am. 2013;21(4):773–89.
11. Cassidy FH, Ishioka KM, McMahon CJ, Chu P, Sakamoto K, Lee KS, et al. MR imaging of scrotal tumors and pseudotumors. Radiographics. 2010;30(3):665–83.
12. Atobatele MO, Oyinloye OI, Nasir AA, Bamidele JO. Posterior urethral valve with unilateral vesicoureteral reflux and patent urachus: a rare combination of urinary tract anomalies. Urol Ann. 2015;7(2):240–3.
13. Lebowitz RL. Voiding cystourethrography in boys: the presence of the catheter does not obscure the diagnosis of posterior urethral valves but prevents estimation of the adequacy of transurethral fulguration. Am J Roentgenol. 1996;166(3):724.
14. Ditchfield MR, GrattanSmith JD, deCampo JF, Hutson JM. Voiding cystourethrography in boys: the presence of the catheter does not obscure the diagnosis of posterior urethral valves but prevents estimation of the adequacy of transurethral fulguration—reply. Am J Roentgenol. 1996;166(3):724–5.
15. Ditchfield MR, Grattansmith JD, Decampo JF, Hutson JM. Voiding cystourethrography in boys—does the presence of the catheter obscure the diagnosis of posterior urethral valves. Am J Roentgenol. 1995;164(5):1233–5.
16. Chauvin NA, Epelman M, Victoria T, Johnson AM. Complex genitourinary abnormalities on fetal mri: imaging findings and approach to diagnosis. Am J Roentgenol. 2012;199(2):W222–W31.
17. Lima M, Manzoni G, editors. Pediatric urology: contemporary strategies from fetal life to adolescence. Milan: Springer; 2015.
18. Levin TL, Han B, Little BP. Congenital anomalies of the male urethra. Pediatr Radiol. 2007;37(9):851–62.
19. Aminsharifi A, Afsar F, Pakbaz S. Laparoscopic management of Müllerian duct cysts in infants. J Pediatr Surg. 2011;46(9):1859–64.
20. Jia W, Liu GC, Zhang LY, Wen YQ, Fu W, Hu JH, et al. Comparison of laparoscopic excision versus open transvesical excision for symptomatic prostatic utricle in children. J Pediatr Surg. 2016;51(10):1597–601.
21. Kato H, Hayama M, Furuya S, Kobayashi S, Islam AM, Nishizawa O. Anatomical and histological studies of so-called Müllerian duct cyst. Int J Urol. 2005;12(5):465–8.
22. Shebel HM, Farg HM, Kolokythas O, El-Diasty T. Cysts of the lower male genitourinary tract: embryologic and anatomic considerations and differential diagnosis. Radiographics. 2013;33(4):1125–43.
23. Krishnaswami S, Fonnesbeck C, Penson D, McPheeters ML. Magnetic resonance imaging for locating nonpalpable undescended testicles: a meta-analysis. Pediatrics. 2013;131(6):E1908–E16.
24. Tasian GE, Copp HL. Diagnostic performance of ultrasound in nonpalpable cryptorchidism: a systematic review and meta-analysis. Pediatrics. 2011;127(1):119–28.
25. Kantarci M, Doganay S, Yalcin A, Aksoy Y, Yilmaz-Cankaya B, Salman B. Diagnostic performance of diffusion-weighted mri in the detection of nonpalpable undescended testes: comparison with conventional MRI and surgical findings. Am J Roentgenol. 2010;195(4):W268–W73.
26. Miyano T, Kobayashi H, Shimomura H, Yamataka A, Tomita T. Magnetic-resonance-imaging for localizing the nonpalpable undescended testis. J Pediatr Surg. 1991;26(5):607–9.
27. Yeung CK, Tam YH, Chan YL, Lee KH, Metreweli C. A new management algorithm for impalpable undescended testis with gadolinium enhanced magnetic resonance angiography. J Urol. 1999;162(3):998–1002.
28. Tonolini M, Ippolito S. Cross-sectional imaging of complicated urinary infections affecting the lower tract and male genital organs. Insights Imaging. 2016;7(5):689–711.
29. Cristoforo TA. Evaluating the necessity of antibiotics in the treatment of acute epididymitis in pediatric patients: a literature review of retrospective studies and data analysis. Pediatr Emerg Care. 2017; https://doi.org/10.1097/PEC.0000000000001018. [Epub ahead of print]
30. Louette A, Krahn J, Caine V, Ha S, Lau TTY, Singh AE. Treatment of acute epididymitis: a systematic review and discussion of the implications for treatment based on etiology. Sex Transm Dis. 2018;45(12):e104–e8.
31. Livingston L, Larsen CR. Seminal vesicle cyst with ipsilateral renal agenesis. AJR Am J Roentgenol. 2000;175(1):177–80.
32. Cascini V, Di Renzo D, Guerriero V, Lauriti G, Lelli Chiesa P. Zinner syndrome in pediatric age: issues in the diagnosis and treatment of a rare malformation complex. Front Pediatr. 2019;7:129.
33. VanderBrink BA, Sivan B, Levitt MA, Pena A, Sheldon CA, Alam S. Epididymitis in patients with anorectal malformations: a cause for urologic concern. Int Braz J Urol. 2014;40(5):676–82.
34. Levenson RB, Singh AK, Novelline RA. Fournier gangrene: role of imaging. Radiographics. 2008;28(2):519–28.
35. Rouzrokh M, Tavassoli A, Mirshemirani A. Fournier's gangrene in children: report on 7 cases and review of literature. Iran J Pediatr. 2014;24(5):660–1.
36. Cundy TP, Boucaut HA, Kirby CP. Fournier's gangrene in a child with congenital genitourinary anomalies. J Pediatr Surg. 2012;47(4):808–11.
37. Bosl GJ, Motzer RJ. Testicular germ-cell cancer. N Engl J Med. 1997;337(4):242–53.
38. Taskinen S, Fagerholm R, Aronniemi J, Rintala R, Taskinen M. Testicular tumors in children and adolescents. J Pediatr Urol. 2008;4(2):134–7.
39. Ahmed HU, Arya M, Muneer A, Mushtaq I, Sebire N. Testicular and paratesticular tumours in the prepubertal population. Lancet Oncol. 2010;11(5):476–83.
40. Nerli RB, Ajay G, Shivangouda P, Pravin P, Reddy M, Pujar VC. Prepubertal testicular tumors: our 10 years experience. Indian J Cancer. 2010;47(3):292–5.
41. Sohaib SA, Koh DM, Barbachano Y, Parikh J, Husband JE, Dearnaley DP, et al. Prospective assessment of MRI for imaging retroperitoneal metastases from testicular germ cell tumours. Clin Radiol. 2009;64(4):362–7.

42. Kok HK, Leong S, Torreggiani WC. Is magnetic resonance imaging comparable with computed tomography in the diagnosis of retroperitoneal metastasis in patients with testicular cancer? Can Assoc Radiol J. 2014;65(3):196–8.

43. Marko J, Wolfman DJ, Aubin AL, Sesterhenn IA. Testicular seminoma and its mimics: from the radiologic pathology archives. Radiographics. 2017;37(4):1085–98.

44. Tsili AC, Tsampoulas C, Giannakopoulos X, Stefanou D, Alamanos Y, Sofikitis N, et al. MRI in the histologic characterization of testicular neoplasms. AJR Am J Roentgenol. 2007;189(6):W331–7.

45. Secil M, Altay C, Basara I. State of the art in germ cell tumor imaging. Urol Oncol-Semin Ori. 2016;34(3):156–64.

46. Tsili AC, Argyropoulou MI, Astrakas LG, Ntoulia EA, Giannakis D, Sofikitis N, et al. Dynamic contrast-enhanced subtraction MRI for characterizing intratesticular mass lesions. AJR Am J Roentgenol. 2013;200(3):578–85.

47. Mohrs OK, Thoms H, Egner T, Brunier A, Eiers M, Kauczor HU, et al. MRI of patients with suspected scrotal or testicular lesions: diagnostic value in daily practice. Am J Roentgenol. 2012;199(3):609–15.

48. Froehlich JM, Metens T, Chilla B, Hauser N, Hohl MK, Kubik-Huch RA. MRI of the female pelvis: a possible pitfall in the differentiation of haemorrhagic vs. fatty lesions using fat saturated sequences with inversion recovery. Eur J Radiol. 2012;81(3):598–602.

49. Epifanio M, Baldissera M, Esteban FG, Baldisserotto M. Mature testicular teratoma in children: multifaceted tumors on ultrasound. Urology. 2014;83(1):195–7.

50. Coley BD, editor. Caffey's pediatric diagnostic imaging, vol. 2. 13th ed. Philadelphia: Elsevier; 2019.

51. Koenigsberg RA, Kelsey D, Friedman AC. Case report: ultrasound and MRI findings in a scrotal epidermoid cyst. Clin Radiol. 1995;50(8):576–8.

52. Hanna NH, Einhorn LH. Testicular cancer—discoveries and updates. N Engl J Med. 2014;371(21):2005–16.

53. Woo LL, Ross JH. The role of testis-sparing surgery in children and adolescents with testicular tumors. Urol Oncol. 2016;34(2):76–83.

54. Moreno CC, Small WC, Camacho JC, Master V, Kokabi N, Lewis M, et al. Testicular tumors: what radiologists need to know-differential diagnosis, staging, and management. Radiographics. 2015;35(2):400–15.

55. Coley BD. Caffey's pediatric diagnostic imaging. 13th. ed. Philadelphia: Elsevier; 2019.

56. Liu S, Koscheski P. Neonatal juvenile granulosa cell tumor of the testis. Appl Radiol. 2016;45(7):32A–B.

57. Yikilmaz A, Lee EY. MRI findings of bilateral juvenile granulosa cell tumor of the testis in a newborn presenting as intraabdominal masses. Pediatr Radiol. 2007;37(10):1031–4.

58. Tsitouridis I, Maskalidis C, Panagiotidou D, Kariki EP. Eleven patients with testicular leydig cell tumors clinical, imaging, and pathologic correlation. J Ultrasound Med. 2014;33(10):1855–64.

59. Shapiro E, Strother D. Pediatric genitourinary rhabdomyosarcoma. J Urol. 1992;148(6):1761–8.

60. Royal SA, Hedlund GL, Galliani CA. Rhabdomyosarcoma of the dome of the urinary bladder: a difficult imaging diagnosis. AJR Am J Roentgenol. 1996;167(2):524–5.

61. Agrons GA, Wagner BJ, Lonergan GJ, Dickey GE, Kaufman MS. From the archives of the AFIP. Genitourinary rhabdomyosarcoma in children: radiologic-pathologic correlation. Radiographics. 1997;17(4):919–37.

62. Shelmerdine SC, Lorenzo AJ, Gupta AA, Chavhan GB. Pearls and pitfalls in diagnosing pediatric urinary bladder masses. Radiographics. 2017;37(6):1872–91.

63. Pai DR, Ladino-Torres MF. Magnetic resonance imaging of pediatric pelvic masses. Magn Reson Imaging Clin N Am. 2013;21(4):751–72.

64. Park K, van Rijn R, McHugh K. The role of radiology in paediatric soft tissue sarcomas. Cancer Imaging. 2008;8:102–15.

65. Van Rijn RR, Wilde JC, Bras J, Oldenburger F, McHugh KM, Merks JH. Imaging findings in noncraniofacial childhood rhabdomyosarcoma. Pediatr Radiol. 2008;38(6):617–34.

66. Stehr M. Pediatric urologic rhabdomyosarcoma. Curr Opin Urol. 2009;19(4):402–6.

67. Aganovic L, Cassidy F. Imaging of the scrotum. Radiol Clin N Am. 2012;50(6):1145–65.

68. Sung T, Riedlinger WF, Diamond DA, Chow JS. Solid extratesticular masses in children: radiographic and pathologic correlation. AJR Am J Roentgenol. 2006;186(2):483–90.

69. Dangle PP, Correa A, Tennyson L, Gayed B, Reyes-Mugica M, Ost M. Current management of paratesticular rhabdomyosarcoma. Urol Oncol. 2016;34(2):84–92.

70. Shah T, Abu-Sanad O, Marsh H. Role of magnetic resonance imaging in the early diagnosis of paratesticular rhabdomyosarcoma. Ann R Coll Surg Engl. 2016;98(5):e74–6.

71. Mason BJ, Kier R. Sonographic and MR imaging appearances of paratesticular rhabdomyosarcoma. AJR Am J Roentgenol. 1998;171(2):523–4.

72. Porter RP, Kaste SC. Imaging findings of recurrent acute lymphoblastic leukemia in children and young adults, with emphasis on MRI. Pediatr Radiol. 2004;34(5):400–8.

73. Chua SC, Rozalli FI, O'Connor SR. Imaging features of primary extranodal lymphomas. Clin Radiol. 2009;64(6):574–88.

74. Simon T, Hero B, Berthold F. Testicular and paratesticular involvement by metastatic neuroblastoma. Cancer. 2000;88(11):2636–41.

75. Bree RL, Hoang DT. Scrotal ultrasound. Radiol Clin N Am. 1996;34(6):1183–205.

76. Sanelli PC, Burke BJ, Lee L. Color and spectral doppler sonography of partial torsion of the spermatic cord. AJR Am J Roentgenol. 1999;172(1):49–51.

77. Terai A, Yoshimura K, Ichioka K, Ueda N, Utsunomiya N, Kohei N, et al. Dynamic contrast-enhanced subtraction magnetic resonance imaging in diagnostics of testicular torsion. Urology. 2006;67(6):1278–82.

78. Gotto GT, Chang SD, Nigro MK. MRI in the diagnosis of incomplete testicular torsion. Br J Radiol. 2010;83(989):e105–7.

79. Trambert MA, Mattrey RF, Levine D, Berthoty DP. Subacute scrotal pain: evaluation of torsion versus epididymitis with MR imaging. Radiology. 1990;175(1):53–6.

80. Maki D, Watanabe Y, Nagayama M, Ishimori T, Okumura A, Amoh Y, et al. Diffusion-weighted magnetic resonance imaging in the detection of testicular torsion: feasibility study. J Magn Reson Imaging. 2011;34(5):1137–42.

81. Woodward PJ, Schwab CM, Sesterhenn IA. From the archives of the AFIP: extratesticular scrotal masses: radiologic-pathologic correlation. Radiographics. 2003;23(1):215–40.

82. Baldisserotto M, de Souza JC, Pertence AP, Dora MD. Color Doppler sonography of normal and torsed testicular appendages in children. AJR Am J Roentgenol. 2005;184(4):1287–92.

83. Behr GG, Johnson C. Vascular anomalies: hemangiomas and beyond—part 1. Fast-flow lesions. AJR Am J Roentgenol. 2013;200(2):414–22.

84. Mulliken JB, Glowacki J. Hemangiomas and vascular malformations in infants and children: a classification based on endothelial characteristics. Plast Reconstr Surg. 1982;69(3):412–22.

85. Kulungowski AM, Schook CC, Alomari AI, Vogel AM, Mulliken JB, Fishman SJ. Vascular anomalies of the male genitalia. J Pediatr Surg. 2011;46(6):1214–21.

86. Drolet BA, Chamlin SL, Garzon MC, Adams D, Baselga E, Haggstrom AN, et al. Prospective study of spinal anomalies in children with infantile hemangiomas of the lumbosacral skin. J Pediatr. 2010;157(5):789–94.

87. Behr GG, Johnson CM. Vascular anomalies: hemangiomas and beyond–part 2, slow-flow lesions. AJR Am J Roentgenol. 2013;200(2):423–36.

Female Genital Tract

15

Sharon W. Gould, Juan S. Calle Toro, Susan J. Back,
Daniel J. Podberesky, and Monica Epelman

Introduction

Transabdominal ultrasound provides an excellent initial evaluation of the female pediatric genital tract; however, MR imaging is superior for detailed evaluation of the ovaries and uterus, as well as surrounding structures. Due to its high spatial resolution and tissue contrast, MR imaging is increasingly being used for pediatric female pelvic imaging.

Although high-resolution imaging may be obtained with transvaginal ultrasound, this technique is not generally appropriate for nonsexually active girls. MR imaging of soft tissue resolution is superior to that of computed tomography (CT), and there is no exposure to ionizing radiation. MR imaging has been shown to decrease the need for diagnostic laparoscopy or additional imaging by providing definitive imaging characterization of pathology [1]. Therefore, MR imaging is an excellent problem-solving tool when transabdominal ultrasound is indeterminate.

This chapter discusses MR imaging techniques for the pediatric female pelvis through review of normal anatomy and development of the female genital tract as well as congenital and acquired disorders.

Magnetic Resonance Imaging Techniques

Patient Preparation

The MR imaging protocol should target suspected pathology identified on prior imaging studies, most commonly ultrasound, keeping in mind the length of the examination. While school-age and adolescent patients can usually tolerate MR imaging, infants, young children, and those with conditions that may limit cooperativity often require sedation. When needed, sedation or anesthesia protocols determine patient preparation including pre-procedure arrival time and withholding of meals. Young infants may tolerate the feed and swaddle technique [2, 3], in which case withholding of both sleep and food is required for at least 4 hours prior to the procedure. The child is then fed and swaddled immediately prior to the examination to promote natural sleep during the examination.

Other patient preparation includes placement of an intravenous (IV) catheter for contrast, best performed prior to feeding and swaddling for infants. In the setting of a complex pelvic anomaly such as a persistent urogenital sinus or cloaca, catheters can be placed into perineal openings with fluid (including dilute contrast) or gel instilled into the body cavities during imaging to better define internal anatomy [4, 5].

MR Imaging Pulse Sequences and Protocols

Protocols vary by institution and MR vendor; however, there are fundamental principles that apply to female pelvic MR imaging (Table 15.1).

T2-weighted sequences without fat suppression performed along oblique coronal and sagittal planes with respect to the uterus are essential for assessment of uterine fundal and zonal anatomy, respectively [6]. If a 3D acquisition is possible, a

S. W. Gould
Department of Medical Imaging, Nemours Children's Health System, A. I. DuPont Hospital for Children, Wilmington, DE, USA

J. S. Calle Toro · S. J. Back
Department of Radiology, The Children's Hospital of Philadelphia, University of Pennsylvania, Philadelphia, PA, USA

D. J. Podberesky · M. Epelman (✉)
Department of Radiology, Nemours Children's Health System, Nemours Children's Hospital, University of Central Florida College of Medicine, Orlando, FL, USA
e-mail: monica.epelman@nemours.org

Table 15.1 Suggested pediatric female pelvic MR imaging protocol

Series	Orientation	Weighting	Comments
1	Multiplanar	T2, no FS	Rapid localizer
2[a]	Axial	T2, no FS	FSE or SSFSE
3[a]	Sagittal oblique	T2, no FS	Aligned to the endometrial canal from series 2
4[a]	Coronal (oblique)	T2 with or without FS	Aligned to the endometrial canal from series 3 for suspected uterine abnormality without FS or straight coronal with FS for adnexal mass
5	Axial	T1, no FS	Routine for landmarks and tissues characterization
6	Axial	In- and out-of-phase, T1 gradient recalled	For tissue characterization
7	Axial	DWI with 2 B-values and ADC map	Highest reasonable B value for one acquisition for improved ADC map
8	Axial	Susceptibility-weighted series	For assessment of blood products or endometriosis
9	Axial or coronal	FS heavily T2-weighted such as STIR	Assessment of musculoskeletal structures for pelvic pain cases
10	Axial	T1 with FS pre- and post-contrast dynamic series	If a pre-contrast series is not included in the protocol, a separate T1-weighted, fat-suppressed series should be obtained Also, subtraction of pre- and post-contrast series should be considered for lesions with hyperintense areas on pre-contrast T1-weighted series
11	Coronal	T1 FS post-contrast delayed	For additional lesion characterization

[a]These series can be obtained without fat suppression as a single 3D acquisition in the coronal or axial plane and then reformatted along the planes of the uterus to decrease overall scan time. 3D acquisitions take longer to acquire and require a higher degree of patient's cooperativity. Decisions regarding 3D series should be made when decisions regarding patient sedation are considered

FS fat suppression, *FSE* fast spin echo, *SSFSE* single-shot fast spin echo, *STIR* short tau inversion recovery

series acquired in the sagittal or axial plane can then be reformatted along the planes of the uterus, reducing the overall study length [7]. Axial T1- and T2-weighted non-fat-suppressed series are useful for identification of anatomic landmarks. Fat-suppressed T1-weighted images are important in the differentiation of fat and blood products, for example, in cases of hemorrhagic cysts, suspected endometriosis, or teratoma. Diffusion-weighted imaging (DWI) may be helpful in inflammatory or ischemic conditions [8, 9], and susceptibility-weighted sequences may be helpful in the evaluation of endometriosis [10, 11]. T1-weighted in- and opposed-phase chemical shift imaging can be highly useful to identify small amounts of fat. Due to the longer echo time of in-phase images, susceptibility artifact from gas or calcium is more noticeable on in-phase images, thus improving detection [6]. Utilization of multipoint Dixon sequences that obtain simultaneous T1-weighted in- and out-of-phase, fat-suppressed, and water-suppressed images or T2-weighted fat-suppressed and water-suppressed images can decrease overall scan time.

Malignant or inflammatory lesions can be better characterized with dynamic post-contrast sequences. In the setting of T1-weighted hyperintense areas on pre-contrast imaging, digital subtraction techniques can aid in identification of subtle areas of contrast enhancement. Bony contusions and muscle strains causing pelvic pain are best seen with fat-suppressed fluid-sensitive sequences such as short tau inversion recovery (STIR) [12].

Although respiratory motion is less of a concern in pelvic imaging than in abdominal imaging, newer techniques that can shorten acquisitions such as parallel imaging, radial or spiral acquisitions, or compressed sensing may help alleviate bulk body motion in awake or restless patients [3, 7, 13]. For some indications, such as complicated pelvic malformations, a technique with high spatial resolution is desirable; however, these sequences have longer acquisition times. The need for high spatial resolution should be considered when determining if a patient requires sedation.

Anatomy

Embryology

Prior to 7 weeks of gestation, the ovaries begin as undifferentiated gonads arising from primordial germ cells, sex cords, and epithelium in the retroperitoneum medial to the developing Wolffian and Müllerian structures [14] (Fig. 15.1). Traction of the round ligament causes the ovaries to ultimately descend into the pelvis due to the change in alignment of the adnexal structures caused by Müllerian duct fusion.

Between 7 and 8 weeks of gestation, ovarian differentiation is influenced by several genes and multiple hormones [14, 15]. Around two million primordial follicles are initially formed that decrease in number to around 400,000 by menarche. The follicles are located in the outer cortex of the ovary surrounded by granulosa cells that arise from sex cord cells.

The uterus, fallopian tubes, and upper two-thirds of the vagina develop from the Müllerian (paramesonephric) ducts, whereas the lower third of the vagina develops from the urogenital (UG) sinus (Fig. 15.2). Müllerian and Wolffian (mesonephric) structures develop in all fetuses during the 6th gestational week [14, 16]. The Wolffian ducts give rise to the ureteric buds and are intimately related to the developing Müllerian structures. In a female fetus with XX chromosomes, the absence of the sex-determining region of the Y chromo-

Fig. 15.1 Differentiation of the ovaries during the development of the female genital tract

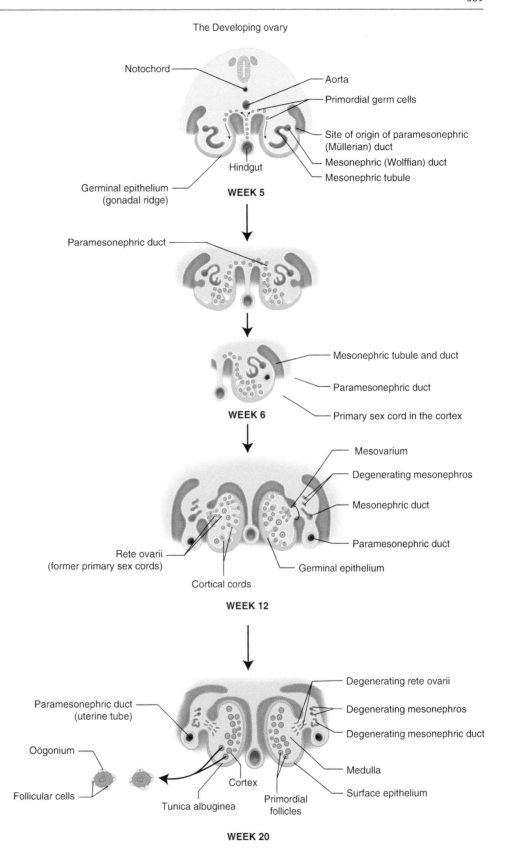

some results in ovarian gonadal differentiation. Without testes to produce testosterone and Müllerian inhibiting substance, the Wolffian structures begin to involute after the 6th gestational week, and the Müllerian ducts persist [14, 17].

Disruption of Müllerian organogenesis results in agenesis or hypoplasia of the uterus, fallopian tubes, and upper vagina on the involved side. Due to the close relationship of the developing Müllerian ducts and ureteric buds, renal and Müllerian

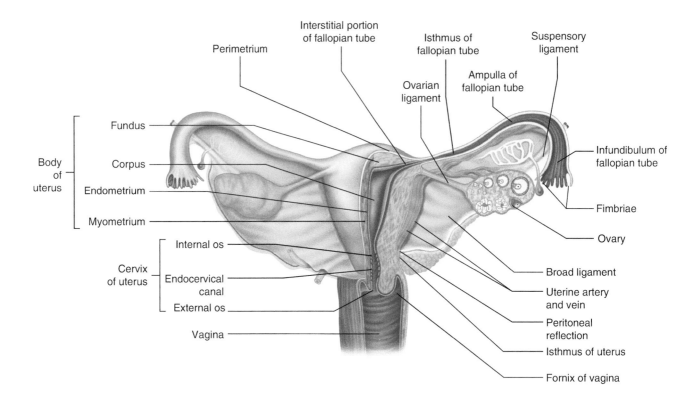

Fig. 15.2 Normal anatomy of the fully formed female genital tract

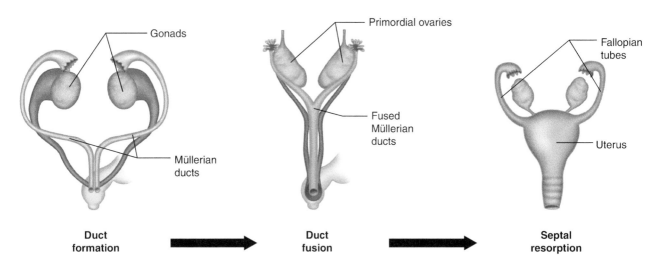

Fig. 15.3 Uterine anomalies during the development of the female genital tract. The female reproductive system develops from the fusion of the Müllerian ducts during embryo development. The septum that separates them eventually disappears. However, if alterations of any kind occur during this process in the fetus, uterine anomalies will develop, including didelphys, septate, or bicornuate uterus, among others

duct anomalies commonly coexist [16–19]. Between the 6th and 11th weeks of gestation, the paired Müllerian ducts fuse in the midline to form the uterus, cervix, and upper vagina [17] (Fig. 15.3). The uterovaginal septum resorbs between 9 and 12 weeks, completing the midline fusion [16, 17].

During the 4th to 6th weeks of gestation, the urorectal septum grows caudally to join the cloacal membrane, dividing the rectum from the urogenital sinus [16, 17, 20, 21]. The distal third of the vagina develops after the Müllerian ducts grow distally to contact the UG sinus. Uterine/upper vaginal and lower vaginal anomalies are not always related due to their different embryologic origins [16–19].

Normal Development and Anatomy

The ovaries are normally located in the ovarian fossae just inferior to the bifurcation of the common iliac arteries and posterior and lateral to the uterine fundus. Both the ovarian arteries and ascending branches of the uterine artery supply the ovaries [22]. The ovaries are covered by epithelium which overlies the compressed stromal layer of tunica albuginea [15].

Table 15.2 Ovarian size and appearance at different developmental stages [23]

Age	Ovarian volume	Follicles	MR appearance
Up to 3 months	1–3.5 mL	<9 mm diameter follicles may be visible	Visible small follicles
Pediatric (<7 years)	0.5–1.5 mL (>4 mL abnormal)	Usually fewer than 6 follicles <9 mm (≥6 follicles abnormal)	May be indiscernible from surrounding pelvic structures
Prepubertal	1–4 mL	Subcentimeter follicles up to 3 cm follicles	More mature appearance with intermediate to slightly T2 hyperintense stroma
Pubertal	2–6 mL	True follicles up to 3 cm	Mature appearance that varies with menstrual cycle and ovulation
Reproductive/ late adolescent	4–16 mL Mean 9.8 mL	True follicles up to 3 cm	Mature appearance that varies with menstrual cycle and ovulation

The medullary region consists of connective tissue and vessels. The cortical region of the ovary in a prepubertal girl consists of submillimeter follicles with granulosa cells forming the intervening stroma. Changes in ovarian size and appearance with age and development are discussed in Table 15.2.

Neonatal ovaries may have identifiable follicles visible on MR imaging as high T2-weighted signal intensity foci of varying size due to the influence of maternal hormones [7, 23]. During early childhood, the ovaries may be hard to differentiate from surrounding pelvic structures on MR imaging due to their small size and intermediate signal intensity. Subcentimeter high T2-weighted signal intensity structures may be seen within the ovaries of young girls, but these may not represent true follicles [18]. In older prepubertal girls, the ovaries are intermediate signal to hyperintense compared to muscle on T2-weighted images and may develop an adult appearance after 7–8 years of age. Because there is substantial overlap in the appearance of pre- and postpubertal ovaries, ovarian features are an unreliable indicator of precocious puberty [24]. However, in a girl under 7 years of age, an ovarian volume of >4 mL with 6 or more follicles should raise the possibility of premature sexual development [23].

Mature ovaries appear heterogeneously hyperintense to muscle on T2-weighted images (Fig. 15.4). The postpubertal ovarian cortex contains follicles in varying stages of maturation as well as corpora lutea and corpora albicans [6]. The stroma is mildly T2-weighted hyperintense to muscle, and immature follicles are quite hyperintense. The corpus luteum develops after mature (Graafian) follicle rupture and expulsion of the oocyte. The wall of the corpus luteum becomes thickened and hyperemic demonstrating high T2-weighted signal intensity and avid contrast enhancement due to enlargement of thecal and granulosa cells (Fig. 15.5). Follicular walls show milder enhancement than that seen in the wall of a corpus luteum. Any hemorrhage within the corpus luteum

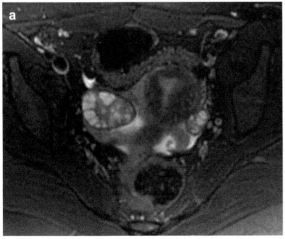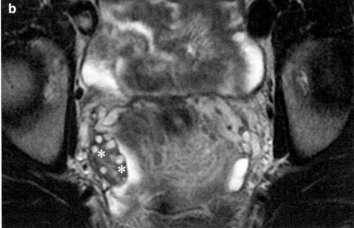

Fig. 15.4 (a) Normal appearance of the ovaries and uterus in a healthy 17-year-old girl. Axial T2-weighted fat-suppressed MR image reveals multiple hyperintense follicles of varying sizes. The uterus is anteverted and its entire length is visible. Notice the flat internal and external fundal contours. (b) Normal appearance of the ovary in another 17-year-old girl. Axial T2-weighted MR image shows cortical follicles in varying stages of maturation. The stroma (∗) is mildly hyperintense to muscle, and immature follicles are quite hyperintense

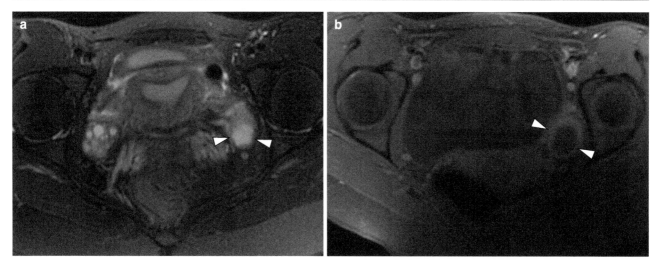

Fig. 15.5 Nonhemorrhagic corpus luteum in a 17-year-old girl. Axial T2-weighted (**a**) and axial T1-weighted fat-suppressed contrast-enhanced (**b**) MR images show a left ovarian cystic structure (*arrow-* *heads*) consistent with a nonhemorrhagic corpus luteum. The wall of the corpus luteum is slightly thickened and shows avid contrast enhancement

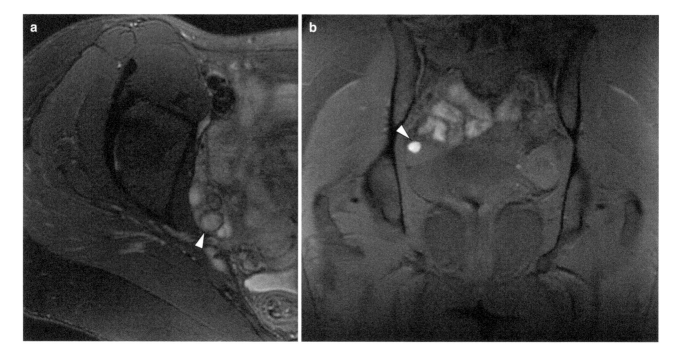

Fig. 15.6 Hemorrhagic corpus luteum (hemorrhagic cyst) in an asymptomatic 17-year-old girl. The images were obtained as part of a right hip MR imaging study. Axial T2-weighted MR image (**a**) shows a right ovarian cyst (*arrowhead*) with walls of intermediate signal intensity. Corresponding coronal T1-weighted fat-suppressed unenhanced MR image (**b**) shows high signal intensity of the ovarian cystic structure (*arrowhead*), a finding consistent with blood products

may appear hyperintense on T1-weighted images [6, 23] (Fig. 15.6). Later, the corpus luteum regresses with loss of T2-weighted hyperintensity and hyperemia. The corpus albicans represents fibrous tissue that replaces the corpus luteum and eventually involutes. Ovarian stroma enhances less than the follicular walls. On DWI, the ovarian stroma does restrict, with low signal intensity on the apparent diffusion coefficient (ADC) maps; however, follicles do not restrict and are bright on ADC maps [8].

Fallopian tubes are paired structures on either side of the pelvis extending from the pelvic sidewalls to the uterine cornua. There are four sections of the fallopian tube: the interstitial portion of the tube is surrounded by myometrium at the uterine corner a long isthmic portion of the tube courses laterally through the mesovarium; the ampullary segment is funnel-shaped and curves anterolateral to the ovary; and the infundibular portion extends posteriorly with its fimbriae covering the posteromedial aspect of the ovary. Normal fallopian tubes measure 10–12 cm in length and 4 mm in diameter in a postpubertal girl and are generally not well seen with any imaging modality unless there is a considerable amount of pelvic ascites [6, 25].

The uterus is a midline structure with the fundus postero-superior to the dome of the bladder with the lower body and cervix located between the posterior bladder wall and rectum. The peritoneum drapes over the uterus along its posterior surface down to the lower uterine segment and then continues posteriorly along the anterior surface of the rectum. This peritoneal reflection creates the pouch of Douglas, a peritoneal recess in which free pelvic fluid may collect. Due to the effect of maternal hormones, the endometrial canal may be seen as a T2-weighted hyperintense stripe in neonates, and a small amount of fluid may be seen in the endometrial cavity [24] (Table 15.3).

At birth, the cervix is approximately twice the length of the uterus [6, 18] (Fig. 15.7). As the effects of maternal hormones subside during the first year of life, the uterus assumes a tubular configuration and uniform T1- and T2-weighted isointensity with muscle with poor definition of the endometrial stripe [7, 24]. At this point, the uterus is the same length as the cervix [6]. During the prepubertal period, the uterus begins to lengthen (Fig. 15.8). At puberty, the uterus develops the pear shape seen in maturity, with the fundus wider than the cervix, and it lengthens becoming longer than the cervix [6, 18, 24].

The zonal anatomy of the uterus is evident on T2-weighted images during puberty (Fig. 15.9). There is considerable cyclical variation of the endometrium, the innermost uterine layer [6, 10]. The T2-weighted hyperintense, mildly enhancing appearance of the endometrium is due to the presence of mucinous glands [7]. During the proliferative phase of the menstrual cycle, estrogen stimulates gradual thickening of the endometrium [18]. After ovulation, during the secretory (luteal) phase, progesterone stimulates further thickening. The endometrium is at its thickest just prior to menstruation, when the endometrium then sloughs and non-enhancing debris and fluid may be seen in the canal. The endometrium is thinnest at the end of menstruation. The next layer is the junctional zone that represents the inner, compact layer of myometrium that measures up to 12 mm in thickness. This layer has low T2-weighted signal intensity due to low water content and normally appears well-marginated [6]. By comparison, the outer myometrial layer is intermediate in signal on T1- and T2-weighted images [23].

The cervix is contiguous with the lower uterine segment or body and the internal os protrudes into the upper third of the vagina in the midline. The cervix has three layers, like the uterus, that are visible on T2-weighted images in postpubertal girls [6]. The endocervix exhibits T2-weighted hyperintensity and enhancement due to the high number of mucinous glands. The inner cervical stroma is compressed and appears low in signal intensity on T2-weighted images, while the outer stromal layer is intermediate in signal intensity [6].

The vagina is situated between the bladder neck and urethra anteriorly and the rectum and anus posteriorly, connecting the cervix with the vulvar vestibule [26]. The vagina also has three layers: the innermost mucosa, the muscularis, and the adventitia [27]. On axial T2-weighted images, the vagina has an H-shaped configuration with a mildly hyperintense

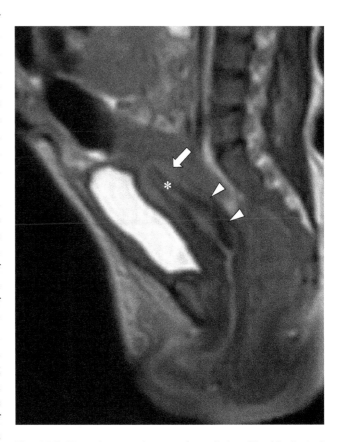

Fig. 15.7 Normal neonatal uterus in a 3-day-old girl. Sagittal T2-weighted MR image shows the normal appearance of the neonatal uterus. The endometrial stripe (*) is well-visualized in most instances. Notice the relative prominence of the cervix (*arrowheads*), which is wider than the fundus (*arrow*)

Table 15.3 Stage of uterine development [23]

Age	Uterine shape	Uterine length (cm)	Endometrium	Uterine length: cervical length
Neonate	Tubular	3.5	Mildly T2-weighted hyperintense	1–1.5:2
Pediatric	Tubular	1–3	Ill-defined	1:1
Prepubertal	Bulbous	3–4.5	Ill-defined – visible stripe	1–1.5:1
Pubertal	Pear-shaped	5–8	Mature zonal anatomy	2:1
Late pubertal/reproductive	Pear-shaped	8–9	Mature zonal anatomy	2:1

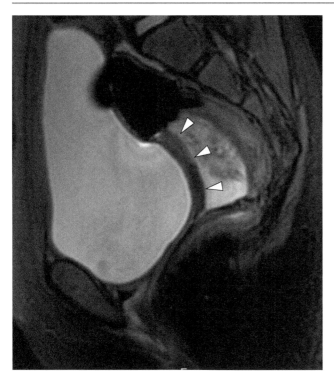

Fig. 15.8 Normal prepubertal uterus in an 8-year-old girl. Sagittal T2-weighted MR image shows the normal prepubertal, tubular appearance of the uterus (*arrowheads*). The uterus is diffusely hypointense and the endometrial stripe is not well seen

inner mucosal layer, a low signal intensity muscularis and a heterogeneously hyperintense perivaginal venous plexus. On sagittal images, the anterior vaginal wall extends superiorly, anterior to the exocervix to form the anterior vaginal fornix. Similarly, the posterior wall extends upward to form the posterior vaginal fornix. Vaginal length can range from 4 to 12 cm in postpubertal girls [26]. The postpubertal vaginal appearance on MR imaging varies with the menstrual cycle under hormonal influence [27]. The mucosal layer is mildly T2-weighted hyperintense and exhibits mild enhancement that appears most prominent during the mid-secretory phase [26]. The hymen is usually an incomplete septation that traverses the junction of the middle and lower thirds of the vagina and is usually not visible on imaging [15]. It represents a vestigial remnant of the vaginal plate that is canalized when the Müllerian ducts extend downward to meet the urogenital sinus.

Anatomic Variants

Müllerian Duct Anomalies Müllerian duct anomalies (MDAs) arise from disrupted development of the Müllerian ductal system as shown in Table 15.4. Because some conditions may be asymptomatic, the true prevalence is unknown [7]. While the incidence

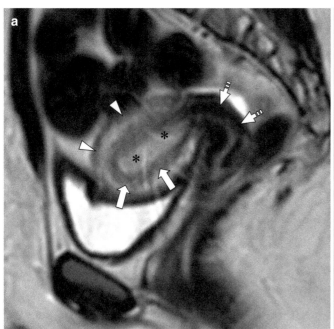
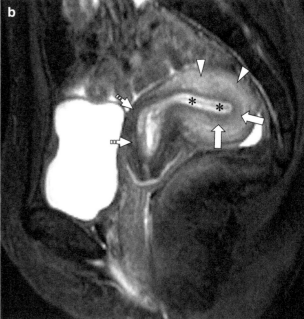

Fig. 15.9 Sagittal T2-weighted MR images obtained in a 14-year-old girl (**a**) and in a 17-year-old girl (**b**) show the normal zonal anatomy of the postpubertal uterus in anteversion (**a**) and retroversion (**b**). The endometrium (∗) is hyperintense, and the subjacent junctional zone

(*arrows*) or inner myometrium has low signal intensity. The inner myometrium is contiguous with the fibromuscular stroma in the cervix (*dashed arrows*), which is also hypointense. The outer myometrium (*arrowheads*) reveals intermediate signal intensity

Table 15.4 Summary of Müllerian duct anomalies (MDAs)

Embryology	Anomaly	Abnormal structures	ASRM class
MD aplasia	Fallopian tube, uterine, cervical, or upper vaginal hypoplasia	Aplasia or hypoplasia of any one or combination of the fallopian tubes, uterus, cervix, and/or vagina	Class I
Unilateral MD hypoplasia/aplasia	Unicornuate uterus	The horn may be absent or rudimentary and may or may not communicate with the primary horn	Class II
Failure of midline fusion of the MDs	Uterus didelphys	Two uterine horns separated by a deep cleft; one may be obstructed. Two cervices Longitudinal vaginal septum is common, and one side may be obstructed as in OHVIRA and Herlyn-Wunder-Werlich	Class III
Incomplete midline fusion of the MDs	Bicornuate uterus	Two uterine horns that fuse at some point above the internal os There is a fundal cleft of at least 10 mm. There may be one (unicollis) or two (bicollis) cervices	Class IV
Persistence of all or part of the midline septum	Septate uterus	Persistence of all or part of the intrauterine septum The fundus may be concave but has no cleft	Class V
Minimal septal persistence	Arcuate uterus	Near complete septal resorption with mild concavity of the fundal contour of the uterine cavity	Class VI

MD Müllerian duct, *ASRM* American Society for Reproductive Medicine, *OHVIRA* Obstructed hemivagina with ipsilateral renal agenesis

in an unselected population has been reported to be 6.7%, the incidence may be as high as 25% in patients with a history of prior miscarriage or infertility [15, 17, 19].

Classification of MDAs is controversial. The most widely accepted system is the classification created by the American Fertility Society, now the American Society of Reproductive Medicine (ASRM), which groups the anomalies based on uterine anatomy and impact on potential pregnancy outcome [28] (Fig. 15.10). However, this system has limited utility in children because it fails to take into account obstructive abnormalities of the cervix and vagina that create symptoms presenting in childhood; and criteria used to describe the morphology of the adult uterus may not be applicable to immature uteri [16, 18, 19].

A segmental approach is therefore recommended in children with careful description of anatomy and abnormalities identified at each anatomic level [17–19]. A search for related urinary tract abnormalities is also warranted in these children due to the high frequency of associated abnormalities including horseshoe kidney, ectopia, dysplasia, and urinary tract dilation [16–19]. Multidisciplinary assessment is best in these cases for thorough evaluation and correct diagnosis because the best chance for preservation or restoration of fertility lies in the initial attempt at repair [16, 19].

Imaging of the neonatal uterus for a suspected MDA may be successful with transabdominal ultrasound due to the temporary uterine stimulation caused by maternal and placental hormones; however, once that effect subsides the small uterine size and lack of definition of the endometrial canal preclude definitive evaluation with any modality [18, 19]. When MR imaging is performed during or after

puberty once the uterus and vagina have a more mature, defined appearance, it is highly useful in the evaluation of MDAs due to its high soft tissue contrast and multiplanar imaging capability [17]. In this setting, MR imaging has a very high diagnostic success rate, approaching 100% [19], and therefore, follow-up imaging is recommended after puberty for patients with a suspected MDA at birth.

Müllerian duct aplasia or hypoplasia results in fallopian tube, uterine, cervical, and/or upper vaginal absence or hypoplasia [17, 18]. This class of anomalies accounts for 5–10% of MDAs and is associated with primary infertility [15, 17–19]. Complete absence of the Müllerian duct structures is known as type 1 Mayer-Rokitansky-Kuster-Hauser (MRKH) syndrome [17, 18]. These patients have normal ovarian function with a normal phenotype, but present with primary amenorrhea (Fig. 15.11). Fertility cannot be restored in these patients, but sexual function can be made possible by vaginal lengthening or creation of a neovagina [16, 17]. The goals of imaging are to assess for rudimentary structures, especially a hypoplastic, obstructed uterus, as well as to assess vaginal length for preoperative planning. Assessment for associated renal abnormalities should be performed, as well. If there are associated renal, ear, or skeletal anomalies, then type II MRKH should be considered, also called MURCS association (Müllerian duct aplasia, unilateral renal agenesis, cervical somite dysplasia association) [18, 19].

Unilateral incomplete or absent Müllerian duct development results in a unicornuate uterus, accounting for approximately 20% of MDAs [17, 19] (Fig. 15.12). The involved horn may be absent, but 65% of cases have a

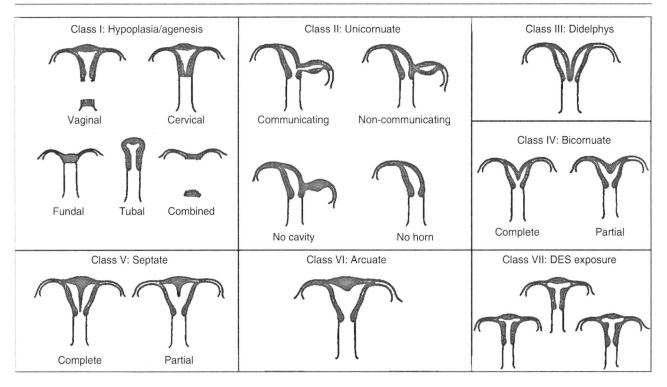

Fig. 15.10 Classification system for Müllerian anomalies developed by the American Society for Reproductive Medicine (formerly known as the American Fertility Society). (Reproduced with permission. Copyright© 2005 by the American Society for Reproductive Medicine). All rights reserved. No part of this presentation may be reproduced or transmitted in any form or by any means, electronic or mechanical, including photocopying, recording, or any information storage and retrieval system without permission in writing from the American Society for Reproductive Medicine, 1209 Montgomery Highway, Birmingham, AL 35216

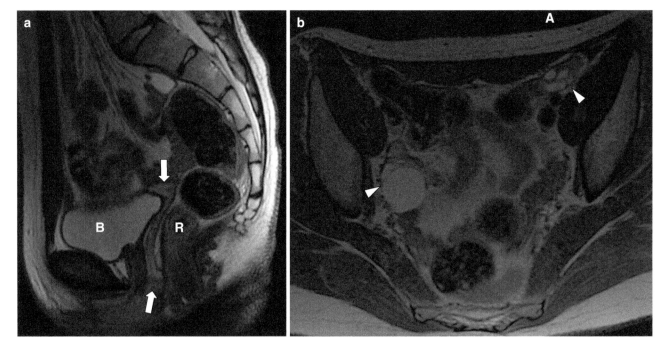

Fig. 15.11 Meyer-Rokitansky-Kuster-Hauser syndrome in a 16-year-old girl. (a) Sagittal T2-weighted MR image shows a hypoplastic, blind-ending vagina (*arrows*) coursing between the rectum (R) and the bladder (B). No normal uterine tissue is identified. (b) Axial T2-weighted MR image shows bilateral normal ovaries (*arrowheads*), which are responsible for the normal female phenotype

hypoplastic horn [16, 19]. Almost 50% of hypoplastic horns have an endometrial canal. Approximately 70% of rudimentary horns do not communicate with the primary,

contralateral horn. As a result, there is an increased incidence of endometriosis in these patients due to retrograde menstruation [16, 19], and affected patients may present with pelvic pain from the obstructed horn (Fig. 15.13). An obstructed rudimentary horn may be seen as a pelvic mass in neonates. Surgical resection of rudimentary horns that contain an endometrial canal is required due to the possibility of both endometriosis and pregnancy implantation in the abnormal horn [17]. MR imaging shows the normally developed horn to be an elongated, banana- or cigar-shaped structure lying off-midline with normal uterine zonal anatomy [16, 17, 19]. The MR imaging appearance of the rudimentary horn varies [17]. If zonal anatomy is present in the rudimentary horn, then an endometrial canal is present. If obstructed, the rudimentary horn can appear as a mass with blood products often appearing hyperintense on T1-weighted series [15, 16, 19]. There is a high incidence of ipsilateral renal anomalies in these patients [16, 17].

Complete failure of fusion of the Müllerian ducts results in a uterus didelphys (Fig. 15.14) with two widely separated horns with a deep fundal cleft, two cervices, and often a longitudinal vaginal septum [17, 18]. This anomaly accounts for 5% of MDAs [15, 19]. There may be a transverse component of the vaginal septum on one side, as well, with unilateral hydro- or hematometrocolpos. These patients typically present with dysmenorrhea, a pelvic mass, and possibly hematosalpinx and endometriosis, as well. However, affected pediatric patients

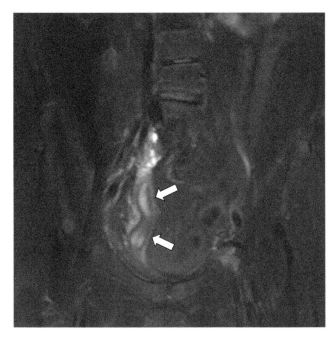

Fig. 15.12 Unicornuate uterus in a peripubertal girl demonstrating a single uterine horn with normal appearance. Coronal T2-weighted fat-suppressed MR image shows the typical banana-shaped appearance of a single, nonobstructed unicornuate uterus (*arrows*). No rudimentary horn is seen in this case

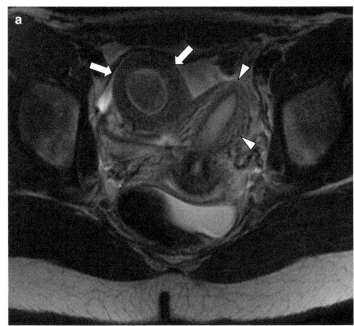

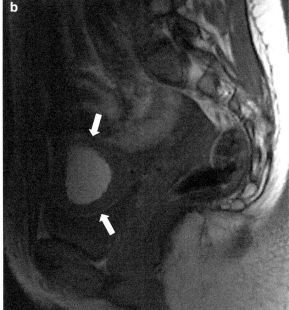

Fig. 15.13 Unicornuate uterus with an obstructed, noncommunicating right uterine horn in a 15-year-old girl who presented with right lower quadrant pain. Axial T2-weighted (**a**) and sagittal T1-weighted (**b**) MR images show retained blood products within the obstructed, noncom-municating right horn (*arrows*). The left uterine horn (*arrowheads*) has the typical banana-shape and shows normal zonal anatomy. It is nonob-structed and functional

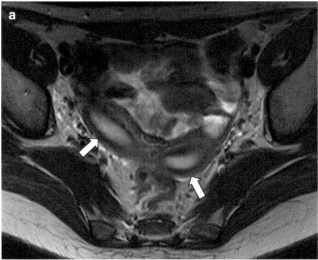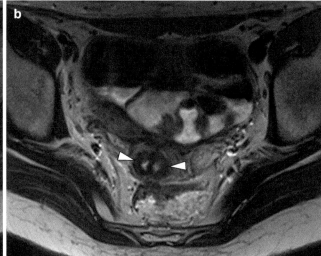

Fig. 15.14 Uterus didelphys in an asymptomatic postpubertal 17-year-old girl. The images are part of a hip study. Axial T2-weighted MR images (**a, b**) show widely divergent uterine horns (*arrows* in **a**) sepa-rated by a very deep fundal cleft caused by failure of Müllerian duct fusion. Two cervices are present (*arrowheads* in **b**), consistent with uterus didelphys

are not amenorrheic due to the patent hemivagina. MR imaging in these pediatric patients shows high signal intensity T1-weighted contents within the dilated, obstructed hemivagina, within the ipsilateral uterine horn, and possibly also in a dilated fallopian tube [17]. Treatment is resection of the vaginal septum relieving the obstruction with careful observation during pregnancy [16]. There is a high association with ipsilateral renal agenesis, a syndrome known as OHVIRA (obstructed hemivagina ipsilateral renal agenesis) or Herlyn-Werner-Wunderlich syndrome [15, 16, 19] (Fig. 15.15). In cases without vaginal obstruction, affected pediatric patients may be asymptomatic. In nonobstructed didelphys uteri, both horns demonstrate normal zonal anatomy [16, 17].

A bicornuate uterus occurs when fusion of the Müllerian ducts is incomplete and accounts for approximately 10% of MDAs [17] (Fig. 15.16). In a bicornuate uterus, there is at least some degree of communication between the endometrial cavities, although there may be two cervices (bicollis) and a vaginal septum. In this setting, differentiation from a didelphys is difficult, although the horns are less widely divergent [16] (Fig. 15.17). According to the ASRM classification, there should be at least a 10 mm cleft in the uterine fundus to classify a uterus as bicornuate [28]; however, this criterion may

be difficult to apply in a small, immature uterus [16, 18, 19] (Fig. 15.18). MR imaging demonstrates two horns that are less splayed than in a didelphys uterus, but the fundal cleft should measure at least 10 mm on coronal imaging [16, 17]. Communication of the endometrial canals may not be appreciable by imaging. Careful assessment should be made to assess for the presence of two cervices and a vaginal septum. Instillation of vaginal gel may help demonstrate a vaginal septum, if appropriate [15–17].

Failure of resorption of the uterovaginal septum gives rise to a septate uterus, the most common MDA comprising 50–55% of cases [16–19] (Fig. 15.19). The septum may be partial or complete and may even extend into the upper vagina. There is a high association with miscarriage in this condition; therefore, recognition and differentiation from a bicornuate uterus is essential [17, 19]. On MR imaging, assessment of the external uterine fundal contour is necessary to exclude the presence of a cleft of 10 mm or more, particularly in the rare co-occurrence of a duplicate cervix [16, 17, 19]. Evaluation of the nature of the septum is required because fibrous septa appear low in signal intensity on T2-weighted sequences and are resectable transvaginally, but septa containing intermediate T2-weighted signal intensity myometrium require a transabdominal approach

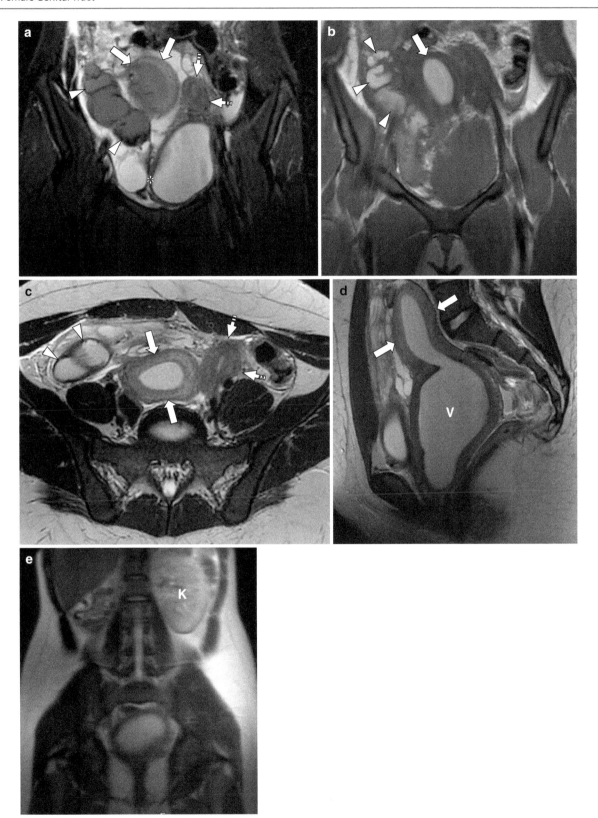

Fig. 15.15 A 14-year-old girl who presented with abdominal pain and distension, but a history of normal, though irregular menstrual periods. Coronal T2-weighted MR image with fat suppression (**a**) coronal T1 (**b**) and axial (**c**) and sagittal (**d**) T2-weighted MR images show a markedly distended right uterine horn (*arrows*) and vagina (V) with blood products consistent with hematometrocolpos. Blood products are also appreciated in the right fallopian tube (*arrowheads* in **a**, **b**), which is markedly distended. These aforementioned findings are consistent with hematosalpinx. The left uterine horn (*dashed arrows*) shows normal zonal anatomy, and it is unobstructed. Coronal T2-weighted MR image (**e**) reveals a solitary left kidney (K) showing compensatory hypertrophy

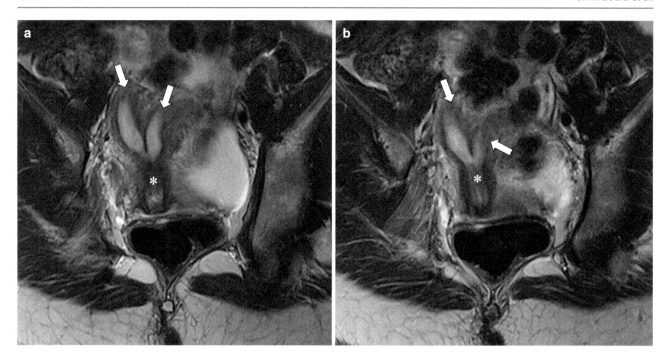

Fig. 15.16 Bicornuate uterus in a 13-year-old girl who presented with vague abdominal pain. Axial T2-weighted MR images (**a, b**) show two widely divergent uterine horns (*arrows*) with two distinct endometrial cavities joining together within the lower uterine segment to form a single cervix (*)

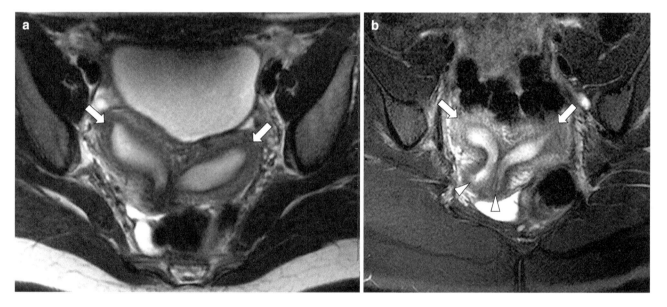

Fig. 15.17 (**a**) Axial T2-weighted and (**b**) coronal-oblique T2-weighted fat-suppressed MR images show widely divergent uterine horns (**a, b**, *arrows*) with a deep fundal cleft. Two cervices (**b**, *arrowheads*) are present. In this setting, differentiation between a bicornuate, bicollis, and a didelphys uterus is difficult

for resection [16, 17, 19]. Due to the smaller size and less developed zonal anatomy of prepubertal uteri, definitive imaging evaluation is best performed after puberty in cases of suspected bicornuate or septate uteri for improved accuracy [19].

An arcuate uterus (Fig. 15.20) is considered a normal variant by some, but represents minimal septal persistence at the fundus resulting in a saddle-shaped indentation of the

fundal aspect of the endometrial canal [16, 19]. The external fundus has a normal convex contour with homogeneous, isointense T2-weighted signal intensity and no hypointense septum [16, 17, 19].

Congenital Vaginal Septa and Imperforate Hymen
Congenital septa in the vagina may be longitudinal due to incomplete Müllerian duct fusion or septal resorption as

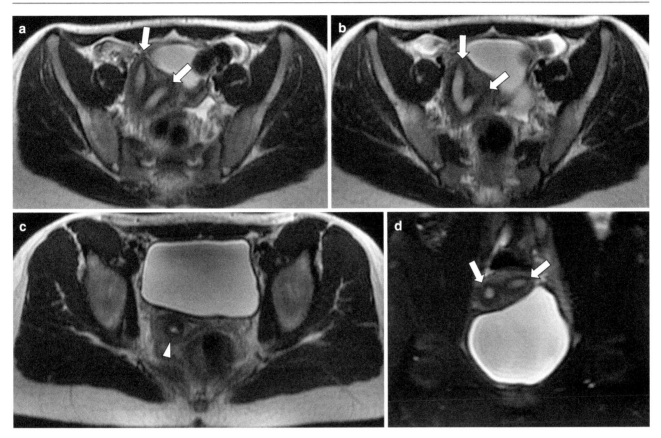

Fig. 15.18 MR imaging obtained in a 10-year-old girl who presented with right lower quadrant pain to exclude appendicitis. Axial T2-weighted (**a–c**) and coronal T2-weighted fat-suppressed (**d**) MR images show an apparent bicornuate unicollis uterus with two divergent uterine horns (*arrows*) and a single cervix (*arrowhead* in **c**). Technically, this uterus does not fulfill the criteria for a bicornuate uterus because the external fundal cleft is not deep enough. This is why in the pediatric population, accurate, descriptive terminology should be used rather than rigid classification system

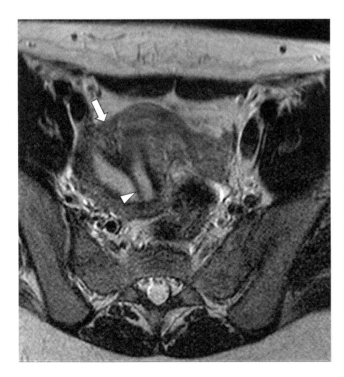

Fig. 15.19 Septate uterus in an 11-year-old girl. Axial T2-weighted MR image shows a separate uterus. The *arrowhead* denotes the hypointense fibrous septum. The *arrow* shows a flattened outer external contour without a fundal cleft

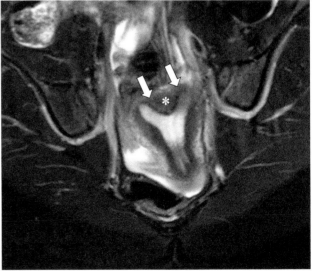

Fig. 15.20 Arcuate uterus in a 17-year-old girl. Axial T2-weighted MR image shows an arcuate uterus which is considered by some to be a normal variant resulting from incomplete resorption of the uterovaginal septum. There is a smooth, mild indentation (*) at the inner fundus and the external fundal contour (*arrows*) is convex, without a cleft

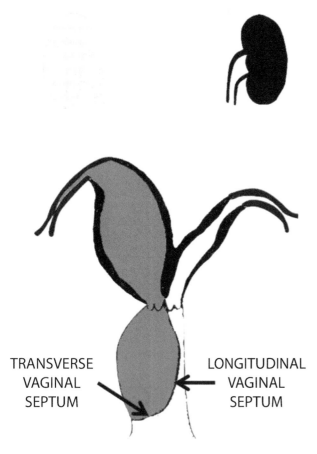

TRANSVERSE
VAGINAL
SEPTUM

LONGITUDINAL
VAGINAL
SEPTUM

Fig. 15.21 Schematic representation of the anatomy of congenital vaginal septa in the setting of OHVIRA (obstructed hemivagina and ipsilateral renal anomaly) or Herlyn-Wunder-Werlich syndrome. The longitudinal vaginal septum, which is the result of failure of lateral fusion of the Müllerian ducts, courses in the craniocaudal dimension. The transverse vaginal septum, which is the result of failed vertical fusion between the Müllerian duct and the urogenital sinus, is typically the source of vaginal obstruction, which characteristically occurs on the same side as the renal agenesis. (Reproduced from Epelman et al. [19] with permission)

described above, transverse due to incomplete fusion of Müllerian duct and urogenital sinus elements, or a combination with obstruction of one hemivagina and uterus as in OHVIRA [15, 18, 19, 26, 29] (Fig. 15.21). Vaginal septa may occur in isolation or along with MDAs, as described above. Transversely oriented septa uncommonly present in infancy as hydrocolpos, seen as T1-weighted hypointense and T2-weighted hyperintense signal in the vagina, and sometimes uterus (hydrometrocolpos). Obstructing septa most commonly present at menarche as primary amenorrhea with hematometrocolpos and pelvic pain [29]. MR imaging shows complex fluid in the vagina and uterus that demonstrates high T1-weighted signal intensity indicative of blood products (Fig. 15.22). This fluid may also distend the fallopian tubes (hematosalpinx).

Imperforate hymen is the result of a completely intact remnant of the vaginal plate and is the most common congenital anomaly of the female genital tract with an incidence of 0.1% [26]. Imperforate hymen is not a MDA, and it is most commonly diagnosed clinically at menarche when the patient develops cyclic pelvic pain and primary amenorrhea, and it has a characteristic appearance on clinical examination [7]. Ultrasound is typically sufficient to confirm the clinical diagnosis. MR imaging may be sporadically helpful if there is suspicion of an MDA (Fig. 15.23). Similar to a vaginal septum, high T1-weighted signal intensity blood products are seen in the vagina and often in the uterus, representing hematometrocolpos. Treatment consists of partial resection of the membrane [15].

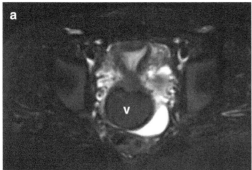
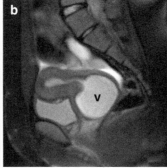
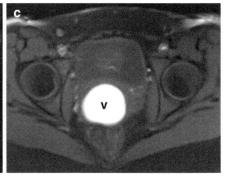

Fig. 15.22 Transverse vaginal septum in a 13-year-old girl who presented with cyclic pelvic pain and primary amenorrhea. Axial STIR (**a**), sagittal T2-weighted fat-suppressed (**b**), and axial T1-weighted fat-suppressed (**c**) MR images show a distended vagina (V) filled with blood products. The most caudal portion of the dilated vagina is not as low as the most caudal aspect of the bladder, a finding that should raise suspicion for a transverse vaginal septum

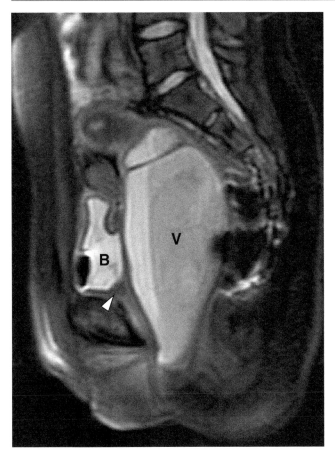

Fig. 15.23 Imperforate hymen in a 13-year-old. Sagittal T2-weighted MR image with fat suppression shows a distended vagina (V) with a fluid level, which extends well below the level of the bladder (B) neck (*arrowhead*)

Spectrum of Female Genital Tract Disorders

Congenital Female Genital Tract Disorders

Congenital Cysts Congenital cysts include fetal/neonatal ovarian cysts, paraovarian cysts, and vaginal cysts. Simple fetal ovarian cysts are round and thin-walled [30, 31]. They typically present in the third trimester and are believed to be the result of exposure to maternal hormones. If the cyst measures 20 mm or less, it is considered to represent a physiologic maturing follicle [31]. The "daughter cyst" sign is reported to be pathognomonic for fetal ovarian cysts [31] (Fig. 15.24). Most of these cysts spontaneously regress. Fetal and/or postnatal cyst aspiration is controversial [31–33]. Neonatal surgery is reserved for complications, which usually occur with cysts larger than 5 cm. If surgery is needed, ovarian function preservation should be attempted. The role for MR imaging is limited in these cases, but may be helpful with fetal evaluation for female genitalia as well as normal urinary and gastrointestinal tracts [31]. MR imaging in the neonatal period cannot reliably differentiate an ovarian cyst from cysts of mesenteric origin or enteric duplication cysts but may confirm the presence of solid or hemorrhagic components. Ovarian neoplasms are rare in neonates [30].

Paraovarian cysts may develop from Wolffian, Müllerian, or mesothelial structures and lie in the adnexa, but are not part of the ovary [34–36]. Because the cysts are not functional, they do not exhibit the cyclic changes expected of ovarian cysts. On MR imaging, there is a defined cyst wall often abutting

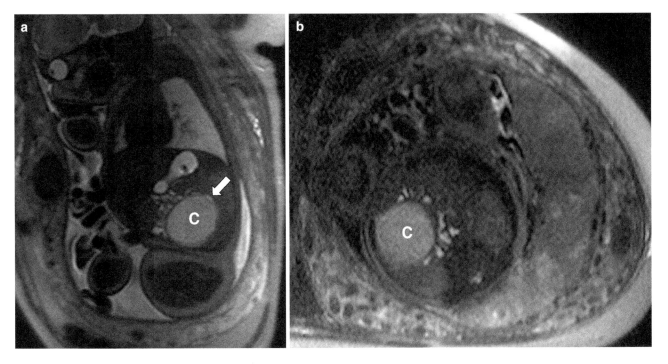

Fig. 15.24 Ovarian cyst in 37 weeks gestation female fetus. Sagittal (**a**) and axial (**b**) T2-weighted MR images show a well-circumscribed cyst (C) inferior to the liver, anterior and inferior to the kidney, and off-midline in the abdomen. A "daughter cyst" sign is indicated by the *arrow* on (**a**)

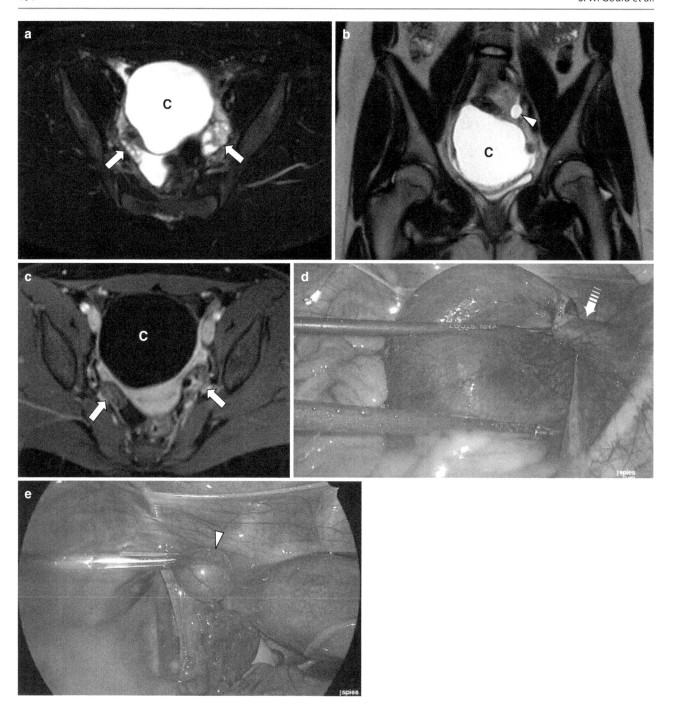

Fig. 15.25 Paraovarian, fallopian tube cyst with associated fallopian tube torsion in a 12-year-old girl who presented with marked right lower quadrant pain. (**a**) Axial T2-weighted, fat-suppressed MR image shows a large simple-appearing cystic (C) structure in close proximity but separate from the right ovary. Both ovaries (*arrows*) are normal in size and MR imaging appearance. (**b**) Coronal T2-weighted MR image redemonstrates the large right hemipelvic cyst and an additional smaller cyst (*arrowhead*) on the left. (**c**) Axial T1-weighted fat-suppressed post-contrast MR image shows adequate enhancement of both ovaries (*arrows*) and enhancement of the thin large cyst wall. (**d**) During laparoscopy, the large, right hemipelvis cystic structure was found to be a right paraovarian, fallopian tube cyst that had resulted in the right fallopian tube being torsed. Note the deep purple color of the cyst and torsed tube (*dashed arrow*). (**e**) The left fallopian tube appeared normal; however, a small cyst (*arrowhead*) was noted around the left fallopian tube

the ovary, with cyst fluid that is T1-weighted hypointense and T2-weighted hyperintense [35, 36]. Paraovarian cysts should not exhibit solid components, wall thickening, enhancement, or hemorrhage. If the cyst can be separated from the ovary, then the diagnosis of paraovarian cyst can be made; however, clear separation may not be possible with large cysts causing mass effect on the adnexa [34, 35]. Paraovarian cysts may act as lead points for tubal torsion [6] (Fig. 15.25).

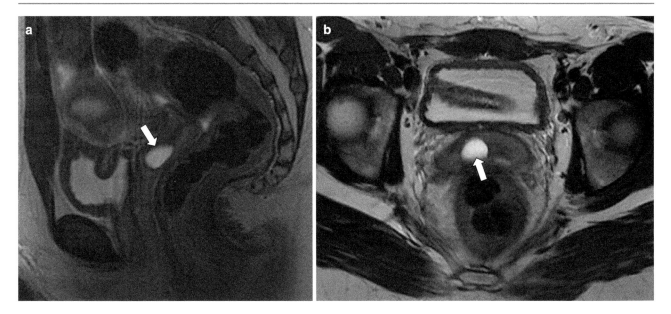

Fig. 15.26 Gartner's duct cyst in a 17-year-old girl. Sagittal (**a**) and axial (**b**) T2-weighted MR images of the pelvis show a Gartner's duct cyst (*arrows*) originating from the right anterior lateral wall of the vagina

Congenital vaginal cysts may arise from Wolffian or Müllerian remnants or can be epidermal inclusion cysts [18, 37]. Gartner's duct cysts are Wolffian remnants that lie along the anterolateral wall of the vagina, often above the pubic symphysis [27, 29] (Fig. 15.26). This differentiates them from Bartholin cysts that arise secondarily within glands located in the lower vagina, along either side, more caudal and posterior [26, 37, 38]. Bartholin gland cysts are formed by obstruction of mucin-secreting glands of the distal vagina, at or below the level of the pubic symphysis. Although MR imaging is rarely used for evaluation of these cysts, they may be found incidentally. Because Gartner's duct cysts are the result of disordered Wolffian duct resorption, they may be associated with ipsilateral renal anomalies and should prompt imaging evaluation of the urinary tract [7, 27]. Vaginal cysts of any origin most commonly have a typical, homogeneous, thin-walled appearance with low T1-weighted and high T2-weighted signal intensity, unless the contents are proteinaceous or hemorrhagic, in which case they may be heterogeneous and bright on T1-weighted images [37]. With secondary infection, the cyst wall may thicken and enhance [18, 26, 27, 29, 37, 38] (Fig. 15.27).

Cloacal Malformations and Urogenital Sinus Disruption of the distal growth of the urorectal septum to meet the cloacal membrane may result in a wide range of abnormalities of the distal gastrointestinal (GI), urinary, and reproductive tracts [18–20, 39, 40]. If two perineal openings are present, a persistent urogenital sinus or cloaca variant should be considered with a single opening for the vagina and urinary tract with a discrete anus [20, 39, 40] (Fig. 15.28). If a single opening is identified, a persistent cloaca should be consid-

ered with communication of all three tracts [39, 40]. Similarly, if a cystic pelvic mass and ascites or hydrometrocolpos are identified on prenatal imaging, a urogenital sinus or cloacal anomaly should be considered [18–21, 39, 40]. Imaging in these children should assess the degree of communication between the respective tracts. There is an increased likelihood of associated Müllerian duct, renal, and spinal anomalies in these children which requires imaging evaluation [21, 39]. Urogenital sinus and cloacal malformations occur in phenotypically female patients; however, male patients with congenital adrenal hyperplasia are included in this group [39]. Some genetically female patients with a cloacal anomaly may exhibit virilization of the external genitalia, although the cause of the virilization is unknown [19, 39].

MR imaging of neonates with a persistent urogenital sinus demonstrates hydrometrocolpos and possibly hydrosalpinx with fluid in the dilated vagina and uterus related to outflow obstruction [18, 19, 39, 40]. Fluid-fluid levels in the bladder and/or vagina may be present due to admixture of urine with uterovaginal secretions [19]. In a cloacal malformation, meconium in the urinary bladder and vagina may create a fluid-fluid level in the bladder and/or vagina, and cloacal stenosis can result in retrograde flow of urine into the vagina and uterus [20, 39]. Imaging assessment of the communication of the reproductive, urinary, and GI tracts is traditionally performed under fluoroscopy; however, MR imaging can be utilized to evaluate communication between structures using instillation of intracavitary gel or dilute contrast combined with high-resolution and multiplanar imaging [21]. MR imaging can simultaneously identify associated Müllerian duct and renal anomalies. High T1-weighted signal intensity meconium below the

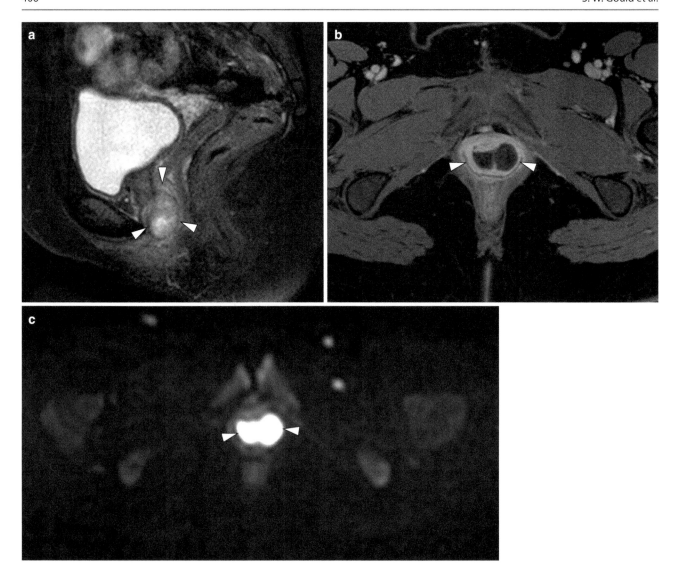

Fig. 15.27 Infected Bartholin's gland cyst in a 16-year-old girl who presented with pelvic and perineal pain. Sagittal T2-weighted fat-suppressed (**a**) and axial T1-weighted post-contrast (**b**) MR images show a thick-walled Bartholin's gland cyst (*arrowheads*) with a thin septation and surrounding inflammatory changes. The cyst shows restricted diffusion on DWI (**c**). Overall findings are consistent with superimposed infection. The patient was taken to the operating room, and purulent material was drained. *N. gonorrhoeae* grew on cultures

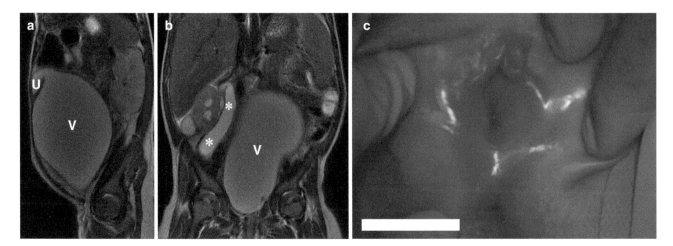

Fig. 15.28 Persistent urogenital sinus with a single orifice for the bladder outflow and vagina in a 20-month-old girl who presented with abdominal distension and pain. (**a**) Sagittal T2-weighted MR image demonstrates a large hydrometrocolpos with fluid distending the uterus (U) and vagina (V). (**b**) Coronal T2-weighted MR image shows the massively fluid distended vagina (V) and right ureteral (*) dilation. (**c**) Examination under anesthesia revealed a persistent urogenital sinus with a single orifice for the bladder outflow and vagina. The urethra drained high in the vagina. There is clitoromegaly, and the rectum is anteriorly positioned

level of the hydrometrocolpos on fetal MR imaging favors a urogenital sinus over a cloacal anomaly [18, 20, 39, 40]; however, a small fistula may not be detected with this technique. In the setting of a larger communication between the urogenital sinus and rectum, the expected T1-weighted hyperintense signal of meconium is less evident due to mixing with urine [39, 40].

Preoperative imaging of urogenital sinus and cloacal anomalies establishes baseline anatomy and imaging appearance in these patients prior to loss of tissue planes post-reconstruction [18, 19, 21]. Initial treatment consists of decompression of the genitourinary tract, diverting colostomy, and relief of ureteral reflux if severe [21, 39]. Eventual repair involves separation of the tracts and creation of discrete perineal openings to provide urinary and fecal continence as well as sexual function. Anatomic findings including the lengths of fistulous connections, associated Müllerian duct, spine, and renal anomalies, the integrity of the pelvic floor musculature, and the functionality of sacral nerves determine the approach to surgical repair [15, 21].

Infectious Female Genital Tract Disorders

Pelvic Inflammatory Disease and Tubo-ovarian Abscess
Pelvic inflammatory disease (PID) is infection of the adnexae as a result of ascending infection from the vagina and cervix [25]. Young age, as opposed to adulthood, as well as an in-dwelling contraceptive device, multiple sexual partners, or high frequency of sexual encounters are all known risk factors [25]. *Neisseria gonorrhoeae* and *Chlamydia trachomatis* are the most common pathogens, although a substantial portion of cases are polymicrobial [6, 25]. The clinical presentation of acute PID usually includes pelvic pain and cervical motion tenderness on examination [6, 25].

Imaging is not often needed as patients are treated based on clinical grounds [25]. Ultrasound is generally the first-line imaging study for patients who have an unclear clinical presentation and fail to respond to initial therapy or when a complication such as pyosalpinx or tubo-ovarian abscess (TOA) is suspected [25]. Ultrasound findings in uncomplicated PID may be unclear, however, and secondary involvement of the adnexa by a regional process such as appendicitis can cause similar findings [6, 25]. Timely diagnosis of PID is important to reduce the likelihood of progression to pyo-

salpinx or TOA as well as the development of adhesions that may increase the risk of chronic pelvic pain, infertility, and ectopic pregnancy [41].

MR imaging is increasingly being used in the assessment of patients with acute and chronic abdominal pain and has been shown to be an effective first-line imaging modality in atypical or complicated PID [6, 42]. The main goal of imaging patients with PID is to identify complications that might require inpatient admission or more invasive treatment options. Uncomplicated PID appears as a loss of tissue planes involving the adnexa with ill-defined intermediate T1-weighted and high T2-weighted signal intensity with diffuse enhancement [6, 41, 42]. Thickening and enhancement of the fallopian tube wall may be seen along with free fluid [6, 25]. The ovary should be identifiable as a discrete structure. Pyosalpinx, a pus-filled fallopian tube, appears as a tortuous, fluid-filled tubular adnexal structure [6, 41] with enhancement and edema of the thickened tubal wall and adjacent pelvic fat. Simple hydrosalpinx, in contrast, has high T2-weighted signal intensity fluid in the lumen, but no tubal wall thickening or surrounding enhancement [25, 41]. In pyosalpinx purulent material within the dilated fallopian tube may appear hyperintense in T1-weighted signal intensity due to proteinaceous or cellular debris. On T2-weighted images, tubal contents are hyperintense to muscle, are often slightly hypointense to urine, and may contain layering debris [6, 41]. The purulent material within the tube restricts on DWI, whereas the simple fluid in hydrosalpinx demonstrates increased diffusion [6].

TOAs result from progression of adnexal infection to form an inflammatory collection involving the fallopian tube, ovary, and surrounding pelvic soft tissues [25]. TOAs may arise in as many as 20% of adolescents with PID [18] and, like pyosalpinx, may require percutaneous, transvaginal, or surgical intervention for effective treatment [41]. Ultrasound may identify a non-specific appearing, complex adnexal mass that could represent a TOA, hemorrhagic cyst, endometrioma, hydro- or pyosalpinx, or neoplasm. On MR imaging, normal adnexal structures including the ovary are obscured by a complex, thick-walled, part solid, and part cystic lesion with enhancing walls and septations [6, 9, 25, 43] (Fig. 15.29). The contents of the abscess appear low to intermediate on T1-weighted images and heterogeneously hyperintense on T2-weighted images, but less intense than urine [25, 35, 41, 43, 44]. A rim of mildly increased T1-weighted sig-

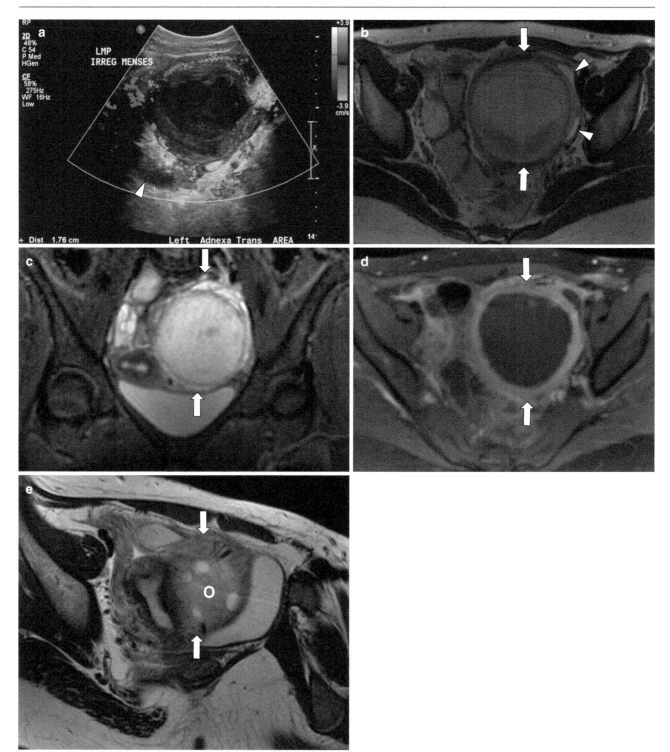

Fig. 15.29 Tubo-ovarian abscess in a nonsexually active 14-year-old girl 2 months after perforated appendicitis with positive cultures for *Bacteroides* and *Streptococcus* sp. (**a**) Ultrasound demonstrates an approximately 8 cm complex fluid collection in the left adnexa with a thick, hypervascular wall. The *arrowheads* and calipers denote a fluid dilated fallopian tube. Axial T2-weighted (**b**) and coronal T2-weighted fat-suppressed (**c**) MR images show a complex fluid collection (*arrows*). The *arrowheads* on (**b**) denote a mildly fluid distended left fallopian tube. Coronal T1-weighted fat-suppressed post-contrast (**d**) MR image shows a thick rim of enhancement. (**e**) An axial-oblique T2-weighted MR image through the left adnexa shows that the left ovary (O) is contained within the complex fluid collection (*arrows*)

nal may be seen along the internal margin of the abscess due to granulation tissue or hemorrhage on unenhanced images [25, 35, 44]. Inflammatory stranding of the pelvic fat might be seen [6, 25, 44]. Abscess contents restrict on DWI due to fluid viscosity [8, 9, 35]. Brisk enhancement is seen in both the abscess wall and septations as well as in the surrounding pelvic inflammatory changes [6, 25, 41], although edema in the pelvic fat is bright on T2-weighted images but non-enhancing [25]. Gas is rarely present but, when seen, confirms the diagnosis of TOA [25, 41].

While TOAs most commonly represent progression of sexually acquired PID in adolescents, when they occur in prepubertal and nonsexually active girls, other etiologies must be considered. If the patient is not sexually active, a primary inflammatory process with secondary adnexal involvement should be sought. Specifically, acute, ruptured appendicitis and inflammatory bowel disease both can result in adnexal involvement and TOA [6, 41] and are relatively common in pediatric patients. A case of TOA has been reported as a result of an appendicolith migrating into the fallopian tube following appendiceal rupture [45]. On MR imaging, evidence of appendicitis and periappendiceal inflammation may be seen contiguous with the adnexal inflammation and abscess. In Crohn disease, transmural inflammation may progress to fistula formation between involved segments of bowel and adjacent structures including the adnexa, uterus, or vagina [46]. On MR imaging, fistulas are best seen on post-contrast T1-weighted fat-suppressed images as enhancing regions extending from inflamed bowel to the involved structure [6, 46]. As with TOAs resulting from ascending infection, prompt diagnosis and therapeutic intervention are needed to reduce the possibility of infertility, ectopic pregnancy, and pelvic adhesions that may result in chronic pelvic pain.

Neoplastic Female Genital Tract Disorders

Ovarian Neoplasms

Ovarian masses are one of the most common gynecologic imaging abnormalities in children, and the majority are benign [47]. MR imaging is useful for preoperative lesion characterization and may influence treatment and surgical decisions in a significant percentage of cases [35, 47].

Germ Cell Tumors Mature ovarian teratomas or dermoids constitute the most common ovarian neoplasm in children [18, 35, 48, 49]. They are also the only benign tumor of germ

cell origin that arise in children. Mature ovarian teratomas are bilateral in 10–15% of cases, and multiple tumors may be present in one ovary. In the experience of Taskinen et al., more than 20% of children with ovarian mature teratoma develop a metachronous benign tumor in the contralateral ovary [50]. These authors recommend annual ultrasound follow-up until pregnancy in order to allow early diagnosis, ovarian preserving surgery, and maintenance of fertility in the case of metachronous tumor development. Because mature teratomas may contain elements from all three germ cell layers, they can have a variable imaging appearance, but commonly contain both macroscopic fat and cystic areas. These lesions may also have a dermoid plug or Rokitansky nodule representing solid components that can include the hair, calcium, or even teeth [49, 51].

The characteristic finding of a benign, mature teratoma on MR imaging is the presence of identifiable fat within the lesion (Fig. 15.30). Fat is seen as high T1-weighted signal intensity on non-fat-suppressed imaging that exhibits signal loss on fat-suppressed images, compared to hemorrhage or protein that remains hyperintense on fat-suppressed T1-weighted sequences [35, 49, 51]. Fluid-fluid levels may be seen with nondependent fat that darkens on fat-suppressed images and with chemical shift artifact at the fat-fluid interface [35, 52]. Calcium may be more difficult to identify on MR imaging than CT, but susceptibility-weighted series may be helpful. Lesion characterization may be more reliable with MR imaging than ultrasound, leading to improved management and surgical planning [47]. Although these lesions are benign, ovarian germ cell tumors are usually removed to avoid complications including torsion, rupture, malignant transformation, and rarely encephalopathy (anti-NMDA-receptor encephalitis) or autoimmune hemolytic anemia [18, 51].

Immature teratomas tend to be larger, occur in younger girls, and carry a worse prognosis [15, 35, 49, 51]. Like other malignant tumors of germ cell origin, they can be associated with elevated beta-human chorionic gonadotropin and alpha-fetoprotein levels prior to resection [51], and these markers can be used for surveillance postoperatively [49]. At imaging, these lesions demonstrate larger solid components, less prominent cystic components, and fewer or smaller fat-containing components [35, 49, 51] (Fig. 15.31). Vaysse et al. proposed a 7.5 cm maximal size above which teratomas should be considered suspicious for malignancy [53].

Dysgerminomas more often occur in older girls and teens [35, 49, 51]. These lesions are similar to seminomas in males and are the least differentiated germ cell tumor [18, 49]. Dysgerminomas are associated with elevated serum lactate

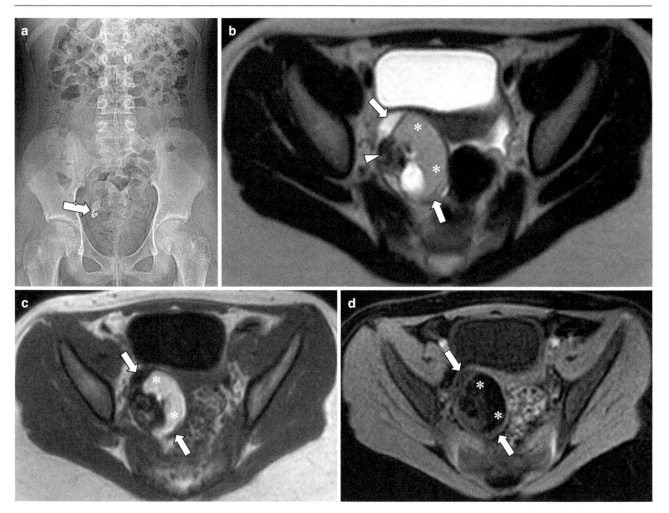

Fig. 15.30 Incidentally found mature ovarian teratoma in an 11-year-old girl being evaluated for abdominal pain. (**a**) Abdominal radiograph shows a cluster of calcific densities (*arrow*) in the right hemipelvis, one of which vaguely resembles a tooth. (**b**) Axial T2-weighted MR image reveals a complex mixed solid and cystic right adnexal lesion (*arrows*). There is focal signal void (*arrowhead*) due to calcification or tooth. Intralesional fat (*) shows intermediate signal. Axial T1-weighted MR images (**c**) without and (**d**) with fat suppression show a focal signal void (*arrows*) due to calcification (or tooth). A vast portion of the mass shows signal loss (*) on the fat-suppressed image (**d**) due to the presence of fat

dehydrogenase and, like seminomas, are radiosensitive [15, 49, 51]. These masses are primarily solid at imaging with T2-weighted hypointense septa that demonstrate contrast enhancement [35, 51] (Fig. 15.32). Small areas of calcification or cystic necrosis may be present, as well. Germ cell tumors, particularly dysgerminoma, may be seen in gonadal dysgenesis, and different cell types may occur in combination. Pelvic and retroperitoneal lymph node spread is more commonly seen than intraperitoneal seeding.

Endodermal sinus tumors or yolk sac tumors are rare germ cell lesions that are usually large with metastatic disease at presentation [35]. These tumors are mixed cystic and solid lesions that characteristically contain dilated vessels that may appear as signal voids on MR imaging. Solid components enhance briskly [35] (Fig. 15.33). Other ovarian germ cell tumors that occur in children include embryonal carcinoma, polyembryoma, and ovarian choriocarcinoma [18, 48]. All of these tumors may metastasize to the lungs, liver, and peritoneum [49] and tend to be solid appearing on MR imaging [35].

Sex Cord-Stromal Neoplasms Granulosa cell tumors are the most common malignant sex cord-stromal tumor, but are uncommon in children except for the juvenile subtype [15, 18, 49]. Juvenile granulosa cell tumors are often large at presentation [49]. These lesions may be multicystic or solid, but are most commonly mixed [15, 24, 35, 51]. On T2-weighted imaging, the tumors often have a sponge-like appearance with intermediate signal intensity solid components and bright fluid [6, 24, 35, 49, 51]. Solid portions of the tumor enhance and up to 70% of lesions contain hemorrhage [35, 49], but the imaging appearance overlaps with other cell types. A distinguishing feature is their common presentation with isosexual precocious puberty due to estrogen secretion [18, 24, 35, 49, 51] (Fig. 15.34). The prognosis for juvenile granulosa

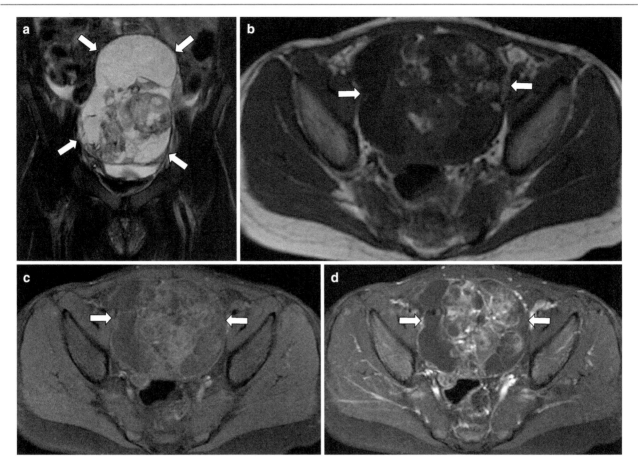

Fig. 15.31 Immature ovarian teratoma in a 7-year-old girl who presented with increasing abdominal pain. (**a**) Coronal T2-weighted fat-suppressed MR image shows a large, complex midline mass (*arrows*). Axial T1-weighted (**b**), axial T1-weighted fat-suppressed MR images obtained pre-contrast (**c**) and post-contrast (**d**) show an immature ovarian teratoma (*arrows*) with a predominantly solid, enhancing appearance with scattered foci of fat and calcification and scant fatty components

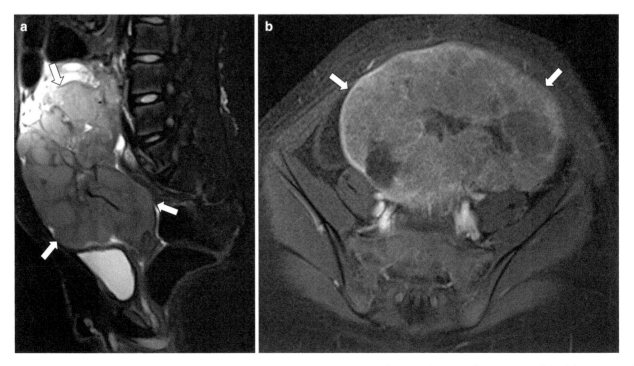

Fig. 15.32 Dysgerminoma in a 15-year-old girl who presented with a pelvic mass. (**a**) Sagittal T2-weighted MR image shows a large, relatively hyperintense mass (*arrows*) with lobulated contours and internal, hypointense, fibrovascular septa. (**b**) Axial T1-weighted fat-suppressed post-contrast MR image shows enhancement of the mass (*arrows*) with more brisk enhancement of the fibrovascular septa

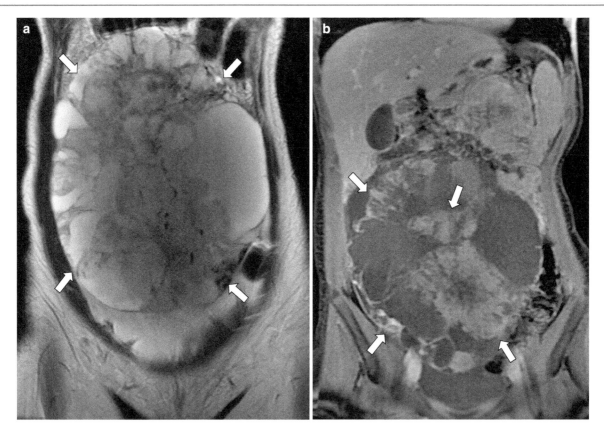

Fig. 15.33 Endodermal sinus tumor in a 14-year-old girl who presented with a right-sided abdominal mass. (**a**) Coronal T2-weighted MR image shows a complex, solid and cystic, space-occupying lesion *(arrows)* with internal flow voids. (**b**) Coronal-enhanced T1-weighted fat-suppressed MR image shows enhancement of the solid components *(arrows)*

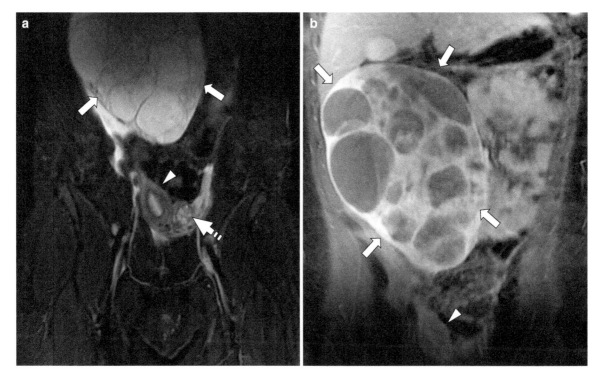

Fig. 15.34 Juvenile granulosa cell tumor in a 9-year-old girl who presented with precocious puberty and a palpable abdominal mass. Coronal T2-weighted (**a**) and T1-weighted fat-suppressed post-contrast (**b**) MR images show a complex, multiloculated cystic mass *(arrows)* with solid, briskly enhancing components. Note the pubertal appearance of the uterus *(arrowheads)*. The left ovary *(dashed arrow on **a**)* is normal in appearance

cell tumors is better than in the adult lesions [54] with resection often curative [51].

Sertoli-Leydig cell tumors present with virilization due to androgen secretion in approximately 30% of patients [18, 35, 49, 51, 54], while the remainder of lesions are nonfunctional [15] (Fig. 15.35). The lesions are frequently malignant and may be associated with other neoplasms associated with the DICER1 mutation [15, 35]. Most tumors are stage 1 at diagnosis [54], although they tend to be large. These tumors are predominantly enhancing solid lesions with intermediate to low signal intensity on T2-weighted imaging due to the fibrous stroma [15, 35, 49, 51, 54]. When cystic components are present, Sertoli-Leydig

tumors may be indistinguishable from juvenile granulosa cell tumors by MR imaging. In girls with virilization, the lesions tend to be very small at presentation [54].

Epithelial Neoplasms Serous and mucinous cystadenomas are the most common epithelial neoplasms in children and are more common than their malignant counterparts [18, 49]. These masses almost always present post menarche [35]. Serous cystadenomas may be unilocular or multilocular with homogeneous cyst contents and fine septations [18, 49, 51] (Fig. 15.36). Mucinous lesions are multilocular with numerous, small locules and variable signal intensity on

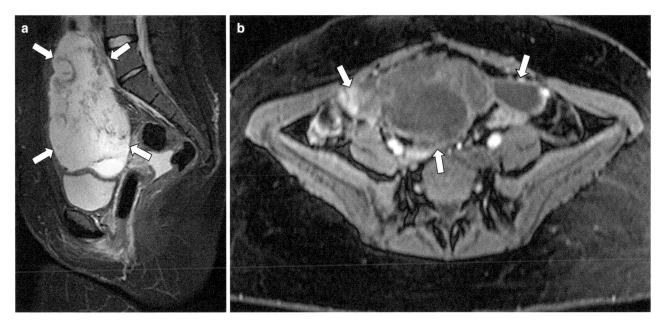

Fig. 15.35 Sertoli-Leydig cell tumor in a 17-year-old girl who presented with abdominal pain. Sagittal T2-weighted fat-suppressed (**a**) and axial enhanced T1-weighted fat-suppressed (**b**) MR images show a

large, complex, cystic and solid lesion (*arrows*) with heterogeneous enhancement. Pathology was consistent with a Sertoli-Leydig cell tumor. Incidentally noted is a tampon within the vagina on (**a**)

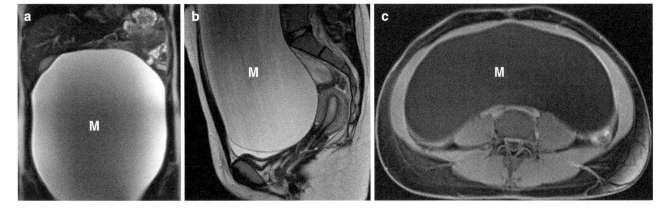

Fig. 15.36 Serous cystadenoma in a 16-year-old girl who presented with increasing abdominal distension. Coronal T2-weighted fat-suppressed (**a**), sagittal T2-weighted (**b**), and axial T1-weighted, fat-suppressed post-contrast (**c**) MR images show a very large abdominopelvic

unilocular cystic mass (M). Incidentally noted are a few cervical nabothian cysts on (**b**). At surgery the cystic mass originated from the right fallopian paratubal region. Pathology was consistent with serous cystadenoma

T2-weighted imaging [51] that may have a "stained glass" appearance [35] (Fig. 15.37). Neither type should have papillary excrescences, a honeycomb appearance, or thick walls, which would suggest a borderline or malignant lesion [35, 49, 51].

Uterine and Vaginal Neoplasms

The most common benign neoplasms of the pediatric uterus and vagina are uterine leiomyomata or fibroids, although these lesions are much less common in children and adolescents than they are in adults [55]. Risk factors include African-Caribbean descent, childbearing age, and family history of fibroids [56]. Uterine leiomyomata or fibroids may be single or multiple, and a case of diffuse leiomyomatosis has been

reported in an adolescent [55]. Generally, the diagnosis is readily made with pelvic ultrasound, although submucosal or pedunculated lesions may be more problematic [56], in which case MR imaging may be helpful. These smooth muscle tumors are often isointense to myometrium on T1-weighted imaging and are most commonly hypointense to isointense on T2-weighted imaging, unless they are hemorrhagic or necrotic [15]. Treatment is usually managed with hormonal therapy, although large lesions may require surgical removal.

Rhabdomyosarcoma is the most common soft tissue sarcoma in children, and the vagina is the most common organ of origin in the female GU tract [29]. The embryonal subtype is most common [57] and is associated with the DICER1 mutation [58]. There is an age peak at 3 years [59] with a 5-year survival rate of approximately 91% [60]. Sarcoma

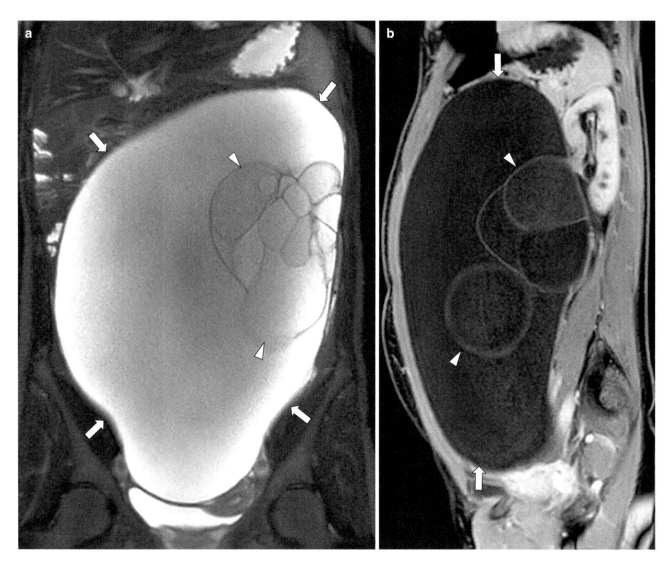

Fig. 15.37 Mucinous cystadenoma in a 15-year-old girl who presented with worsening abdominal distension and bloating. Coronal T2-weighted fat-suppressed (**a**) and sagittal T1-weighted fat-suppressed post-contrast (**b**) MR images show a massive cystic lesion (*arrows*) occupying the majority of the abdomen and pelvis containing a cluster of smaller, variable-size cysts (*arrowheads*) adherent to the left posterolateral wall. Mild enhancement of the smaller cysts' walls is seen. However, no solid or fatty component is seen within the lesion. The left ovary could not be identified; therefore, it was inferred that the lesion originated from the left ovary, which was confirmed at surgery. Pathology revealed mucinous cystadenoma

botryoides may present clinically as a mass resembling a "bunch of grapes" protruding from the introitus [57]. These patients may have obstructive hydronephrosis if there is distal ureteral involvement. MR imaging may be helpful in assessing the extent of tumor as well as to search for metastatic disease. The primary tumor also resembles a "bunch of grapes" with high internal T2-weighted signal intensity [57, 59] and heterogeneous contrast enhancement [29] (Fig. 15.38). Blood products are commonly seen [57].

Traumatic Female Genital Tract Disorders

Trauma to the perineum in females most commonly occurs as the result of a straddle injury, but may also be due to non-straddle blunt or penetrating trauma [37, 38]. Injuries are usually confined to the labia, and treatment is supportive, although hematomas of the vulva can expand rapidly [37]. More extensive injury extending deeper into the perineum is uncommon but is more frequently seen with penetrating or non-straddle injuries.

CT imaging is the first-line modality in evaluating the extent of acute injury [37] with intravenous contrast utilized for evaluation of active hemorrhage [38]. MR imaging may be helpful if further anatomic delineation is needed due to its superior soft tissue contrast [37]. Vaginal laceration can occur secondary to blunt pelvic or perineal trauma and may be associated with pelvic fracture [61] and concurrent with urologic injuries [62]. Lacerations have also been reported secondary to waterskiing and water slide-related incidents [63]. Undetected vaginal laceration can lead to pelvic abscess; therefore, clinical evidence of lower urinary tract, and perineal injury should raise suspicion for possible vaginal injury [61]. If imaging is required, the superior tissue contrast and anatomic definition of MR imaging would be ideal for high-resolution pelvic imaging in this setting. Because vaginal and perineal injuries may also result from sexual trauma, appropriate patient evaluation is required in these cases.

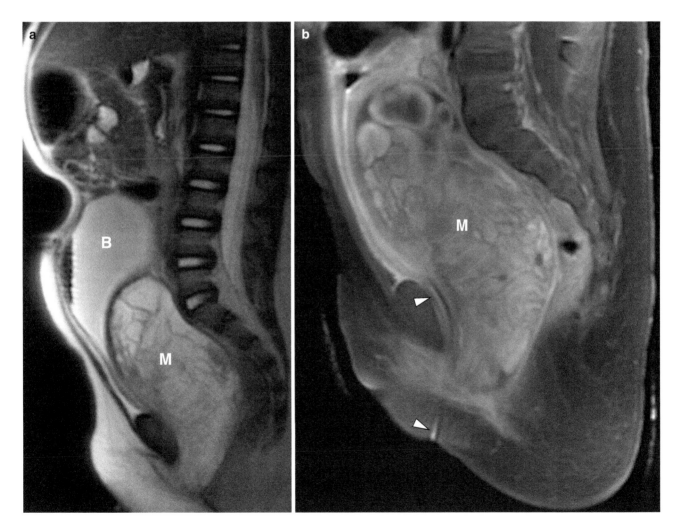

Fig. 15.38 Vaginal rhabdomyosarcoma in a 2-year-old girl who presented with pelvic pain, vaginal bleeding, and a mass extruding from the introitus. (**a**) Sagittal T2-weighted MR image shows a markedly dilated vagina secondary to a hyperintense, multiseptated vaginal mass (M) displacing the bladder (B), which is catheterized and markedly displaced anteriorly and superiorly. (**b**) Sagittal T1-weighted fat-suppressed post-contrast MR image shows heterogeneous enhancement of the vaginal mass (M). *Arrowheads* indicate the patient's bladder catheter

Foreign bodies in the vagina result in persistent, foul-smelling, dark or bloody discharge, occasionally accompanied by pelvic or abdominal pain [18, 64]. The most common foreign bodies in children are retained fragments of toilet tissue that lodge in the posterior fornix. Soft foreign bodies may take approximately 2 weeks to present clinically when vaginal bleeding is noted [6]. Small, hard objects such as crayons, coins, stones, toy fragments, or metallic foreign bodies such as hairpins may result in bright red blood if vessel erosion occurs [64]. Forgotten tampons also can result in discharge or infection. If the foreign object is not known to have been inserted by the girl herself, sexual abuse must be considered [6, 18]. If there is a question about the diagnosis, imaging can be performed (Fig. 15.39), although MR imaging is less commonly utilized than ultrasound.

Miscellaneous Female Genital Tract Disorders

Acquired Ovarian Cysts In a peripubertal girl, a simple cyst measuring less than or equal to 3 cm most likely represents a mature follicle and requires no further investigation

[23, 34, 36, 48] (Fig. 15.40) (Table 15.5). Nonfunctioning, simple cysts between 3 and 5 cm generally also do not require follow-up in an asymptomatic postpubertal girl because they are likely due to failed ovulation or a persistent corpus luteum [23, 36]. Failed ovulation can result in a functional cyst that appears simple [34] but may continue to grow and cause pain [18], however, and symptomatic cases may require further evaluation or follow-up. Simple cysts between 5 and 7 cm in postpubertal girls can be followed and should involute over one to two menstrual cycles [23, 36]; however, cysts larger than 5 cm may require aspiration or resection due to the increased risk of torsion. A cyst measuring more than 7 cm requires further imaging for characterization [23, 36]. In a girl with precocious puberty, an ovarian cyst measuring 9 mm or more should raise the possibility of an autonomously functioning cyst or hormone-producing tumor [24], and imaging may be helpful for lesion characterization. MR imaging is well suited to demonstrating simple cyst characteristics including homogeneous hyperintensity on T2-weighted imaging with no enhancement or appreciable T1-weighted signal intensity. The walls should be imperceptibly thin, and there should be no solid or nodular components.

Hemorrhagic ovarian cysts develop from corpora lutea and may cause acute pelvic pain. Typically, hemorrhagic

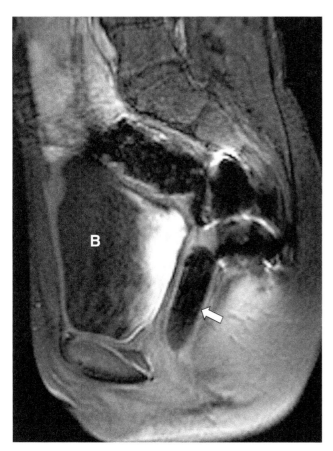

Fig. 15.39 Vaginal foreign body in a 5-year-old girl who presented with vaginal discharge. Coronal-enhanced T1-weighted fat-suppressed MR image shows a well-delineated, low signal intensity, cylindrical-shaped structure (*arrow*) within the vagina consistent with a foreign body. A crayon was removed during vaginoscopy. B, bladder

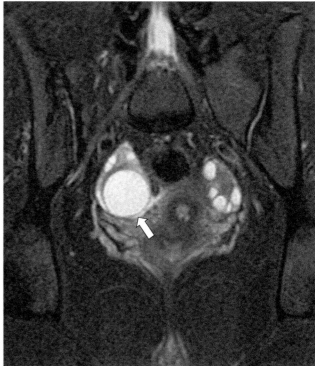

Fig. 15.40 Coronal T2-weighted fat-suppressed MR image in a 17-year-old girl obtained as part of a hip study shows a simple-appearing, thin-walled cyst in the right ovary, measuring less than 3 cm in diameter consistent with a mature follicle (*arrow*). This is a normal, expected finding and requires no further investigation

Table 15.5 Ovarian cysts – simple cysts only, no clinical signs of hormonal abnormality [23]

Developmental stage	Size	Management
Fetal/neonatal	<2.5 cm	No follow-up needed
	>2.5 cm or complex	Follow-up imaging required
	>4 cm	Increased risk of torsion, follow-up, and management are controversial
Pediatric	>3 cm	Unusual prior to puberty – consider follow-up imaging to assess for growth
		May represent paraovarian cyst, neoplasm, or abnormal follicle. Malignancy rare
	>6 follicles and ovarian volume > 4 mL	Consider premature ovarian development
Pubertal	<3 cm	Likely follicle, no follow-up needed
	3–5 cm	Failed ovulation/follicular cyst/corpus luteum cyst, no follow-up needed if asymptomatic
	5–6.9 cm	Failed ovulation/follicular cyst. Lesions greater than 5 cm show increased risk of torsion
		Surgical aspiration/resection vs follow-up to resolution after 1–2 cycles
	>7 cm	Requires further characterization – increased chance of neoplasm

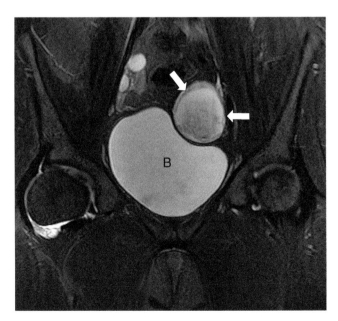

Fig. 15.41 Hemorrhagic ovarian cyst in an 11-year-old girl incidentally found on hip MR imaging. Coronal T2-weighted fat-suppressed MR image shows a cystic lesion (*arrows*) with mild, diffuse low signal intensity when compared with the adjacent T2-weighted hyperintense fluid in the bladder (B). The lesion resolved on 3-month follow-up study, confirming its functional nature

cysts are diagnosed on ultrasound, and the follow-up examination showing resolution of the lesion is considered sufficient to confirm the diagnosis. Occasionally, on ultrasound, the appearance can be confusing as these lesions can appear as complex cysts or solid lesions, although they should not show evidence of internal flow on color Doppler evaluation. MR imaging is seldom obtained but can be useful in cases of a potential associated pathology, possible complication, or unusual sonographic appearance. Hemorrhagic ovarian cysts can have a variable appearance depending upon the age of the hemorrhage on both, ultrasound and MR imaging [6, 18, 34, 36]. In addition, their appearance depends on several additional factors, such as the form and breakdown of hemoglobin, hematocrit, clot formation and retraction, red blood cell membrane integrity, and ambient oxygen level. While classic teaching is that hemorrhagic ovarian cysts manifest as hyperintense lesions on both T1- and T2-weighted images, their MR imaging appearance is quite variable. For example, in the published series by Kanso et al., the vast majority of hemorrhagic ovarian cysts show low signal intensity on T1-weighted images [65].

MR imaging is a valuable tool in differentiating hemorrhagic ovarian cysts from ovarian torsion or neoplasms. In the acute/subacute setting, T1-weighted imaging may reveal hyperintense signal that does not darken on fat-suppressed images [6, 7, 9]. On T2-weighted images, the internal signal is variable depending upon the age of the hemorrhage, in the acute/subacute setting hemorrhagic cysts are usually hyperintense, However, these may become hypointense when hemosiderin deposition takes place (Fig. 15.41). A lacy pattern of low signal internal reticulation may be seen [36], and a hematocrit effect may be present [23]. The cyst walls may enhance slightly, but there should be no nodularity or internal enhancement. Unlike endometriomata, the "T2-shading" effect from repeated episodes of hemorrhage is less commonly seen [6]. The internal components should never enhance following the administration of intravenous contrast. The cyst should involute over one to two cycles [18, 36, 66], and MR imaging is also useful in assessing cysts that fail to involute.

If imaging is performed in the setting of acute, painful cyst rupture, the collapsed cyst may be visible with increased T2-weighted signal, possibly with blood products and a variable amount of free pelvic fluid that also may appear heterogeneous on T1- and T2-weighted images due to blood products [6, 15] (Fig. 15.42).

Polycystic Ovarian Syndrome Polycystic ovarian syndrome (PCOS) includes infrequent ovulation or anovulation, hyperandrogenism, and enlarged, polycystic ovaries [6, 67, 68]. Many affected patients may also have insulin resistance [68, 69]. Menstrual irregularity, hirsutism, and obesity are frequent clinical manifestations. The syndrome is common,

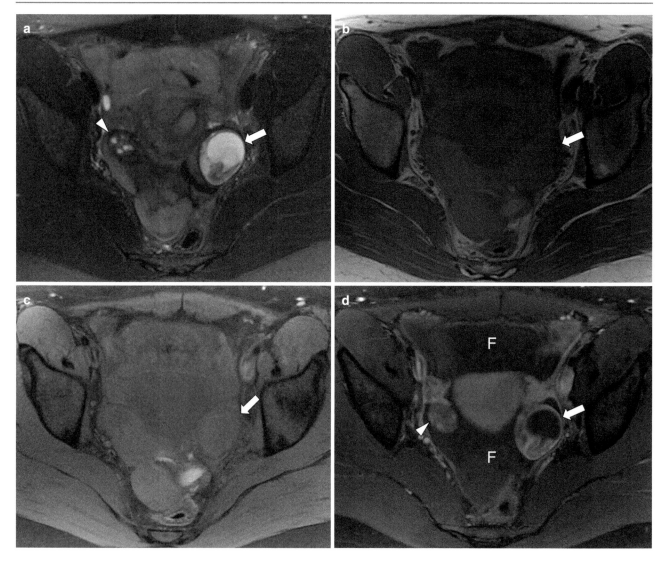

Fig. 15.42 Ruptured hemorrhagic ovarian cyst in a 17-year-old girl who presented with a few days of persistent lower abdominal and pelvic pain without associated guarding or rebound. (**a**) Axial T2-weighted fat-suppressed MR image shows a complex left ovarian cyst (*arrow*) with a crenulated appearance. The right ovary (*arrowhead*) is normal. There is a moderate amount of complex free abdominal fluid, which is hard to adequately discern from the adjacent bowel loops due to its relatively high signal. Axial T1-weighted (**b**) and axial T1-weighted fat-suppressed (**c**) MR images show a predominantly hypointense left ovarian cyst (*arrows*) with a few hyperintense foci posteriorly. Axial enhanced T1-weighted fat-suppressed MR image (**d**) shows to better advantage the complex left ovarian cyst (*arrow*) with a crenulated appearance. A moderate amount of complex free pelvic fluid (F) is now better appreciated. The relatively high signal intensity of the fluid is most consistent with hemoperitoneum. The overall appearance is most consistent with a ruptured hemorrhagic ovarian cyst. Normal appearing right ovary (*arrowhead*) is seen. The findings completely resolved on follow-up exam obtained a few weeks later

affecting 5–10% of teens and women of reproductive age [6, 67]. There is overlap in the appearance of normal adolescent ovaries and polycystic ovarian morphology. Normal adolescent ovaries may contain numerous follicles [67, 70], and conversely, the ovaries may appear normal in cases of PCOS. Clinical and laboratory evidence of PCOS is necessary for definitive diagnosis [6, 54, 68, 69].

The Rotterdam criteria were developed using transvaginal ultrasound for assessment of polycystic ovarian morphology with greater than 12 follicles in each ovary measuring 2–9 mm or ovarian volume more than 10 ml being considered abnormal [71]. Because transvaginal ultrasound often cannot be used in most children and adolescents, and due to the limitations of transabdominal ultrasound, MR imaging may be helpful in investigation of suspected polycystic ovaries in teens [6, 67, 72]. On T2-weighted images, the ovaries demonstrate numerous follicles with central T2-weighted hypointense stroma (Fig. 15.43). Due to the normal presence of multiple follicles in adolescent ovaries, Rosenfeld has suggested utilization of ovarian volume rather than number of cysts be used to assess ovaries for PCOS [69, 73] with either a mean ovarian volume of >12 mL or a single ovarian volume of >15 mL considered abnormally enlarged. Fondin et al. have suggested an even lower ovarian volume of greater than 10 mL as suspicious for PCOS by MR imaging [72].

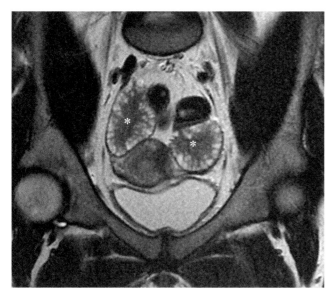

Fig. 15.43 Polycystic ovarian syndrome in an 18-year-old female who presented with irregular menstrual cycles and hirsutism. Coronal T2-weighted MR image shows enlarged ovaries with prominent hypointense central stroma (*asterisks*) and multiple peripherally arranged, tiny follicles. These imaging findings are typical of polycystic ovarian syndrome; however, elevated androgen levels are needed to confirm the diagnosis

Endometriosis Endometriosis exists when endometrial tissue is found outside the uterus [18, 74, 75]. Multiple etiologies have been proposed for the occurrence of ectopic endometrial tissue, but the most commonly accepted explanation is retrograde menstruation [18, 76]. Endometriosis causes significant morbidity and should always be considered in the differential diagnosis of chronic pelvic pain. The most common finding on imaging is an endometrioma; a chronic cyst-like collection of blood products in the adnexa or pelvis due to repeated hemorrhage of endometrial rests during menstruation [74].

On MR imaging, endometriomas have bright signal intensity on T1-weighted images and low signal intensity on T2-weighted images due to degraded, proteinaceous blood products [6, 36, 75]. With repeated hemorrhage, layering may result in fluid-fluid levels or even T2 "shading," a gradual decrease in signal in the dependent portion of the collection [75, 77] (Fig. 15.44). While T2 shading is classically associated with endometriomas, this finding may less commonly be seen in hemorrhagic cysts, and differentiation between these entities may be challenging. Corwin et al. have reported finding T2 dark spots, small very low T2-weighted signal intensity foci within the endometriomas that represent chronic hemorrhage (Fig. 15.45) and are not typically seen in hemorrhagic cysts [75]. In the experience of Outwater et al. [78], endometriomas tend to demonstrate higher T1-weighted and lower T2-weighted signal intensities when compared to hemorrhagic ovarian cysts. Endometriomas tend to have lower ADC values on DWI than hemorrhagic ovarian cysts,

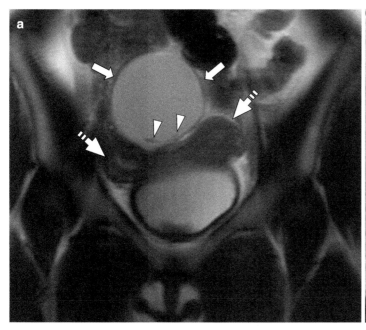

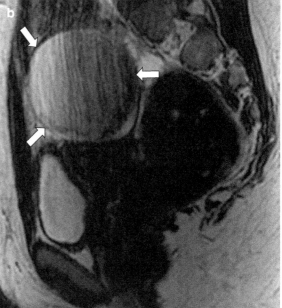

Fig. 15.44 Endometrioma in a 14-year-old girl with a history of OHVIRA (obstructed hemivagina ipsilateral renal agenesis) or Herlyn-Werner-Wunderlich syndrome who presented with worsening dysmenorrhea and an adnexal endometrioma. (**a**) Coronal T2-weighted MR image shows a uterus didelphys with widely splayed uterine horns (*dashed arrows*) and approximately 7 cm adnexal endometrioma (*arrows*) with a few T2-weighted hypointense spots (*arrowheads*). (**b**) Sagittal T2-weighted MR image shows T2 shading within the endometrioma (*arrows*) with fluid-fluid levels related to repeated hemorrhagic episodes. (**c**) Axial T1-weighted fat-suppressed MR image shows high signal intensity within the adnexal endometrioma (*arrows*), a finding that helps confirm that the lesion does not contain fat and contains blood products

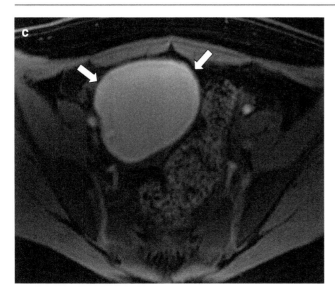

Fig. 15.44 (continued)

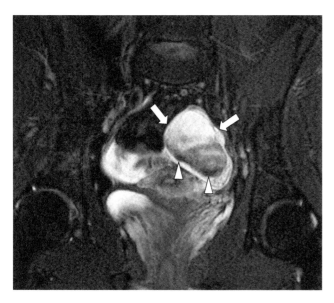

Fig. 15.45 Left adnexal endometrioma in an 18-year-old girl who presented with worsening pelvic pain. Coronal T2-weighted MR image shows a cystic lesion (*arrows*) with T2-shading and a few T2-weighted dark spots (*arrowheads*)

but there is some overlap, and distinction between the two entities can be problematic [66, 74].

The deep, infiltrative form of endometriosis is defined as peritoneal implants of endometrial tissue with invasion greater than 5 mm in depth [79]. Any pelvic structures may be involved including organs, ligaments, peritoneal reflections, and recesses [74]. Infiltrative endometriosis causes fibrotic and hyperplastic fibromuscular changes that are seen on MR imaging as ill-defined or nodular regions of intermediate T1-weighted signal intensity and abnormal low T2-weighted signal intensity [74, 79]. MR imaging findings in endometriosis may be quite subtle and difficult to detect.

T2-weighted hypointense tethering of structures, wall invasion or thickening, and deformity of affected organs may be found with small foci of T1- and T2-weighted hyperintensity sometimes scattered within the ill-defined signal abnormality [74, 79]. Adhesions may cause anteflexion or retroflexion of the uterus as well [6].

Adenomyosis Adenomyosis is defined as the invasion of endometrial glandular and stromal tissue into the myometrium with associated smooth muscle hypertrophy, and it may be diffuse or focal [80–82]. An adenomyoma is a mass-like form of adenomyosis [81, 82]. Both entities commonly coexist with endometriosis and are also associated with pelvic pain. Adenomyosis is rare in children; however, complications of adenomyotic cysts have been reported in adolescent patients [80, 83] (Fig. 15.46).

The classic imaging finding of adenomyosis is a widened and indistinct uterine junctional zone on T2-weighted images, often associated with uterine enlargement [81, 82]. There may also be foci of bright T1- and T2-weighted signal within the abnormal myometrium representing endometrial glands with hemorrhage [80, 81] as well as punctate T1- and T2-weighted hypointense foci representing hemosiderin [82]. When focal, adenomyosis may resemble a leiomyoma or uterine contraction; however, contractions are transient [81]. Adenomyomata appear mass-like and have low signal intensity on both T1- and T2- weighted images with internal high signal foci [81, 82].

Ovarian/Adnexal Torsion Ovarian torsion is twisting of the vascular pedicle of the ovary that results in ovarian ischemia. Prompt diagnosis and surgical reduction are necessary to preserve ovarian viability [22, 84]. Torsion most commonly involves both the ovary and ipsilateral fallopian tube but may involve either structure in isolation. Right-sided torsion is more common, likely due to the anchoring effect of the sigmoid mesentery on the left adnexa [18, 22, 84, 85]. While ovarian torsion may occur de novo particularly in neonates and perimenarchal girls [9, 18, 22, 85, 86], ovarian or adnexal cysts and masses may act as lead points for torsion. Oltmann et al. found that torsion occurred more commonly without an underlying lesion in perimenarchal girls aged 9–14 [85]. If the volume ratio of the affected ovary to contralateral side is greater than or equal to 20:1, an underlying adnexal mass should be sought [87]. Ovarian or adnexal lesions larger than 5 cm are associated with an increased risk of torsion [22, 85].

While ultrasound remains the first-line modality for assessment of acute pelvic pain, differentiating adnexal torsion from nonsurgical entities such as hemorrhagic ovarian cysts is often problematic when transvaginal technique cannot be used, as in nonsexually active girls. MR imaging provides an excel-

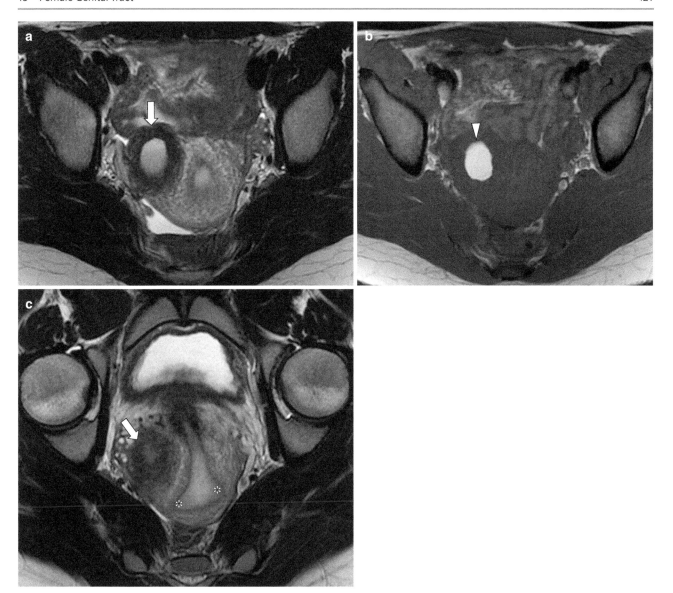

Fig. 15.46 Adenomyotic cyst in an 18-year-old girl who presented with chronic pelvic pain, with MR imaging performed for evaluation of uterine lesion seen on ultrasound. (**a**) Axial T2-weighted MR image shows a thick-walled cyst (*arrows*) with surrounding hypointense signal, likely representing a combination of myometrial hypertrophy and hemosiderin deposition. (**b**) Axial T1-weighted MR image demonstrates high-signal fluid (*arrowhead*), likely representing hemorrhagic/proteinaceous fluid contained within the lesion. (**c**) Axial oblique T2-weighted MR image shows the presence of two uterine horns (*), distinct from the adenomyotic cyst (*arrow*)

lent problem-solving tool for further imaging when transabdominal ultrasound is inconclusive [6] and clinical evidence is not convincing enough to proceed to laparoscopy. Beranger-Gilbert et al. found a 77% sensitivity and 86% specificity of MR imaging for ovarian torsion [88]. In addition, intermittent vascular compression may result in a more subacute presentation, reducing the clinical suspicion for ovarian torsion [88]. MR imaging is becoming more widely utilized in this setting due to faster techniques, avoidance of exposure to ionizing radiation, and superior tissue contrast.

Ipsilateral ovarian enlargement is a consistent finding in ovarian torsion in children [22, 89]; however, there is overlap in the sizes of normal and torsed ovaries [88]. Torsion should be considered in the appropriate clinical setting when the ipsilateral ovary measures three times greater in volume than the normal side [22] or 5 cm or more in diameter [85]. A twisted vascular pedicle or "whirlpool" sign is highly associated with ovarian torsion [88, 89]. A thickened fallopian tube of >10 mm is also strongly associated with ovarian torsion [86, 88], and the tube may contain hemorrhage demonstrating T1-weighted hyperintensity and variable T2-weighted hypointensity depending upon the stage of blood products [9, 86, 90]. The thickened, twisted pedicle may have a spiral appearance, or may have a solid, "beak-like" configuration [9]. Uterine deviation toward the involved side is specific for ovarian torsion [86, 88], as is enlargement of the ovarian vas-

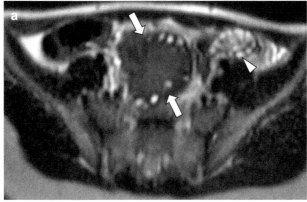 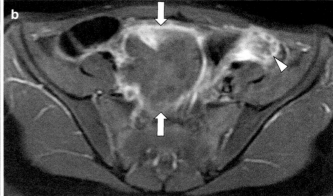

Fig. 15.47 Ovarian torsion in a 9-year-old girl who presented with right lower quadrant abdominal pain. (**a**) Axial T2-weighted MR image shows an abnormally hypointense, enlarged right ovary (*arrows*) with numerous peripherally arranged follicles, which is displaced toward the midline. Compare the abnormal right ovarian parenchyma to the normal left ovary (*arrowhead*). (**b**) Axial enhanced T1-weighted fat-suppressed MR image shows no enhancement of the torsed right ovary (*arrows*), in contrast to the normal enhancement exhibited by the left ovary (*arrowhead*)

cular pedicle [88]. Intra-ovarian findings including peripheral follicles and ovarian stromal edema have been reported by some authors [22, 86, 90], while others have found these findings to be less specific [88]. Displacement of the torsed ovary may occur toward the midline. Asymmetrically decreased enhancement of the involved ovary and tube may be seen [9, 89] and may represent ischemia or infarction (Fig. 15.47). Ovarian hemorrhage is associated with decreased ovarian viability [86, 88]. Abnormal diffusion can be seen in the fallopian tube wall and involved ovary [9].

The incidence of adnexal and/or ovarian torsion in girls is low at approximately 0.02%, similar to the rate of testicular torsion in boys at 0.03% [91]; however, the incidence of testicular torsion in boys with testicular pain is higher than the incidence of ovarian torsion in girls with abdominopelvic pain. Only 30% of patients with suspected ovarian torsion are found to have torsed ovaries at the time of surgery [85]. Ovarian salvage rates are much lower than testicular salvage rates (14.4% versus 30.3%, respectively), likely due to the greater difficulty in accurately differentiating torsion from other etiologies of acute pelvic pain [91]. Piper et al. [91] and Oltmann et al. [85] advocate early use of laparoscopy to improve the rate of ovarian salvage.

At the authors' institution, evaluation of girls with acute abdominopelvic pain and unclear ultrasound results involves a brief, 15–25-min limited MR imaging protocol utilizing an axial Dixon T2-weighted turbo spin-echo sequence, axial DWI, and axial and coronal multipoint Dixon T1-weighted sequences without and with a gadolinium-based contrast agent [6]. This imaging approach has not only increased specificity in identification of ovarian torsion, it has improved the ability to exclude other potential processes such as appendicitis. Because even dusky or hemorrhagic torsed ovaries respond well to detorsion with normal follicu-

lar development and reperfusion on follow-up imaging [92, 93], a brief MR imaging examination may reduce the need for diagnostic laparoscopy and improve the specificity of the imaging diagnosis of adnexal torsion.

Conclusion

The excellent contrast resolution, lack of ionizing radiation, and multiplanar capability of MR imaging are well suited to imaging of pediatric genital tract abnormalities. Newer techniques and shortened acquisition times have increased the utility of MR imaging in the pediatric population. As a result, MR imaging is increasingly being used for pediatric gynecologic imaging particularly for lesion/cyst characterization and assessment of congenital anomalies and even in the assessment of acute lower abdominal and pelvic pain. Although ultrasound remains the first-line modality in assessment of pediatric gynecologic disorders, MR imaging is an increasingly powerful tool for further investigation of these conditions when needed.

References

1. Ratner E, Staib L, Cross S, Raji R, Schwartz P, McCarthy S. The clinical impact of gynecologic MRI. AJR Am J Radiol. 2015;204(3):674–80.
2. Tsiflikas I, Obermayr F, Werner S, Teufel M, Fuchs J, Schafer J. Functional magnetic resonance urography in infants: feasibility of a feed-and-sleep technique. Pediatr Radiol. 2019;49(3): 351–7.
3. Ahmad R, Hu HH, Krishnamurthy R, Krishnamurthy R. Reducing sedation for pediatric body MRI using accelerated and abbreviated imaging protocols. Pediatr Radiol. 2018;48(1):37–49.
4. Baughman S, Richardson R, Podberesky D, Dalrymple N, Yerkes E. 3-Dimensional magnetic resonance genitography: a different look at cloacal malformation. J Urol. 2007;178(4. Pt 2):1675–8.

5. Podberesky DJ, Towbin AJ, Eltomey MA, Levitt MA. Magnetic resonance imaging of anorectal malformations. Magn Reson Imaging Clin N Am. 2013;21(4):791–812.

6. Cox M, Gould SW, Podberesky DJ, Epelman M. Magnetic resonance imaging of acquired disorders of the pediatric female pelvis other than neoplasm. Pediatr Radiol. 2016;46(6):806–17.

7. Son JK, Ali S, Khouri NA, Lee EY. MR imaging evaluation of pediatric genital disorders: MR technologic overview and interpretation. Magn Reson Imaging Clin N Am. 2019;27(3):201–321.

8. Chavhan GB, AlSabban Z, Babyn PS. Diffusion-weighted imaging in pediatric body MR imaging: principles, technique and emerging applications. Radiographics. 2014;34(3):E73–88.

9. Iraha Y, Okada M, Iraha R, Azama K, Yamashiro T, Tsubakimoto M, et al. CT and MR imaging of gynecologic emergencies. Radiographics. 2017;37(5):1569–86.

10. Takeuchi M, Matsuzaki K, Harada M. Susceptibility-weighted MRI of extra-ovarian endometriosis: preliminary results. Abdom Imaging. 2015;40(7):2512–6.

11. Cimsit C, Yoldemir T, Guclu M, Akpinar IN. Susceptibility-weighted magnetic resonance imaging for the evaluation of deep infiltrating endometriosis: preliminary results. Acta Radiol. 2015;57(7):878–85.

12. DelGrande F, Santini F, Herzka DA. Fat-suppression techniques for 3-T imaging of the musculoskeletal system. Radiographics. 2014;34(1):217–33.

13. Jaimes C, Kirsch JE, Gee MS. Fast, free-breathing and motion-minimized techniques for pediatric body magnetic resonance imaging. Pediatr Radiol. 2018;48(9):1197–208.

14. Chavhan GB, Parra DA, Oudjhane K, Miller SF, Babyn PS, Salle JLP. Imaging of ambiguous genitalia: classification and diagnostic approach. Radiographics. 2008;28:1891–904.

15. Gould SW, Servaes S, Lee EY, Lipsich J, Loya VMT, Epelman MS. Female genital tract. In: Lee EY, editor. Pediatric radiology practical imaging evaluation of infants and children. Philadelphia: Wolters Kluwer; 2018. p. 973–1010.

16. Li Y, Phelps A, Zapala MA, MacKenzie JD, MacKenzie TC, Courtier J. Magnetic resonance imaging of Mullerian duct anomalies in children. Pediatr Radiol. 2016;46(6):796–805.

17. Behr SC, Courtier JL, Qayyum A. Imaging of Mullerian duct anomalies. Radiographics. 2012;32(6):E233–50.

18. Servaes S, Victoria T, Lovrenski J, Epelman MS. Contemporary pediatric gynecologic imaging. Semin Ultrasound CT MRI. 2010;31(2):116–40.

19. Epelman M, Dinan D, Gee MS, Servaes S, Lee EY, Darge K. Müllerian duct and related anomalies in children and adolescents. Radiol Clin N Am. 2013;21(4):773–89.

20. Furey EA, Bailey AA, Twickler DM. Fetal MR imaging of gastrointestinal abnormalities. Radiographics. 2016;36(3):904–17.

21. Podberesky DJ, Towbin AJ, Eltorney MA, Levitt MA. Magnetic resonance imaging of anorectal malformations. Magn Reson Imaging Clin N Am. 2013;21(4):791–812.

22. Sintim-Damoa A, Majmudar AS, Cohen HL, Parvey LS. Pediatric ovarian torsion: spectrum of imaging findings. Radiographics. 2017;37(6):1892–908.

23. Langer JE, Oliver ER, Lev-Toaff AS, Coleman BG. Imaging of the female pelvis through the life cycle. Radiographics. 2012;32(6):1575–97.

24. Chung EM, Biko DM, Schroeder JW, Cube R, Conran RM. From the radiologic pathology archives: precocious puberty: radiologic-pathologic correlation. Radiographics. 2012;32(7):2071–99.

25. Rezvani M, Shaaban AM. Fallopian tube disease in the nonpregnant patient. Radiographics. 2011;31(2):527–48.

26. Walker DK, Salibian RA, Salibian AD, Belen KM, Palmer SL. Overlooked diseases of the vagina: a directed anatomic-pathologic approach for imaging assessment. Radiographics. 2011;31(6):1583–98.

27. Siegelman ES, Outwater EK, Banner MP, Ramchandani P, Anderson TL, Schnall MD. High-resolution MR imaging of the vagina. Radiographics. 1997;17(5):1183–203.

28. The American Fertility. Society classifications of adnexal adhesions, distal tubal occlusion, tubal occlusion secondary to tubal ligation, tubal pregnancies, Mullerian anomalies, and intrauterine adhesions. Fertil Steril. 1988;49(6):944–55.

29. Matos J, Orazi C, Sertorio F, Magnano G, Toma P, Granata C. Imaging of diseases of the vagina and external genitalia in children. Pediatr Radiol. 2019;49(6):827–34.

30. Schmahmann S, Haller JO. Neonatal ovarian cysts: pathogenesis, diagnosis, and management. Pediatr Radiol. 1997;27(2):101–5.

31. Trinh TW, Kennedy AM. Fetal ovarian cysts: review of imaging spectrum, differential diagnosis, management, and outcome. Radiographics. 2015;35(2):621–35.

32. Enriquez G, Duran C, Toran N, Piqueras J, Gratacos E, Aso C, et al. Conservative versus surgical treatment for complex neonatal ovarian cysts: outcomes study. AJR Am J Radiol. 2004;185(2):501–8.

33. Kessler A, Nagar H, Graif M, Ben-Sira L, Miller E, Fisher D, et al. Percutaneous drainage as the treatment of choice for neonatal ovarian cysts. Pediatr Radiol. 2006;36(9):954–8.

34. Laing FC, Allison SJ. US of the ovary and adnexa: to worry or not to worry. Radiographics. 2012;32(6):1621–39.

35. Lam CZ, Chavhan GB. Magnetic resonance imaging of pediatric adnexal masses and mimics. Pediatr Radiol. 2018;48(9):1291–306.

36. Ackerman S, Irshad A, Lewis M, Anis M. Ovarian cystic lesions a current approach to diagnosis and management. Radiol Clin N Am. 2013;51(6):1067–85.

37. Choe J, Wortman JR, Sodickson AD, Khurana B, Uyeda JW. Imaging of acute conditions of the perineum. Radiographics. 2018;38(4):1111–30.

38. Hosseinzadeh K, Heller MT, Houshmand G. Imaging of the female perineum in adults. Radiographics. 2012;32(4):E129–68.

39. Chauvin NA, Epelman M, Victoria T, Johnson AM. Complex genitourinary abnormalities on fetal MRI: imaging findings and approach to diagnosis. AJR Am J Radiol. 2012;199(2):W222–31.

40. Dannull KA, Browne LP, Meyers MZ. The spectrum of cloacal malformations: how to differentiate each entity prenatally with fetal MRI. Pediatr Radiol. 2019;49(3):387–98.

41. Dohke M, Watanabe Y, Okumura A, Amoh Y, Hayashi T, Yoshizako T, et al. Comprehensive MR imaging of acute gynecologic diseases. Radiographics. 2000;20(6):1551–66.

42. Czeyda-Pommersheim F, Kalb B, Costello J, Liau J, Meshksar A, Tiwari HA, et al. MRI in pelvic inflammatory disease: a pictorial review. Abdom Radiol. 2017;42(3):935–50.

43. Uyeda JW, Gans BS, Sodickson A. Imaging of acute and emergent genitourinary conditions: what the radiologist needs to know. AJR Am J Radiol. 2015;204:W631–W9.

44. Kim SH, Kim SH, Yang DM, Kim KA. Unusual causes of tubo-ovarian abscesses: CT and MR imaging findings. Radiographics. 2004;24(6):1575–89.

45. Vyas RC, Sides C, Klein DJ, Reddy SY, Santos MC. The ectopic appendicolith from perforated appendicitis as a cause of tubo-ovarian abscess. Pediatr Radiol. 2008;38(9):1006–8.

46. Towbin AJ, Sullivan J, Denson LA, Wallihan DB, Podberesky DJ. CT and MR enterography in children and adolescents with inflammatory bowel disease. Radiographics. 2013;33(7):1843–60.

47. Marro A, Allen LM, Kives SL, Moineddin R, Chavhan GB. Simulated impact of pelvic MRI in treatment planning for pediatric adnexal masses. Pediatr Radiol. 2016;46(9):1249–57.

48. Anthony EY, Caserta MP, Singh J, Chen MYM. Adnexal masses in female pediatric patients. AJR Am J Radiol. 2012;198(5):W426–31.

49. Epelman M, Chikwava KR, Chauvin N, Servaes S. Imaging of pediatric ovarian neoplasms. Pediatr Radiol. 2011;41(9):1085–99.

50. Taskinen S, Urtane A, Fagerholm R, Lohi J, Taskinen M. Metachronous benign ovarian tumors are not uncommon in children. J Pediatr Surg. 2014;49(4):543–5.

51. Heo SH, Kim JW, Shin SS, Jeong SI, Lim HS, Choi YD, et al. Review of ovarian tumors in children and adolescents: radiologic-pathologic correlation. Radiographics. 2014;34(7):2039–55.

52. Park E-A, Cho JY, Lee MW, Kim SH, Seong CK, Kim SH. MR features of fluid-fluid levels in ovarian masses. Eur Radiol. 2007;17:3247–54.

53. Vaysse C, Delsol M, Carfagna L, Bouali O, Combelles S, Lemasson F, et al. Ovarian germ cell tumors in children. Management, survival and ovarian prognosis. A report of 75 cases. J Pediatr Surg. 2010;45(7):1484–90.

54. Tanaka YO, Tsunoda H, Kitagawa Y, Ueno T, Yoshikawa H, Saida Y. Functioning ovarian tumors: direct and indirect findings at MR imaging. Radiographics. 2004;24(Suppl 1):S147–66.

55. Pai D, Coletti MC, Elkins M, Ladino-Torres M, Caoili E. Diffuse uterine leiomyomtosis in a child. Pediatr Radiol. 2012;42(1):124–8.

56. Moyle PL, Kataoka MY, Nakai A, Takahata A, Reinhold C, Sala E. Nonovarian cystic lesions of the pelvis. Radiographics. 2010;30(4):921–38.

57. Agrons GA, Wagner BJ, Lonergan GJ, Dickey GE, Kaufman MS. From the archives of the AFIP. Genitourinary rhabdomyosarcoma in children: radiologic-pathologic correlation. Radiographics. 1997;17(4):919–37.

58. Dehner LP, Jarzembowski JA, Hill DA. Embryonal rhabdomyosarcoma of the uterine cervix: a report of 14 cases and a discussion of its unusual clinicopathological associations. Mod Pathol. 2012;25(4):602–14.

59. Parikh JH, Barton DPJ, Ind TEJ, Sohaib SA. MR imaging features of vaginal malignancies. Radiographics. 2008;28(1):49–63.. quiz 322

60. Garel L, Dubois J, Grignon A, Filiatrault D, Vliet GV. US of the pediatric female pelvis: a clinical perspective. Radiographics. 2001;21(6):1393–407.

61. Niemi TA, Norton LW. Vaginal injuries in patients with pelvic fractures. J Trauma. 1985;25(6):547–51.

62. Goldman HB, Idom CB, Dmochowski RR. Traumatic injuries of the female external genitalia and their association with urological injuries. J Urol. 1998;159(3):956–9.

63. Laufer MR, Makai G. Evaluation and management of female lower genital tract trauma. In: Post TW, editor. UpToDate. Waltham: UpToDate Inc. https://www.uptodate.com. Accessed 13 Aug 2019.

64. Stricker T, Navratil F, Sennhauser FH. Vaginal foreign bodies. J Paediatr Child Health. 2004;40(4):205–7.

65. Kanso HN, Hachem K, Aoun NJ, Haddad-Zebouni S, Klein-Tomb L, Atallah D, et al. Variable MR findings in ovarian functional hemorrhagic cysts. J Magn Reson Imaging. 2006;24(2):356–61.

66. Lee NK, Kim S, Kim KH, Suh DS, Kim TU, Han GJ, et al. Diffusion-weighted magnetic resonance imaging in the differentiation of endometriomas from hemorrhagic cysts in the ovary. Acta Radiol. 2016;57(8):998–1005.

67. Brown M, Park AS, Shayya RF, Wolfson T, Su HI, Chang RJ. Ovarian imaging by magnetic resonance in adolescent girls with polycystic ovary syndrome and age-matched controls. J Magn Reson Imaging. 2013;38(3):689–93.

68. Bremer AA. Polycystic ovary syndrome in the pediatric population. Metab Syndr Relat Disord. 2010;8(5):375–94.

69. Rosenfeld RL. The polycystic ovary morphology-polycystic ovary syndrome spectrum. J Pediatr Adolesc Gynecol. 2015;28(6):412–9.

70. Lakhani K, Seifalian AM, Atiomo WU, Hardiman P. Polycystic ovaries. Br J Radiol. 2002;75(889):9–16. Review

71. ESHRE/ R. ASRM-sponsored PCOS consensus workshop group. Revised 2003 consensus on diagnostic criteria and long-term health risks related to polycystic ovary syndrome (PCOS). Hum Reprod. 2004;19(1):41–7. Review

72. Fondin M, Rachas A, Huynh V, Franchi-Abella S, Teglas J-P, Duranteau L, et al. Polycystic ovary syndrome in adolescents: which MR imaging-based diagnostic criteria? Radiology. 2017;285(3):961–70.

73. Rosenfeld RL. The diagnosis of polycystic ovary syndrome in adolescents. Pediatrics. 2015;136(6):1154–65.

74. Siegelman ES, Oliver ER. MR imaging of endometriosis: ten imaging pearls. Radiographics. 2012;32(6):1675–91.

75. Corwin MT, Gerscovich EO, Lamba R, Wilson MD. Differentiation of ovarian endometriomas from hemorrhagic cysts at MR imaging: utility of the T2 dark spot sign. Radiology. 2014;271(1):126–32.

76. Jensen JR, Charles C, Coddington I. Evolving spectrum: the pathogenesis of endometriosis. Clin Obstet Gynecol. 2010;53(2):379–88.

77. Glastonbury CM. The shading sign. Radiology. 2002;224(1):199–201.

78. Outwater E, Schiebler ML, Owen RS, Schnall MD. Characterization of hemorrhagic adnexal lesions with MR imaging: blinded reader study. Radiology. 1993;186(2):489–94.

79. Antonio Coutinho J, Bittencourt LK, Pires CE, Junqueira F, Lima CM, Coutinho E, et al. MR imaging in deep pelvic endometriosis: a pictorial essay. Radiographics. 2011;31(2):549–67.

80. Brosens I, Gordts S, Habiba M, Benagiano G. Uterine cystic adenomyosis: a disease of younger women. J Pediatr Adolesc Gynecol. 2015;28(6):420–6.

81. Byun JY, Kim SE, Choi BG. Diffuse and focal adenomyosis: MR imaging findings. Radiographics. 1999;19(Spec No):S161–S170.

82. Takeuchi M, Matsuzaki K. Adenomyosis: usual and unusual imaging manifestations, pitfalls, and problem-solving MR imaging techniques. Radiographics. 2011;31(1):99–115.

83. Ho ML, Raptis C, Hulett R. Adenomyotic cyst of the uterus in an adolescent. Pediatr Radiol. 2008;38(11):1239–42.

84. Huchon C, Fauconnier A. Adnexal torsion: a literature review. Eur J Obstet Gynecol Reprod Biol. 2010;150(1):8–12.

85. Oltmann SC, Fischer A, Barber R. Cannot exclude torsion--a 15 year review. J Pediatr Surg. 2009;44(6):1212–6.

86. Rha SE, Byun JY, Jung SE. CT and MR findings of adnexal torsion. Radiographics. 2002;22(2):283–94.

87. Servaes S, Zurakowski D, Laufer MR. Sonographic findings of ovarian torsion in children. Pediatr Radiol. 2007;37(5):446–51.

88. Beranger-Gibert S, Sakly H, Ballester M, Rockall A, Bornes M, Bazot M, et al. Diagnostic value of MR imaging in the diagnosis of adnexal torsion. Radiology. 2015;279(2):461–70.

89. Duigenan S, Olivia E, Lee SI. Ovarian torsion: diagnostic features on CT and MRI with pathologic correlation. AJR Am J Radiol. 2012;198(2):W122–31.

90. Lourenco AP, Swenson D, Tubbs RJ, Lazarus E. Ovarian and tubal torsion: imaging findings on US, CT and MRI. Emerg Radiol. 2014;21(2):179–87.

91. Piper HG, Oltmann SC, Xu L, Adusumilli S, Fischer AC. Ovarian torsion: diagnosis of inclusion mandates earlier intervention. J Pediatr Surg. 2012;47(11):2071–6.

92. Cohen SB, Oelsner G, Seidman DS, Admon D, Mashiach S, Goldenberg M. Laparoscopic detorsion allows sparing of the twisted ischemic adnexa. J Am Assoc Gynecol Laparasc. 1999;6(2):139–43.

93. Selim MF, Haggag MS, Hassan MA. Detorsion or adnexectomy for adnexal torsion and MRI for assessment of necrosis. J Gynecol Surg. 2015;31(6):336–41.

Peritoneum and Retroperitoneum

16

Archana Malik

Introduction

Peritoneal and retroperitoneal disorders are commonly encountered in the pediatric population. Recent advances in technology have led to increasing use of magnetic resonance (MR) imaging for evaluating the pediatric abdomen and pelvis, given its lack of ionizing radiation and superior contrast resolution compared to computed tomography (CT). This chapter reviews fundamental anatomy of the peritoneum and retroperitoneum, MR imaging techniques and protocols, as well as MR imaging findings across a range of peritoneal and retroperitoneal disease processes presenting in the pediatric population.

Magnetic Resonance Imaging Techniques

MR imaging is a standard part of evaluation of the pediatric abdomen and pelvis. Advances in MR imaging techniques such as faster pulse sequences with higher image signal and contrast, multichannel phased array coils allowing parallel imaging and other MR acceleration techniques, and improved gradients have resulted in decreased scan times and improved image quality of MR imaging in pediatric patients [1–3].

Patient Preparation and Coil Selection

Obtaining a high-quality abdominopelvic MR imaging study in young children can be challenging. Patient motion is the primary cause of image degradation, which may be involuntary secondary to respiratory or bowel motion or voluntary from conscious patient movement. Involuntary motion can be decreased or eliminated using specialized MR techniques

that are discussed under MR pulse sequences and protocols. Voluntary motion artifacts can be reduced by awake imaging in conjunction with a child life specialist or through the use of sedation or general anesthesia [4].

Generally, pediatric patients older than 6 years of age who understand verbal commands can lie still for the duration of the exam after explanation of the procedure and reassurance. Child life specialist preparing and coaching the pediatric patient in the scanner room, along with the use of distraction techniques such as MR compatible music/videos, can reduce patient anxiety and help pediatric patients undergo MR imaging awake [5]. For younger children or patients who are claustrophobic or cannot lie still, MR imaging examinations are performed with sedation or general anesthesia. These pediatric patients are evaluated by the anesthesiologist or sedation team physician prior to the procedure [4, 6].

Commonly used sedation medications include oral chloral hydrate, intravenous propofol or dexmedetomidine, and inhaled anesthetic agents. Neonates and young infants usually can be safely imaged without sedation using a "feed and swaddle" technique.

The patient should have nothing by mouth (NPO) for a period of time prior to MR imaging, particularly if sedation is used. Oral contrast agents are not necessary. To ensure patient comfort, the patient is instructed to empty their bladder immediately prior to the exam.

Selection of the appropriate coil is critical and depends on the patient size. It is desired to use the smallest coil that covers the region of interest, to ensure a high signal to noise ratio and improved spatial resolution. The head coil usually suffices for infants and younger children, with a phased array body or torso coil used for older children and adolescents [7].

A. Malik (✉)
Department of Radiology, St. Christopher's Hospital for Children,
Drexel University College of Medicine, Philadelphia, PA, USA
e-mail: archana.malik@americanacademic.com

© Springer Nature Switzerland AG 2020
E. Y. Lee et al. (eds.), *Pediatric Body MRI*, https://doi.org/10.1007/978-3-030-31989-2_16

MRI Pulse Sequences and Protocols

Unenhanced Spin-Echo Sequences T1-weighted MR images obtained with either spin-echo or gradient-echo techniques provide good anatomical detail and are sensitive to pathology associated with fat or blood products. T2-weighted fast spin-echo MR images obtained with and without fat suppression are sensitive to fluid and cellular lesions. T2-weighted MR images can be obtained using single-shot techniques (e.g., HASTE, SSH-TSE, or SSFSE) with short acquisition times (<30 seconds) and produce motion-free images in children who cannot suspend respiration, which is a key advantage in the pediatric population [8, 9]. Obtaining T2-weighted sequences with fat suppression improves contrast between the disease process and underlying tissues by eliminating signal from background fat.

Sequences are obtained with 3–5 mm slice thickness with minimal spacing depending on patient size. Respiratory triggering is typically used for fast spin-echo T2-weighted MR images, with single-shot images acquired ideally as a breath-hold but also acceptable as a free-breathing acquisition.

Unenhanced Gradient-Echo Sequences Axial Dixon dual-echo (in- and opposed-phase) gradient-echo T1-weighted sequences have shorter acquisition time when compared to the T1 FSE images and therefore can be performed within short breath-hold times [8–10]. Loss of signal on opposed-phase imaging is helpful for detection of intracellular lipid within lesions (e.g., adrenal adenomas). Balanced steady-state free precession sequences (e.g., FIESTA, B-FFE, TrueFISP) are gradient-echo sequences with mixed weighting (signal intensity α T2/T1) that have similar imaging times with single-shot imaging and generate high-quality anatomic images in a single breath-hold. These image exhibit hypointense chemical shift artifacts outlining the interfaces between water and fat is particularly useful for evaluating lymph nodes and blood vessels within the small-bowel mesentery and omentum.

Contrast-Enhanced Sequences Gadolinium-based contrast agents are used on pediatric MR imaging to characterize focal lesions, at typical dose of 0.1 mmol/kg. There is increasing use of three-dimensional gradient recalled echo (GRE) fat-suppressed T1-weighted (e.g., LAVA, THRIVE, VIBE) pre- and post-contrast sequences as these can be acquired in multiple planes in substantially less time than conventional T1-weighted SE sequences with fat suppression, also allowing improved contrast detection in pediatric patients with small volume of contrast dose [10].

Anatomy

Embryology

The primitive gut within the abdominal cavity is suspended by two peritoneal reflections called the primitive mesenteries which contain vessels, lymphatic channels, and nerves. The various mesenteries are generated from the common dorsal mesentery, while the falciform ligament and lesser sac arise from the ventral mesentery (Fig. 16.1). The majority of ventral portion of the mesentery at the level of the midgut is lost during evolution in the fetal life. Specialized development including rotation, descent, and resorption of the mesenteric plane occurs throughout fetal life [11].

Fig. 16.1 Embryological development of the peritoneal spaces, schematic diagram. (**a**) The ventral mesentery contains the liver bud (liver), and the dorsal mesentery contains the splenic bud (S), superior to the transverse mesocolon. St = stomach, R = right, L = left. (**b**) With continued development, these organs migrate counterclockwise and take the attached mesenteries with them. (**c**) This migration divides the right peritoneal cavity into the right perihepatic space and the lesser sac (*blue area*). The left peritoneal space forms the left subphrenic space (*purple area*)

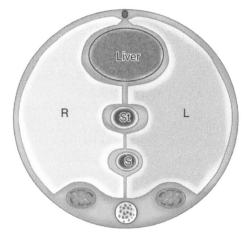

Fetus 5th week

a

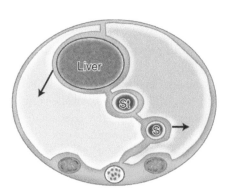

Fetus 10th week

b

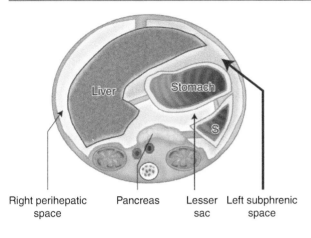

Right perihepatic   Pancreas   Lesser   Left subphrenic
    space   sac   space

Post-Natal

c

Fig. 16.1 (continued)

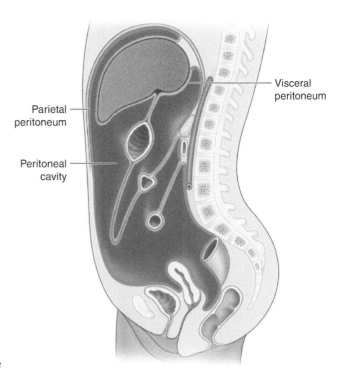

Fig. 16.2 The structure of the peritoneum and the peritoneal cavity. The parietal peritoneum (*red outline*) outlines the inner abdominal wall, diaphragm, and the posterior abdominal wall. The visceral peritoneum (*blue outline*) invaginates to cover the organs

Normal Development and Anatomy

The peritoneum is an epithelial-lined thin serous membrane and includes two components, the parietal peritoneum that covers the innermost surface of the abdominal wall and inferior surface of the diaphragm and the visceral peritoneum that outlines the majority of the visceral organs (Fig. 16.2). The peritoneal cavity is the potential space between the parietal and visceral peritoneum which contains a few mL of serous fluid. It is a closed sac in males and is open in females to the extraperitoneal space via the ostia of the fallopian tubes [12, 13].

The peritoneal ligaments, mesentery, and omentum are specialized peritoneal infoldings comprising double layer of peritoneum, blood vessels, lymphatics, and variable amount of fat, which divide the peritoneal cavity into the greater sac and the lesser sac. The lesser sac is situated posterior to the stomach and communicates with the greater sac via the epiploic foramen or foramen of Winslow. The peritoneum and its reflections can be involved by various disease processes of infectious, inflammatory, neoplastic, and traumatic etiologies. The peritoneal fluid flows superiorly from the pelvis to the subhepatic and subphrenic spaces through the paracolic gutters, following the negative intra-abdominal pressure gradient. Peritoneal tumors and infection follow the peritoneal fluid circulation. Knowledge of the anatomy is helpful in understanding the disease process localization and spread.

The retroperitoneum is the space between the posterior parietal peritoneum and the posterior body wall, extending from the diaphragm to the pelvic inlet. The duodenum, portions of the colon, pancreas, adrenal glands, kidneys, abdominal aorta, and inferior vena cava are located in the retroperitoneum, and these are separated from the peritoneum

Table 16.1 Contents of the peritoneal and retroperitoneal spaces

Intraperitoneal organs (suspended by mesentery)	Primary retroperitoneal organs (no mesentery)	Secondary retroperitoneal organs (lost mesentery during development)
Stomach	Adrenal glands	Duodenum, second and third parts
Liver and gallbladder	Kidneys and ureters	Pancreas: head, neck, and body
Spleen	Inferior vena cava	Ascending and descending colon
Pancreas: tail	Aorta	Upper two thirds rectum
Duodenum, first part	Distal third rectum	
Jejunum		
Ileum		
Appendix	Anal canal	
Transverse and sigmoid colon		

anteriorly by the posterior peritoneal fascia (Table 16.1) [13]. The retroperitoneum can be divided into three compartments, the anterior and posterior pararenal spaces and the perirenal space by the anterior and posterior renal fascia and the latero-conal fascia (Fig. 16.3). A newer classification system categorizes the perirenal space into the retromesenteric, retrorenal, and latero-conal spaces which are potentially contiguous [14].

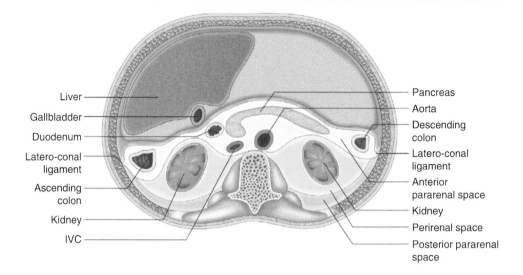

Fig. 16.3 The retroperitoneal spaces. Schematic transverse section through the kidneys shows the perirenal and pararenal spaces and the latero-conal ligaments. IVC inferior vena cava

Spectrum of Peritoneal and Retroperitoneal Disorders

Congenital Peritoneal and Retroperitoneal Disorders

Gastroschisis and Omphalocele Gastroschisis and omphalocele comprise the two main types of ventral abdominal wall defects. Fetal MR imaging is a useful adjunct to ultrasound for detailed evaluation of these entities. Gastroschisis is herniation through a paraumbilical abdominal wall defect, with normal insertion of the cord, and absence of a covering sac. As the herniated bowel loops are free floating and subject to the amniotic fluid, there is propensity for bowel wall thickening and adhesions and complications of bowel atresia [15]. The exact etiology of gastroschisis is unclear. There is an association with young maternal age. On MR imaging, freely floating bowel loops are seen herniating through an anterior abdominal wall defect adjacent to an intact umbilical cord (Fig. 16.4). Intraluminal fluid and meconium within bowel loops appear hyperintense on T2-weighted and T1-weighted MR images, respectively.

Omphalocele is herniation of abdominal viscera at the base of the umbilical cord through an enlarged umbilical ring, with insertion of the cord on the covering membrane. Herniating organs can include bowel loops, liver, and other viscera and are covered by a hernia sac. Etiological factors include failure of bowel loops to return to the abdominal cavity after normal physiologic herniation (occurs during 11 and 13 weeks of gestation) and failure of the abdominal wall closure. Unlike gastroschisis, there is a high association with other congenital abnormalities, with cardiac, central nervous system, and urogenital abnormalities are the most common. Omphalocele can also be a part of more complex abdominal wall defects such as pentalogy of Cantrell, cloacal exstrophy, and limb-body wall complex [16, 17]. On fetal MR imaging, a central anterior abdominal wall defect with herniation of the abdominal organs into a thin-walled sac is seen (Fig. 16.5). The herniating liver is hypointense on T2-weighted and slightly hyperintense on T1-weighted MR images (see Fig. 16.5).

Omental and Mesenteric Cysts Omental and mesenteric cysts are uncommon developmental intra-abdominal lesions that result due to migration of a small-bowel or colonic diverticulum into the small-bowel mesentery or mesocolon [18]. Clinical presentation is variable ranging from asymptomatic to acute abdomen [19–21].

On MR imaging, these cystic lesions are thin-walled, T1-weighted hypointense and T2-weighted hyperintense with no or minimal wall enhancement, as opposed to enteric duplication cysts that typically have an enhancing wall. The imaging findings of various cystic lesions can overlap, with histology typically required for definitive diagnosis (Table 16.2) [18].

Mesothelial Cyst Mesothelial cyst is a rare congenital lesion that arises from coelomic remnants and is lined by mesothelial cells. Mesothelial cysts can occur in the mesentery, spleen, adrenal gland, ovary, falciform ligament, processus vaginalis, and diaphragm.

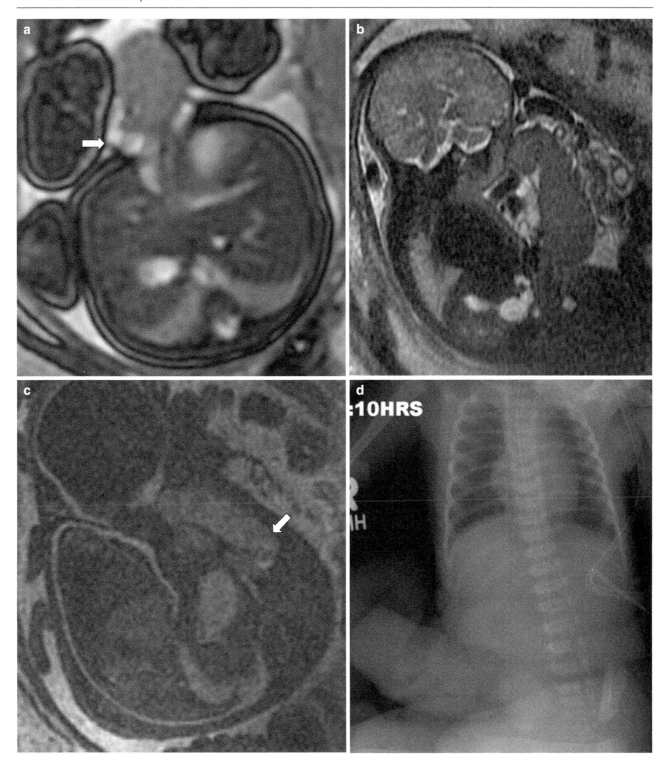

Fig. 16.4 Pre- and postnatal imaging appearance of gastroschisis. Prenatal MR imaging of a 36-weeks gestation female fetus (**a**) axial steady-state free precession (SSFP) MR image demonstrates a midline abdominal defect (*arrow*) and herniation of intra-abdominal contents. (**b**, **c**) Sagittal single-shot T2-weighted (**b**) and T1-weighted fat-suppressed (**c**) MR images show high T1-weighted signal within the herniated bowel confirming the presence of meconium (*arrow*) within colon. Postnatal imaging with preoperative (**d**) and postoperative (**e**) abdominal radiographs, as well as postoperative photograph (**f**) noting silo placement

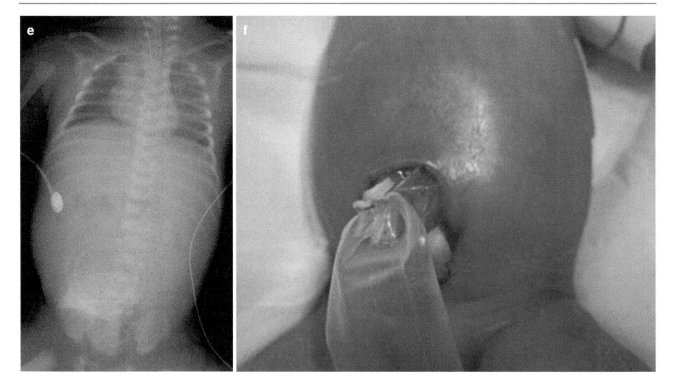

Fig. 16.4 (continued)

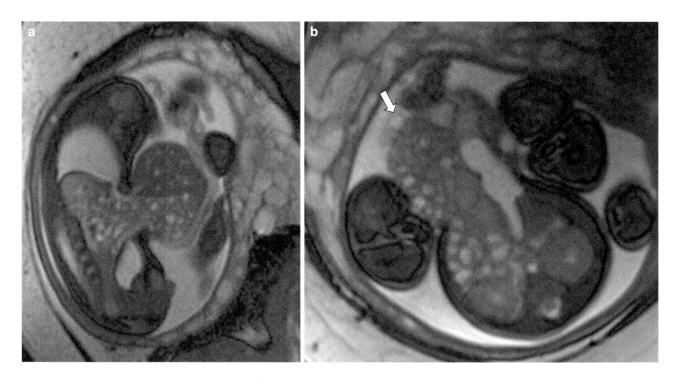

Fig. 16.5 Fetal MR imaging appearance of an omphalocele in a 23-weeks gestation male fetus. Sagittal (**a**) and axial (**b**) SSFP MR images show a contained herniation of liver and bowel loops through a midline abdominal wall defect. The umbilical cord (*arrow*) inserts at the apex of the herniating mass differentiating it from a gastroschisis

On MR imaging, the cysts are T1-weighted hypointense and T2-weighted hyperintense with no discernible wall (Fig. 16.6). Unlike lymphatic malformations, these are unilocular cystic lesions which lack internal septations and intrinsic T1-weighted signal. Diaphragmatic mesothelial cysts have been described as bilobed cystic lesions located between the posterolateral aspect of the right liver lobe and the diaphragm [22, 23].

Meconium Peritonitis and Pseudocyst Meconium peritonitis is the most common cause of peritoneal calcifications in the neonate. It is a sterile, chemical peritonitis that occurs due to intrauterine intestinal perforation [24]. This can also result in scrotal calcifications in neonates with patent processus vaginalis (Fig. 16.7).

Lymphatic Malformation Lymphatic malformations are developmental anomalies in which focal lymphatic channels fail to establish connections with the central lymphatic system. Most common location is the head, neck, or axilla. Intra-abdominal location is uncommon but can occur within the mesentery and retroperitoneum [22, 23]. Clinical presentation is variable, including progressive abdominal distention and acute or chronic abdominal pain.

On imaging, these are multiseptated, cystic collections insinuating multiple planes. Ultrasound is a sensitive modality and shows cystic or multicystic mass with internal septations. MR imaging is the preferred imaging modality

Table 16.2 Histologic classification for peritoneal and retroperitoneal congenital cystic masses

Omental and mesenteric cyst	Enteric lining (mucosa)
Enteric duplication cyst	Enteric lining (mucosa), dual muscle lining with neural elements
Mesothelial cyst	Mesothelial lining
Lymphatic malformation	Endothelial lining
Pseudocyst (non-pancreatic)	No lining

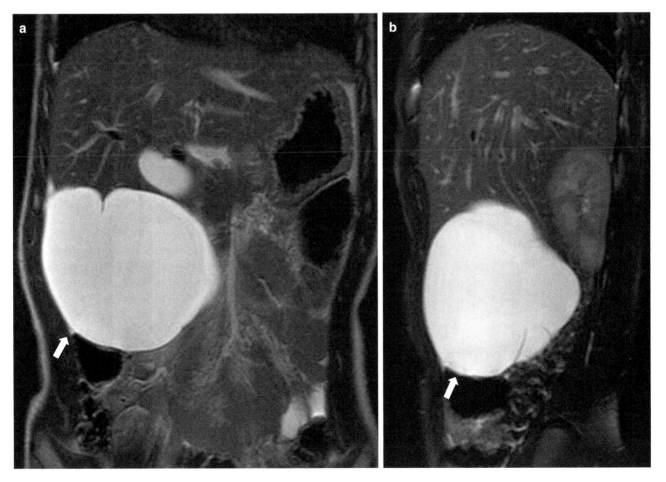

Fig. 16.6 Mesothelial cyst in a 15-year-old boy. Coronal (**a**) and sagittal (**b**) T2-weighted MR images of the abdomen show a well-circumscribed, fluid intensity mass (*arrows*) in the right upper quadrant, inferior to and abutting the liver. Axial-enhanced T1-weighted fat-suppressed MR image (**c**) shows minimal peripheral enhancement confirming the lesion's cystic nature. This was found to be a mesothelial cyst on histology

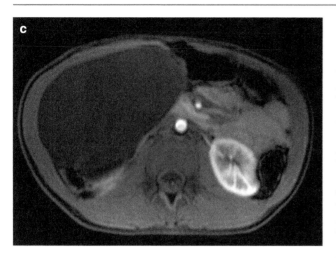

Fig. 16.6 (continued)

for preoperative assessment, as it provides better anatomic delineation of the cystic mass with surrounding organs. MR imaging findings include T1-weighted hypointense and T2-weighted hyperintense multilocular cystic lesions with peripheral and septal enhancement. Intrinsic T1-weighted signal intensity can be seen in some lymphatic malformations from proteinaceous elements (Fig. 16.8).

Bronchogenic Cyst Bronchogenic cyst is a benign congenital anomaly secondary to aberrant budding of the developing tracheobronchial tree between 26th and 40th days of gestation. The abnormal bud differentiates into a blind ending, fluid-filled pouch, lined by respiratory epithelium with bronchial glands, smooth muscle, and cartilage [25]. Bronchogenic cyst most commonly occurs in the mediastinum, typically near the carina; however extra-mediastinal locations such as lung parenchyma

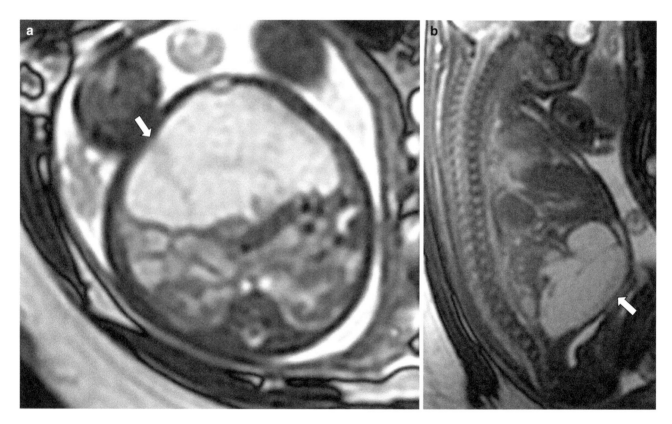

Fig. 16.7 Pre- and postnatal imaging findings of meconium peritonitis and pseudocyst. Axial (**a**) and sagittal (**b**) SSFP MR images of a 30-week gestation female fetus from a prenatal MR imaging demonstrate a large, complex cystic lesion (*arrows*) in the peritoneal cavity with mildly dilated proximal bowel loops. The cystic lesion demon-strates high T1-weighted signal on the sagittal T1-weighted fat-sup-pressed MR image (**c**), similar to adjacent bowel loops. Postnatally, abdomen radiograph (**d**) and abdominal ultrasound (**e**) at day 1 of life confirm the findings of meconium peritonitis and a calcified mass in the midline and right hemiabdomen consistent with pseudocyst

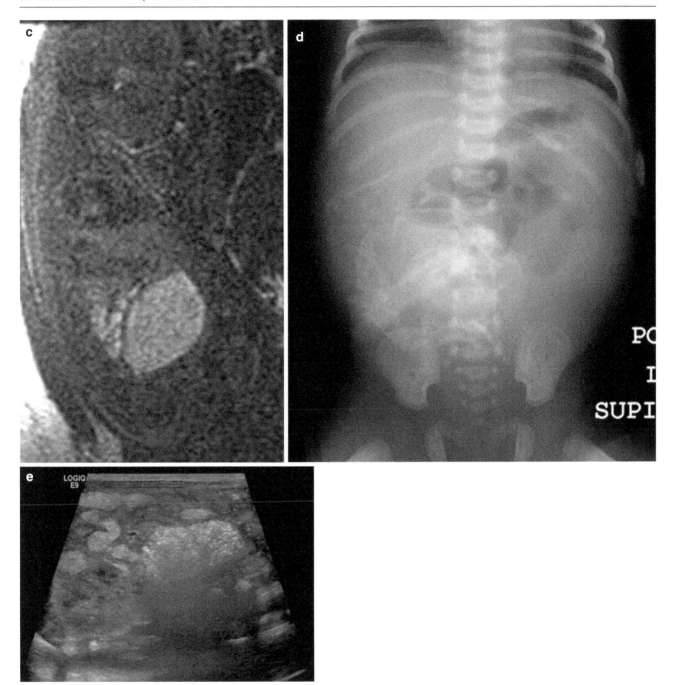

Fig. 16.7 (continued)

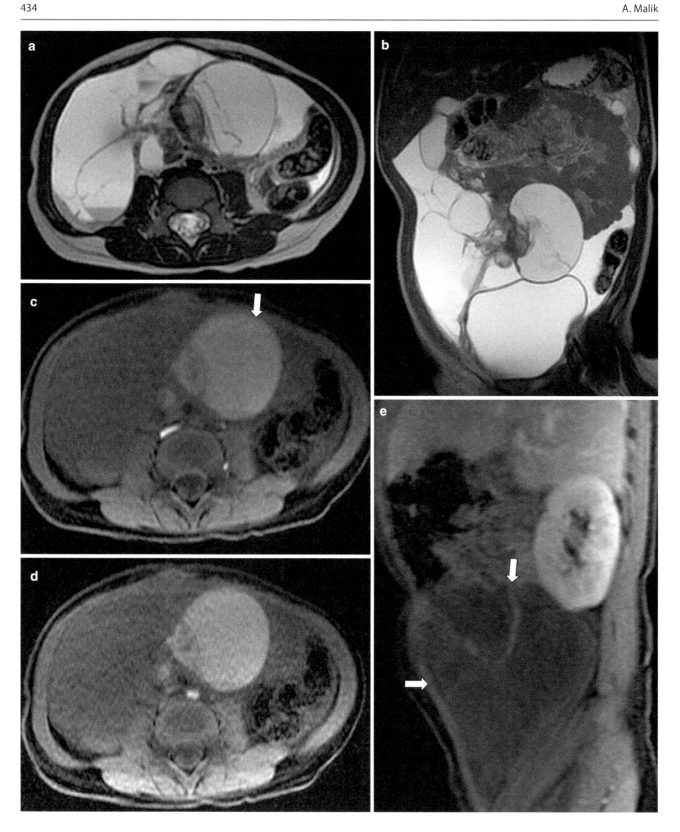

Fig. 16.8 Lymphatic malformation in a 20-month-old boy who presented with progressively worsening abdominal distention and discomfort. Axial (**a**) and coronal (**b**) radial T2-weighted MR images show a predominantly hyperintense, multiloculated cystic lesion with fluid-fluid levels. Axial-unenhanced T1-weighted fat-suppressed MR image (**c**) shows T1-weighted hyperintensity within a large locule (*arrow*), suggesting proteinaceous component. Axial- (**d**) and sagittal- (**e**) enhanced T1-weighted fat-suppressed MR images show peripheral and septal enhancement (*arrows*). The extent of the lesion and relationship with surrounding structures is better evaluated by MR imaging

and pleura have been described, with rare occurrence in the retroperitoneum [26, 27]. Presentation is usually within first few decades of life and varies with size and location of the cyst. Symptoms when present usually occur secondary to compression of adjacent organs.

MR imaging shows a sharply marginated, rounded cystic lesion with no enhancement. MR imaging has supe-rior soft tissue contrast resolution compared to CT and is therefore helpful in characterization of bronchogenic cysts which do not follow homogenous or fluid attenuation on CT. Signal characteristics depend upon the nature of the fluid and are typically T1-weighted hypointense and T2-weighted hyperintense. T1-weighted signal can be seen with proteinaceous material (Fig. 16.9). Both

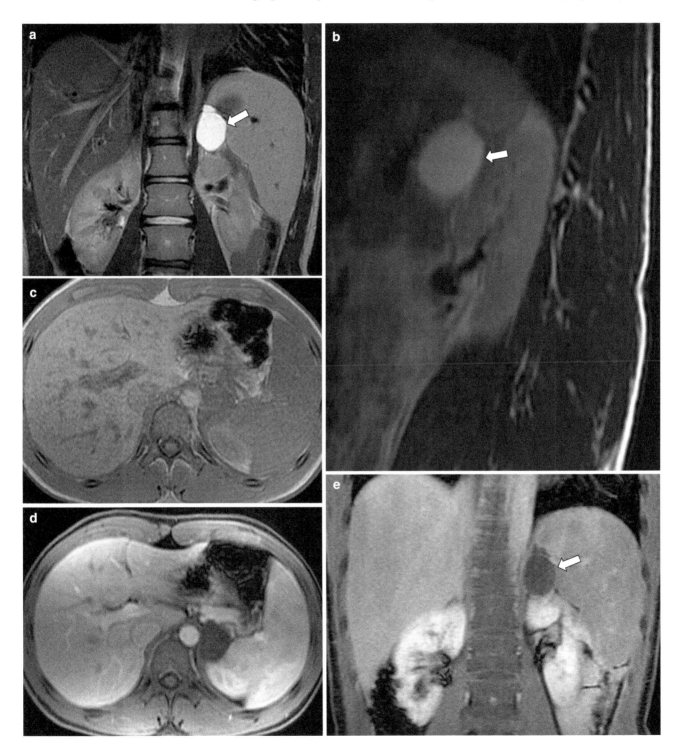

Fig. 16.9 Retroperitoneal bronchogenic cyst in a 16-year-old boy on MR imaging. Coronal (**a**) and sagittal (**b**) T2-weighted MR images show a cystic lesion (*arrows*) in the left retroperitoneum, immediately anterior to the upper pole of the left kidney. Axial-unenhanced T1-weighted MR image (**c**) shows hypointensity, while axial- (**d**) and coronal- (**e**) enhanced T1-weighted fat-suppressed MR images show peripheral enhancement (*arrow*). This lesion was found to be a bronchogenic cyst by histology

subdiaphragmatic and retroperitoneal locations have also been described for bronchogenic cysts [28].

Infectious and Inflammatory Peritoneal and Retroperitoneal Disorders

Mesenteric Adenitis MR imaging of the acute abdomen, particularly for suspected appendicitis, is emerging as an alternative to CT when ultrasound is equivocal [29]. Mesenteric lymph nodes in children are often considered abnormal if they are greater than 5 mm in diameter. Mesenteric lymphadenopathy can be seen with infectious, inflammatory, or neoplastic etiologies. Mesenteric adenitis is benign inflammation of the mesenteric lymph nodes, seen as an isolated finding in the absence of other infectious, inflammatory, or neoplastic etiologies [30]. The clinical presentation can mimic other common acute abdominal processes such as appendicitis, including nausea, vomiting, right lower quadrant abdominal pain and tenderness, fever, and leukocytosis.

On MR imaging, multiple prominent right lower quadrant mesenteric lymph nodes are seen adjacent to the ileocecal valve, sometimes with associated mild ileocecal wall thickening but in the absence of other pathologic features (Fig. 16.10).

Omental Infarction Omental infarction is vascular compromise of the greater omentum and can either be primary or secondary to surgical trauma. The right lateral edge of the omentum has a more tenuous blood supply than the rest of the omentum, making it more prone to infarction. Clinical presentation typically is subacute onset of right lower quadrant pain, often with a mildly elevated white blood cell count, mimicking other entities such as acute appendicitis. Other GI symptoms such as vomiting, nausea, and fever are uncommon. Imaging plays a useful role in establishing the diagnosis.

On MR imaging, omental infarction presents typically as a large (>5 cm) fatty encapsulated mass, with soft tissue stranding adjacent to the ascending colon (Fig. 16.11). Early or mild infarction may manifest as mild fat stranding and haziness anterior to the colon. Swirling of vessels in the omentum suggests omental torsion [31, 32].

Peritoneal Inclusion Cyst Peritoneal inclusion cyst, also known as peritoneal pseudocysts, typically occur in females of reproductive age. There are known association with prior abdominal or pelvic surgery, pelvic inflammatory disease, and endometriosis. The most common presenting symptom is lower abdominal or pelvic pain. Although these can be diagnosed by ultrasound, MR imaging can be helpful in equivocal cases as it allows improved characterization of the lesion and delineation of adjacent anatomic structures.

On MR imaging, peritoneal inclusion cysts are regular- or irregular-shaped cystic lesions which abut and envelop the

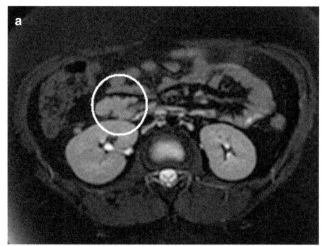

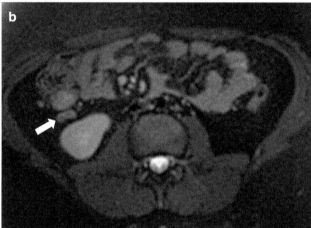

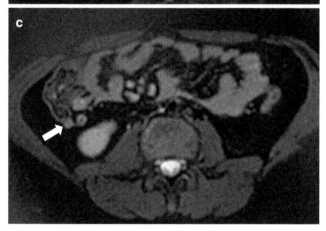

Fig. 16.10 Mesenteric adenitis in a 10-year-old boy who presented with acute abdominal pain and increased inflammatory markers. Axial (**a–c**) T2-weighted fat-suppressed MR images of the abdomen and pelvis demonstrate a cluster of enlarged mesenteric lymph nodes (*circle*) in the right hemiabdomen with a normal appendix (*arrows*)

surrounding structures (often an ovary) and typically have low signal intensity on T1-weighted MR images and high signal intensity on T2-weighted MR images. Internal heterogeneity of the lesion on T1- and T2-weighted sequences with "spider web" appearance can be noted. There is no enhancement on post-contrast T1-weighted fat-suppressed MR images (Fig. 16.12) [33, 34].

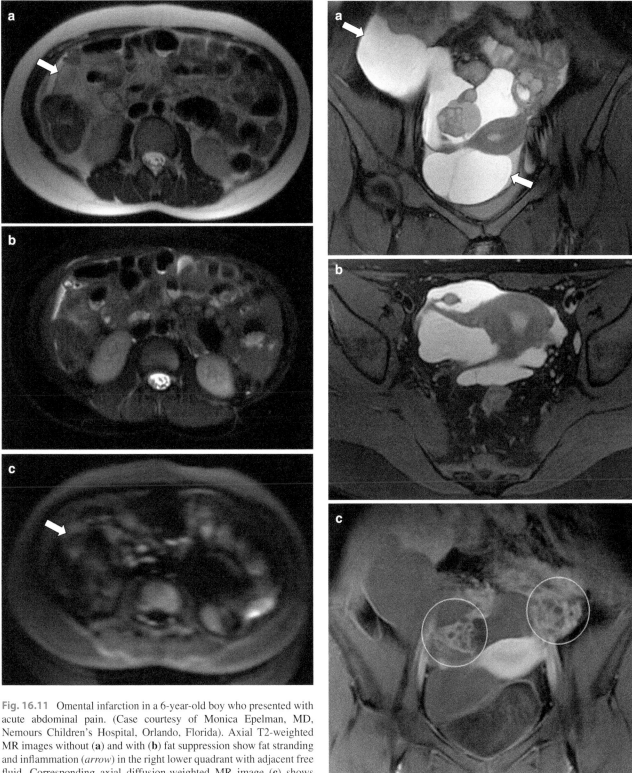

Fig. 16.11 Omental infarction in a 6-year-old boy who presented with acute abdominal pain. (Case courtesy of Monica Epelman, MD, Nemours Children's Hospital, Orlando, Florida). Axial T2-weighted MR images without (**a**) and with (**b**) fat suppression show fat stranding and inflammation (*arrow*) in the right lower quadrant with adjacent free fluid. Corresponding axial diffusion-weighted MR image (**c**) shows associated restricted diffusion (*arrow*)

Abdominal Cerebrospinal Fluid (CSF) Pseudocyst Ventriculoperitoneal shunt placement is a commonly performed procedure for management of hydrocephalus. Shunt-related complications include infection of the shunt, malfunction due to mechanical disruption or blockage, and formation of intra-

Fig. 16.12 Peritoneal inclusion cyst in a 19-year-old woman with prior abdominal surgeries who presented with pelvic discomfort. Coronal (**a**) and axial (**b**) T2-weighted fat-suppressed MR images demonstrate a complex, irregular cystic lesion (*arrows*) in the pelvis with internal septations giving a "spider web" appearance. Mild peripheral and septal enhancement is noted on corresponding coronal-enhanced T1-weighted fat-suppressed MR image (**c**). Both ovaries appear "entrapped" within cystic lesion (*circles*), consistent with a peritoneal inclusion cyst

abdominal CSF pseudocyst, most commonly occurring at the distal tip of the shunt [35]. Development of pseudocyst is attributed to inflammatory response usually secondary to an infectious process. As the name implies, the pseudocyst is lined by a fibrous wall that is non-epithelial and may include inflamed serosa [36, 37].

Pediatric patients with abdominal pseudocysts most commonly present with signs and symptoms of increased intracranial pressure due to shunt malfunction and acute abdominal signs such as abdominal pain, distention, and bowel obstruction depending upon the size of the cyst. Although plain radiographs and ultrasound are the first-line imaging modalities for investigation of a suspected pseudocyst, cross-sectional imaging may be required when patients present with acute abdomen mimicking other common acute pathologies [37, 38]. On MR imaging, the pseudocysts are low T1-weighted/high T2-weighted signal unilocular or multiseptated lesions that occur at the distal tip of the shunt catheter, with variable peripheral enhancement.

If infection is present, treatment includes temporary externalization of the shunt, systemic antibiotics, and repositioning or revising the shunt either as ventriculoperitoneal or alternate routes such as ventriculoatrial or ventriculopleural locations [36]. Ultrasound-guided percutaneous aspiration may be helpful in guiding antibiotic treatment.

Intraperitoneal and Retroperitoneal Abscess Abdominal and pelvic abscesses can be seen in pediatric patients due to infectious and inflammatory etiologies, such as perforated appendicitis, inflammatory bowel disease, enterocolitis, pelvic inflammatory disease, and tubo-ovarian infection (female patients). Retroperitoneal abscesses can be seen with hematogenous or musculoskeletal infections such as discitis-osteomyelitis (Fig. 16.13) [39].

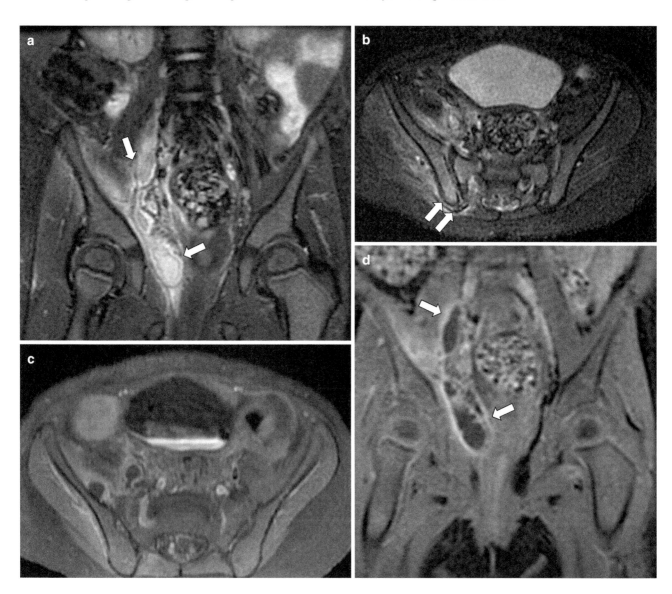

Fig. 16.13 Retroperitoneal and pelvic abscesses in a 17-month-old girl with septic sacroiliitis and osteomyelitis. Coronal (**a**) and axial (**b**) STIR MR images show multiloculated fluid collections in the right retroperitoneal soft tissues and right iliacus and extending inferiorly into the pelvis with rim enhancement on axial- (**c**) and coronal- (**d**) enhanced T1-weighted fat-suppressed MR images, consistent with abscesses (*arrows*). Abnormal high STIR signal is noted in the right ischium and sacroiliac joint (**b**; *paired arrows*)

Neoplastic Peritoneal and Retroperitoneal Disorders

Benign and malignant peritoneal and retroperitoneal masses are sometimes encountered in the pediatric population. These masses can be mesodermal, ectodermal, neurogenic, or lymphatic in origin.

Peritoneal masses are much less common in children compared to adults, given the decreased prevalence of neoplasms with peritoneal spread [40]. When peritoneal malignancy is present, metastatic disease is much more common than primary peritoneal neoplasms in the pediatric population [40, 41].

Desmoid tumor, inflammatory myofibroblastic tumor, Castleman disease, and other mesenchymal masses can present as localized peritoneal masses, whereas diffuse peritoneal disease can be seen with malignant tumors such as rhabdomyosarcoma, non-Hodgkin lymphoma, and desmoplastic small round cell tumors (DSRCT) [41].

Benign Neoplasms The majority of the benign peritoneal solid masses appear as focal lesions.

Desmoid Tumor or Mesenteric Fibromatosis Desmoid tumor or mesenteric fibromatosis is a benign but locally aggressive neoplasm of mesenchymal origin, seen in association with familial adenomatous polyposis (FAP) and Gardner syndrome [42]. Desmoid tumor can be intra-abdominal (mesenteric location most common), in the abdominal wall, or extraabdominal.

Intra-abdominal desmoids seen in association with FAP and Gardner syndrome are often located in the small-bowel mesentery, are more infiltrative, and have less well-defined margins compared to non-FAP-associated desmoids [43, 44]. Desmoids can also be mass-like and result in local compression or infiltration and present as intestinal obstruction or hydronephrosis. Signal characteristics vary with the proportion of collagen, spindle cells, and extracellular matrix [45]. Most commonly, desmoid tumor is usually intermediate to hyperintense relative to skeletal muscle on T2-weighted MR images and isointense on T1-weighted MR images. T2-weighted hypointensity suggests the presence of increasing collagen and decreasing cellularity. Higher T2-weighted signal is reflective of higher cellularity and can suggest active growth or recurrence. Contrast enhancement is variable [44, 45].

Inflammatory Myofibroblastic Tumor Inflammatory myofibroblastic tumor (IMT) is a rare mesenchymal tumor that can arise in any anatomic location, but most often seen in the lung, mesentery, and omentum [46]. With more recent data, this is now considered a neoplasm of borderline biologic behavior rather than an inflammatory process as previously thought. It is most commonly seen in children and young adults. Clinical presentation varies with location of the lesion and may include systemic signs and symptoms mimicking an infectious process. Abdominal pain is the most common symptom [46, 47].

The imaging findings are variable and nonspecific, although the presence of a well-circumscribed, solid mass with central calcifications is suggestive of IMT. On MR imaging, the tumor appears hypointense relative to skeletal muscle on T1-weighted sequences and hyperintense on T2-weighted sequences, noting that tumors with a large fibrous component can appear hypointense on both sequences. Enhancement pattern is variable and mostly heterogeneous. Larger lesions may have areas of central necrosis [47, 48]. Imaging appearance can vary with histologic composition of inflammatory cell infiltrate and fibrosis. Treatment of choice is complete surgical excision [46].

Castleman Disease Castleman disease is an idiopathic benign lymphoproliferative disorder that most commonly arises in the chest but can involve the lymphatic tissues in the neck and mesentery [49]. It is primarily seen in young adults with rare occurrence in pediatric population. There are two recognized clinical forms, unicentric and multicentric [49, 50].

In children, Castleman disease is usually unicentric, appearing as a well-circumscribed, intensely enhancing discrete mass or dominant mass with satellite nodules in the mesentery [51]. Hepatosplenomegaly, ascites, and diffuse lymphadenopathy are seen in the multicentric form [52].

On MR imaging, Castleman disease is hypointense on T1-weighted MR images and heterogeneously hyperintense on T2-weighted MR images relative to skeletal muscle. Peripheral flow voids representing feeding vessels may be seen. Enhancement pattern is typically early and intense, with delayed washout. A characteristic feature of Castleman disease is a T2-weighted hypointense stellate scar, which is also hypointense on early phase-enhanced T1-weighted fat-suppressed MR images [50, 52].

Lipoblastoma Lipoblastoma is an uncommon benign mesenchymal tumor seen exclusively in infants and young children, with almost 90% of the cases diagnosed before the age of 3 years [53]. Presentation depends upon size and location of the lesion. It usually involves soft tissues of the extremities and trunk and is rarely seen in the face, neck, buttock, perirectal area, and abdomen. In the abdomen, mesenteric, omental, and retroperitoneal locations have been described. Lipoblastoma is the primary differential for a fat-containing retroperitoneal tumor in the pediatric population [53, 54].

MR imaging demonstrates a soft tissue lobulated mass which is hyperintense on T1- and T2-weighted MR images and demonstrates characteristic signal loss on fat-suppressed sequences, consistent with a fat-containing lesion (Fig. 16.14). Signal intensity of the mass is relative to the amounts of lipoblasts and myxocollagenous stromal tissue

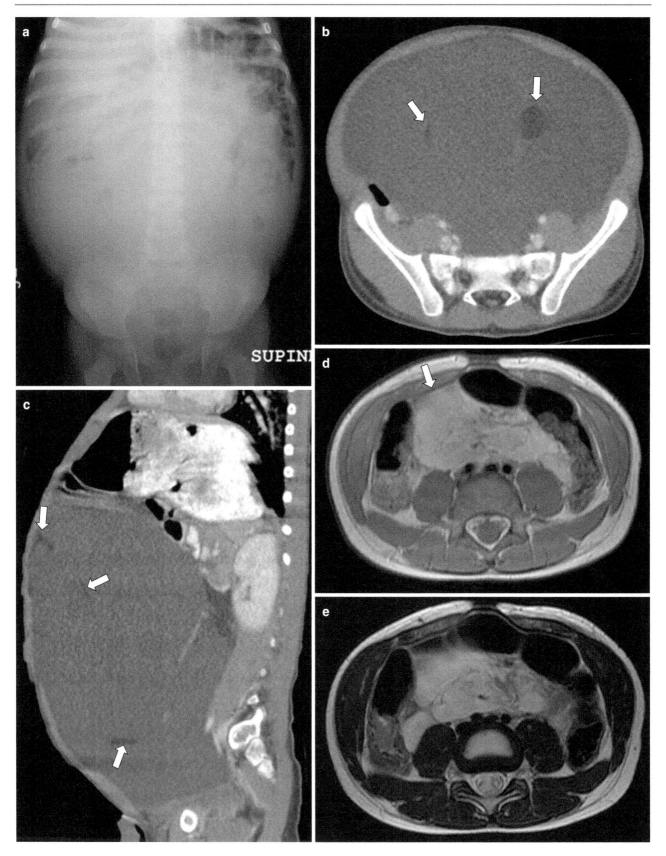

Fig. 16.14 Lipoblastoma in a 3-year-old boy who presented with progressively worsening abdominal distention and discomfort. Initial abdomen radiograph (**a**) shows large central mass in the abdomen and pelvis with peripheral displacement of the bowel loops. Axial (**b**) and sagittal (**c**) CT images show a large cystic mass in the abdomen and pelvis with scattered foci of fat attenuation (*arrows*). MR imaging better demonstrates the fatty nature of the mass with high signal intensity on axial T1-weighted (**d**), as well as axial (**e**) and coronal (**f**) T2-weighted MR images. The mass demonstrates signal loss (*arrow*) following fat suppression (**g**)

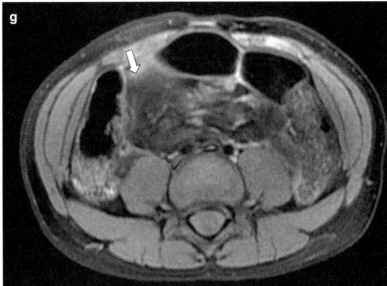

Fig. 16.14 (continued)

within it [53]. Treatment is complete excision. Recurrence can occur if there are positive surgical margins [54].

Nerve Sheath Tumor Neurofibromas and plexiform neurofibromas are benign peripheral nerve sheath tumors and the hallmark lesion of neurofibromatosis type-1 (NF-1), a genetic multisystem neurocutaneous disorder [55]. In patients with NF-1, involvement of the gastrointestinal organs and associated mesenteric and peritoneal soft tissues is much less common than cutaneous manifestations [55, 56]. Symptoms are nonspecific and may include abdominal pain, intestinal obstruction, or other symptoms from mass effect. The paraspinal and presacral region in the distribution of the lumbosacral plexus are the most common abdominal locations for neurofibromas. Mesenteric plexiform neurofibromas may appear as multiple, discrete nodular masses or infiltrating lesions.

MR imaging is the modality of choice for imaging patients with NF-1, as the findings are characteristic and multiplanar capabilities allow in delineating the extent of the tumors. Neurofibromas demonstrate hypointensity on T1-weighted MR images and heterogeneous hyperintensity on T2-weighted MR images, with characteristic central T2-weighted hypointensity (also known as the "target" sign) secondary to central fibrocollagenous tissue and surrounding myxoid matrix. The central T2-weighted hypointense areas also show corresponding enhancement on post-contrast sequences (Fig. 16.15) [55]. Plexiform neurofibromas can cause diffuse enlargement of the nerve and neural plexus, resulting in a "bag of worms" appearance.

Paraganglioma Paraganglioma, or extra-adrenal pheochromocytoma, arises from neuroendocrine cells and most commonly occurs in the head and neck [57]. The retroperitoneum is the second most common primary tumor site in the pediatric age group [58]. The patient may present with symptoms related to excessive catecholamine production, such as headache, sweating, palpitations, and hypertension.

MR imaging is the preferred modality for investigation of suspected paraganglioma. Signal characteristics are hypointense or isointense compared with the liver parenchyma on T1-weighted MR images and markedly hyperintense on T2-weighted MR images (the "light bulb" sign). There is avid enhancement on arterial phase-enhanced T1-weighted fat-suppressed sequences (Fig. 16.16) [58].

Malignant Neoplasms

Desmoplastic Small Round Cell Tumor Desmoplastic small round cell tumor (DSRCT) is a highly aggressive soft tissue tumor which most commonly presents in adolescents and young adults with male predominance [59]. Clinical presentation may be late and may include abdominal distention, pain, anemia, weight loss, and change in bowel habits. The peritoneal cavity is the most common site of involvement [60]. The most typical imaging appearance is that of a large, heterogeneous pelvic (retrovesical) mass with multiple rounded peritoneal and nodal metastases, with or without ascites.

On MR imaging, the masses are hypointense on T1-weighted MR images, intermediate in signal on T2-weighted

MR images with central necrotic hyperintense areas, and heterogeneous enhancement on post-contrast MR images (Fig. 16.17). Restricted diffusion can be seen on diffusion-weighted MR images. The tumor spreads directly via the mesentery or via lymphatic and hematogenous routes. Involvement of the liver, lungs, bones, and the brain can be seen. PET/CT is useful in detection of early tumor relapse [60, 61].

Differential diagnosis for diffuse peritoneal disease includes lymphoma, germ cell tumor (testicular tumor in male patients), other soft tissue sarcomas in adolescents, and

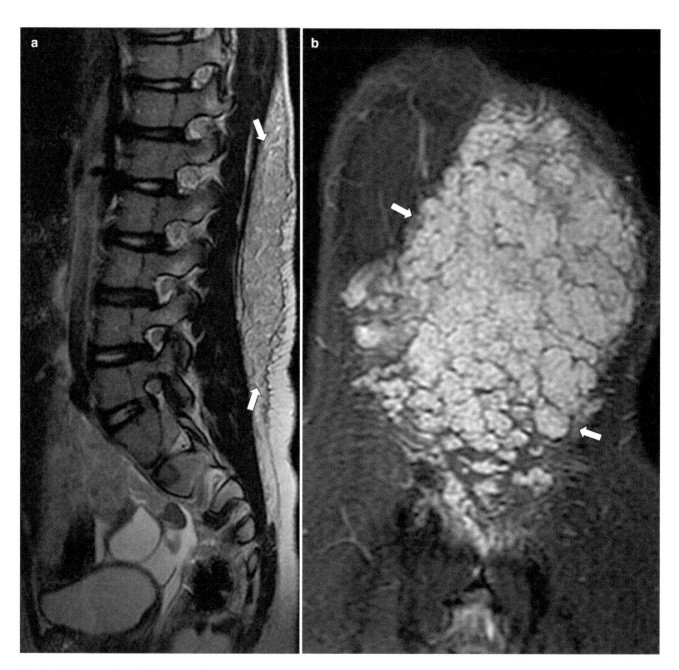

Fig. 16.15 Mesenteric plexiform neurofibroma in a 5-year-old boy with neurofibromatosis-type I. Sagittal T2-weighted (**a**) and coronal STIR (**b**) MR images from thoracolumbar spine MR imaging show a large plexiform neurofibroma (*arrows*) along the superficial dorsal paraspinal soft tissues. Incidentally seen is an additional neurofibroma (*arrows*) in the small-bowel mesentery on axial T2-weighted MR image (**c**) with corresponding enhancement on axial-enhanced T1-weighted fat-suppressed (**d**) MR image. Coronal (**e**) and axial (**f**) CT images subsequently show the entire extent of the mesenteric plexiform neurofibroma

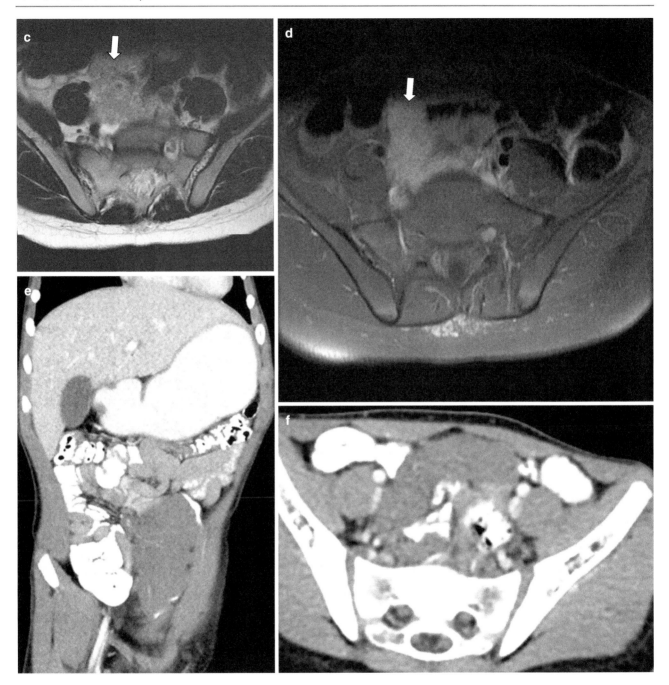

Fig. 16.15 (continued)

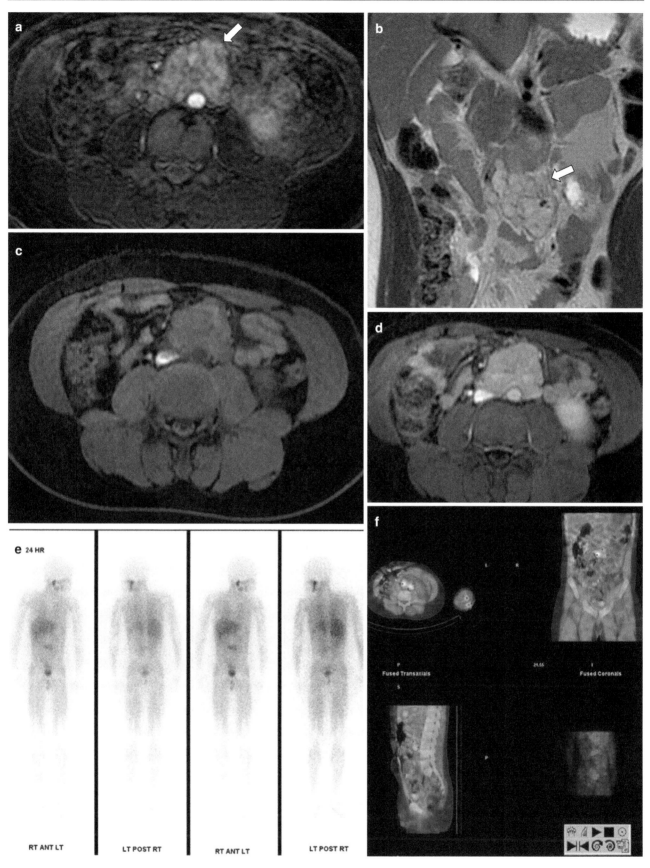

Fig. 16.16 Paraganglioma in an 11-year-old boy with solitary left kidney who presented with hypertension. MR angiography performed to evaluate for renal artery stenosis shows a lobulated retroperitoneal soft tissue mass (*arrows*) on axial noncontrast MR angiogram (**a**) and coronal T2-weighted (**b**) sequences. Axial GRE T1-weighted fat-suppressed pre-contrast (**c**) and post-contrast (**d**) MR images show avid enhancement within this retroperitoneal mass. Additional imaging with I-123 MIBG scan demonstrates increased tracer uptake in the midline retroperitoneal region on planar (**e**) and fused SPECT (**f**) images, consistent with paraganglioma

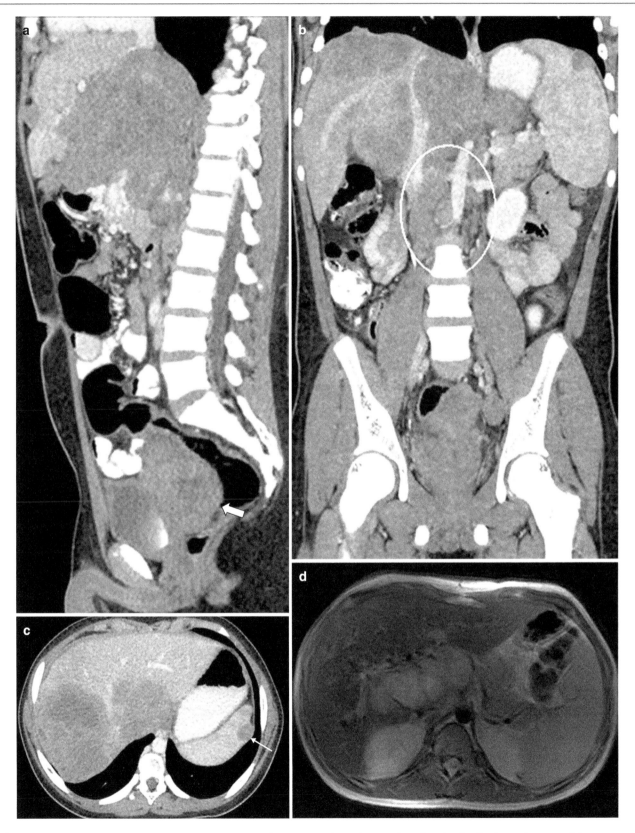

Fig. 16.17 Desmoplastic small round cell tumor (DSRCT) in a 14-year-old boy who presented with 20-pound weight loss. Sagittal (**a**), coronal (**b**), and axial (**c**) images from initial CT show a heterogeneous mass (*thick arrow*) in the retrovesical region with additional soft tissue masses involving the omentum and serosal surfaces (*thin arrow*) with concurrent liver and lymph node (*circle*) metastases. Post-chemotherapy, there is reduction in size and extent of these masses which demonstrate heterogeneous hyperintense and hypointense signal on axial T2-weighted (**d**, **e**) and T1-weighted fat-suppressed (**f**) MR images, respectively. Axial-enhanced GRE T1-weighted fat-suppressed MR images (**g**, **h**) show heterogeneous enhancement by the mass

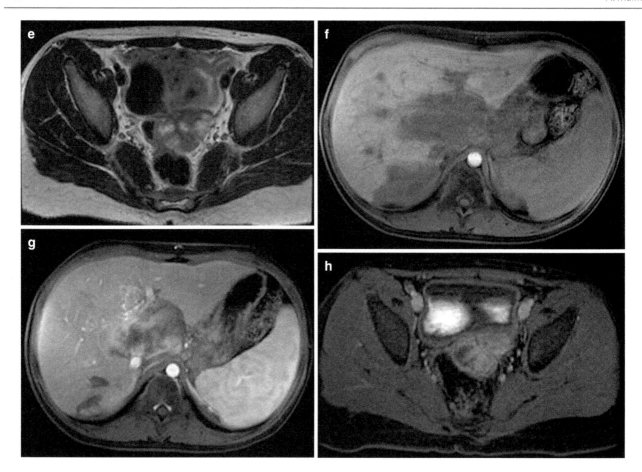

Fig. 16.17 (continued)

metastatic rhabdomyosarcoma or neuroblastoma in younger patients.

Retroperitoneal (Extra-Adrenal) Neuroblastic Tumors Neuroblastic tumors are the most common extracranial solid neoplasms in children and include neuroblastoma, ganglioneuroblastoma, and ganglioneuroma [62]. These tumors vary in the degree of cellular and extracellular maturity, of which neuroblastoma is the most malignant tumor. While adrenal location is most common, it can arise anywhere along the sympathetic chain from the neck through the pelvis. The organ of Zuckerkandl is a mass of neural crest tissue adjacent to the mid- to distal abdominal aorta and is another recognized site of disease [62, 63]. Neuroblastomas occur in early childhood with up to 95% diagnosed by 7 years of age. Presenting features are diverse and vary with the anatomical location and size of the tumor.

MR imaging allows assessment of the primary tumor regardless of the location and extent of the disease, noting superior evaluation for metastatic marrow disease and spinal canal involvement when compared to CT. Tumor typically demonstrates hypo- to isointense signal on T1-weighted MR images and hyperintense signal on T2-weighted MR images, with variable contrast enhancement (Fig. 16.18). Heterogeneity can be seen with areas of calcification and hemorrhage [63]. These tumors tend to encase the major vessels rather than invade them.

Lymphoma Lymphoma is the most common malignant neoplasm to involve the mesentery and peritoneal cavity in children. Mesenteric and peritoneal disease is much more common in non-Hodgkin lymphoma than in Hodgkin lymphoma [64, 65]. The bowel and adjacent mesentery are commonly involved with Burkitt lymphoma, which typically manifests with extensive disease because of its short doubling time [66]. Peritoneal infiltration has been described in up to 24% of patients and ascites in 39% [65].

On MR imaging, lymphoma presents as round or oval, heterogeneously hypointense masses on both T1- and T2-weighted MR images with variable enhancement and diffusion restriction (Fig. 16.19) [65, 67].

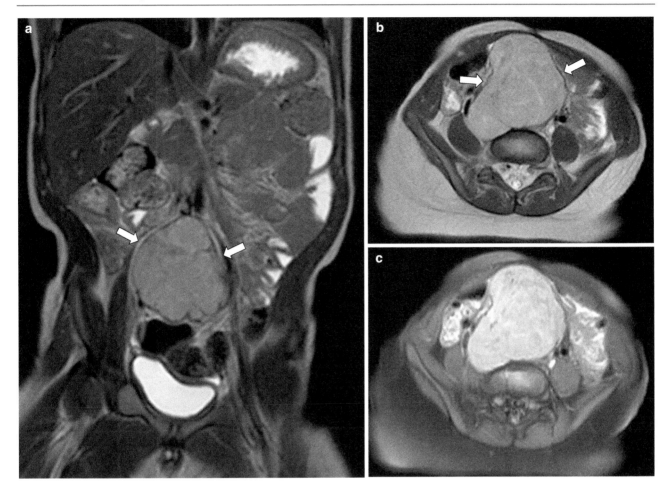

Fig. 16.18 Neuroblastoma arising from organ of Zuckerkandl in a 20-month-old boy who presented with palpable abdominal mass. Coronal (**a**) and axial (**b**) T2-weighted MR images show a heteroge- neously hyperintense mass (*arrows*) in the midline splaying the aortic bifurcation, which exhibits avid enhancement on axial enhanced T1-weighted fat-suppressed MR image (**c**)

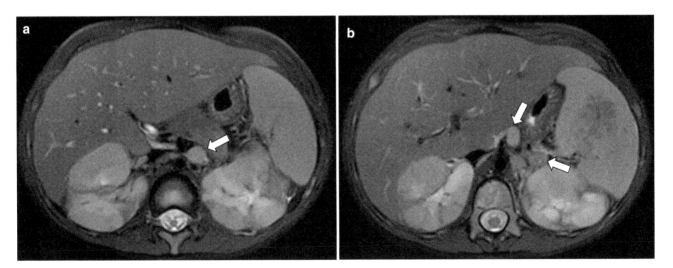

Fig. 16.19 Diffuse large B-cell lymphoma multiorgan involvement in a 7-year-old girl who presented with intermittent fevers and lymphade- nopathy. Axial (**a**, **b**) T2-weighted MR images show multiple enlarged gastrohepatic and para-aortic lymph nodes (*arrows*), multiple interme- diate to mildly hypointense bilateral renal masses, as well as a lobulated splenic mass with hepatosplenomegaly. Renal and splenic masses are hypoenhancing on enhanced GRE T1-weighted fat-suppressed axial (**c**) and coronal (**d**) MR images

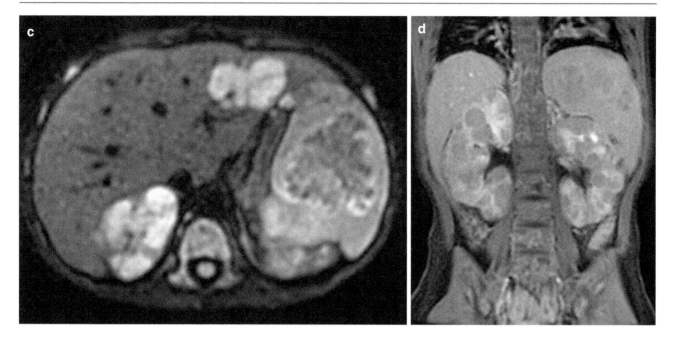

Fig. 16.19 (continued)

Rhabdomyosarcoma Rhabdomyosarcoma (RMS) is the most common soft tissue sarcoma in pediatric patients and accounts for 5–15% of all solid tumors [68]. RMS most commonly occurs in the head and neck, with other reported sites such as genitourinary organs, extremity, biliary tract, and retroperitoneum [68, 69]. Omental location is very rare. Clinical presentation is variable depending upon the location and extent of the tumor. RMS generally is a rapidly growing, malignant mesenchymal tumor with high propensity for hematogenous and lymphatic spread. It can be classified into embryonal, alveolar, botryoid, and anaplastic subtypes, of which embryonal is the most common type in pediatric patients [69]. Intraperitoneal involvement is uncommon and includes findings of ascites, enhancing nodules, omental caking, and pseudomyxoma peritonei. Secondary intra-abdominal extension can be seen with retroperitoneal and pelvic RMS.

MR imaging features of rhabdomyosarcoma are nonspecific and can mimic other soft tissue tumors. The tumor is isointense to skeletal muscle on T1-weighted MR images and heterogeneously hyperintense on T2-weighted MR images, with enhancement on post-contrast imaging. Larger lesions may show areas of hemorrhage or necrosis (Fig. 16.20). Complete surgical excision is the treatment of choice, with chemotherapy that also plays an important role because of its high chemosensitivity [69].

Peritoneal Metastases Peritoneal metastases are very uncommon in pediatric patients, given the decreased frequency of primary gastrointestinal, ovarian, and uterine neoplasms in young patients compared to adults [70]. Neuroblastoma and intracranial neoplasms are reported to metastasize to the peritoneum in children.

MR imaging shows nodular masses with intermediate to hyperintense signal on T2-weighted MR images and hypointense signal on T1-weighted MR images. Contrast enhancement is variable (Fig. 16.21). MR imaging is gaining increased acceptance as a primary modality for imaging surveillance of patients with testicular cancer, given its lack of ionizing radiation exposure and the relatively young patient demographic. In this context, MR surveillance consists of axial T1- and T2-weighted MR images of the retroperitoneum to evaluate for lymphadenopathy, from the level of the renal vessels through the pelvis.

Traumatic Peritoneal and Retroperitoneal Disorders

Peritoneal and retroperitoneal injuries include visceral, solid organ, and vascular injuries [71]. Abdominal trauma can result in hemoperitoneum or retroperitoneal hemorrhage. Retroperitoneal hematoma can also be seen with spinal injury [71, 72].

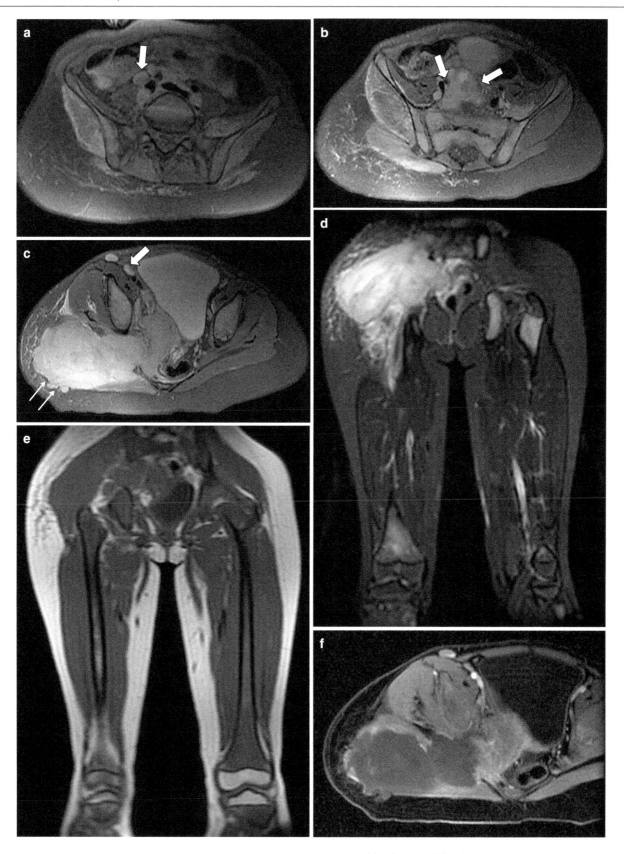

Fig. 16.20 Metastatic rhabdomyosarcoma in a 6-year-old girl who presented with history of prolonged right hip and back pain. Axial T2-weighted fat-suppressed MR images (**a**, **b**) through the lower abdomen and pelvis show multiple enlarged retroperitoneal and right iliac lymph nodes (*arrows*). Axial (**c**) and coronal (**d**) T2-weighted fat-suppressed MR images of the pelvis demonstrate a large mass (*double* *arrows*) arising from the right gluteal musculature with extension into the pelvis as well as right iliac lymph nodes (*single arrow*), and diffuse marrow signal abnormality as manifested by low signal on coronal T1-weighted MR imaging (**e**), consistent with bone metastasis. The gluteal mass is largely necrotic on axial-enhanced T1-weighted fat-suppressed MR image (**f**)

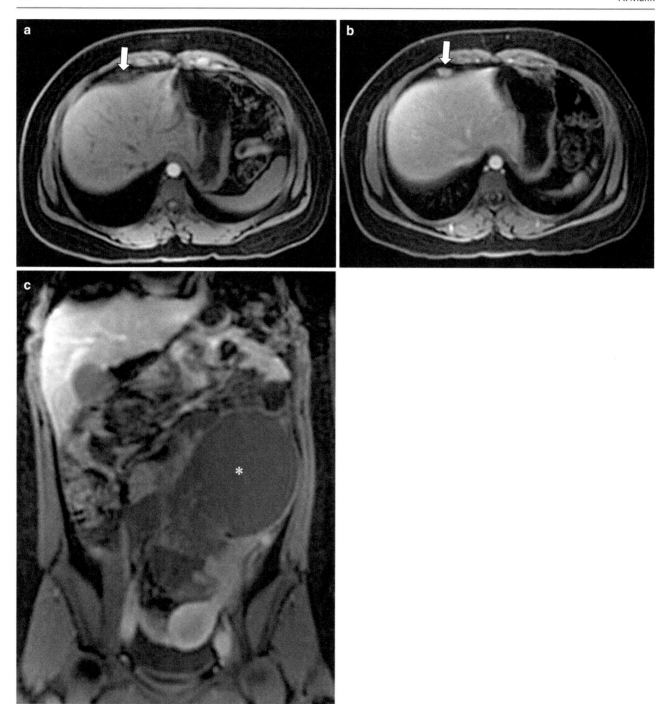

Fig. 16.21 Peritoneal metastases in a 17-year-old girl with malignant left ovarian mucinous cystadenocarcinoma. Axial GRE T1-weighted fat-suppressed MR images pre- (**a**) and post- (**b**) contrast show enhancing peritoneal nodularity (*arrows*) along the liver. Coronal-enhanced T1-weighted fat-suppressed MR image (**c**) shows the large heterogeneous left ovarian mass (*asterisk*) extending superiorly into the abdomen, consistent with the primary malignancy

MR imaging appearance of blood products vary with the stage of bleeding. For example, acute blood or deoxyhemoglobin is isointense on T1-weighted and hypointense on T2-weighted MR images. Subacute blood or intracellular methemoglobin is hyperintense on T1-weighted MR images, while late subacute blood (extracellular methemoglobin) is also hyperintense on T2-weighted MR images. Chronic blood or hemosiderin is hypointense on both T1- and T2-weighted MR images. Pneumoperitoneum appears as areas of low signal intensity on both T1- and T2-weighted MR images.

Conclusion

MR imaging is valuable in evaluation and characterization of pediatric peritoneal and retroperitoneal disorders, given its superior soft tissue contrast resolution, lack of ionizing radiation, and multiplanar capabilities. With use of optimized protocols which include faster and specialized techniques and appropriate coils and select use of sedation or anesthesia, MR imaging evaluation of the peritoneum and retroperitoneum in young patients is gaining wider acceptance.

References

1. Chavhan GB, Babyn PS, Vasanawala SS. Abdominal MR imaging in children: motion compensation, sequence optimization, and protocol organization. Radiographics. 2013;33(3):703–19.
2. Vasanawala SS, Lustig M. Advances in pediatric body MRI. Pediatr Radiol. 2011;41(Suppl 2):549–54.
3. Chavhan GB, Babyn PS, Singh M, Vidarsson L, Shroff M. MR imaging at 3.0 T in children: technical differences, safety issues, and initial experience. Radiographics. 2009;29(5):1451–66.
4. Edwards AD, Arthurs OJ. Paediatric MRI under sedation: is it necessary? What is the evidence for the alternatives? Pediatr Radiol. 2011;41(11):1353–64.
5. Harned RK 2nd, Strain JD. MRI-compatible audio/visual system: impact on pediatric sedation. Pediatr Radiol. 2001;31(4):247–50.
6. Rappaport B, Mellon RD, Simone A, Woodcock J. Defining safe use of anesthesia in children. N Engl J Med. 2011;364(15):1387–90.
7. Anupindi S, Jaramillo D. Pediatric magnetic resonance imaging techniques. Magn Reson Imaging Clin N Am. 2002;10(2):189–207.
8. Mackenzie JD, Vasanawala SS. Advances in pediatric MR imaging. Magn Reson Imaging Clin N Am. 2008;16(3):385–99.
9. Jaimes C, Gee MS. Strategies to minimize sedation in pediatric body magnetic resonance imaging. Paediatr Radiol. 2016;46(6):916–27.
10. Jaimes C, Kirsch JE, Gee MS. Fast, free breathing and motion-minimizing techniques for pediatric body magnetic resonance imaging. Paediatr Radiol. 2018;48(9):1197–208.
11. Healy JC, Reznek RH. The peritoneum, mesenteries and omenta: normal anatomy and pathological processes. Eur Radiol. 1998;8(6):886–900.
12. Tirkes T, Sandrasegaran K, Patel AA, Hollar MA, Tejada JG, Tann M, et al. Peritoneal and retroperitoneal anatomy and its relevance for cross-sectional imaging. Radiographics. 2012;32(2):437–51.
13. Goenka AH, Shah SN, Remer EM. Imaging of the retroperitoneum. Radiol Clin North Am. 2012;50(2):333–55.
14. Dillman JR, Smith EA, Morani AC, Trout AC. Imaging of the pediatric peritoneum, mesentery and omentum. Pediatr Radiol. 2017;47(8):987–1000.
15. Kronfli R, Bradnock TJ, Sabharwal A. Intestinal atresia in association with gastroschisis: a 26-year review. Pediatr Surg Int. 2010;26(9):891–4.
16. Stoll C, Alembik Y, Dott B, Roth MP. Omphalocele and gastroschisis and associated malformations. Am J Med Genet A. 2008;146A(10):1280–5.
17. Daltro P, Fricke BL, Kline-Fath BM, Werner H, Rodrigues L, Fazecas T, et al. Prenatal MRI of congenital abdominal and chest wall defects. AJR Am J Roentgenol. 2005;184(3):1010–6.
18. Ros PR, Olmsted WW, Moser RP Jr, Dachman AH, Hjermstad BH, Sobin LH. Mesenteric and omental cysts: histologic classification with imaging correlation. Radiology. 1987;164(2):327–32.
19. Stoupis C, Ros PR, Abbitt PL, Burton SS, Gauger J. Bubbles in the belly: imaging of cystic mesenteric or omental masses. Radiographics. 1994;14(4):729–37.
20. Chung MA, Brandt ML, St-Vil D, Yazbeck S. Mesenteric cysts in children. J Pediatr Surg. 1991;26(11):1306–8.
21. Vanek VW, Phillips AK. Retroperitoneal, mesenteric, and omental cysts. Arch Surg. 1984;119(7):838–42.
22. Estaun JE, Alfageme AG, Banuelos JS. Radiologic appearance of diaphragmatic mesothelial cysts. Pediatr Radiol. 2003;33:855–8.
23. Akinci D, Akhan O, Ozmen M, Ozkan OS, Karcaaltincaba M. Diaphragmatic mesothelial cysts in children: radiologic findings and percutaneous ethanol sclerotherapy. AJR Am J Roentgenol. 2005;185(4):873–7.
24. Eckoldt F, Heling KS, Woderich R, Kraft S, Bollmann R, Mau H. Meconium peritonitis and pseudo-cyst formation: prenatal diagnosis and post-natal course. Prenat Diagn. 2003;23(11):904–8.
25. Stocker JT. The respiratory tract. In: Stocker JT, Dehner LP, editors. Pediatric pathology, vol. 1. Philadelphia: Lippincott; 1992. p. 517–8.
26. McAdams HP, Kirejczyk WM, Rosado-de-Christenson ML, Matsumoto S. Bronchogenic cyst: imaging features with clinical and histopathologic correlation. Radiology. 2000;217(2):441–6.
27. Siegelman ES, Birnbaum BA, Rosato EF. Bronchogenic cyst appearing as a retroperitoneal mass. AJR Am J Roentgenol. 1998;171:527–8.
28. Murakami R, Machida M, Kobayashi Y, Ogura J, Ichikawa T, Kumazaki T. Retroperitoneal bronchogenic cyst: CT and MR imaging. Abdom Imaging. 2000;25:444–7.
29. Koning JL, Naheedy JH, Kruk PG. Diagnostic performance of contrast-enhanced MR for acute appendicitis and alternative causes of abdominal pain in children. Pediatr Radiol. 2014;44(8):948–55.
30. Macari M, Hines J, Balthazar E, Megibow A. Mesenteric adenitis: CT diagnosis of primary versus secondary causes, incidence, and clinical significance in pediatric and adult patients. AJR Am J Roentgenol. 2002;178:853–8.
31. Kamaya A, Federle MP, Desser TS. Imaging manifestations of abdominal fat necrosis and its mimics. Radiographics. 2011;31:2021–34.
32. McClure MJ, Khalili K, Sarrazin J, Hanbidge A. Radiological features of epiploic appendagitis and segmental omental infarction. Clin Radiol. 2001;56(10):819–27.
33. Moyle PL, Kataoka MY, Nakai A, Takahata A, Reinhold C, Sala E. Nonovarian cystic lesions of the pelvis. Radiographics. 2010;30:921–38.
34. Jain KA. Imaging of peritoneal inclusion cysts. AJR Am J Roentgenol. 2000;174:1559–63.
35. Hahn YS, Engelhard H, McLone DG. Abdominal CSF pseudocyst: clinical features and surgical management. Pediatr Neurosci 1985–1986;12:75–79.
36. Harsh GR. Peritoneal shunt for hydrocephalus utilizing the fimbria of the fallopian tube for entrance to the peritoneal cavity. J Neurosurg. 1954;11:284–94.
37. Rainov N, Schobess A, Heidecke V, et al. Abdominal CSF pseudocyst in patients with ventriculo-peritoneal shunts: report of fourteen cases and review of literature. Acta Neurochir. 1994;127:73–8.
38. Chung J, Yu J, Kim JH, Nam SJ, Kim MJ. Intraabdominal complications secondary to ventriculoperitoneal shunts: CT findings and review of the literature. AJR Am J Roentgenol. 2009;193(5):1311–7.
39. Brook I. Intra-abdominal, retroperitoneal, and visceral abscesses in children. Eur J Pediatr Surg. 2004;14(4):265–73.
40. Chung EM, Biko DM, Arzamendi AM, Meldrum JT, Stocker JT. Solid tumors of the peritoneum, omentum, and mesentery in children: radiologic-pathologic-correlation. Radiographics. 2015;35(2):521–46.
41. Levy AD, Rimola J, Mehrotra AK, Sobin LH. From the archives of the AFIP: benign brous tumors and tumorlike lesions of the

mesentery—radiologic-pathologic correlation. Radiographics. 2006;26(1):245–64.

42. Einstein DM, Tagliabue JR, Desai RK. Abdominal desmoids: CT findings in 25 patients. AJR Am J Roentgenol. 1991;157:275–9.

43. Shinagare AB, Ramaiya NH, Jagannathan JP, Krajewski KM, Giardino AA, Butrynski JE, Raut CP. A to Z of desmoid tumors. AJR Am J Roentgenol. 2011;197:W1008–14. Review.

44. McCarville MB, Hoffer FA, Adelman CS, Khoury JD, Li C, Skapek SX. MRI and biologic behavior of desmoid tumors in children. AJR Am J Roentgenol. 2007;189(3):633–40.

45. Azizi L, Balu M, Belkacem A, Lewin M, Tubiana JM, Arrivé LMRI. Features of mesenteric desmoid tumors in familial adenomatous polyposis. AJR Am J Roentgenol. 2005;184(4):1128–35. Review

46. Karnak I, Senocak ME, Ciftci AO, Cağlar M, Bingöl-Koloğlu M, Tanyel FC, Büyükpamukçu N. Inflammatory myofibroblastic tumor in children: diagnosis and treatment. J Pediatr Surg. 2001;36(6):908–12.

47. Kim SJ, Kim WS, Cheon JE, Shin SM, Youn BJ, Kim IO, Yeon KM. Inflammatory myofibroblastic tumors of the abdomen as mimickers of malignancy: imaging features in nine children. AJR Am J Roentgenol. 2009;193(5):1419–24.

48. Sedlic T, Scali EP, Lee WK, Verma S, Chang SD. Inflammatory pseudotumours in the abdomen and pelvis: a pictorial essay. Can Assoc Radiol J. 2014;65(1):52–9.

49. Farruggia P, Trizzino A, Scibetta N, Cecchetto G, Guerrieri P, D'Amore ES, D'Angelo P. Castleman's disease in childhood: report of three cases and review of the literature. Ital J Pediatr. 2011;37:50. Review

50. Zhou LP, Zhang B, Peng WJ, Yang WT, Guan YB, Zhou KR. Imaging findings of Castleman disease of the abdomen and pelvis. Abdom Imaging. 2008;33(4):482–8.

51. Li FF, Zhang T, Bai YZ. Mesenteric Castleman's disease in a 12-year-old girl. J Gastrointest Surg. 2011;15(10):1896–8.

52. Bonekamp D, Horton KM, Hruban RH, Fishman EK. Castleman disease: the great mimic. Radiographics. 2011;31(6):1793–807.

53. Reiseter T, Nordshus T, Borthne A, Roald B, Naess P, Schistad O. Lipoblastoma: MRI appearances of a rare paediatric soft tissue tumour. Pediatr Radiol. 1999;29(7):542–5.

54. Gentimi F, Tzovaras AA, Antoniou D, Moschovi M, Papandreou E. A giant mesenteric lipoblastoma in an 18-month old infant: a case report and review of the literature. African J Paediatr Surg. 2011;8(3):320–3.

55. Levy AD, Patel N, Dow N, Abbott RM, Miettinen M, Sobin LH. From the archives of the AFIP: abdominal neoplasms in patients with neurofibromatosis type 1: radiologic-pathologic correlation. Radiographics. 2005;25(2):455–80.

56. Basile U, Cavallaro G, Polistena A, Giustini S, Orlando G, Cotesta D, et al. Gastrointestinal and retroperitoneal manifestations of type 1 neurofibromatosis. J Gastrointest Surg. 2010;14(1):186–94.

57. Lack EE. Paraganglioma. In: Sternberg SS, editor. Diagnostic surgical pathology. 2nd ed. New York: Raven Press; 1994. p. 599–621.

58. Lee KY, Oh YW, Noh HJ, Lee YJ, Yong HS, et al. Extraadrenal paragangliomas of the body: imaging features. AJR Am J Roentgenol. 2006;187(2):492–504.

59. Kis B, O'Regan KN, Agoston A, Javery O, Jagannathan J, Ramaiya NH. Imaging of desmoplastic small round cell tumour in adults. Br J Radiol. 2012;85(1010):187–92.

60. Bellah R, Suzuki-Bordalo L, Brecher E, Ginsberg JP, Maris J, Pawel BR. Desmoplastic small round cell tumor in the abdomen and pelvis: report of CT findings in 11 affected children and young adults. AJR Am J Roentgenol. 2005;184(6):1910–4.

61. Tateishi U, Hasegawa T, Kusumoto M, Oyama T, Ishikawa H, Moriyama N. Desmoplastic small round cell tumor: imaging findings associated with clinicopathologic features. J Comput Assist Tomogr. 2002;26(4):579–83.

62. Lonnergan GJ, Schwab CM, Suarez ES, Carlson CL. Neuroblastoma, ganglioneuroblastoma, and ganglioneuroma: radiologic-pathologic correlation. Radiographics. 2002;22(4):911–34.

63. Berdon WE, Stylianos S, Ruzal-Shapiro C, Hoffer F, Cohen M. Neuroblastoma arising from the organ of Zuckerkandl: an unusual site with a favorable biologic outcome. Pediatr Radiol. 1999;29(7):497–502.

64. Sandlund JT, Downing JR, Crist WM. Non-Hodgkin's lymphoma in childhood. N Engl J Med. 1996;334(19):1238–48.

65. Biko DM, Anupindi SA, Hernandez A, Kersun L, Bellah R. Childhood Burkitt lymphoma: abdominal and pelvic imaging findings. AJR Am J Roentgenol. 2009;192(5):1304–15.

66. Hamrick-Turner JE, Saif MF, Powers CI, Blumenthal BI, Royal SA, Iyer RV. Imaging of childhood non-Hodgkin lymphoma: assessment by histologic subtype. Radiographics. 1994;14(1):11–28.

67. Ng YY, Healy JC, Vincent JM, Kingston JE, Armstrong P, Reznek RH. The radiology of non-Hodgkin's lymphoma in childhood: a review of 80 cases. Clin Radiol. 1994;49(9):594–600.

68. Miller RW, Young JL Jr, Novakovic B. Childhood cancer. Cancer. 1995;75(1 Suppl):395–405.

69. Chung CJ, Fordham L, Little S, Rayder S, Nimkin K, Kleinman PK, Watson C. Intraperitoneal rhabdomyosarcoma in children: incidence and imaging characteristics on CT. AJR Am J Roentgenol. 1998;170(5):1385–7.

70. Pickhardt PF, Bhalla S. Primary neoplasms of peritoneal and subperitoneal origin: CT findings. Radiographics. 2005;25(4):983–95.

71. Bagley LJ. Imaging of spinal trauma. Radiol Clin N Am. 2006;44(1):1–12.

72. Madiba TE, Muckart DJ. Retroperitoneal hematoma and related organ injury: management approach. S Afr J Surg. 2001;39(2):41–5.

Whole-Body MR Imaging

Mary-Louise C. Greer

Introduction

In the past decade, there has been a rapid increase in the utilization of whole-body magnetic resonance imaging (whole-body MR imaging) in the pediatric population [1–3]. This has been facilitated by technical developments enabling large field of view (FOV) imaging in clinically feasible timeframes while achieving high contrast and spatial resolution [2, 4, 5]. Whole-body MR imaging has become a valuable tool in assessing diffuse, multifocal, and/or multisystem disease processes with an ever-expanding range of indications, both oncologic and non-oncologic [3, 6–11]. It can facilitate diagnosis, document disease burden and treatment response, and guide invasive procedures such as biopsy. The additional appeal of whole-body MR imaging in the pediatric population relates to its lack of ionizing radiation in comparison with alternative large FOV imaging techniques such as computed tomography (CT), with or without positron emission tomography (FDG-PET), and even to a small degree skeletal surveys [12].

In this chapter, whole-body MR imaging techniques and protocols are discussed (both generic and disease-specific protocols) with consideration of a systematic approach to image analysis and standardized reporting. These help to optimize disease detection while minimizing false positive and false negative interpretations [7, 13]. A false positive screening test can be detrimental, particularly in children if leading to radiologic investigations involving ionizing radiation or unnecessary invasive procedures [14–16]. In addition, the application of pediatric whole-body MR imaging across a spectrum of diseases is reviewed, including clinical features, characteristic imaging findings, and management. These include cancer predisposition syndromes (CPS), other neoplastic disorders, and treatment-related complications such as osteonecrosis, infectious and noninfectious inflam-

matory disorders, myopathies, and postmortem imaging as an adjunct to autopsy.

Magnetic Resonance Imaging Techniques

Patient Preparation

There is no preparation for most pediatric patients undergoing whole-body MR imaging unless requiring sedation or general anesthesia (GA), when institutional fasting policies should be followed. Defining risks related to GA in pediatrics is beyond the scope of this chapter, although its impact on CPS surveillance should be considered [7]. A range of techniques can be employed to minimize need for GA and alleviate anxiety in pediatric MR imaging, especially beneficial for patients aged 4 to 6 years or in older developmentally delayed children, improving compliance and reducing motion artifacts. These include MR scanner simulation, child life specialists, video goggles, headphones for music, and animal-assisted therapy [17–19].

MR Imaging Pulse Sequences and Protocols

Standard MR Imaging Pulse Sequences and Protocols

No one standard pediatric whole-body MR imaging protocol currently exists, most recently illustrated in a 2016 multi-center survey conducted through the Society for Pediatric Radiology (SPR); however, there are some techniques that are commonly utilized [2, 20]. The SPR survey confirmed that coronal short tau inversion recovery (STIR) is the most frequently employed imaging plane and sequence, used by 90% of responders, and non fat-suppressed coronal T1-weighted and axial diffusion-weighted MR imaging (DWI) sequences used by almost 50% [2]. Wide variability in whole-body MR imaging protocols exists among institutions and for different

M.-L. C. Greer (✉)
Department of Diagnostic Imaging, The Hospital for Sick Children, University of Toronto, Toronto, ON, Canada
e-mail: mary-louise.greer@sickkids.ca

© Springer Nature Switzerland AG 2020
E. Y. Lee et al. (eds.), *Pediatric Body MRI*, https://doi.org/10.1007/978-3-030-31989-2_17

Table 17.1 Whole-body MR imaging protocols for pediatric oncology

Authors	Imaging planes	Pulse sequences	Approximate imaging time (min)
Gottumukkala et al. 2019 [10]	Coronal	STIR, T1W in-phase and opposed-phase GRE[a]	45 (variable, depending on specific indication)
	Axial	SSFSE/HASTE, DWI	
	Sagittal	STIR (if LCH evaluation)	
Villani et al. 2016 [21]	Coronal	STIR	18
Eutsler and Khanna 2016 [8]	Coronal	STIR	40
	Axial	STIR, HASTE, DWI	
Davis et al. 2016 [6]	Coronal	STIR, HASTE, T1W (optional MR angiography)	Not available
	Axial	STIR, HASTE	
Nievelstein and Littooij 2016 [22]	Coronal	STIR, T1W TSE	32
	Axial	DW1, T2W SPAIR	
Anupindi et al. 2015 [16]	Coronal	STIR, T1W, HASTE	72 (average)
	Axial	STIR (head, neck, lower extremities, T2W fat-suppressed) (chest, abdomen, ± pelvis), HASTE	
	Sagittal	HASTE	

From Gottumukkala et al. [10], with permission. Reprinted with permission from Radiological Society of North America© RSNA
Abbreviations: *DWI* diffusion-weighted imaging, *GRE* gradient echo, *HASTE* half-Fourier acquisition single-shot turbo spin echo, *LCH* Langerhans cell histiocytosis, *SPAIR* spectrally adiabatic inversion recovery, *SSFSE* single-shot fast spring echo, *T1W* T1-weighted, *T2W* T2-weighted, *TSE* turbo spin echo
[a]T1-weighted fat-suppressed post-contrast sequence optional for targeted characterization of known lesions or at-risk organs; plane(s) best suited to region of interest

indications. Table 17.1 summarizes some recently published protocols for pediatric oncology [6, 8, 10, 16, 21, 22].

Coronal STIR imaging, either alone or combined with other sequences, is the mainstay of whole-body MR imaging due to its robust fat suppression, shorter acquisition time in the coronal plane, and excellent depiction of pathology as high signal intensity lesions [2–4, 7, 20]. Acquired as individual stations from head to toe (or sometimes vertex to heels), the number of stations is dependent on patient height [1, 4, 10]. As few as two stations may be needed in infants and up to seven in adult-sized adolescents, with an average of 4–5.

Sample per station coronal STIR acquisition parameters at 1.5 Tesla (T) are TE 95 ms, TR 5270 ms, TI 150 ms, slice thickness 5 mm, slice gap 1 mm, matrix 384 x 269, and field of view (FOV) 500 mm and at 3 Tesla are TE 70 ms, TR 9126 ms, TI 230 ms, slice thickness 6 mm, slice gap 1 mm, matrix 308 x 303, and FOV 460 mm. Acquisition time per

station is approximately 3 minutes for 40 slices, acquired free breathing with 25–30% phase oversampling.

Automated post-processing tools available on most MR scanners allow these stations to be merged at the scanner console, displayed as a series of whole-body images from anterior to posterior (Fig. 17.1). Large-bore (70 cm) higher field strength MR scanners may require a smaller maximum FOV (e.g., 300–350 mm) head to foot to avoid distortion artifacts, necessitating extra stations for full coverage (Fig. 17.2).

Coronal T1-weighted turbo spin echo (TSE) or gradient echo (GRE) sequences provide anatomic information, particularly useful for the bone marrow [2, 6, 10, 13, 23]. Typically acquired as a two-dimensional (2D) sequence without fat suppression, coronal stations are merged and displayed as above. T1-weighted MR imaging with Dixon technique is an alternative, generating non fat-suppressed and robust fat-suppressed images from a single acquisition (along with in- and opposed-phase images), other options

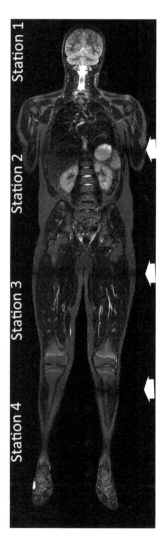

Fig. 17.1 Whole-body MR surveillance image from a 12-year-old boy with Li-Fraumeni syndrome. Coronal STIR image acquired on a 1.5 Tesla scanner in four stations merged into a whole-body image (*digital stitch artifact indicated by arrows*)

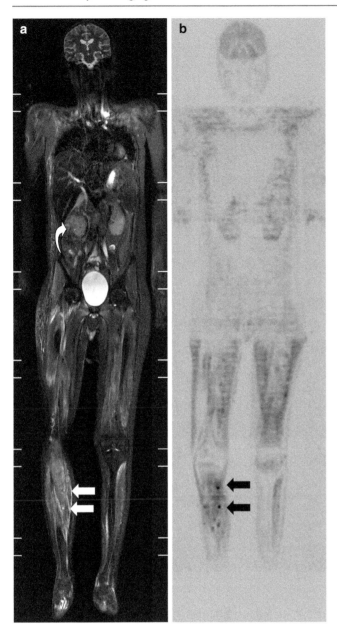

Fig. 17.2 Pre-B-cell acute lymphoblastic leukemia (ALL) in a 12-year-old boy with pyomyositis. Coronal whole-body (**a**) STIR and (**b**) inverted diffusion-weighted imaging (DWI) ($b = 1000$ s/mm^2) on a 3 Tesla scanner requiring seven stations to achieve whole-body anatomic coverage. Diffuse T2-weighted hyperintensity in muscles and subcutaneous tissues (**a**) is present from edema. There are also numerous intramuscular foci demonstrating high STIR signal intensity with thin hypointense rims (**a**, *white arrows*) and (**b**) low signal intensity on inverted DWI (**b**, *black arrows*), in keeping with multiple tiny fungal abscesses, with renal involvement (*curved arrow* in **a**)

being 3D T1-weighted TSE and faster GRE sequences [5, 9]. Pasoglou et al. [24] performed 3D whole-body T1-weighted TSE MR imaging in adult prostate cancer patients, showing equal sensitivity to 2D imaging for detecting skeletal metas-

tases ($p = 0.317$), with greater sensitivity for detection of abnormal nodes ($p < 0.001$).

Axially acquired diffusion-weighted whole-body imaging with background suppression (DWIBS) has recently been incorporated into pediatric whole-body MR imaging protocols, primarily for oncologic indications, complementing STIR in lesion detection and providing functional information [2, 8, 10, 16, 23, 25]. DWIBS improves lesion conspicuity and helps characterize lesions by directly comparing DWI (trace) images with apparent diffusion coefficient (ADC) maps. Cysts and necrotic lesions are bright on both image sets from "T2 shine-through" fluid signal intensity, while solid lesions selectively demonstrate low signal intensity on ADC maps (low ADC values), helping minimize false positive and negative findings in CPS surveillance [1, 23, 26]. Detection can be hampered at sites of respiratory and cardiac motion and in organs with long T2 relaxation times such as the spleen, leading to false negative findings, although splenic lesions have been detected reliably in lymphoma on DWI [27–29]. Its utility in evaluating inflammatory disorders is unclear, potentially aiding distinction of equivocal inflammatory and neoplastic lesions [30]. This may also have value in defining disease activity in chronic recurrent multifocal osteomyelitis (CRMO)/chronic non-bacterial osteomyelitis (CNO), the focus of a European Society of Pediatric Radiology (ESPR) MSK Taskforce developing whole-body MR imaging guidelines for CRMO in children [30, 31].

A minimum of two *b*-values are obtained at 50–100 s/mm^2 for liver lesions and between 600 and 1000 s/mm^2 for solid organ and osseous lesions. Both b-values are useful for evaluating lymph nodes [23]. Sample per station axial DWI acquisition parameters at 1.5 Tesla for b-value 800 s/mm^2 are TE 70 ms, TR 6100 ms, slice thickness 5 mm, slice gap 1 mm, matrix 208 x 204, FOV 520 mm, number of excitations = 2, free breathing with spectral fat suppression, and parallel imaging reducing acquisition times.

Post-processing tools enable axial DWI images to be reconstructed coronally, merged automatically into whole-body displays, and inverted for improved lesion conspicuity and direct coronal DWI acquisitions are increasingly performed (Fig. 17.3a, b). Comparison with whole-body ADC maps and axial source images is essential for lesion characterization [1] (Fig. 17.3c, d). Quantitative lesion analysis using ADC values is not yet in the clinical realm but is likely to be as standardization between different scanners evolves.

Less commonly acquired sequences and imaging planes include axial and sagittal T2-weighted MR imaging (with or without fat suppression) as TSE or single-shot T2-weighted

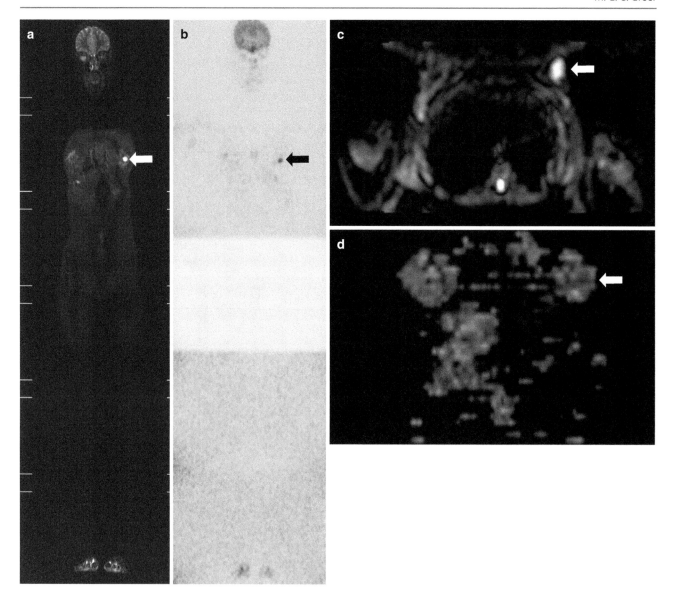

Fig. 17.3 Li-Fraumeni syndrome in a 15-year-old girl. Surveillance whole-body MR Image on a 3 Tesla scanner shows a phyllodes tumor in the left breast. Coronal whole-body STIR sequence (**a**) shows a left breast lesion of high signal intensity (*white arrow*). On diffusion-weighted whole-body imaging with background suppression (DWIBS) trace images (b value = 1000 s/mm²) – axially acquired and then recon-structed coronally (**b**) and inverted – the lesion is of low signal (*black arrow*), corresponding to the high signal focus on the native non-inverted DWIBS image (**c**, *white arrow*). On reconstructed coronal apparent diffusion coefficient (ADC) map imaging (**d**), the lesion demonstrates low signal intensity (*white arrow*), consistent with diffusion restriction in a solid mass

sequences and axial STIR and axial T1-weighted MR imaging, variably employed in indication-specific protocols (Table 17.1 and see Table 17.2).

Acquisition times for a generic whole-body MR imaging protocol range from 30 to 60 minutes, increasing as more sequences and/or imaging planes are employed [2, 10, 32]. Advanced MR imaging techniques such as compressed sensing and multislice excitation are increasingly being adopted into routine practice and are likely to decrease whole-body MR imaging scan times substantially [10].

Supplementary MR Imaging Pulse Sequences and Protocols

A major benefit of MR imaging is its flexibility in performing large and small field of view (FOV) imaging in the same examination. Regional imaging complements whole-body MR imaging by providing comprehensive, small FOV evaluation with higher spatial resolution for body parts of particular interest. Examples include brain MR imaging in LFS due to the high incidence of cerebral tumors with this condition [7, 33, 34].

Table 17.2 Pediatric whole-body MR Imaging: single institution indication-based protocols

Disease spectrum	Specific indications	Sequence	Imaging plane and coverage	Optional/others
Congenital disorders – Cancer predisposition syndromes	LFS	STIR	Coronal WB	Coronal WB T1 GRE ± FS
		DWI	*Axial WB	Axial WB SS T2 FS
				+ dedicated brain MRI
				First MRI Gd + then Gd-
	HPPS	STIR	Coronal NCAP/CAP WB	Coronal WB T1 GRE ± FS
		DWI	*Axial NCAP/CAP WB	Axial WB SS T2 FS
				If CAP + dedicated neck MRI
	HRB	STIR	Coronal WB	Coronal WB T1 GRE ± FS
		DWI	*Axial WB	Axial WB SS T2 FS
	CMMRD	STIR	Coronal WB	Coronal WB T1 GRE ± FS
		DWI	*Axial WB	Axial WB SS T2 FS
				+ dedicated brain MRI
	NF1/2/schwannomatosis	STIR	Coronal WB	NF2: brain +IAM, spine +/−WB;
		DWI	*Axial WB	Schwannomatosis: brain + spine +/− WB if symptomatic
Other neoplastic and related disorders	Lymphoma	STIR	Coronal WB	Coronal WB T1 GRE ± FS
		DWI	*Axial WB	Axial WB SS T2 FS
	LCH	STIR	Coronal WB, sagittal spine	Coronal WB T1 GRE ± FS
		DWI	*Axial WB	
	Other neoplasms	STIR	Coronal WB	Coronal WB T1 GRE ± FS
		DWI	*Axial WB	
	Osteonecrosis	STIR	Coronal WB	Limited coverage of shoulders and hips, coronal DWI
		T1 GRE	Coronal WB	
Infectious and noninfectious inflammatory disorders	FUO	STIR	Coronal WB	ROI axial T1 FSE, T2 FSE FS
	CRMO/CNO	STIR	Coronal WB, sagittal spine	WB axial T1+/− T2 FSE FS
	ERA	STIR	Coronal WB, sagittal spine, axial pelvis, coronal oblique SIJ, sagittal knees, sagittal ankles	
Miscellaneous	Inflammatory myopathy – PM/JDM	STIR	Axial WB	Neck to hands/feet
		T1 FSE	Axial WB	5 mm slice, 15 mm gap
	Inherited neuromuscular disorder	STIR	Axial WB	Neck to hands/feet,
		T1 FSE	Axial WB	5 mm slice, 0.5 mm gap
	Postmortem	T2 FSE FS	Coronal and axial CAP WB	3D T2 FSE FS cardiac MRI
				Dedicated brain MRI
		T1 FSE	Coronal and axial CAP WB	

Abbreviations: *MRI* magnetic resonance imaging, *LFS* Li-Fraumeni syndrome, *HPPS* hereditary paraganglioma-pheochromocytoma syndrome, *HRB* hereditary retinoblastoma, *CMMRD* combined mismatch repair deficiency syndrome, *NF 1/2* neurofibromatosis types 1 and 2, *IAM* internal auditory meati, *FUO* fever of unknown origin, *CRMO* chronic recurrent multifocal osteomyelitis, *CNO* chronic non-bacterial osteomyelitis, *ERA* enthesitis-related arthritis, *LCH* Langerhans cell histiocytosis, *NAI* non-accidental injury, *PM* polymyositis, *JDM* juvenile dermatomyositis, *STIR* short tau inversion recovery, *DWI* diffusion-weighted imaging, *WB* whole-body, *Axial* axially acquire then coronally reconstruct and merge trace and ADC map, invert to display OR direct coronal acquisition, merge and invert to display, *T1* T1-weighted, *GRE* gradient echo, *FS* fat-suppressed, *FSE* fast spin echo, *SSH* single shot, *T2* T2-weighted, *3D* three-dimensional, *Gd* gadolinium-based contrast agent, (+) with, (−) without, *SIJ* sacroiliac joints, *ROI* region of interest, *CAP* chest, abdomen, pelvis, *NCAP* neck, chest, abdomen, pelvis

Targeted imaging is less comprehensive and can form part of a standard whole-body MR imaging protocol. Limited extra sequences may be acquired routinely to improve lesion detection in areas more commonly affected by a disease process or performed ad hoc problem-solving an abnormality identified on standard whole-body sequences [1]. One example is in CRMO, where targeted sagittal spine STIR (or T2-weighted) sequences complement coronal whole-body STIR sequences to better visualize vertebrae [1, 32, 35] (Fig. 17.4). By comparison, targeted imaging in LFS may help resolve a non-specific bone marrow T2-weighted hyperintensity by adding limited fat-suppressed T2-weighted MR

imaging in an optimal plane, guiding the need for more comprehensive imaging or intervention.

MR Scanners

Pediatric whole-body MR imaging can be satisfactorily performed on 1.5 and 3T scanners, contrast-to-noise and signal-to-noise ratio (SNR) gains at 3T balanced against increased susceptibility and motion artifacts and dielectric effects degrading image quality, with multi-transmit technology potentially reducing the latter [9, 36]. In assessing anatomy, artifacts, and overall image quality, Mohan et al. found pedi-

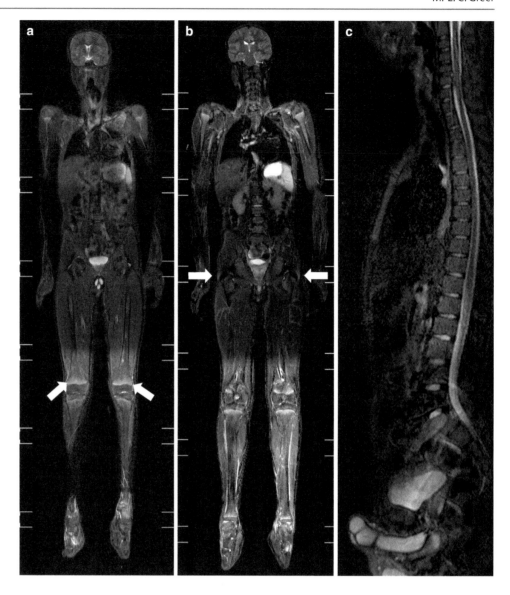

Fig. 17.4 Chronic recurrent multifocal osteomyelitis (CRMO) in a 12-year-old boy with fever and pain. Coronal whole-body STIR MR images acquired on a 3 Tesla scanner in seven stations (**a**, **b**) show bilateral symmetric distal femoral metaphyseal T2-weighted hyperintensities (**a**, *arrows*), greater than expected for hematopoietic marrow and mild enthesitis with increased T2-weighted signal (**b**, *arrows*) abutting the greater trochanters bilaterally. (**c**) Sagittal STIR MR image (three stations merged) better demonstrates normal MR appearance of the vertebral bodies

atric whole-body MR imaging to be superior at 1.5T, with 3T imaging still acceptable. Koh et al. [36] found DWI to be less robust at 3T, while Ahlawat et al. [37] found no significant difference in detection of tumors in neurofibromatosis on whole-body MR imaging at both field strengths.

Sliding or step-by-step table movement is usually employed for whole-body MR imaging, continuous table movement (CTM) mostly reserved for MR angiography. Although CTM offers greater patient throughput, artifacts such as stair-step artifact are more prominent when reformatting primary axial images into other planes. Advantages include improved imaging in the isocenter, which is associated with reduced field heterogeneity and peripheral field distortions [9, 36, 38].

Coils

Choice of coils in whole-body MR imaging is vendor dependent, with a variety of coils used to achieve full anatomic coverage while minimizing delays associated with coil

exchange. Where available, in-table quadrature body coils are used in combination with surface coils for the torso to improve patient comfort, with possible mild loss of SNR compared with body coils containing anterior and posterior elements. Flexible phased array coils in the extremities and dedicated head coils for the head and neck typically complete the whole-body MR imaging coil configuration, with multichannel coils combined with parallel imaging to decrease scan times [4, 9, 10, 36].

Anatomic Coverage

Defining "whole-body" MR imaging (contiguous and multiregional scanning) is important for consistency among different imaging centers and serial scans. By convention, anatomic coverage of whole-body MR imaging is head-to-toes or vertex-to-heels and if less should be specified [7]. For example, if limiting coverage to the torso (chest, abdomen, and pelvis), this could be defined as "CAP whole-body MRI" and if including the neck and proximal upper and lower extremities "NCAPPE whole-body MRI."

Use of Intravenous Contrast

Whole-body MR imaging is almost exclusively performed without intravenous contrast [23]. Gadolinium-based contrast agents (GBCA) are usually reserved for specific clinical scenarios such as tumor detection on initial regional brain MR imaging in LFS surveillance or targeted imaging in osteomyelitis to define an abscess potentially amenable to drainage [1, 33]. Discussion of GBCA-related risks is beyond the scope of this chapter.

Newer intravenous contrast agents showing promise in whole-body MR imaging include ultrasmall particle iron oxide (USPIO) agents (e.g., ferumoxytol), clinically approved as an iron replacement therapy in Europe and North America and used off-label as an MR imaging contrast agent. These agents initially are imaged in the blood pool phase where they are used for MR angiography, followed by a delayed (~24 hours postinjection) lymphotropic phase in which contrast is taken up by macrophages and transported into lymph nodes. Normal lymph nodes demonstrate decreased T2-weighted signal intensity due to immune cell infiltration, while malignant lymph nodes retain their high signal intensity. Concerns regarding anaphylaxis have limited clinical

adoption of USPIO as MR imaging contrast agents [10, 39, 40]. Whole-body MR imaging acquired concurrently with 18F-fluorodeoxyglucose (FDG) PET (PET-MRI) is emerging as an appealing alternative to FDG-PET/CT in Hodgkin lymphoma based on current data, and with ongoing research, many applications in oncologic imaging are anticipated with increasing availability of tissue-specific tracers [23, 41].

Anatomy

Anatomic Considerations for Whole-Body MR Imaging

Patient Position

Patient positioning is important for optimizing image quality. Usually imaged supine for greater comfort, patients are placed close to the scanner isocenter in anatomic position. Their hands and forearms are typically aligned by their sides oriented sagittally, but these may be obscured by distortion artifact in larger patients. Improved visualization may be achieved by imaging with arms extended overhead hands together while prone, but requires an extra station, increasing study time [1]. Alternatively, improved visualization can be achieved without time penalty or artifact to adjacent structures by resting the hands on the upper thighs anteriorly or tucked behind the buttocks posteriorly, oriented coronally [31] (Fig. 17.5).

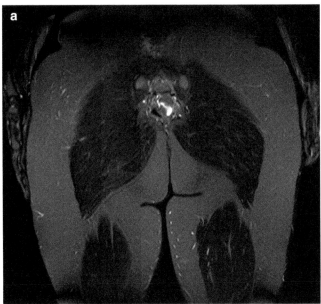
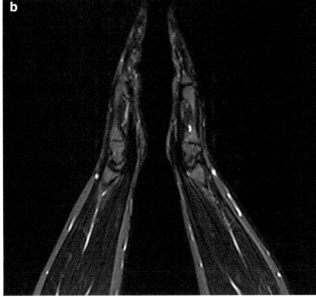

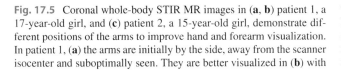

Fig. 17.5 Coronal whole-body STIR MR images in (**a**, **b**) patient 1, a 17-year-old girl, and (**c**) patient 2, a 15-year-old girl, demonstrate different positions of the arms to improve hand and forearm visualization. In patient 1, (**a**) the arms are initially by the side, away from the scanner isocenter and suboptimally seen. They are better visualized in (**b**) with

the arms extended overhead, necessitating an extra station acquisition. Patient 2 (**c**) has both hands and forearms resting on the upper thighs anteriorly, better visualized without causing artifact or requiring a separate anatomic station. Subcutaneous edema in the left forearm (*arrow*) relates to the presence of an intravenous cannula

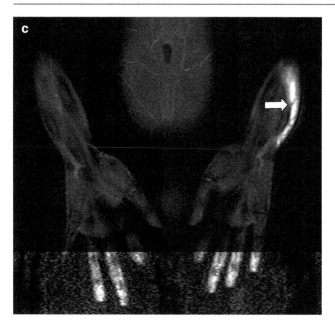

Fig. 17.5 (continued)

Indication-Specific Anatomic Coverage

Modifications to standard whole-body MR imaging coverage and addition of regional or targeted supplementary sequences vary with the pathology under investigation [1, 10] (see Table 17.2).

Spectrum of Disorders

Congenital Disorders: Cancer Predisposition Syndromes

Whole-body MR imaging is central to surveillance in a number of pediatric cancer predisposition syndromes (CPS) to detect primary and recurrent tumors and subsequent malignant neoplasms [7, 16, 25, 42]. CPS patients may initially present prior to tumor development with a known germline pathogenic mutation or positive family history or may present with a tumor either at an earlier age than expected or with multiple synchronous lesions suggestive of a CPS [43, 44].

Recent data suggest that the rate of inherited pathogenic mutations in pediatric patients with cancer is as high as 14%. This number is expected to rise with future results of ongoing multicenter studies such as the St. Jude Children's Research Hospital–Washington University Pediatric Cancer Genome Project [45–47]. Although rare, awareness of CPS is important for early cancer detection and improved outcomes, as demonstrated in LFS [21].

Surveillance benefits, not validated for all CPS, must be balanced against considerations such as the time and financial costs associated with serial imaging as well as potential risks related to general anesthesia and GBCA [13, 16, 25, 48–52].

Studies suggest that the psychological burden of having a CPS can be improved by active surveillance leading to a feeling of patient/family empowerment [52, 53]. In 2016, a multidisciplinary expert panel convened by the American Association for Cancer Research (AACR) proposed a surveillance threshold for pediatric CPS where risk of malignancy in the first two decades is greater than 5%. It can be lower if highly aggressive and amenable to treatment such as rhabdoid tumors [44]. Those syndromes in which whole-body MR imaging is considered most beneficial are reviewed here [7, 10]. Table 17.2 summarizes their indication-specific protocols.

Li-Fraumeni Syndrome

Li-Fraumeni syndrome (LFS) is an autosomal dominant condition resulting from a pathogenic variant of the TP53 tumor suppressor gene. It has a high penetrance, almost 50% by 30 years, prevalence of 1:5000, and near 100% lifetime risk of malignancy (4% by 1-year-old), affecting females slightly earlier than males [33, 54]. In Brazil, a variant founder mutation (p.R337H) has a higher prevalence (1:375) but lower penetrance (15–20% by 30 years) [54]. Clinical presentation, varying with tumor type, includes mass, pain, or seizures.

Core LFS-associated childhood tumors are osteosarcoma, soft tissue sarcoma, adrenocortical carcinoma (4% in classic LFS, 8–10% with p.R337H), and brain tumors, including choroid plexus carcinoma, astrocytoma, and medulloblastoma, and in late adolescence leukemia and premenopausal breast cancer (later onset with p.R337H) [21, 33, 55]. Less common malignancies include melanoma; malignant fibrous histiocytoma; colorectal, renal, and lung carcinoma; and papillary thyroid cancer [21, 34, 54] (Fig. 17.6).

Whole-body MR imaging includes coronal STIR and axial DWI. The key review sites are suprarenal regions for adrenocortical carcinomas and the bone marrow for osseous sarcomas [10, 56]. Sagittal or axial fat-suppressed T2-weighted sequences are optional for solid organs and coronal T1-weighted MR imaging for bone metastases, with Dixon fat suppression increasingly applied. Subtle marrow T2-weighted hyperintensities warrant careful interrogation due to high risk of osteosarcoma and leukemia.

Whole-body and dedicated brain MR imaging scans are recommended annually from diagnosis. From 6 years, or when GA is no longer required, these are usually scheduled as annual brain and whole-body MR imaging staggered at

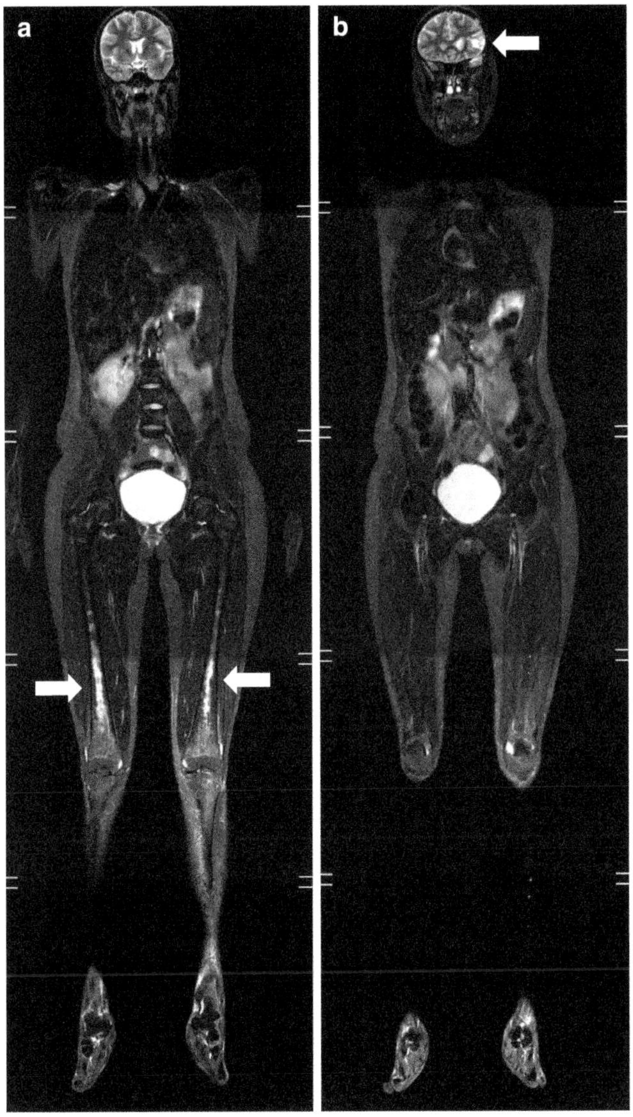

Fig. 17.6 Li-Fraumeni syndrome in a 17-year-old girl. New diagnosis of leukemia demonstrated on coronal whole-body STIR (**a**) with T2-weighted hyperintensities (*white arrows*) in the bone marrow of both distal femora as well as an anaplastic astrocytoma (**b**), with T2-weighted hyperintense signal (*white arrow*) in the left parietal lobe consistent with gliosis

6-month intervals, with focused abdominopelvic ultrasound also performed every 3–4 months [33]. Integration of equivocal or positive findings across different surveillance arms is essential to stratify risk and avoid unnecessary investigations (Fig. 17.7). The performance of whole-body MR surveillance imaging for detecting malignant and premalignant lesions has been demonstrated in a number of recent studies [14, 32, 46]. Discussion of treatment options is beyond the scope of this chapter given the broad spectrum of tumors encountered.

Hereditary Paraganglioma-Pheochromocytoma Syndrome

Hereditary paraganglioma-pheochromocytoma (HPP) syndrome is autosomal dominant with a penetrance of 90%, resulting from *SDHx* and non-*SDHx* (e.g., *MAX*) gene pathogenic variants [57, 58]. Characterized by succinate dehydrogenase subunit B/fumarate hydratase (SDHB/FH)-related tumors, most are of neural crest origin, usually benign with increased risk of malignant transformation [59]. 10–20% metastasize, with risk factors including size > 4.5 cm and hormonal inactivity [59, 60]. Catecholamine-secreting sympathetic trunk lesions in the lower mediastinum, abdomen, and pelvic can cause hypertension or tachycardia, while non-secreting parasympathetic trunk lesions from skull base to upper mediastinum cause mass effect such as cranial nerve palsies [57, 59]. Rare SDHB-related tumors include gastrointestinal stromal tumors (GIST), oncocytomas, renal cell carcinomas, and pituitary adenomas [57, 58, 61, 62].

Whole-body MR imaging in HPP syndrome consists of coronal STIR and axial DWI sequences with limited coverage (NCAP) alternating biannually with CAP coverage whole-body MR imaging and regional neck MR imaging from 6 to 8 years when GA is not needed [7, 57]. The paraspinal regions from the skull base to pelvis, specifically the sympathetic trunk, organ of Zuckerkandl, aortocaval region, vas deferens, carotid body, and kidneys, are key review sites [25] (Fig. 17.8). GIST occurs rarely, often in stomach and multiple, and while the gastrointestinal tract is poorly evaluated on whole-body MR imaging, dedicated imaging is not justified due to its low incidence [57]. Whole-body MR imaging has a higher sensitivity than biochemistry for lesion detection, 87.5% versus 37.5%, with mass effect on adjacent structures aiding larger lesion localization [57, 61].

Benign secreting tumors can be managed perioperatively with alpha-blocking agents and beta-blockers +/− tyrosine hydroxylase inhibitors and larger lesions by site-dependent open or laparoscopic curative surgical resection. Disease control for malignant lesions includes radioisotopes including [1]I-MIBG or ^{111}In-pentetreotide scintigraphy or chemotherapy [63].

Hereditary Retinoblastoma

Retinoblastoma (RB) is the most common pediatric intraocular malignancy, with an incidence of 1/15,000 in infancy. 40% of cases are inheritable with an *RB1* pathogenic germline mutation [64, 65]. Hereditary RB is associated with higher ocular bilaterality, with early onset of subsequent malignant neoplasms (SMN) in up to 20%, especially following external beam radiotherapy. SMN include pineoblastoma, osteosarcoma, soft tissue sarcoma, malignant

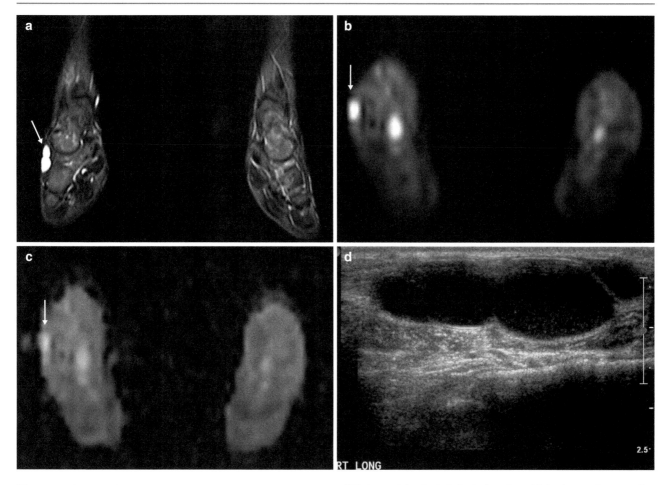

Fig. 17.7 Li-Fraumeni syndrome in a 12-year-old boy undergoing surveillance, whole-body MR imaging (merged whole-body MR image is shown in Fig. 17.1). Single station coronal STIR MR image of the lower extremity (**a**) shows a high signal intensity lesion (*white arrows*) in the right ankle, which also exhibits high signal intensity (**b**) on axial diffusion-weighted whole-body imaging with background suppression (DWIBS) trace image (b = 800 s/mm²) and (**c**) high signal intensity on the apparent diffusion coefficient (ADC) map consistent with a cyst. Follow-up ultrasound (**d**) confirmed a 4.6 cm cyst with some internal debris most consistent with a ganglion that resolved spontaneously

melanomas, and more rarely breast, bladder, lung, and uterine tumors. These SMN appear increasingly in different decades; now 5-year survivals exceed 95% in North America [66, 67]. Surveillance involves clinical assessment including annual skin checks for melanoma, laboratory, and imaging studies [67].

There is debate about the value of whole-body MR imaging for surveillance of SMN, primarily for detection of osteosarcoma, which may be asymptomatic rather than presenting with pain and swelling [66]. With this caveat, whole-body MR imaging is recommended by the AACR consensus group, acquiring coronal STIR with axial DWI sequences annually from 8 to 10 years, with the relatively late starting age for surveillance reflecting the later age of osteosarcoma occurrence in RB [7, 67]. Targeted imaging of suspicious bone marrow T2-weighted hyperintensities should be performed. In addition, dedicated brain MRI begins at diagnosis and

ends at 5 years of age, while imaging for other SMN using whole-body MR imaging typically continues into adulthood [25, 64, 67, 68] (Fig. 17.9). Osseous and soft tissue sarcomas in hereditary RB are managed the same as sporadic tumors, with regional MR imaging for local staging and chest CT and bone scans for distant metastases, usually to lung.

Constitutional Mismatch Repair Deficiency (CMMRD)

Constitutional mismatch repair deficiency (CMMRD) is a rare, autosomal recessive CPS with biallelic *MMR* germline mutations in one of four genes. It has a relatively high risk of early tumor onset with median age 7.5 years [69, 70]. Three key tumor groups occur: (1) hematologic malignancies such as non-Hodgkin lymphoma (NHL) and T-lymphoblastic leukemia (T-ALL) most frequently; (2) malignant brain and spinal tumors, with high-grade glio-

Fig. 17.8 Hereditary
paraganglioma-
pheochromocytoma (HPP)
syndrome in a 13-year-old
boy with a right carotid body
paraganglioma. The patient
presented with 2 cm right
neck mass since birth and a
positive family history of
sibling with a malignant
glioma. Coronal whole-body
STIR merged MR image (**a**)
and single station MR image
(**b**) show low to intermediate
signal intensity 3 cm mass
(*arrow*) in right carotid space
at level of carotid bifurcation,
suboptimally visualized due
to distortion artifact related to
dental braces (*arrowheads*).
Coronal image from cropped
contrast-enhanced CT neck
(**c**) better demonstrates the
peripherally enhancing
necrotic mass (*arrow*)
consistent with a
paraganglioma

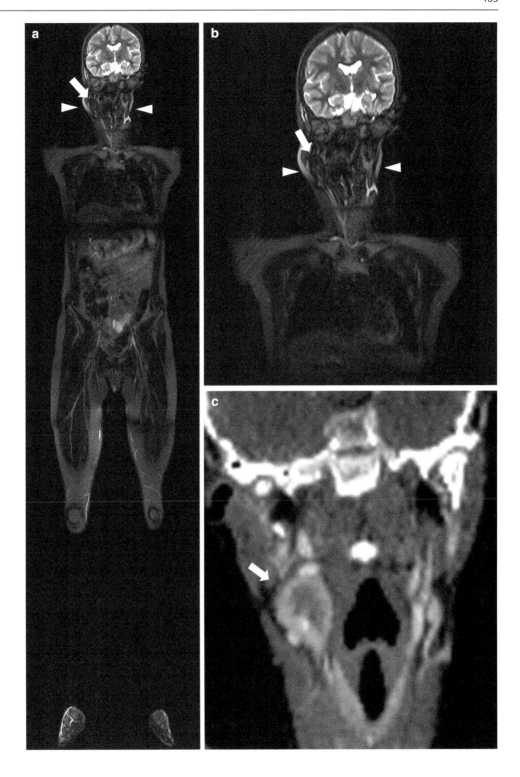

mas, PNET, and medulloblastoma; and (3) gastrointestinal tract tumors (commonly colorectal and small bowel carcinomas). It is associated with but distinct from Lynch syndrome, both of which are associated with the formation of colonic adenomas that can undergo malignant transforma-

tion to adenocarcinoma [69, 70]. Symptomatology is broad including café au lait spots reminiscent of NF1, occasionally leading to misdiagnosis [69].

Standard coverage whole-body MR imaging using coronal STIR and axial DWI sequences is advocated annually

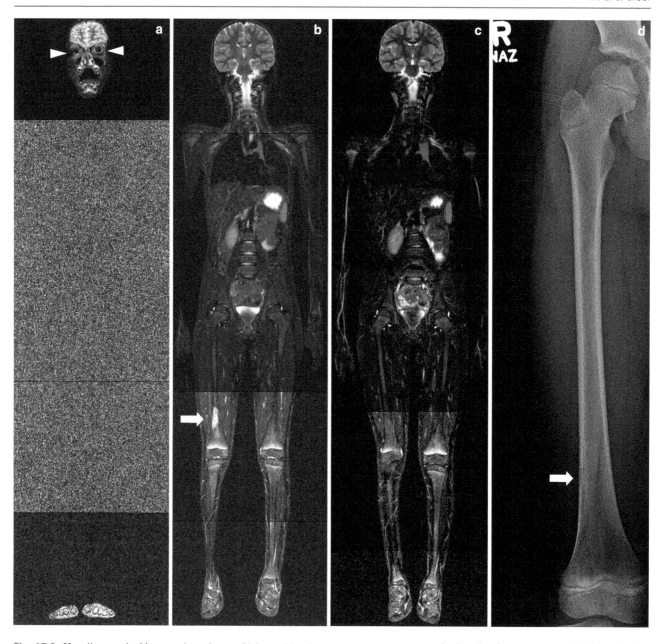

Fig. 17.9 Hereditary retinoblastoma in a 6-year-old boy with prior bilateral enucleations. Coronal whole-body STIR surveillance MR images show (**a**) orbital prostheses with low T2-weighted signal (*arrowheads*) and (**b**) a new focus of high T2-weighted signal intensity (*arrow*) in the right distal femur confirmed on biopsy as an osteosar- coma, not present on prior imaging from a year ago (**c**). Frontal radio- graph of the right femur (**d**) shows slightly coarsened trabecular pattern in the distal diaphysis (*arrow*) but no discrete lytic or sclerotic lesion, periosteal reaction, or soft tissue mass, demonstrating the greater sensi- tivity of MR imaging for tumor detection

from the age of 6 or when GA is no longer required, with optional supplementary sequences listed in Table 17.2 [7, 70] (Fig. 17.10). AACR recommendations also include regional brain MR imaging from diagnosis, abdomino-pelvic ultrasound from 1 year, each performed every 6 months. Imaging findings are typical for brain, gut, and bone tumors, with genitourinary tumors in the late first decade [70].

Neurofibromatosis 1, Neurofibromatosis 2, and Schwannomatosis

These three entities are distinct but related autosomal domi-nant entities associated with mutations on chromosomes 17 and 22 [71, 72]. Symptoms vary with lesions such as pain and increasing tumor size concerning in peripheral nerve sheath tumors in NF-1 and hearing loss and imbalance with vestibular schwannomas in NF-2 [71, 72].

In NF-1, a single standard coverage whole-body MR imaging scan using coronal STIR and axial DWI is advocated in late adolescence/pre-adulthood as per the AACR recommendation, to establish the baseline number, size, sig-nal, and distribution of plexiform neurofibromas (PN). They typically show a target pattern on STIR, brighter peripherally than centrally [7, 37, 71].

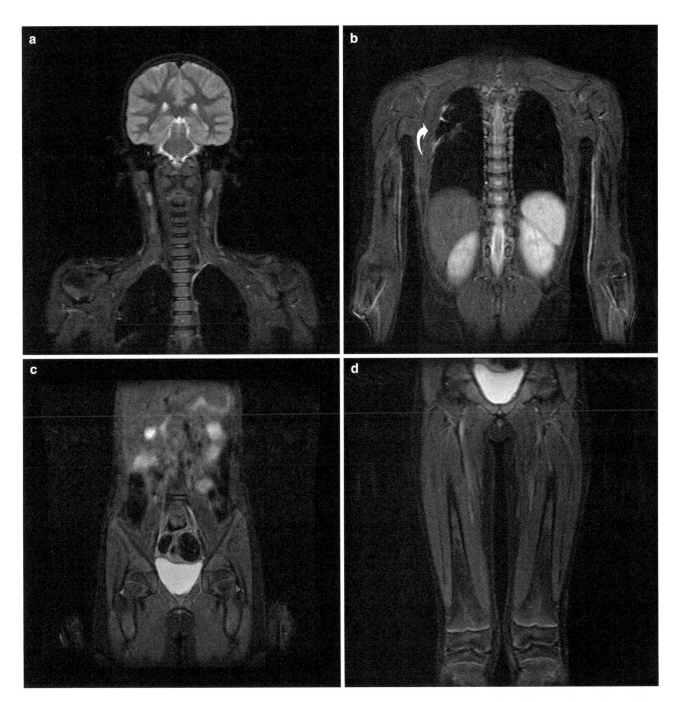

Fig. 17.10 Constitutional mismatch repair deficiency syndrome (CMMRD) in a 9-year-old boy with past history of colonic adenomas and an anaplastic astrocytoma. Coronal STIR images of individual anatomic stations (**a–e**) acquired separately show T2-weighted hyperintensity in the marrow of the proximal right tibia (**e**, *arrow*), a non-specific finding. Scarring in the right upper lobe is seen from previous biopsies (**b**, *curved arrow*). Coronal STIR sequences as part of whole-body MR imaging performed 9 years later (**f**) with improved spatial resolution. Targeted imaging of the liver was required to assess small liver nodules – the largest measuring 1.5 cm that is hypointense on axial (**g**) single-shot T2-weighted and (**h**) balanced steady-state free precession sequences (*arrows*) and confirmed by biopsy to be focal nodular hyperplasia

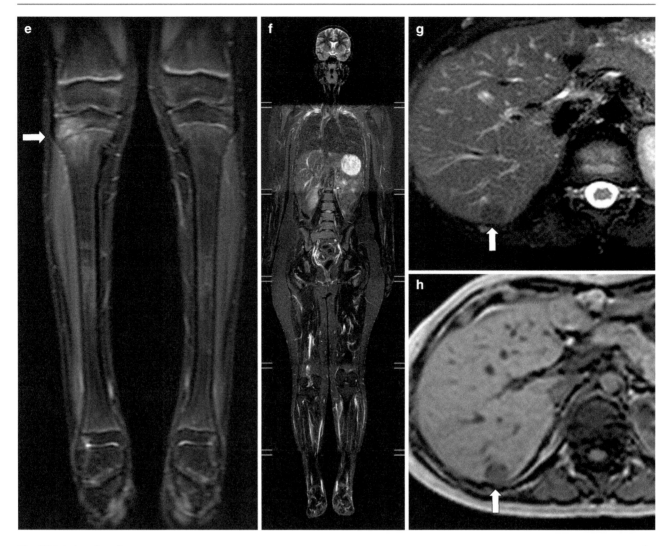

Fig. 17.10 (continued)

Internal PN sites warrant closer review due to their higher propensity for malignant degeneration to peripheral nerve sheath tumors [10]. Targeted imaging (+/− GBCA) is indicated when symptomatic to detect change in PN size and signal characteristics that could suggest malignant degeneration, as well as mass effect on adjacent structures (Fig. 17.11). In NF-2 and schwannomatosis, whole-body MR imaging is advocated if symptomatic to assess sites of discomfort or mass effect, supplementing regional brain and spine MR imaging, with high-resolution imaging of the internal auditory meati in NF-2 and craniocervical region in schwannomatosis [7, 37, 72].

Management is multidisciplinary. For more aggressive tumors, microsurgery is balanced against radiotherapy. Monoclonal antibodies such as bevacizumab newly offer potential to shrink schwannomas [72].

Other Neoplastic and Related Disorders

Lymphoma

Pediatric lymphoma includes Hodgkin lymphoma (HL) and non-Hodgkin lymphoma (NHL). HL is characterized by nodal and extranodal disease, the most common tumor in adolescence and representing 10–15% of childhood malignancies but is highly curable.

Non-Hodgkin lymphoma (NHL) is more common under 10 years, with sub-types Burkitt, diffuse large B-cell, and anaplastic and lymphoblastic lymphoma [73, 74]. HL can present with classic "B" symptoms of fever, night sweats, and weight loss. It can be associated with immunosuppression and Epstein-Barr virus infections. NHL presents more variably, with chest and/or abdominal masses [73].

Fig. 17.11 Neurofibromatosis type 1 in a 10-year-old boy with previous history of malignant nerve sheath tumors. (**a**) Coronal whole-body STIR at 1.5 Tesla and (**b**) a single station image through the torso demonstrate a retroperitoneal target lesion (*arrow*) left of the L4/5 intervertebral disc in keeping with a plexiform neurofibroma, showing a target sign of low signal centrally and high signal peripherally. There is associated levoscoliosis as well as small hepatic lesions (*curved arrows*), presumed metastases

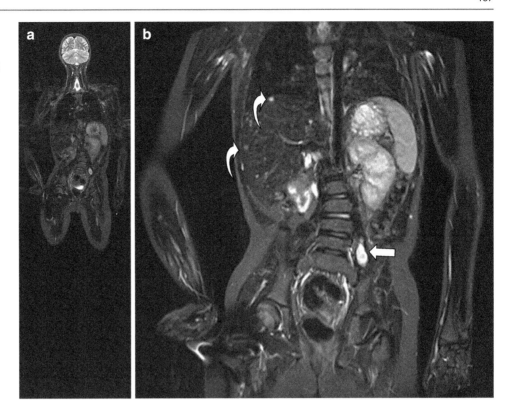

With a potential for widespread disease, whole-body MR imaging is an attractive imaging option offering excellent soft tissue detail and increasingly functional information for tumor viability. Value adding of DWI in pediatric whole-body MR imaging is largely based on HL staging and treatment response data in children and adolescents. Littooij et al. [75] reported a high sensitivity (100%) but lower specificity (62%) for detection of residual disease compared with FDG-PET/CT, whereas other studies reported a mix of lower sensitivities and higher specificities [9, 23, 29, 76]. As such, whole-body MR imaging is increasingly considered a viable alternative to PET/CT, alone or in conjunction with PET imaging, at each stage of HL [10, 76]. Whole-body MR imaging includes standard coverage coronal STIR and axial DWI. Optional sequences include coronal T1-weighted gradient echo (with or without fat suppression) and axial fat-suppressed single-shot T2-weighted sequences.

HL can manifest with a single enlarged node or confluent nodal masses in the neck, chest, abdomen, and/or pelvis. NHL can present with splenomegaly and bowel wall involvement. Lung involvement from HL and NHL is less common and less well seen on MRI. As previously discussed, DWI remains reasonably accurate for detecting splenic lesions in HL, despite intrinsic limitations [10, 26, 28]. Lower spatial resolution of large FOV imaging and affected nodes not enlarging has prompted consideration of ultrasmall particle iron oxide (USPIO) agents in lymphoma [39, 40] (Fig. 17.12). Predicated by the tumor type and tailored to the specific patient, treatment options include chemotherapy alone or in combination with radiotherapy. Surgery is reserved for GIT complications of NHL such as bowel obstruction or perforation.

Langerhans Cell Histiocytosis

Langerhans cell histiocytosis (LCH) is a myeloid neoplasia of dendritic cells with three distinct disease patterns: (1) single focus (~70%) in 5–15 year-olds, affecting bones and occasionally lung; (2) multifocal (~20%) in 1–5 year-olds, involving the liver, spleen, lymph nodes (mostly cervical), skin and bones, and infrequently posterior pituitary gland resulting in diabetes insipidus; and (3) fulminant multifocal (10%) in infants under 2, causing anemia and thrombocytopenia, affecting the reticuloendothelial system, and can be fatal [77, 78]. Skeletal sites are most common, especially skull, ribs, spine, mandible, pelvis, and long bones [77]. Whole-body MR imaging, more sensitive in detecting bone lesions than skeletal survey and bone scans, is now used for diagnosis and follow-up of osseous and extraskeletal lesions [79]. It is complementary to ultrasound for evaluating nodal or soft tissue masses, liver, and splenic disease. Regional brain MR imaging is for evaluation of pituitary stalk involvement. However, it is currently not used for assessing cystic lung disease, which is more common in adults and better characterized by CT [77, 79].

Whole-body coronal STIR and DWI and sagittal spine STIR sequences are standard for evaluation of LCH.

Fig. 17.12 Diffuse B-cell lymphoma in a 16-year-old girl. Unmerged coronal STIR (**a**, **b**) MR images and coronal diffusion-weighted MR imaging (b = 800 s/mm^2) (**c**) of the torso and proximal upper and lower extremities demonstrate multiple bone marrow STIR hyperintense lesions (*arrows*) in the humeri, vertebrae, pelvis, and femora with left axillary lymph node involvement (**a**, *arrowhead*; **c**, *curved arrow*). (**d**) Positron emission tomography (PET) with 18-FDG performed 2 weeks later demonstrates similar distribution of PET-avid lesions in the axial and appendicular bone marrow (*arrows*) and left axilla (*curved arrow*)

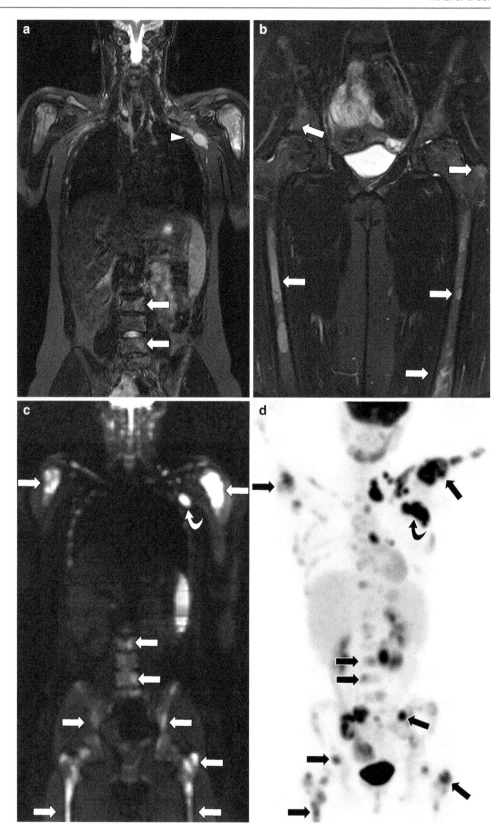

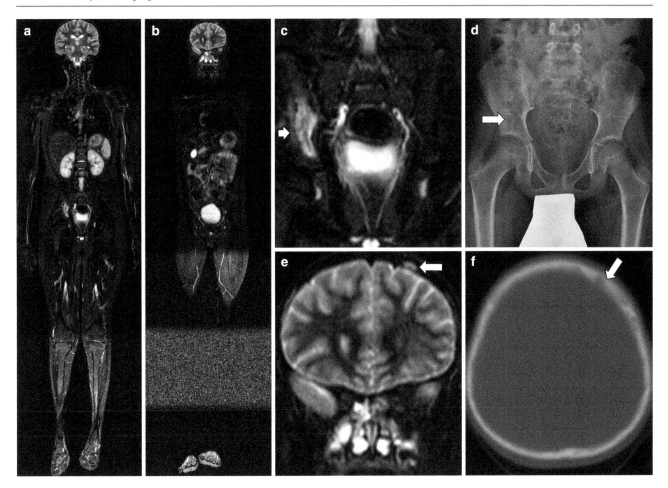

Fig. 17.13 Langerhans cell histiocytosis (LCH) in a 10-year-old boy who presented with pelvic pain. Coronal whole-body STIR sequences (**a**, **b**) and single station images (**c**, **e**) show bone marrow STIR hyperintense lesions, respectively, in the right iliac and left frontal bones (*arrows*), consistent with LCH lesions. On the pelvic radiography obtained at presentation (**d**), this lesion was barely perceptible as a subtle lucency (*arrow*) obscured by bowel gas. Axial bone window setting CT image (**f**) confirms the presence of the calvarial lesion (*arrow*) is seen on bone windows

T1-weighted whole-body sequences are optional with targeted imaging of abdominal organs as required. Osseous lesions can be indolent or aggressive. They can be variable with perilesional edema, endosteal scalloping (of inner and outer diploe), periosteal reactions, soft tissue masses, and in the spine often presenting as vertebra plana [77, 80]. Often seen as discrete, round, or geographic T2-weighted hyperintensities, they are iso- to hypointense on T1-weighted MR imaging and can enhance [80] (Fig. 17.13). Hepatic involvement can present as diffuse enlargement, focal lesions, and periportal fibrosis, progressing to cirrhosis and splenomegaly, which has a worse outcome [77].

Depending on symptoms, follow-up may be annual or biannual, with PET/MRI likely to have an expanded role in evaluation and monitoring as it becomes more widely available [10]. Lesion site, extent, global burden, and activity determine suitability for local treatment such as surgical curettage, excision, or intralesional steroid injection or need for chemotherapy [79]. With recent recognition of underlying somatic mutations in LCH, B-Raf-MEK pathway inhibition may be an option for those unresponsive to standard therapy [78].

Other Neoplasms

Whole-body MR imaging is infrequently used to evaluate solid tumors in children and adolescents, typically representing only 5–10% of whole-body MR studies [1–3] (Fig. 17.14). It may help characterize a known primary lesion detected by another modality while simultaneously performing local and distant staging [1, 10, 81]. Examples include rhabdomyosarcoma, Ewing sarcoma, primitive neuroectodermal tumor, and neuroblastoma (Fig. 17.15).

Whole-body coronal STIR and axial DWI sequences are standardly acquired for evaluation of LCH. Optional sequence includes coronal T1-weighted MR imaging with or without fat suppression, with targeted imaging for primary tumor delineation as required. More comprehensive regional imaging may be warranted for tumor staging neuroblastoma or Wilms tumor. Detection of osseous metastases is a key focus in whole-body MR imaging. The performance of whole-body MR imaging relative to CT or 99 m Tc bone scintigraphy was recently studied in a systematic review of

osseous metastases in pediatric patients by Smets et al. [82, 83]. These were variably described as focal or diffuse marrow lesions, hypointense on T1-weighted MR imaging, and/or hyperintense on T2-weighted MR imaging, with sensitivities compared with reference standards ranging from 82% to 100% [82]. Utility of whole-body MR imaging in detection of lung nodules remains a focus of active investigation, with newer MR imaging techniques using ultrashort echo times that show promise, with reliable detection of 4 mm nodules in combination with PET [84]. Formal guidelines do not currently exist for whole-body MR imaging of sporadic solid tumors. Utilization is likely to keep pace with technologic advances, especially as PET/MR imaging becomes more accessible and economically feasible.

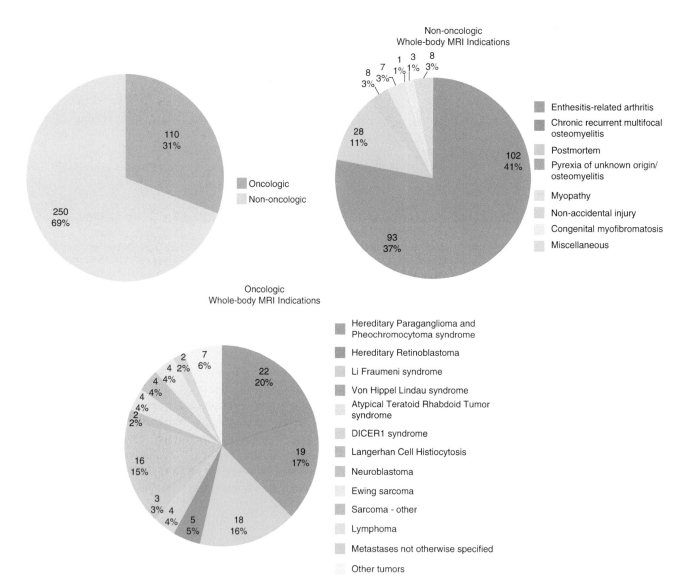

Fig. 17.14 Non-oncologic and oncologic whole-body MR imaging referrals over a 12-month period in 2017 at a single tertiary pediatric institution. (From Greer [1], with permission)

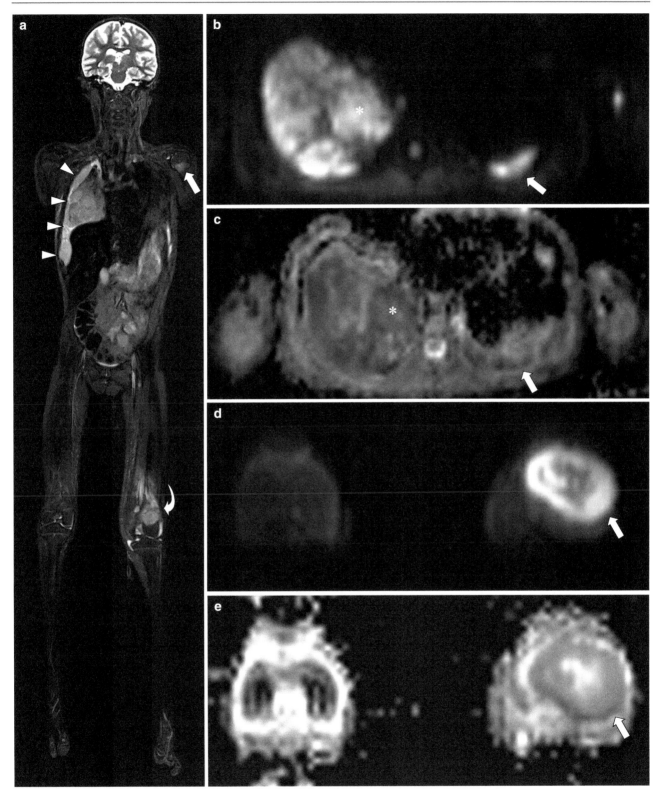

Fig. 17.15 Metastatic rhabdomyosarcoma in a 9-year-old girl post-stem cell transplant and radiotherapy. Coronal whole-body STIR (**a**) MR image demonstrates extensive right pleural/lung metastases (*arrowheads*), as well as metastases in the left proximal humerus (*straight arrow*) and left distal femur (*curved arrow*). Axial diffusion-weighted MR imaging with background suppression (DWIBS) (**b**, **d**) trace images ($b = 1000$ s/mm^2) and (**c**, **e**) apparent diffusion coefficient (ADC) maps are displayed. (**b**, **c**) The extensive disease in the right hemithorax (*) and a small left pleural metastatic nodule (*arrows*) all restrict with high signal intensity on the DWI trace image and low signal intensity on the ADC map. (**d**, **e**) The left distal femoral metastasis (*arrows*) also demonstrates diffusion restriction

Chemotherapy-Induced Osteonecrosis

Osteonecrosis or avascular necrosis (AVN) is a sequela of oncotherapy, especially high-dose corticosteroids. AVN is increasingly demonstrated when surveilling asymptomatic patients in up to 42% of newly diagnosed Hodgkin lymphoma. Patients with leukemia and sickle cell disease are other at-risk groups [85, 86]. If undetected, AVN can progress. Metadiaphyseal involvement is less problematic. However, epiphyseal AVN in weight-bearing joints is subject to articular surface collapse and fragmentation, with resultant pain and immobility. Over time, secondary degenerative arthropathy develops [87].

Coronal whole-body STIR and T1-weighted gradient echo sequences are acquired with standard coverage to identify lesion number, distribution, and extent of articular surface involvement/collapse if epiphyseal [85]. Targeted imaging limited to shoulder and pelvic girdles may be sufficient with GBCA rarely required. DWI in sickle cell disease can help differentiate marrow ischemia from infection [86]. Usually

involving long bones, osteonecrosis is seen as geographic areas of yellow marrow bound by rings of low signal on T1- and T2-weighted sequences, with or without an inner band of high T2 signal ("double line" sign) [85]. Radiographs can monitor subchondral fragmentation or collapse for progression or resolution. MR imaging follow-up may be needed if more symptomatic (Fig. 17.16). Early detection and treatment change and/or temporary immobilization may avert progression, particularly in weight-bearing regions such as femoral heads, knee, and ankle joints. This may prevent joint replacement [87].

Infectious and Noninfectious Inflammatory Disorders

Fever of Unknown Origin

Fever of unknown origin (FUO) is episodic pyrexia above 38.0 °C (100.4 °F) lasting 8 or more days (previously

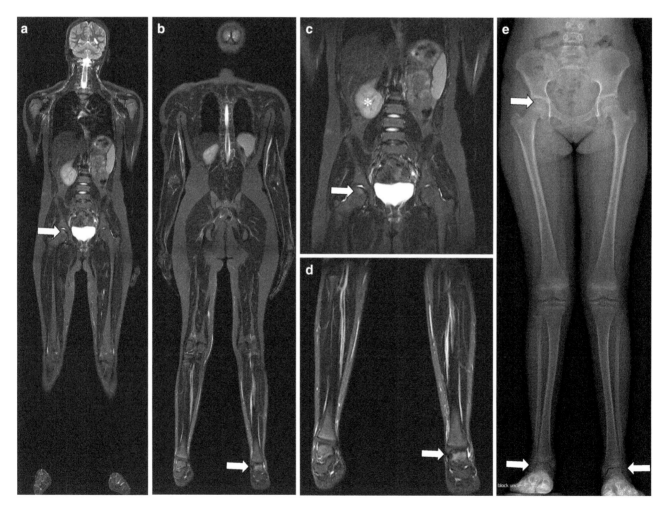

Fig. 17.16 Osteonecrosis in an 11-year-old girl. Coronal STIR (**a, b**) whole-body MR images and (**c, d**) single station MR images demonstrate subtle subchondral STIR hyperintense foci in the right hip and bilateral talar domes, with marginal low signal intensity and irregularity of the articular surface in the left talus suggesting more advanced osteochondral lesions with minor collapse (*arrows*). (**e**) Radiographic changes (*arrows*) are less well seen on lower extremity survey radiography compared to MR images

>3 weeks) with no defined cause, independent of laboratory testing [88]. Although not a first-line investigation, whole-body MR imaging may identify a source, inflammatory or oncologic, where baseline laboratory and imaging tests have proven unhelpful, especially in younger patients [88]. Lindsay et al. [89] found whole-body MR imaging, combined with targeted imaging as needed, identified an infection source or an alternate diagnosis in almost 22% of patients under 6 years with suspected osteomyelitis with

little time penalty. Coronal whole-body STIR, with targeted axial T1- and fat-suppressed T2-weighted MR imaging of focal abnormalities, permits delineation of one or more sites of osteomyelitis, septic arthritis, and/or myositis, guiding biopsy or abscess drainage (Fig. 17.17).

Chronic Recurrent Multifocal Osteomyelitis

Chronic recurrent multifocal osteomyelitis (CRMO), also known as chronic non-bacterial osteomyelitis (CNO), is an

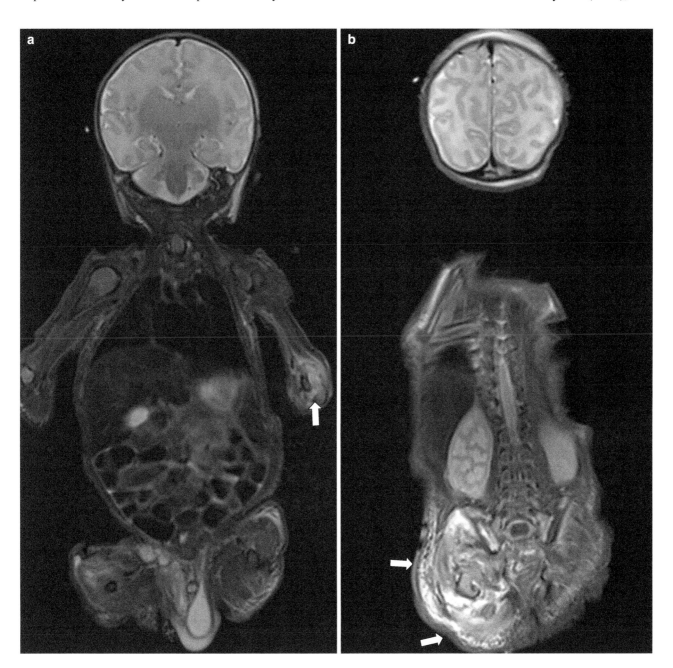

Fig. 17.17 *Staphylococcus aureus* abscesses and septic arthritis in a 21-day-old boy with persistent fevers. Coronal whole-body STIR sequences acquired in two stations on a 3 Tesla scanner demonstrate a left elbow joint effusion (**a**, *arrow*) and a right gluteal muscle abscess (**b**, *arrows*) with more generalized high signal subcutaneous edema.

Targeted STIR MR imaging in (**c**) the sagittal plane through the left elbow better demonstrates the effusion (*arrows*). An axial STIR MR image through the pelvis (**d**) shows the abscess (*straight arrow*) as well as iliac wing osteomyelitis (*curved arrow*)

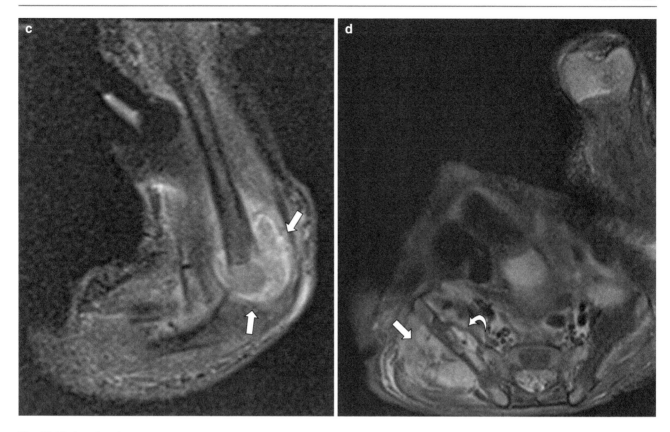

Fig. 17.17 (continued)

autoimmune skeletal disorder affecting children and adolescents, more commonly females. It is characterized by 6 or more months of pain and occasional reduced range of movement, sometimes also affecting the skin and bowel [90, 91]. With no clear etiology, CRMO is a diagnosis of exclusion; serologic inflammatory markers are often elevated without a clear source [91]. Whole-body MR imaging with coronal STIR, sagittal spine STIR, or T2-weighted fat-suppressed sequences and optional axial sequences is now central to the diagnosis of CRMO [1, 35]. Multifocal bone marrow T2-weighted hyperintense lesions are often bilaterally symmetric, geographic, or ill-defined in pediatric patients with CRMO. To date, there is limited data validating DWI for grading CRMO lesion activity [30, 35, 91].

Key sites of CRMO are the lower extremities (femurs and tibias more common than feet), pelvis and sacroiliac joints, spine, sternum, and clavicles, with perimetaphyseal location in 79–90% of cases. CRMO can also present as juxtaphyseal nodules, periosseous edema, myositis, and joint effusions [90]. Vertebral lesions are limited to the vertebral body and can progress to collapse (vertebra plana). Overlap occurs with spondyloarthritis (Fig. 17.18).

Treatment is usually with nonsteroidal anti-inflammatory medications. However, 20–25% of adolescents fail to respond, developing relapsing disease [91]. Usually annual whole-body MR imaging is performed to monitor CRMO, sooner with symptomatic progression [1]. Development of a whole-body MR imaging-based CRMO scoring system is an area of active research, to enable standardized reporting of disease burden, capture activity, and assess treatment response [31, 35].

Enthesitis-Related Arthritis

Enthesitis-related arthritis (ERA) or spondyloarthritis is a subset of juvenile idiopathic arthritis. It manifests with joint pain and swelling in late childhood/early adolescence, with 60–80% HLA-B27 positivity, and a slight male predominance [8, 32, 92]. Whole-body MR imaging is now integral to diagnosis and management of ERA. Coronal whole-body STIR and targeted STIR sequences can be acquired as follows: sagittal spine, axial pelvis, coronal oblique sacroiliac joints, sagittal knees, and ankles [1, 32]. Bone marrow T2-weighted hyperintense lesions are usually perienthesal with adjacent soft tissue edema and swelling, characteristically at the Achilles tendon. It can be accompanied by synovitis, joint or bursal fluid, and arthritis such as tarsitis and sacroiliitis. Vertebral or "corner" lesions abut the vertebral

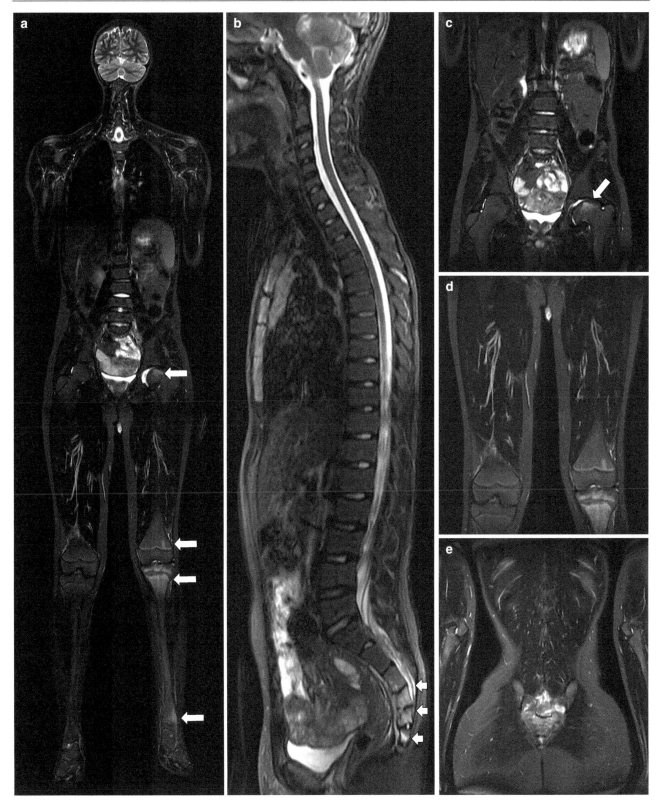

Fig. 17.18 Chronic recurrent multifocal osteomyelitis (CRMO) in a 13-year-old boy with a past history of left hip Perthes disease. Coronal whole-body (**a**) and sagittal whole spine (**b**) STIR sequences demonstrate periphyseal and vertebral body STIR hyperintensities (*arrows*) in keeping with CRMO lesions in the bone marrow. (**c**) Single station small field of view (FOV) STIR MR image shows bone marrow edema in the left femoral head with associated flattening and mild joint space widening from past Perthes disease (*arrow*). Single station coronal STIR MR images (**d**) redemonstrate lesions seen in (**a**) in the left distal femoral metaphysis and proximal tibial metaphysis and epiphysis, and (**e**) the sacrum, better seen on dedicated sagittal spine imaging (**b**)

endplates extending to the posterior elements with no collapse (Fig. 17.19).

Anti-inflammatory therapies are used along with conventional and newer biologic agents [92]. Standardization of core anatomic sites, sequences, and whole-body MR imaging planes is underway, which is a component of the OMERACT (Outcomes Measures in Rheumatology) scoring system that is used to evaluate inflammatory arthritis and ultimately guide treatment regimens [93].

Traumatic Disorder

Non-accidental Trauma

The few studies comparing whole-body MR imaging and skeletal surveys for suspected child abuse have shown whole-body MR imaging to be insensitive for detection of high specificity injuries such as rib and metaphyseal fractures, with no established role to assess non-accidental imaging at this time [94, 95]. Skeletal survey remains the reference standard for identifying skeletal injuries, regional CT, and MR imaging of the brain and abdomen used for suspected intracranial and solid organ injury.

Miscellaneous Disorders

Polymyositis, Juvenile Dermatomyositis, and Neuromuscular Disorders

Autoimmune inflammatory myopathies including polymyositis (PM) and juvenile dermatomyositis (JDM) cause rapid onset symmetric, proximal muscle weakness [96]. JDM also

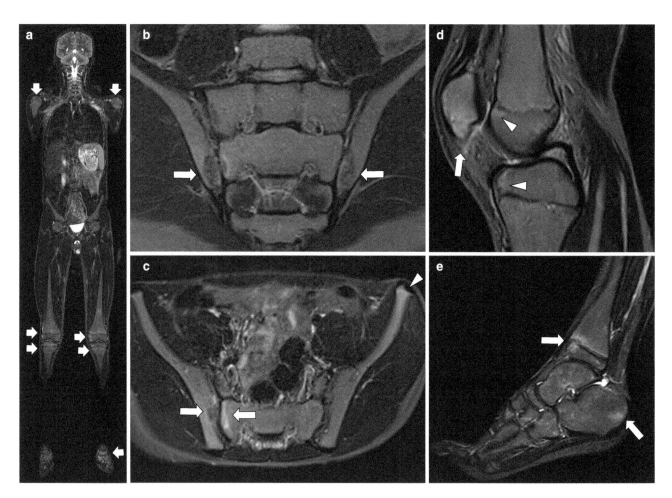

Fig. 17.19 Juvenile spondyloarthropathy or enthesitis-related arthritis (ERA), in an HLA-B27-positive 13-year-old boy. Coronal whole-body STIR sequence (**a**) shows a number of subtle areas of STIR hyperintense bone marrow edema (*arrows*) in the epiphyses and metaphyses around the shoulders and knees bilaterally and left hindfoot. (**b**) Angled coronal STIR MR image of the sacroiliac joints and (**c**) axial STIR MR image of the pelvis show bilateral sacroiliitis, with right greater than left marrow edema with low signal subchondral sclerosis (*arrows*) and left anterior superior iliac spine apophysitis with mild edema (*arrowhead*). Targeted sagittal STIR MR imaging of the left knee (**d**) shows patellar apophysitis with bone marrow and soft tissue edema (*arrow*) at the inferior patellar pole and mild perimetaphyseal edema (*arrowheads*) abutting the distal femoral and proximal tibial physes anteriorly. (**e**) More striking periphyseal edema (*arrows*) in the distal left tibia and calcaneus is present on sagittal STIR MR imaging of left ankle, in keeping with ERA

has a characteristic skin rash (papules over extensor surfaces and heliotrope rash of eyelids). Diagnosis is dependent on the rash plus 3–4 of the following: muscle weakness, characteristic findings on muscle biopsy, EMG abnormalities, and elevated muscle enzymes. Interstitial lung disease can be also seen in 35–40% [97, 98]. Patients with inherited neuromuscular (NM) disorders including spinal muscular atrophy and congenital muscular dystrophy have gradual onset diffuse muscle weakness with a variable pattern, hypotonia, and often skeletal, cardiorespiratory, and neurologic complications [99].

Whole-body MR imaging is now routinely used in both groups. STIR and T1-weighted sequences are more often acquired axially than coronally, with extended coverage from neck to hands and feet, not just limited to the shoulder and pelvic girdles as previously [1]. Wider slice gaps (10–15 mm) are sufficient in PM and JDM to distinguish proximal from distal muscle group involvement and evaluate neck and trunk muscles. Minimal or no gap is required in NM disorders for precise delineation of affected muscles groups. Anatomic distribution of disease can suggest the specific genetic defect [99, 100]. Active changes include intramuscular T2-weighted hyperintensity, with or without perifascial edema, while chronic changes include muscle atrophy, fatty infiltration, and occasionally calcinosis [96, 97, 100] (Fig. 17.20).

PM and JDM are usually treated with corticosteroids, which carries an increased risk of AVN that can also be assessed by MR imaging [98]. For inherited NM disorders, the focus is primarily on diagnosis with symptomatic support [99]. In both groups, whole-body MR imaging scoring systems are under development and/or validation, to act as biomarkers of disease severity and guide therapy [97, 100].

Postmortem

There is an emerging role for whole-body MR imaging to supplement conventional autopsy or facilitate minimally invasive autopsy [101, 102]. Often performed in conjunction with whole-body CT and skeletal surveys, whole-body MR imaging can be limited to the torso ("CAP") acquiring coronal and axial T1- and fat-suppressed T2-weighted sequences, with regional cardiac and brain MR imaging. Normal postmortem findings are still being established, and use will be influenced by access to MR scanners and local expertise, uptake only likely to increase in the pediatric realm (Fig. 17.21).

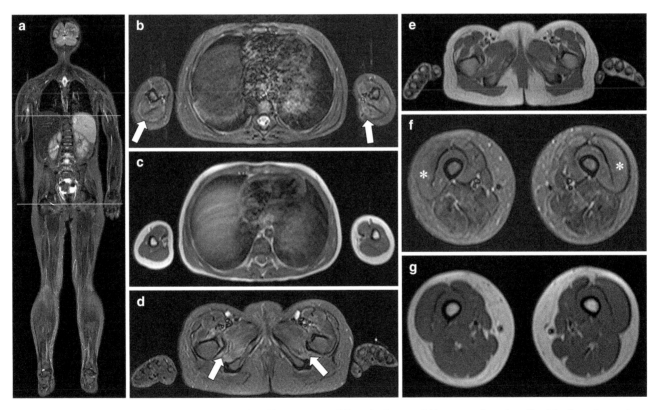

Fig. 17.20 Juvenile dermatomyositis in a 6-year-old girl with new onset muscle weakness. Coronal whole-body STIR MR image (**a**) demonstrates increased T2-weighted signal intensity in the proximal upper and lower extremity muscles consistent with edema, with lines indicating axial imaging positions. Affected upper (**b**, **c**) and lower (**d–g**) extremity muscle groups are better demonstrated on axial imaging. On STIR MR image, (**b**) bilateral triceps and biceps muscle and perifascial edema (*arrows*) are more diffuse and severe on the right and medial on the left, with bilaterally symmetric muscle edema involving the (**d**) adductors (*arrows*), (**f**) quadriceps and hamstring musculature, particularly the vastus lateralis (*asterisks*). (**c**, **e**, **f**) On T1-weighted MR imaging, there is no fatty replacement or muscle atrophy, in keeping with acute-onset active disease

478   M.-L. C. Greer

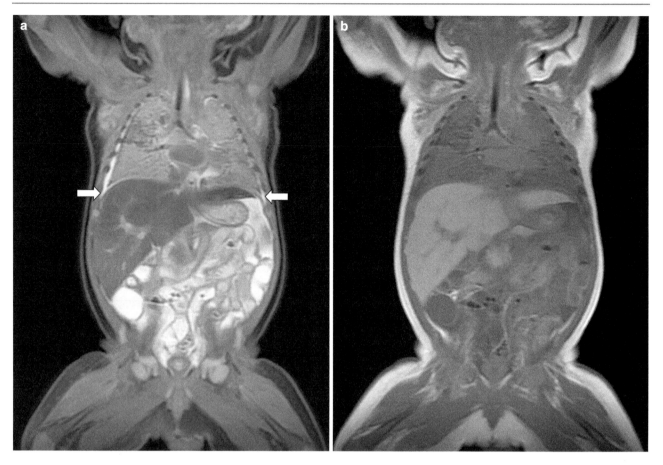

Fig. 17.21 Postmortem MR imaging of a 7-week-old boy found non-responsive. Coronal MR imaging covering neck to pelvis (NCAP) with (**a**) fat-suppressed T2-weighted fast spin echo and (**b**) non-fat-suppressed T1-weighted spin echo sequences shown. No cause was identified, with patchy lung consolidation, bilateral pleural effusions (*arrows*), and fluid-filled bowel loops all attributed to postmortem state

Image Analysis and Standardized Reporting

Coronal imaging is the workhorse of whole-body MR imaging, whether alone or in conjunction with other imaging sequences and planes. Pitfalls can be technical with inadequate oversampling resulting in signal loss where stations merge impacting interpretation. In addition, pathology can mimic normal anatomy such as axillary lymph nodes versus rib lesions in the coronal plane [1]. Lecouvet [13] advocates close interrogation of the sternum, ribs, and vertebrae on all coronal sequences, use of small FOV stations, and direct correlation of different sequences and imaging planes, especially for DWI to minimize false negative interpretations. Anatomic checklists highlighting lesion locations in a range of different CPS may improve detection of significant pathology while reducing overcalls or false positive interpretations, which can range up to 35% [7, 14, 15]. Standardized reporting templates can add value by highlighting key review areas prompting image analysis, flagging important findings for subsequent radiology review and clinical correlation.

Conclusion

Whole-body MR imaging is a rapidly evolving technique and now an important step in the diagnostic imaging paradigm for a range of oncologic and non-oncologic pediatric disorders. It has unique challenges relating to acquisition and analysis; however, it is most effective when optimized for the clinical indication and likely to be of even greater value as functional elements become more robust.

References

1. Greer MC. Whole-body magnetic resonance imaging: techniques and non-oncologic indications. Pediatr Radiol. 2018;48(9):1348–63.
2. Schooler GR, Davis JT, Daldrup-Link HE, Frush DP. Current utilization and procedural practices in pediatric whole-body MRI. Pediatr Radiol. 2018;48(8):1101–7.
3. Damasio MB, Magnaguagno F, Stagnaro G. Whole-body MRI: non-oncological applications in paediatrics. Radiol Med. 2016;121(5):454–61.

4. Chavhan GB, Babyn PS. Whole-body MR imaging in children: principles, technique, current applications, and future directions. Radiographics. 2011;3(6):1757–72.

5. Pasoglou V, Michoux N, Larbi A, Van Nieuwenhove S, Lecouvet F. Whole body MRI and oncology: recent major advances. Br J Radiol. 2018;91(1090):20170664. Review

6. Davis JT, Kwatra N, Schooler GR. Pediatric whole-body MRI: a review of current imaging techniques and clinical applications. J Magn Reson Imaging. 2016;44(4):783–93.

7. Greer MC, Voss SD, States LJ. Pediatric cancer predisposition imaging: focus on whole-body MRI. Clin Cancer Res. 2017;23(11):e6–e13.

8. Eutsler EP, Khanna G. Whole-body magnetic resonance imaging in children: technique and clinical applications. Pediatr Radiol. 2016;46(6):858–72.

9. Goo HW. Whole-body MRI in children: current imaging techniques and clinical applications. Korean J Radiol. 2015;16(5):973–85.

10. Gottumukkala RV, Gee MS, Hampilos PJ, Greer MC. Current and emerging roles of whole-body mri in evaluation of pediatric cancer patients. Radiographics. 2019;39(2):516–34.

11. Teixeira SR, Elias Junior J, Nogueira-Barbosa MH, Guimarães MD, Marchiori E, Santos MK. Whole-body magnetic resonance imaging in children: state of the art. Radiol Bras. 2015;48(2):111–20.

12. Mathews JD, Forsythe AV, Brady Z, Butler MW, Goergen SK, Byrnes GB, et al. Cancer risk in 680,000 people exposed to computed tomography scans in childhood or adolescence: data linkage study of 11 million Australians. BMJ. 2013;346:f2360.

13. Lecouvet FE. Whole-body MR imaging: musculoskeletal applications. Radiology. 2016;279(2):345–65.

14. Mai PL, Khincha PP, Loud JT, DeCastro RM, Bremer RC, Peters JA, et al. Prevalence of cancer at baseline screening in the National Cancer Institute Li-Fraumeni Syndrome Cohort. JAMA Oncol. 2017;3(12):1640–5.

15. Saya S, Killick E, Thomas S, Taylor N, Bancroft EK, Rothwell J, et al. Baseline results from the UK SIGNIFY study: a whole-body MRI screening study in TP53 mutation carriers and matched controls. Familial Cancer. 2017;16(3):433–40.

16. Anupindi SA, Bedoya MA, Lindell RB, Rambhatla SJ, Zelley K, Nichols KE, Chauvin NA. Diagnostic performance of whole-body mri as a tool for cancer screening in children with genetic cancer-predisposing conditions. AJR Am J Roentgeno. 2015;205(2):400–8.

17. Carter AJ, Greer ML, Gray SE, Ware RS. Mock MRI: reducing the need for anaesthesia in children. Pediatr Radiol. 2010;40(8):1368–74.

18. Jaimes C, Gee MS. Strategies to minimize sedation in pediatric body magnetic resonance imaging. Pediatr Radiol. 2016;46(6):916–27.

19. Perez M, Cuscaden C, Somers JF, Simms N, Shaheed S, Kehoe LA, et al. Easing anxiety in pediatric magnetic resonance imaging: a pilot study using animal assisted therapy. Pediatr Radiol. 2019;49(8):1000–9.

20. Ley S, Ley-Zaporozhan J, Schenk JP. Whole-body MRI in the pediatric patient. Eur J Radiol. 2009;70(3):442–51.

21. Villani A, Shore A, Wasserman JD, Stephens D, Kim RH, Druker H, et al. Biochemical and imaging surveillance in germline TP53 mutation carriers with Li-Fraumeni syndrome: 11 year follow-up of a prospective observational study. Lancet Oncol. 2016;17(9):1295–305.

22. Nievelstein RA, Littooij AS. Whole-body MRI in paediatric oncology. Radiol Med. 2016;121(5):442–53.

23. Lecouvet FE, Van Nieuwenhove S, Jamar F, Lhommel R, Guermazi A, Pasoglou VP. Whole-body MR imaging: the novel, "intrinsically hybrid," approach to metastases, myeloma, lymphoma, in bones and beyond. PET Clin. 2018;13(4):505–22.

24. Pasoglou V, Michoux N, Peeters F, Larbi A, Tombal B, Selleslagh T, et al. Whole-body 3D T1-weighted MR imaging in patients with prostate cancer: feasibility and evaluation in screening for metastatic disease. Radiology. 2015;275(1):155–66.

25. Greer MC. Imaging of cancer predisposition syndromes. Pediatr Radiol. 2018;48(9):1364–75.

26. Chavhan GB, Alsabban Z, Babyn PS. Diffusion-weighted imaging in pediatric body MR imaging: principles, technique, and emerging applications. Radiographics. 2014;34(3):E73–88.

27. Albano D, La Grutta L, Grassedonio E, Patti C, Lagalla R, Midiri M, et al. Pitfalls in whole body MRI with diffusion weighted imaging performed on patients with lymphoma: what radiologists should know. Magn Reson Imaging. 2016;34(7):922–31.

28. Littooij AS, Kwee TC, Barber I, Granata C, de Keizer B, Beek FJ, et al. Accuracy of whole-body MRI in the assessment of splenic involvement in lymphoma. Acta Radiol. 2016;57(2):142–51.

29. Regacini R, Puchnick A, Luisi FAV, Lederman HM. Can diffusion-weighted whole-body MRI replace contrast-enhanced CT for initial staging of Hodgkin lymphoma in children and adolescents? Pediatr Radiol. 2018;48(5):638–47.

30. Leclair N, Thörmer G, Sorge I, Ritter L, Schuster V, Hirsch FW. Whole-body diffusion-weighted imaging in chronic recurrent multifocal osteomyelitis in children. PLoS One. 2016;11(1):e0147523.

31. Andronikou S. Invited lecture 60: MRI in the diagnosis of CNO/CRMO. Pediatr Radiol. 2018;48(Suppl 2):S432.

32. Aquino MR, Tse SM, Gupta S, Rachlis AC, Stimec J. Whole-body MRI of juvenile spondyloarthritis: protocols and pictorial review of characteristic patterns. Pediatr Radiol. 2015;45(5):754–62.

33. Kratz CP, Achatz MI, Brugières L, Frebourg T, Garber JE, Greer MC, et al. Cancer screening recommendations for individuals with li-Fraumeni syndrome. Clin Cancer Res. 2017;23(11):e38–45.

34. Ballinger ML, Best A, Mai PL, Khincha PP, Loud JT, Peters JA, et al. Baseline surveillance in li-fraumeni syndrome using whole-body magnetic resonance imaging: a meta-analysis. JAMA Oncol. 2017;3(12):1634–9.

35. Arnoldi AP, Schlett CL, Douis H, Geyer LL, Voit AM, Bleisteiner F, et al. Whole-body MRI in patients with non-bacterial osteitis: radiological findings and correlation with clinical data. Eur Radiol. 2017;27(6):2391–9.

36. Koh DM, Blackledge M, Padhani AR, Takahara T, Kwee TC, Leach MO, Collins DJ. Whole-body diffusion-weighted MRI: tips, tricks, and pitfalls. AJR Am J Roentgenol. 2012;199(2):252–62.

37. Ahlawat S, Fayad LM, Khan MS, Bredella MA, Harris GJ, Evans DG, et al. Whole body MRI committee for the REiNS International Collaboration; REiNS International Collaboration Members 2016. Current whole-body MRI applications in the neurofibromatoses: NF1, NF2, and schwannomatosis. Neurology. 2016;87(7 Suppl 1):S31–9.

38. Weckbach S, Michaely HJ, Stemmer A, Schoenberg SO, Dinter DJ. Comparison of a new whole-body continuous-table-movement protocol versus a standard whole-body MR protocol for the assessment of multiple myeloma. Eur Radiol. 2010;20(12):2907–16.

39. Klenk C, Gawande R, Uslu L, Khurana A, Qiu D, Quon A, et al. Ionising radiation-free whole-body MRI versus (18)F-fluorodeoxyglucose PET/CT scans for children and young adults with cancer: a prospective, non-randomised, single-Centre study. Lancet Oncol. 2014;15(3):275–85.

40. Muehe AM, Feng D, von Eyben R, Luna-Fineman S, Link MP, Muthig T, et al. Safety report of ferumoxytol for magnetic resonance imaging in children and young adults. Investig Radiol. 2016;51(4):221–7.

41. Ponisio MR, McConathy J, Laforest R, Khanna G. Evaluation of diagnostic performance of whole-body simultaneous PET/MRI in pediatric lymphoma. Pediatr Radiol. 2016;46(9):1258–68.

42. Tijerin Bueno M, Greer ML, Malkin D, Villani A, Moineddin R. Whole body MRI in children with cancer predisposition syndromes (abstract). Pediatr Radiol. 2015;45(Suppl 1):S71.

43. Jongmans MC, Loeffen JL, Waanders E, Hoogerbrugge PM, Ligtenberg MJ, Kuiper RP, Hoogerbrugge N. Recognition of genetic predisposition in pediatric cancer patients: an easy-to-use selection tool. Eur J Med Genet. 2016;59(3):116–25.

44. Brodeur GM, Nichols KE, Plon SE, Schiffman JD, Malkin D. Pediatric cancer predisposition and surveillance: an overview, and a tribute to Alfred G. Knudson Jr. Clin Cancer Res. 2017;23(11):e1–5.

45. Zhang J, Walsh MF, Wu G, Edmonson MN, Gruber TA, Easton J, et al. Germline mutations in predisposition genes in pediatric cancer. N Engl J Med. 2015;373(24):2336–46.

46. Oberg JA, Glade Bender JL, Sulis ML, Pendrick D, Sierci AN, Hsiao SJ, et al. Implementation of next generation sequencing into pediatric hematology-oncology practice: moving beyond actionable alterations. Genome Med. 2016;8(1):133.

47. Downing JR, Wilson RK, Zhang J, Mardis ER, Pui CH, Ding L, et al. The pediatric cancer genome project. Nat Genet. 2012;44(6):619–22.

48. Sadowski EA, Bennett LK, Chan MR, Wentland AL, Garrett AL, Garrett RW, Djamali A. Nephrogenic systemic fibrosis: risk factors and incidence estimation. Radiology. 2007;243(1):148–57.

49. Tibussek D, Rademacher C, Caspers J, Turowski B, Schaper J, Antoch G, Klee D. Gadolinium brain deposition after macrocyclic gadolinium administration: a pediatric case-control study. Radiology. 2017;285(1):223–30.

50. Davidson AJ, Disma N, de Graaff JC, Withington DE, Dorris L, Bell G, et al. Neurodevelopmental outcome at 2 years of age after general anaesthesia and awake-regional anaesthesia in infancy (GAS): an international multicentre, randomised controlled trial. Lancet. 2016;387(10015):239–50.

51. Druker H, Zelley K, McGee RB, Scollon SR, Kohlmann WK, Schneider KA, Wolfe Schneider K. Genetic counselor recommendations for cancer predisposition evaluation and surveillance in the pediatric oncology patient. Clin Cancer Res. 2017;23(13):e91–7.

52. Schmidt CO, Sierocinski E, Hegenscheid K, Baumeister SE, Grabe HJ, Völzke H. Impact of whole-body MRI in a general population study. Eur J Epidemiol. 2016;31(1):31–9.

53. McBride KA, Ballinger ML, Schlub TE, Young MA, Tattersall MHN, Kirk J, et al. Psychosocial morbidity in TP53 mutation carriers: is whole-body cancer screening beneficial? Familial Cancer. 2017;16(3):423–32.

54. Achatz MI, Zambetti GP. The inherited p53 mutation in the Brazilian population. Cold Spring Harb Perspect Med. 2016;6(12). pii: a026195.

55. Ballinger ML, Ferris NJ, Moodie K, Mitchell G, Shanley S, James PA, Thomas DM. Surveillance in germline TP53 mutation carriers utilizing whole-body magnetic resonance imaging. JAMA Oncol. 2017;3(12):1735–6.

56. Schooler GR, Davis JT, Daldrup-Link H, Frush DP. Variability in billing practices for whole-body magnetic resonance imaging: reply to Degnan et al. Pediatr Radiol. 2019;49(1):154.

57. Rednam SP, Erez A, Druker H, Janeway KA, Kamihara J, Kohlmann WK, et al. Von Hippel-Lindau and hereditary pheochromocytoma/paraganglioma syndromes: clinical features, genetics, and surveillance recommendations in childhood. Clin Cancer Res. 2017;23(12):e68–75.

58. Ricketts CJ, Forman JR, Rattenberry E, Bradshaw N, Lalloo F, Izatt L, et al. Tumor risks and genotype-phenotype-proteotype analysis in 358 patients with germline mutations in SDHB and SDHD. Hum Mutat. 2010;31(1):41–51.

59. Turkova H, Prodanov T, Maly M, Martucci V, Adams K, Widimsky J Jr, et al. Characteristics and outcomes of metastatic SDHB and sporadic pheochromocytoma/paraganglioma: an National Institutes of Health Study. Endocr Pract. 2016;22(3):302–14.

60. Assadipour Y, Sadowski SM, Alimchandani M, Quezado M, Steinberg SM, Nilubol N, et al. SDHB mutation status and tumor size but not tumor grade are important predictors of clinical outcome in pheochromocytoma and abdominal paraganglioma. Surgery. 2017;161(1):230–9.

61. Jasperson KW, Kohlmann W, Gammon A, Slack H, Buchmann L, Hunt J, et al. Role of rapid sequence whole-body MRI screening in SDH-associated hereditary paraganglioma families. Familial Cancer. 2014;13(2):257–65.

62. Ricketts CJ, Shuch B, Vocke CD, Metwalli AR, Bratslavsky G, Middelton L, et al. Succinate dehydrogenase kidney cancer: an aggressive example of the Warburg effect in cancer. J Urol. 2012;188(6):2063–71.

63. Bholah R, Bunchman TE. Review of pediatric pheochromocytoma and paraganglioma. Front Pediatr. 2017;5:155.

64. Yamanaka R, Hayano A, Takashima Y. Trilateral retinoblastoma: a systematic review of 211 cases. Neurosurg Rev. 2019;42(1):39–48.

65. Draper GJ, Sanders BM, Brownbill PA, Hawkins MM. Patterns of risk of hereditary retinoblastoma and applications to genetic counselling. Br J Cancer. 1992;66(1):211–9.

66. Friedman DN, Lis E, Sklar CA, Oeffinger KC, Reppucci M, Fleischut MH, et al. Whole-body magnetic resonance imaging (WB-MRI) as surveillance for subsequent malignancies in survivors of hereditary retinoblastoma: a pilot study. Pediatr Blood Cancer. 2014;61(8):1440–4.

67. Kamihara J, Bourdeaut F, Foulkes WD, Molenaar JJ, Mossé YP, Nakagawara A, et al. Retinoblastoma and neuroblastoma predisposition and surveillance. Clin Cancer Res. 2017;23(13):e98–e106.

68. de Jong MC, Kors WA, de Graaf P, Castelijns JA, Kivelä T, Moll AC. Trilateral retinoblastoma: a systematic review and meta-analysis. Lancet Oncol. 2014;15(10):1157–67.

69. Wimmer K, Kratz CP, Vasen HF, Caron O, Colas C, Entz-Werle N, et al. Diagnostic criteria for constitutional mismatch repair deficiency syndrome: suggestions of the European consortium 'care for CMMRD' (C4CMMRD). J Med Genet. 2014;51(6):355–65.

70. Tabori U, Hansford JR, Achatz MI, Kratz CP, Plon SE, Frebourg T, Brugières L. Clinical management and tumor surveillance recommendations of inherited mismatch repair deficiency in childhood. Clin Cancer Res. 2017;23(11):e32–7.

71. Evans DGR, Salvador H, Chang VY, Erez A, Voss SD, Druker H, et al. Cancer and central nervous system tumor surveillance in pediatric neurofibromatosis 2 and related disorders. Clin Cancer Res. 2017;23(12):e54–61.

72. Evans DGR, Salvador H, Chang VY, Erez A, Voss SD, Schneider KW, et al. Cancer and central nervous system tumor surveillance in pediatric neurofibromatosis 1. Clin Cancer Res. 2017;23(12):e46–53.

73. Averill LW, Acikgoz G, Miller RE, Kandula VV, Epelman M. Update on pediatric leukemia and lymphoma imaging. Semin Ultrasound CT MR. 2013;34(6):578–99.

74. Kelly KM. Hodgkin lymphoma in children and adolescents: improving the therapeutic index. Blood. 2015;126(22):2452–8.

75. Littooij AS, Kwee TC, de Keizer B, Bruin MC, Coma A, Beek FJ, et al. Whole-body MRI-DWI for assessment of residual disease after completion of therapy in lymphoma: a prospective multicenter study. J Magn Reson Imaging. 2015;42(6):1646–55.

76. Littooij AS, Kwee TC, Barber I, Granata C, Vermoolen MA, Enriquez G, et al. Whole-body MRI for initial staging of paediatric lymphoma: prospective comparison to an FDG-PET/CT-based reference standard. Eur Radiol. 2014;24(5):1153–65.

77. Zaveri J, La Q, Yarmish G, Neuman J. More than just Langerhans cell histiocytosis: a radiologic review of histiocytic disorders. Radiographics. 2014;34(7):2008–24.

78. Tran G, Huynh TN, Paller AS. Langerhans cell histiocytosis: a neoplastic disorder driven by Ras-ERK pathway mutations. J Am Acad Dermatol. 2018;78(3):579–90.e4.

79. Goo HW, Yang DH, Ra YS, Song JS, Im HJ, Seo JJ, et al. Whole-body MRI of Langerhans cell histiocytosis: compari-

son with radiography and bone scintigraphy. Pediatr Radiol. 2006;36(10):1019–31.

80. Samet J, Weinstein J, Fayad LM. MRI and clinical features of Langerhans cell histiocytosis (LCH) in the pelvis and extremities: can LCH really look like anything? Skelet Radiol. 2016;45(5):607–13.

81. Guiomar R, Pereira da Silva S, Conde P, Cristóvão P, Maia AC, Pechirra P, et al. Cross-protection to new drifted influenza a(H3) viruses and prevalence of protective antibodies to seasonal influenza, during 2014 in Portugal. Vaccine. 2017;35(16):2092–9.

82. Smets AM, Deurloo EE, Slager TJE, Stoker J, Bipat S. Whole-body magnetic resonance imaging for detection of skeletal metastases in children and young people with primary solid tumors – systematic review. Pediatr Radiol. 2018;48(2):241–52.

83. Guimarães MD, Noschang J, Teixeira SR, Santos MK, Lederman HM, Tostes V, et al. Whole-body MRI in pediatric patients with cancer. Cancer Imaging. 2017;17(1):6.

84. Burris NS, Johnson KM, Larson PE, Hope MD, Nagle SK, Behr SC, Hope TA. Detection of small pulmonary nodules with ultra-short echo time sequences in oncology patients by using a PET/MR system. Radiology. 2016;278(1):239–46.

85. Littooij AS, Kwee TC, Enríquez G, Verbeke JI, Granata C, Beishuizen A, et al. Whole-body MRI reveals high incidence of osteonecrosis in children treated for Hodgkin lymphoma. Br J Haematol. 2017;176(4):637–42.

86. Pratesi A, Medici A, Bresci R, Micheli A, Barni S, Pratesi C. Sickle cell-related bone marrow complications: the utility of diffusion-weighted magnetic resonance imaging. J Pediatr Hematol Oncol. 2013;35(4):329–30.

87. Albano D, Patti C, Sconfienza LM, Galia M. Whole-body MRI in the early detection of multifocal osteonecrosis. Br J Radiol. 2017;90(1077):20170240.

88. Antoon JW, Potisek NM, Lohr JA. Pediatric fever of unknown origin. Pediatr Rev. 2015;36(9):380–90; quiz 391

89. Lindsay AJ, Delgado J, Jaramillo D, Chauvin NA. Extended field of view magnetic resonance imaging for suspected osteomyelitis in very young children: is it useful? Pediatr Radiol. 2019;49(3):379–86.

90. von Kalle T, Heim N, Hospach T, Langendörfer M, Winkler P, Stuber T. Typical patterns of bone involvement in whole-body MRI of patients with chronic recurrent multifocal osteomyelitis (CRMO). Rofo. 2013;185(7):655–61.

91. Voit AM, Arnoldi AP, Douis H, Bleisteiner F, Jansson MK, Reiser MF, et al. Whole-body magnetic resonance imaging in chronic recurrent multifocal osteomyelitis: clinical longterm assessment may underestimate activity. J Rheumatol. 2015;42(8):1455–62.

92. Weiss PF. Update on enthesitis-related arthritis. Curr Opin Rheumatol. 2016;28(5):530–6.

93. Østergaard M, Eshed I, Althoff CE, Poggenborg RP, Diekhoff T, Krabbe S, et al. Whole-body magnetic resonance imaging in inflammatory arthritis: systematic literature review and first steps toward standardization and an OMERACT scoring system. J Rheumatol. 2017;44(11):1699–705.

94. Perez-Rossello JM, Connolly SA, Newton AW, Zou KH, Kleinman PK. Whole-body MRI in suspected infant abuse. AJR Am J Roentgenol. 2010;195(3):744–50.

95. Merlini L, Carpentier M, Ferrey S, Anooshiravani M, Poletti PA, Hanquinet S. Whole-body MRI in children: would a 3D STIR sequence alone be sufficient for investigating common paediatric conditions? A comparative study. Eur J Radiol. 2017;88:155–62.

96. Zhen-Guo H, Min-Xing Y, Xiao-Liang C, Ran Y, He C, Bao-Xiang G, et al. Value of whole-body magnetic resonance imaging for screening multifocal osteonecrosis in patients with polymyositis/dermatomyositis. Br J Radiol. 2017;90(1073): 20160780.

97. Thyoka M, Adekunle O, Pilkington C, Walters S, Arthurs OJ, Humphries P, et al. Introduction of a novel magnetic resonance imaging-based scoring system for assessing disease activity in children with juvenile dermatomyositis. Rheumatology (Oxford). 2018;57(9):1661–8.

98. Huang ZG, Gao BX, Chen H, Yang MX, Chen XL, Yan R, et al. An efficacy analysis of whole-body magnetic resonance imaging in the diagnosis and follow-up of polymyositis and dermatomyositis. PLoS One. 2017;12(7):e0181069.

99. Quijano-Roy S, Avila-Smirnow D, Carlier RY. WB-MRI muscle study group. Whole body muscle MRI protocol: pattern recognition in early onset NM disorders. Neuromuscul Disord. 2012;22(Suppl 2):S68–84.

100. Hollingsworth KG, de Sousa PL, Straub V, Carlier PG. Towards harmonization of protocols for MRI outcome measures in skeletal muscle studies: consensus recommendations from two TREAT-NMD NMR workshops, 2 May 2010, Stockholm, Sweden, 1–2 October 2009, Paris, France. Neuromuscul Disord. 2012;22(Suppl 2):S54–67.

101. Arthurs OJ, van Rijn RR, Whitby EH, Johnson K, Miller E, Stenzel M, et al. ESPR postmortem imaging task force: where we begin. Pediatr Radiol. 2016;46(9):1363–9.

102. Shruthi M, Gupta N, Jana M, Mridha AR, Kumar A, Agarwal R, et al. Comparative study of conventional and virtual autopsy using postmortem MRI in the phenotypic characterization of stillbirths and malformed fetuses. Ultrasound Obstet Gynecol. 2018;51(2):236–45.

Index

© Springer Nature Switzerland AG 2020
E. Y. Lee et al. (eds.), *Pediatric Body MRI*, https://doi.org/10.1007/978-3-030-31989-2